AFTER THE KIDNEY TRANSPLANT – THE PATIENTS AND THEIR ALLOGRAFT

Edited by **Jorge Ortiz** and **Jason André**

After the Kidney Transplant – The Patients and Their Allograft
Edited by Jorge Ortiz and Jason André

Published by InTech
Janeza Trdine 9, 51000 Rijeka, Croatia

Publishing Process Manager Davor Vidic

Technical Editor Teodora Smiljanic

Cover Designer InTech Design Team

Additional hard copies can be obtained from orders@intechopen.com

After the Kidney Transplant – The Patients and Their Allograft,
Edited by Jorge Ortiz and Jason André
p. cm.
ISBN 978-953-307-807-6

For EU product safety concerns:
IN TECH d.o.o., Prolaz Marije Krucifikse Kozulić 3, 51000 Rijeka, Croatia,
info@intechopen.com or visit our website at intechopen.com.

Meet the editors

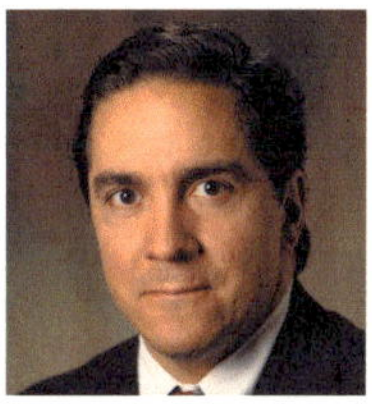

Dr. Jorge Ortiz completed the General Surgery Residency Program at North Shore University Hospital in New York, NY from 1991-1996. Following the completion of his residency he completed an Organ Transplant Fellowship at University of Miami Medical Center from 1996 – 1998 following which he joined the staff in the Division of Transplantation at UC Irvine Medical Center at the University of California and was appointed Director, Renal Transplant Program from 1998-2000 when he left to join the medical staff at Einstein. Today, Dr. Ortiz is the Director of Liver Transplantation and Hepatobiliary Surgery and the Director of Surgical Transplant Fellowship at Albert Einstein Medical Center and has over ten years experience in liver transplantation and research.

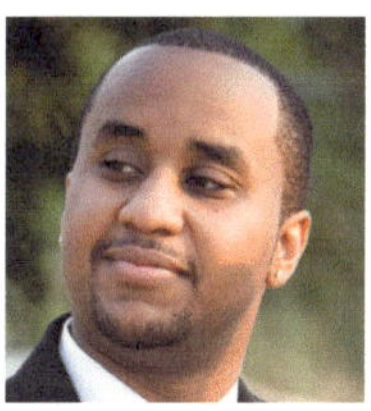

Dr. Jason André is currently a surgery resident at Albert Einstein Medical Center. Raised in Virginia, Dr. André began his path to become a surgeon at the University of Virginia (UVA) where he majored in Psychology. During his time at UVA, Dr. André spent time working with inner city kids and educating men about the effects of sexual abuse on women. Once he completed his training at UVA, Dr. André received his doctorate of medicine at Howard University College of Medicine where his passion for surgery grew. Dr. André is now completing his training at Albert Einstein Medical Center.

Contents

Preface XI

Part 1 Infections and Transplantation 1

Chapter 1 **Infectious Complications in Kidney Transplantation 3**
Amr El-Husseini and Rashad Hassan

Chapter 2 **Handling of Fungal Infections in Patients with Chronic Immunosuppression Post Renal Transplant 47**
Ewa Swoboda-Kopec, Irina Netsvyetayeva, Magdalena Sikora, Mariusz Jasik and Piotr Fiedor

Chapter 3 **CMV Infection in CMV-Seropositive Kidney Transplant Recipients 67**
Jong Man Kim and Sung Joo Kim

Chapter 4 **Posttransplant Lymphoproliferative Disorders Following Kidney Transplantation 79**
Daan Dierickx

Chapter 5 **Post-Trasplant Lymphoproliferative Disorders (PTLD) in Adult Kidney Trasplantated Patients 109**
Savina Aversa, Silvia Stragliotto, Fabio Canova, Boso Caterina and Marino Dario

Part 2 Glomerulonephritis 125

Chapter 6 **Focal Segmental Glomerulosclerosis (FSGS) Recurrence in Kidney Allograft Recipients 127**
Oktawia Mazanowska and Dorota Kamińska

Chapter 7 **Therapeutic Approach to Focal and Segmental Glomerulosclerosis (FSGS) Recurrence in Kidney Transplant Recipients 141**
Guillaume Canaud, Frank Martinez and Christophe Legendre

Chapter 8 **Post-Transplant Glomerulonephritis in Live-Donor Renal Transplant Recipients: Clinical Course and Risk Factors 151**
Ahmed Akl, Hany Adel and Ehab Wafa

Part 3 Transplant Associated Disease 169

Chapter 9 **Psychological Aspects of Kidney Transplantation 171**
Magdalena Trzcinska and Zbigniew Włodarczyk

Chapter 10 **Characteristics of Anaemia Management in Patients with Chronic Kidney Disease 181**
Zvonimir Puretic

Chapter 11 **Post Transplant Anaemia 195**
Bhadran Bose and David Mudge

Chapter 12 **New Onset Diabetes After Solid Organ Transplantation 205**
Phuong-Thu T. Pham, Phuong-Mai T. Pham, Parikh S, Son V. Pham, Phuong-Anh T. Pham and Phuong-Chi T. Pham

Chapter 13 **Sexual and Reproductive Function in Chronic Kidney Disease and Effect of Kidney Transplantation 229**
Mahboob Lessan-Pezeshki and Shirin Ghazizadeh

Chapter 14 **Management of Bone Disease in Kidney Transplant Recipients 253**
Rubin Zhang and Brent Alper

Chapter 15 **Hypertension in the Kidney Transplant Recipient 267**
Heather H. Jones and Daniel J. Salzberg

Chapter 16 **Diagnosis and Treatment of Status Epilepticus in a Pediatric Renal Recipient 279**
Gao Hong-jun, Luo xiangdong, Liang Taisheng, Liang Fangfang et al.

Part 4 Graft Function 295

Chapter 17 **Chronic Allograft Nephropathy 297**
Harzallah Kais

Chapter 18 **Antibody-Mediated Kidney Allograft Rejection 323**
Xu Haiyan and He Xiaozhou

Chapter 19 **Pathogenesis and Preventive Strategies of Chronic Dysfunction of Renal Allograft 335**
Wenqian Huo, Keqin Zhang, Chengguo Ge, Gang Wu, Fengshuo Jin, Gang Yuan and Qiansheng Li

Chapter 20 **Delayed Graft Function 357**
Qiansheng Li, Wenqian Huo, Keqin Zhang, Gang Wu, Fengshuo Jin, Xi Lin, Xiaojiang Jiang and Dong Gao

Chapter 21 **Factors Related to Graft Outcome in Pediatric Renal Transplantation: a Single Center Study 367**
Jean Herman and Rita Van Damme-Lombaerts

Preface

There are many obstacles in kidney transplantation. For the transplant team, there is the balance between immunosuppression to aid in the recipient's tolerance of the allograft and the infection risk of a suppressed immune system. These potential long term complications of kidney transplantation are relatively well known, but there are several more complications that patients and families do not consider when preparing themselves for a kidney transplant.

A few of the more common opportunistic infections are investigated in this book to discuss the workup and treatment for these pathogens. These include viral infections like CMV and fungal infections like Cryptococcus. Special attention is also paid to the phenomenon of Posttransplant Lymphoproliferative Disorder (PTLD) and the incidence after kidney transplantation. This is a devastating disease that has serious implications on the transplant recipient. A great deal of research has been devoted to PTLD and its treatment. This book helps the reader to understand the importance of PTLD and its causes, implications, and possible future direction of research.

Unfortunately, some of the original problems that patient's have that required a kidney transplant are not cured by the transplantation. As a result, these very same causes of kidney dysfunction in the native kidneys affect the new allograft. A prime example of this is focal segmental glomerulonephritis (FSGS). This is a topic of great interest because recurrent FSGS can lead to allograft failure and the need for a new kidney after transplantation. From this book, the reader will understand why FSGS in particular is such an important disease, and what recurrent FSGS means for the patient and the transplant team.

To have a successful kidney transplantation, the patient's body must be fooled into believing the allograft is not foreign tissue. This requires powerful immunosuppression therapy which can greatly affect the overall homeostasis of the recipient. New onset diabetes, depression, sexual dysfunction, seizures, anemia and bone disease are a few of the examples that are investigated in this book. From reading this, the reader will begin to understand the sacrifices that must be made by the patient in transplantation.

The final hurdle for the transplant patient is dealing with chronic issues with his or her allograft. The kidney that the patient received over time will start to fail due to several factors that contribute to allograft dysfunction. This book delineates the work up as well as the causes for chronic allograft dysfunction. Finally, there is some time spent on pediatric allograft function as well as delayed graft function to give the reader the full spectrum of potential allograft complications for the recipient.

After reading this book, the reader will understand some of the sacrifices that the transplant recipient makes in order to receive his or her kidney and the long term dedication that is needed for success. Although the benefits of attempting a kidney transplant far outweigh downfalls of the long term sequelae, kidney transplantation is not a benign procedure. It is the hope of these authors that the reader will leave with a sense of understanding towards the kidney recipients.

Dr. Jorge Ortiz
Albert Einstein Medical Center
Philadelphia, PA
USA

Dr. Jason André
Albert Einstein Medical Center
Philadelphia, PA
USA

Part 1

Infections and Transplantation

1

Infectious Complications in Kidney Transplantation

Amr El-Husseini[1] and Rashad Hassan[2]
[1]*University of South Florida*
[2]*Mansoura Urology and Nephrology Center*
[1]*USA*
[2]*Egypt*

1. Introduction

Kidney transplantation is associated with lower risk for infection than other solid organ transplantations, reflecting the elective nature of kidney transplantation and clinical and nutritional status of recipients. Infection, however, remains a significant cause of morbidity and mortality in renal transplant recipients. Infections related to transplant surgical complications, acquisition of health care-associated pathogens, and reactivation of latent disease can affect graft function and transplant outcome. Graft dysfunction or chronic rejection leads to augmented immunosuppression, increasing the risk for infection with immunomodulating viruses. Although rare, donor-derived infections can arise by delayed donor seroconversion of unidentified pathogens in the organ donor at the time of organ procurement.

Despite prophylactic therapy against common pathogens; infections are the second most common cause of death after cardiovascular disease in renal transplant recipients. According to the U.S. Renal Data System (USRDS), infections occurred at a rate of 45 per 100 patient-years during the first 3 years after transplantation (Snyder et al., 2009).

2. Viral infections

2.1 Introduction

Viral infections are a major problem in allograft recipients, most commonly 1 to 6 months after transplantation. Clinical disease can occur later, especially after intensification of immunosuppression or physiologic insults that increase the net state of immunosuppression.

Notably, cytomegalovirus (CMV) and herpes simplex virus (HSV) infection rates have decreased since the mid-1990s as a result of effective antiviral prophylaxis; hepatitis B virus (HBV) and hepatitis C virus (HCV) infection rates increased during the same period for unclear reasons.

2.2 Cytomegalovirus (CMV)

2.2.1 Background and clinical presentation

CMV is the most important pathogen in transplant recipients.

CMV infection occurs primarily after the first month of transplantation with an estimated incidence of 30% to 78% if antiviral prophylaxis is not administered, depending on the serologic status of the donor and recipient.

- CMV disease is an important cause of morbidity and mortality and is defined by the presence of clinical signs and symptoms attributable to CMV infection, and the presence of CMV in plasma by Nucleic Acid Testing (NAT) or pp65 antigenemia (KDIGO, 2009).

It has a variety of direct and indirect effects (Fishman & Rubin, 1998; Reinke et al., 1994) which include the following:

1. non-specific febrile syndrome:
   - Fever and neutropenia syndrome with features of infectious mononucleosis, including hepatitis, nephritis, leukopenia, or thrombocytopenia
2. Tissue-invasive CMV disease (defined as CMV disease and CMV detected in tissue with histology, NAT or culture) presented with:
   - Pneumonitis: is the most serious manifestation of CMV disease and is characterized by dyspnea, hypoxemia, interstitial infiltrates, and the detection of CMV antigens, nucleic acids, or inclusion bodies on Broncho-Alveolar Lavage (BAL).
   - Gastrointestinal invasion with colitis, gastritis, ulcers, bleeding, or perforation: Diagnostic endoscopy can reveal solitary or multiple mucosal ulcerations with hemorrhage. Tissue specimens should be stained for CMV using immunofluorescent anti-CMV antibody and examined for inclusion bodies.
   - Hepatitis, pancreatitis
   - Chorioretinitis
   - Central nervous system CMV disease (e.g., meningitis, encephalitis, myelitis): may be more difficult to diagnose. Neurologic disease caused by other neurotropic opportunistic pathogens, and drug toxicities, should be simultaneously investigated.
   - Multiorgan involvement can be observed in disseminated CMV disease.

With the exception of chorioretinitis, the direct clinical manifestations of CMV infection usually occur 1 to 4 months after transplantation; chorioretinitis usually does not occur until later in the transplant course.

Although CMV is a common cause of clinical infectious disease syndromes, the indirect effects of viral infection are equally important. CMV infection produces a profound suppression of a variety of host defenses, predisposing to secondary invasion by such pathogens as P. carinii (jiroveci), Candida, Aspergillus, and some bacteria. CMV also contributes to the risk for graft rejection (through induction of anti-endothelial cell antibodies that contribute to both acute and chronic rejection), post-transplant lymphoproliferative disease (PTLD), Human Herpes Virus-6 (HHV-6) and HHV-7 infections, and acceleration of Hpatits C Virus (HCV) infection.

2.2.2 Routes of transmission

CMV can be transmitted by the allograft, through blood products, or by sexual contact and establishes lifelong latency after primary infection (Hartmann et al., 2006).

2.2.3 Patterns of transmission

Transmission of CMV in the transplant recipient occurs in one of three patterns: primary infection, reactivation, and superinfection (Fishman & Rubin, 1998).

2.2.3.1 Primary Cytomegalovirus Infection

Primary infection occurs most often when seronegative individuals receive grafts from latently infected, seropositive donors, with subsequent reactivation of the virus and systemic dissemination after transplantation. Forty percent to 50% of these patients experience direct infectious disease manifestations of CMV, whereas most are viremic, often without symptoms. Primary CMV infection also may occur in seronegative individuals after transfusion or exposure in the community. This disease may be severe.

2.2.3.2 Secondary Cytomegalovirus Infection

Secondary Cytomegalovirus Infection represents infection in a previously infected seropositive host caused by either:

a. Reactivation Cytomegalovirus Infection. In reactivation infection, seropositive individuals reactivate endogenous virus after transplantation.
   When conventional immunosuppressive therapy is used, approximately 10% to 15% experience direct infectious disease syndromes, with a higher rate with the use of induction antilymphocyte therapy. Fifty percent of these individuals are viremic, often without symptoms.
b. Cytomegalovirus Superinfection. Virus may be reactivated in the setting of an allograft from a seropositive donor transplanted into a seropositive recipient with superinfection with new virus strain.

2.2.4 Risk factors

- Specific risk factors include CMV donor-recipient mismatching and the use of lymphocyte-depleting preparations induction for rejection therapy.
- Other risk factors include episodes of allograft rejection, comorbid illnesses, neutropenia, and, potentially, coinfection with HHV-6 and -7(Hartmann et al., 2006).
- MMF has also been variably reported to be associated with an increased incidence of CMV viremia and CMV disease with increased risk in patients receiving MMF 3 g/day (Fishman & Davis, 2008).

2.2.5 Diagnosis

Clinical management of CMV, including prevention and treatment, is important for the transplant recipient. It is based on an understanding of the causes of CMV activation and the available diagnostic techniques.

Culture-based methods include conventional tissue culture and shell vial centrifugation and can be performed on blood, buffy coat blood fraction, urine, cerebrospinal fluid (CSF), respiratory secretions, or other tissue specimens. Tissue culture is most commonly employed for antiviral resistance testing; although polymerase chain reaction (PCR)-based methods are available those do not require isolation of virus from culture (Pegues et al., 2010).

Staining conventional cell culture or shell vial culture with monoclonal antibody against early CMV viral antigens at 48 hours can decrease the time to diagnosis but is not as sensitive as traditional viral culture.

Serological tests are useful before transplantation to predict risk but are of little value after transplantation in defining clinical disease (this statement includes measurements of anti-CMV IgM levels). Interpretation of CMV serologies may be confounded by the presence of passive antibody that may have been acquired from a blood or body-fluid contamination (KDIGO, 2009).

The demonstration of CMV inclusions in tissues in the setting of a compatible clinical presentation is the "gold standard" for diagnosis.

Quantitation of the intensity of CMV infection has been linked to the risk for infection in transplant recipients (Caliendo et al., 2000; Humar et al., 2002).

Two types of quantitative assays have been developed: molecular and antigen detection assays.

1-The antigenemia assay is a semiquantitative fluorescent assay in which circulating neutrophils are stained for CMV early antigen (pp65) that is taken up nonspecifically as a measure of the total viral burden in the body.

2-The molecular assays (direct DNA polymerase chain reaction, hybrid capture, amplification assays) are highly specific and sensitive for the diagnosis of CMV disease associated with viremia and to monitor response to antiviral therapy.

The most commonly used assays include plasma-based polymerase chain reaction testing and the whole-blood hybrid capture assay. Whole-blood and plasma-based PCR assays cannot be directly compared. The highest viral loads often are associated with tissue-invasive disease, with the lowest in asymptomatic CMV infection. Either assay can be used in management.

The advent of quantitative assays for the diagnosis and management of CMV infection has allowed noninvasive diagnosis in many patients with two important exceptions:

- Neurological disease, including chorioretinitis
- Gastrointestinal disease, including invasive colitis and gastritis

In these syndromes, the CMV assays are often negative, and tissue diagnosis may be required.

Qualitative CMV DNA detection by PCR is extremely sensitive but cannot differentiate active disease or latent infection (Humar et al., 2002).

2.2.6 Prevention of CMV infection

In the absence of antiviral prophylaxis, symptomatic CMV disease can be seen in approximately 8% of kidney transplant recipients (Paya & Razonable, 2003), although older estimates placed it at 10–60% (Hibberd et al., 1992a). Accordingly, strategies that can prevent CMV infection and disease should lead to improved outcomes following kidney transplantation.

Prevention of CMV infection must be individualized for immunosuppressive regimens and the patient.

Two strategies are commonly used for CMV prevention: **universal prophylaxis** and **preemptive therapy**. Randomized controlled trials have demonstrated that the incidence of CMV disease can be reduced by prophylaxis and preemptive therapies in solid-organ transplant recipients (Hodson et al., 2007; Strippoli et al., 2006).

Universal prophylaxis involves giving antiviral therapy to all at-risk patients beginning at or immediately after transplantation for a defined period.

There is high-quality evidence from a large systematic review that CMV prophylaxis in solid-organ transplant recipients significantly reduces all-cause mortality, CMV disease mortality, CMV disease, but not acute rejection or graft loss. (Hodson et al., 2007)

In **preemptive therapy**, quantitative assays are used to monitor patients at predefined intervals to detect early disease with administration of therapy in case of positive assay.

Preemptive therapy incurs extra costs for monitoring and coordination of outpatient care, while reducing the cost of drugs and the inherent toxicities.
At the present time, the use of viral load monitoring to prompt preemptive therapy is not recommended for high-risk kidney transplant recipients.
The basis for this concern is both a lack of data in CMV D+/R− kidney transplant recipients, the implications of a failure to comply with the preemptive monitoring approach and the relative safety and efficacy of universal chemoprophylaxis in high-risk organ transplant recipients (Hodson et al., 2007).
The approach of universal prophylaxis may be more useful for patients at high risk for CMV disease, whereas preemptive therapy may be more useful for patients at low or intermediate risk for CMV disease.
Prophylaxis has the possible advantage of preventing not only CMV infection during the period of greatest risk but also diminishing infections secondary to HHV-6, HHV-7, and Epstein-Barr Virus (EBV). The indirect effects of CMV (i.e. graft rejection, opportunistic infection) also may be reduced by routine prophylaxis.
In practice, neither universal prophylaxis nor preemptive therapy is perfect. Infrequently, breakthrough disease and ganciclovir resistance have been observed with both approaches (Kalil et al., 2005).
Given the risk for invasive infection, patients at risk for primary infection are generally given prophylaxis for 3 to 6 months after transplantation (especially in patients receiving depleting anti–T lymphocyte antibodies). There is strong evidence linking the use of antibody treatment of rejection with increased risk of CMV infection and disease. The use of these agents results in activation of CMV from latency to active infection and studies in this high-risk population have shown that antiviral chemoprophylaxis reduces the incidence of CMV disease by about 60% (Hodson et al., 2005). Other groups are candidates for preemptive therapy if an appropriate monitoring system is in place, and patient compliance is good. Current data support the use of universal prophylaxis (not preemptive therapy), however, in the prevention of indirect effects of CMV infection, including PTLD, opportunistic infections, allograft rejection, and mortality (Kalil et al., 2005).
The currently used antiviral agents for universal prophylaxis include intravenous or oral ganciclovir, oral valganciclovir, valacyclovir, CMV immunoglobulin (CMVIG), and a combination of antiviral therapy and CMVIG.
Although oral ganciclovir is more convenient to administer than its intravenous formulation, it is substantially less bioavailable (4% to 6%) and achieves significantly lower serum levels.
Valganciclovir, the L-valine ester of ganciclovir, is administered in a dose of 450 to 900 mg per day by mouth for CMV prophylaxis and produces similar area under the curve values to intravenous ganciclovir (5 mg/kg per day) and much higher values than oral ganciclovir (3 g per day) and is more effective than ganciclovir in preventing CMV disease at 6 months among kidney transplant recipients. (Asberg et al., 2007).
Some recent studies failed to demonstrate a benefit of CMVIG administered prophylactically (Hodson et al., 2007) although in nonblinded, nonrandomized trials, CMVIG reduced the incidence of virologically confirmed CMV-associated syndromes and secondary opportunistic infections in D+/R- renal transplants.
Ganciclovir, valganciclovir, and valacyclovir require dosage adjustment for decreased creatinine clearance.

2.2.7 Treatment of CMV infection

Effective antiviral agents for CMV prophylaxis and treatment have substantially decreased the morbidity and mortality associated with CMV disease.

Oral valganciclovir (900 mg twice daily) has been demonstrated to have comparable safety and efficacy to intravenous ganciclovir for clearing CMV viremia and resolving clinical disease in solid organ transplant patients with mild to moderate CMV disease(Paya et al., 2004).

Patients with high CMV viral loads or severe tissue invasive disease, and those who fail to achieve a reduction in viral load after 7 or more days of oral valganciclovir treatment should be treated with intravenous ganciclovir (5 mg/kg twice daily, with dosage adjustments for renal dysfunction) for at least 2 to 3 weeks with a reduction in the immunosuppression if the disease is severe until a quantitative assay for CMV is negative (Sia & Patel, 2000).

Experience in treating refractory CMV disease suggests that the addition of CMV hyperimmune globulin (150 mg/kg/dose intravenously given every 3 to 4 weeks) or intravenous pooled gammaglobulin (IVIG) to ganciclovir may improve the clinical response.

Patients with CMV disease should receive at least weekly monitoring of blood viral load and the presence of CMV in plasma, detected by NAT or pp65 antigenemia, at the end of treatment is a major predictor of recurrent CMV disease (1).

The use of completely oral regimens for treatment appears to be effective with the exception of invasive gastrointestinal disease.

It is worth noting that similar data are not available for pediatric kidney transplant recipients or other children undergoing solid-organ transplantation.

Accordingly, while the use of oral valganciclovir may be appropriate for some adult kidney transplant recipients experiencing mild to moderate CMV disease, all pediatric kidney transplant recipients should receive intravenous ganciclovir for the treatment of CMV disease (KIDGO, 2009).

Further, concern also exists with regards to the use of oral valganciclovir in patients in whom there are questions regarding adequate absorption of this medication.

Adverse effects of ganciclovir include reversible, dose-related granulocytopenia and thrombocytopenia, fever, rash, seizures, nausea, myalgias, abnormalities in liver enzyme determinations, and, rarely, pancreatitis (Paya et al., 2004).

Drug interactions include an increased seizure risk when used in combination with acyclovir and imipenem, and additive marrow suppression with azathioprine, mycophenolate, and TMP-SMX (Paya et al., 2004).

Renal transplant recipients with ongoing risk factors for CMV should receive long-term maintenance therapy with oral ganciclovir (1000 mg 3 times daily), valganciclovir (450 to 900 mg once daily) or valacyclovir (2 g, 4 times daily) (Paya et al., 2004). Relapses occur, primarily in patients not treated beyond the achievement of a negative quantitative assay.

Some relapses occur in gastrointestinal disease because the assays used to follow disease are unreliable in this setting. Repeat endoscopy should be considered to ensure the clearance of infection (Kalil et al., 2005).

Alternative therapies are available in intravenous form only, including foscarnet and cidofovir which can be used to treat disease associated with ganciclovir-resistant CMV strains (Mylonakis et al., 2002).

Although it is active against most ganciclovir-resistant strains of CMV, combination therapy (ganciclovir and foscarnet) for organ transplant recipients is preferred given the toxicities of high-dose, single-agent therapy, and given the antiviral synergy that has been reported (Mylonakis et al., 2002).

Cidofovir has been used in renal transplant recipients, often with nephrotoxicity.
Foscarnet and cidofovir may exhibit synergistic nephrotoxicity with calcineurin inhibitors.
leflunamide also seems to have useful activity against both CMV and BK polyomavirus (Fishman & Davis, 2008).
The anti-CMV activity and safety of maribavir in CMV-seropositive patients were evaluated in a randomized RCT in allogeneic stem-cell transplant recipients but not in KTRs. The results showed that maribavir can reduce the incidence of CMV infection and, unlike ganciclovir, does not cause myelosuppression (Winston et al., 2008).

2.2.8 Chemoprophylaxis

Chemoprophylaxis is defined as the use of an antimicrobial agent in the absence of evidence of active infection, to prevent the acquisition of infection and the development of disease.
A variety of potential antiviral agents have been evaluated.
Ganciclovir, valganciclovir, acyclovir and valacyclovir were demonstrated to be effective in the preventing CMV infection and disease (Hodson et al., 2007). However, head-to-head comparisons demonstrated that ganciclovir was more effective than acyclovir in preventing both CMV infection and CMV disease. Oral valganciclovir was as effective as intravenous ganciclovir in the prevention of both CMV infection and disease. Oral and intravenous ganciclovir yielded similar results. The use of acyclovir and valacyclovir should be restricted to situations where ganciclovir/valganciclovir cannot be used (Hodson et al., 2007).
Randomized controlled trials (RCTs) evaluated oral antiviral agents for the prevention of CMV disease have treated patients for 3 months after transplantation (Hodson et al., 2007). A recent meta-analysis did not find a difference in treatment efficacy for patients receiving less or more than 6 weeks of therapy (KDIGO, 2009). So, Chemoprophylaxis with ganciclovir or valganciclovir for at least 3 months after transplantation reduces CMV infection and disease in high-risk patients.
The impetus behind prolonged treatment is an increasing recognition of late CMV disease. Two studies evaluated ganciclovir in patients who received antilymphocyte antibody therapy demonstrated a reduction in CMV disease (Hibberd et al., 1995; KDIGO, 2009).
Accordingly, the use of intravenous ganciclovir or oral valganciclovir has been recommended for CMV prophylaxis during antilymphocyte antibody therapy (1). The use of oral ganciclovir should be avoided for patients with high level CMV viremia (1). The use of acyclovir or famciclovir is not recommended, given the absence of data supporting the efficacy of these agents. It is also suggested that CMV serologies be repeated for patients CMV-seronegative prior to transplant, who require antibody therapy as treatment for rejection to decide their current risk status.
Lastly, chemoprophylaxis is associated with improved graft survival compared to preemptive antiviral therapy initiated in response to increased CMV load (KDIGO, 2009).

2.2.9 CMV viral load testing

While resolution of clinical signs and symptoms are critical in the management of CMV disease, measurement of the CMV viral load provides additional useful information.
The use of viral load monitoring identifies both virologic response (guiding duration of therapy) as well as the possible presence of antiviral resistance. The presence of detectable CMV load at the end of therapy is associated with an increased rate of recurrent disease (Humar et al., 2002). The time to clearance of CMV in plasma as measured by NAT may be

prolonged compared to pp65, and may be associated with an increase risk of recurrent CMV disease (Weinberg et al., 2000).

2.2.10 Immunosuppression and graft function monitoring during CMV disease

The reduction of immunosuppression used as part of the treatment of CMV disease places patients at some risk for the development of rejection. The presence of CMV infection and disease has been associated with the development of rejection independent of reduction of immunosuppression.

Accordingly, careful monitoring of kidney allograft function is warranted during treatment of CMV disease to guide the use of immunosuppression (KDIGO, 2009).

2.3 Epstein-Barr virus (EBV)

2.3.1 Introduction

EBV is associated with an array of disorders ranging from infectious mononucleosis to nasopharyngeal carcinoma, Burkitt lymphoma, and B-cell lymphomas in immunocompromised patients.

EBV disease is defined by signs and symptoms of active viral infection and increased EBV load.

The EBV viral load is defined as the amount of viral genome that is detectable in the peripheral blood by NAT.

Primary EBV (human herpes virus 4) infection is associated with an increased incidence of post-transplant lymphoproliferative disease (PTLD) in kidney transplant recipients (KTRs). An EBV-negative KTR from an EBV-positive donor is at increased risk for developing PTLD (Cockfield et al., 1993; McDonald et al., 2008). A newly detectable or rising EBV load often precedes EBV disease and PTLD (Rowe et al., 2001). Identification of seronegative patients with a rising EBV load offers the opportunity to preemptively intervene and potentially prevent progression to EBV disease including PTLD (Paya et al., 1999).

Primary EBV infection in EBV-seronegative organ transplant recipients occurs most frequently in the first 3–6 months following organ transplantation (Breinig et al., 1987). This is most likely due to the fact that the source of the EBV infection is attributable to either the donor organ or blood products received by the patient at or near the time of transplant. Serial measurement of EBV loads in previously seronegative patients allows the identification of onset of infection (Rowe et al., 2001).

Continued observation of EBV loads in newly infected patients identifies those patients with rapidly rising viral loads who are likely to be at greatest risk of progressing to EBV disease. Because the most likely sources of EBV infection in KTRs are either passenger leukocytes from the donor allograft or blood products exposure (which are more likely at or near the time of transplantation), the likelihood that they will develop primary EBV infection is reduced with time after transplantation. Accordingly, EBV load monitoring should be performed most frequently during the first 3–6 months after transplant. Because the risk of developing EBV infection after this time period is diminished, but not eliminated, continued surveillance of EBV load is recommended, albeit at less frequent intervals (KDIGO, 2009).

2.3.2 EBV disease diagnosis

EBV virus disease can present with varied manifestations, including nonspecific febrile illness, gastroenteritis, hepatitis and other manifestations that may be attributable to CMV or other pathogens. Although biopsy to detect the presence of EBV infection within affected tissue is the most definitive way to confirm the diagnosis of EBV disease, histological confirmation may not be feasible for patients with some nonspecific clinical syndromes that may not localize to specific tissue (e.g. febrile syndromes) (2).

Because the EBV viral load is detectable and elevated in the vast majority of KTRs with EBV disease, including PTLD, the combination of the presence of a compatible clinical syndrome in association with a high EBV load provides a sensitive and specific approach to the diagnosis of EBV disease (Green et al., 2006). However, it is still necessary to be cautious in considering this diagnosis, as many patients may have asymptomatic elevations of EBV load. Accordingly, such patients may be misdiagnosed as having EBV disease, if they develop intercurrent infections due to an alternative pathogen at a time that they are having an asymptomatic elevation in their EBV load. In such patients, a tissue diagnosis may be the only method of confirming the presence or absence of EBV disease (KDIGO, 2009).

2.3.3 EBV-associated PTLD

EBV plays a central role in the pathogenesis of PTLD (Nalesnik, 2001; Preiksaitis & Keay, 2001).

The most clearly defined risk factor for PTLD is primary EBV infection, which increases the risk for PTLD by 10-fold to 76-fold.

PTLD are clinical syndromes associated with EBV and lymphoproliferation, which range from self-limited, polyclonal proliferation to malignancies containing clonal chromosomal abnormalities (2).

The approach to the management of PTLD can vary according to the PTLD disease classification.

Furthermore, EBV-negative PTLD lesions have been reported and these lesions may behave differently then EBV-positive lesions and may warrant alternative therapeutic options. In addition, lesions with a characteristic clinical appearance on physical examination or imaging studies may be due to alternative pathogens (e.g. pulmonary nodules attributable to fungal pathogens). Because of all these concerns, it is imperative that suspected PTLD lesions be biopsied and undergoes histolopathologic evaluation by a pathologist experienced with the diagnosis of PTLD (2).

Observational studies have suggested KTRs with EBV disease are at high risk of developing PTLD (Dharnidharka et al., 2001b). Observational studies have also shown that mortality from EBV-associated PTLD is over 50% (Caillard et al, 2006; Opelz & Dohler, 2004). The presence of immunosuppression is major risk factor for the development of EBV disease, including PTLD, in KTRs (Dharnidharka & Harmon, 2001a; McDonald et al., 2008).

High EBV loads have been found at the time of diagnosis of PTLD. Because the EBV load becomes positive 4–16 weeks prior to development of PTLD, the presence of a rising EBV load identifies patients in whom intervention may prevent PTLD (Rowe et al., 2001).

The clinical presentations of EBV-associated PTLD vary and include the following (Paya et al., 1999):

- Unexplained fever (fever of unknown origin)
- A mononucleosis-type syndrome, with fever and malaise, with or without pharyngitis or tonsillitis (often diagnosed incidentally in tonsillectomy specimens).
- Most are non-Hodgkin lymphomas (Hodgkin disease is the most common lymphoma in age-matched controls), are of B-cell origin, and are $CD20^+$.
- Gastrointestinal bleeding, obstruction, or perforation

- Abdominal mass lesions
- Infiltrative disease of the allograft with dysfunction of the transplanted organ that may be confused histologically with severe rejection.
- Hepatocellular or pancreatic dysfunction
- Central nervous system disease

The prolonged or repeated administration of lymphocytic-depleting antibody preparations is a significant risk factor for the development of PTLD. Predictors of poor survival from PTLD include increased age, elevated lactic acid dehydrogenase values, severe organ dysfunction, multiorgan involvement, and constitutional symptoms (fever, night sweats, weight loss) (Fishman, 2007).

2.3.4 Management

Clinical management depends on the stage of disease. In the initial stages, particularly in children, re-establishment of immune function may be sufficient to cause PTLD to regress. At this stage, it is possible that antiviral therapy might have some utility given the viremia and role of EBV as an immunosuppressive agent. With the progression of disease to extranodal and monoclonal malignant forms, reduction in immunosuppression may be useful, but alternative therapies are often required. In kidney transplantation, the failure to regress with significant reductions in immunosuppression may suggest the need to sacrifice the allograft for patient survival. Combinations of anti–B cell therapy (anti-CD20, rituximab), chemotherapy (CHOP: cyclophosphamide, hydroxydaunomycin, vincristine [Oncovin], prednisone), or adoptive immunotherapy with stimulated T cells have been used (Haque et al., 2002; Straathof et al., 2002).

2.4 Hepatitis C Virus (HCV)

2.4.1 Introduction

KTRs infected with HCV have worse patient- and allograft-survival rates and are at increased risk for several complications, including worsening liver disease, new-onset diabetes after transplantation (NODAT) and glomerulonephritis than KTRs without HCV infection.

2.4.2 Patient and graft survival

Controversy exists regarding the impact of pre-transplant HCV infection on the outcome of renal transplantation.

Initially, studies of short follow-up periods suggested that neither patient nor graft survival was altered after transplantation despite an increase in HCV RNA levels (Lau et al., 1993; Lee et al., 2001; Orloff et al., 1995).

In contrast, studies with lengthier follow-up after transplantation have found decreased patient and graft survival in HCV-positive renal transplant recipients (Legendre et al., 1998; Mahmoud et al., 2004; Sezer et al., 2004).

Post-transplantation HCV-related liver disease is often progressive in renal transplant recipients. Factors implicated in more rapid progression of HCV include alcohol abuse and HBV co-infection (Martin & Fabrizi, 2008).

HCC and liver cirrhosis were more frequent causes of mortality in HCV-positive than HCV-negative recipients (Hanafusa et al., 1998).

The Transplant Guideline Work Group determined that liver enzymes should be checked every month for the first 6 months of the post-transplant period, and every 3 months thereafter. The detection of clinically worsening liver enzymes should prompt referral for hepatologic evaluation. Annual liver ultrasound and alpha-fetoprotein level to screen for hepatocellular carcinoma should be considered in patients with cirrhosis on liver biopsy (KDIGO, 2009).

Most studies regarding post-transplant HCV outcomes comprise chronically infected recipients, usually those who acquired HCV during hemodialysis. However, the subsets of solid organ transplant recipients who become infected with HCV in the peri-operative period have a markedly different course with some studies suggest that HCV acquired at the time of transplantation may have a particularly aggressive course (Delladetsima et al., 2006; Sypsa et al, 2004) most probably because they develope an acute hepatitis at a time of maximum immunosuppression.

2.4.3 Hepatitis C virus and post-transplant diabetes in kidney transplant recipients

The association of diabetes mellitus and HCV has become increasingly apparent more recently in the immunocompetent HCV population and particularly after solid organ transplantation in HCV-infected patients. The overall incidence of post-transplant diabetes mellitus has been reported to vary from 10% to 54% (Fabrizi et al., 2005).

Tacrolimus increases the risk for NODAT, and might be expected to impart at least an additive risk for NODAT to HCV-infected KTRs (KDIGO, 2009; van Duijnhoven et al., 2002). This association also was observed by Bloom and colleagues, who found that among the HCV-positive patients, there was an eight times increased incidence of post-transplant diabetes mellitus in patients treated with tacrolimus (58%) compared with cyclosporine (7.7%) (Bloom et al., 2002).

2.4.4 Hepatitis C virus and post-transplant nephropathy

Hepatitis C virus infection has been implicated in the pathogenesis of glomerulonephritis and mixed cryoglobulinemia in both native and transplanted kidneys and can lead to graft loss. Therefore, the Hepatitis C and Transplant Guideline Work Groups concluded that HCV-infected KTRs should be tested for proteinuria every 3–6 months (KDIGO, 2009).

Membranoproliferative glomerulonephritis (MPGN) is the most common pathological finding likely to arise in patients infected with HCV, followed by membranous nephropathy, minimal change disease, and renal thrombotic microangiopathy. These may be recurrent or manifest as de novo disease (Meyers et al., 2003).

MPGN has been reported in 45% of HCV-positive renal transplant recipients who underwent renal biopsy for worsened renal function. In the HCV-negative group, the incidence was only 5.9% (Meyers et al., 2003). De novo disease was found in 18% of the MPGN patients, and chronic renal allograft nephropathy was similar in HCV-positive and HCV-negative recipients (Cruzado et al., 2001). Initially, MPGN and chronic allograft nephropathy may have similar presentation with proteinuria and can be a diagnostic dilemma requiring electron microscopy to differentiate the two.

As recommended for all KTRs, patients who develop new-onset proteinuria (either urine protein/creatinine ratio >1 or 24-hour urine protein greater than 1 g on two or more occasions) should have an allograft biopsy with immunofluorescence and electron microscopy.

Interferon-based therapies may be effective in treating HCV-related glomerulopathy in native kidney disease. However, interferon use in KTRs is associated with an increased risk of rejection. Ribavirin can reduce proteinuria in HCV-associated glomerulopathy, although its impact on kidney function is unknown and it does not lead to viral clearance (KDIGO, 2009).

2.4.5 Immunosuppressive protocols in HCV infected renal transplant recipients

No randomized prospective study has been done to determine optimal immunosuppressive regimens in renal transplant recipients infected with HCV. As mentioned earlier, studies have shown tacrolimus as an additive risk in HCV patients for the development of NODAT. Azathioprine and antilymphocyte agents to treat rejection have been implicated in more severe liver disease in HCV-infected recipients. Administration of high-dose steroids and antilymphocyte antibodies should be avoided and only used after a critical evaluation of potential risk and benefit, especially the risk for accelerating the course of liver disease (Pegues et al., 2010).

A liver biopsy should be performed to assess underlying activity and stage of HCV-related liver disease. This information can help guide expected response rates and aggressiveness of therapy. Patients with advanced fibrosis or cirrhosis or both need to be considered for combined liver-kidney transplantion.

2.4.6 Anti-HCVviral therapy

2.4.6.1 Pretransplant antiviral therapy

As mentioned above, HCV is associated with worse patient and graft survivals, increased risk of post-transplant diabetes mellitus and de novo glomerulopathy. So, eradication of HCV before transplantation might mitigate some of these adverse outcomes (Cruzado et al., 2003; Huraib et al., 2001; Kamar et al., 2003b).

Interferon is effective for viral eradication in HCV-infected patients, especially when combined with ribavirin. However, the administration of interferon after kidney transplantation can be deleterious to the allograft and should generally be avoided in KTRs, unless there is indication of worsening hepatic injury (Rostaing et al., 1995).

It would be best if treatment could be undertaken before proceeding to the solid organ transplant.

Results of treatment of HCV in dialysis patients varies, with sustained virological rates ranging from 16% to 68% (Fabrizi et al., 2004b).

Post-transplantation improvements in hepatic activity index were seen to persist in patients treated with interferon while on the waiting list compared with patients who were not given interferon before renal transplantation (Huraib et al., 2001). Post-transplant glomerulopathy also is reduced by pretransplant interferon therapy.

Most studies report treatment regimens including interferon monotherapy administered for 6 to 12 months.

Ribavirin is renally excreted and its metabolites are not cleared by dialysis, and it needs to be used very cautiously if at all in dialysis patients because of the fear of hemolytic anemia that may occur despite low doses of 200 mg three times a week in dialysis patients and can be severe enough to mandate discontinuation of the drug (Tan et al., 2001).

Some pilot studies have reported ribavirin use in addition to interferon in patients on dialysis (Bruchfeld et al., 2001) but there was no evidence that adding ribavirin in dialysis patients provided any added therapeutic benefit.

There is considerable clinical experience, although few studies, using pegylated interferon monotherapy in dialysis patients with chronic HCV (Russo et al., 2006) with an increase in side effects in this population and response rates that are not better than with standard interferon because the half-life of regular interferon is increased in patients on dialysis.

2.4.6.2 Antiviral therapy for HCV after transplantation

Post-transplantation interferon therapy generally is contraindicated in organ transplant recipients other than recipients of liver allografts; this is due to multiple reports of precipitation of renal failure and organ rejection owing to interferon therapy (Said et al., 2008). Interferon alfa therapy should be limited to patients with severe recurrence of HCV, such as advanced fibrosis/cirrhosis or fibrosing cholestatic HCV.

Ribavirin monotherapy has been associated with reduction in aminotransferases and necroinflammation in renal transplant recipients (may be due to decreased lymphocytic proliferation, decreased synthesis of proinflammatory cytokines, and a decrease of T helper type 2 cytokine production favoring a T helper type 1 profile) but no virological response (Said et al., 2008). On the contrary, Karmer and colleagues found biochemical improvement without histological or virological improvement in these patients (Kamar et al., 2003a).

2.5 Hepatitis B Virus (HBV)

2.5.1 Introduction

The incidence and prevalence of HBV infection among patients awaiting renal transplantation have declined in recent years largely as a result of vaccination of patients on dialysis and improved infection control measures during dialysis. With these measures, the incidence of HBV infection in dialysis patients has decreased considerably in recent years to approximately 1%.

Hepatitis B virus infected patients are at risk of exacerbation of the infection, progressive liver disease, development of hepatocellular carcinoma and decreased survival after kidney transplantation (Aroldi et al., 2005).

Immunosuppression following kidney transplantation leads to increased replication of HBV and results in progressive liver disease.

2.5.2 Liver Biopsy: its role before transplantation

It is difficult; on clinical grounds alone, to estimate the severity of liver disease in chronic kidney disease (CKD) patients. For this reason, liver biopsy should be incorporated in the evaluation of renal transplant candidates with HBsAg and both liver histology and evaluation of HBV replication by serum markers (i.e., HBeAg and HBV DNA) should be concerned before deciding transplant candidacy in HBsAg-positive patients.

In patients with histologically mild liver disease, renal transplantation is not contraindicated. If the initial liver biopsy shows extensive fibrosis and there is active HBV replication, repeat liver biopsy should be considered after a year or more of antiviral therapy to determine whether regression of liver fibrosis has occurred (Pegues et al., 2010).

2.5.3 Disease progression after kidney transplantation

HBV infection in transplant recipients may be associated with only minor elevations of aminotransferase levels despite histologic progression. Known risk factors for progression of HBV-related liver disease include alcohol use; longer duration of infection; high serum

levels of HBV DNA; genotype C; coinfection with hepatitis C and D; HIV infection; and immunosuppression (Pegues et al., 2010).
The patient survival in renal transplant recipients is a well established adverse effect of HBsAg positivity while the effect of HBsAg status on graft survival is less clear, although it might be enhanced in HBV-infected recipients as a result of a diminished immune response resulting from chronic viral infection (Pegues et al., 2010).

2.5.4 Pretransplant management of hepatitis B virus–positive dialysis patients

Lamivudine monotherapy is associated with viral suppression in most patients with end-stage renal disease (Lapinski et al., 2005).
The problems with lamivudine include development of resistance with prolonged antiviral therapy, which can result in virological and clinical breakthrough.

2.5.5 Antiviral Therapy of Chronic Hepatitis B Virus in Renal Transplant Recipients

2.5.5.1 Timing of initiation

Data on optimal timing of initiation of antiviral therapy are scarce.
However, renal transplant recipients with active HBV (HBsAg positive) should be started on antiviral therapy at the time of transplantation irrespective of HBV DNA levels (Han et al., 2001; Filik et al., 2006) or even during dialysis to prevent worsening of liver disease after transplantation.
The primary goals of management are maximal suppression of viral replication, while minimizing development of resistance and prevention of hepatic fibrosis.
Cessation of antiviral therapy in the immunocompromised host is associated with an increased risk of flare of liver disease and rarely decompensated liver disease in transplant recipients (Chan et al., 2002; Liaw et al., 1999).
Indefinite therapy carries its own risks, including that of antiviral toxicity (rare) and of drug resistance.
Although interferon (IFN) and pegylated IFN are efficacious in the treatment of chronic HBV, their use is contraindicated in renal transplant recipients because the immunomodulatory actions of IFN may lead to the precipitation of severe and often irreversible graft dysfunction.
The introduction of lamivudine was a major advance in the management of post-transplantation HBV-related liver disease. A dose of 100 mg/day orally has been shown to be highly effective in suppression of HBV replication and normalization of aminotransferases in greater than 80% of patients (Fabrizi et al., 2004a;, Kletzmayr et al., 2000; Rostaing et al., 1997).
Because lamivudine is metabolized by the kidney, the dose should be reduced in patients with impaired renal function to 50 mg daily for a creatinine clearance of 30 to 49 mL per minute.
Lamivudine is well tolerated, and has no adverse immunomodulatory activity.

2.5.5.2 Duration of therapy

The optimal duration of therapy that ensures long-term remission of viremia and maintenance of normal liver function and minimizes the development of resistance is not known and in an immunocompromised host may need to be indefinite.
At least 24 months of prophylactic treatment has been recommended (Wirth, 2006).

Withdrawal of antiviral therapy may be associated with a relapse and increased viral replication, even resulting in liver failure (Rostaing et al., 1997).
The risk of resistance increases with duration of lamivudine therapy. This is usually reflected by a secondary increase in the HBV DNA titers. A commonly used definition is demonstration of >5 log10 copies/mL rebound of HBV DNA.
The clinical presentation varies. While some patients show no significant biochemical changes or clinical symptoms, others develop deterioration in liver function (Gane & Pilmore, 2002).

2.5.6 Newer agents

Other nucleotide and nucleoside analogues are now available for use in HBV-infected individuals, including adefover, entecavir, telbivudine and tenofovir (Chang et al., 2006; Marcellin et al., 2008; van Bommel et al., 2006). Advantages include potency, low rates of resistance allowing prolonged therapy without breakthrough, and efficacy in lamivudine-resistant patients. No data exist in renal transplant recipients; however, dose reductions may be necessary if renal insufficiency is present.

2.6 Human Immunodeficiency Virus (HIV)

2.6.1 HIV and kidney transplantation

- Patients with HIV require specialized care in centers with appropriate expertise.
- Screening for HIV infection should be carried out on all kidney transplant recipients (ideally before transplantation) in order to identify those kidney transplant recipients that will require specialized care.
- Antiretroviral therapy is necessary to maintain virologic suppression and normal immunologic function in HIV patients undergoing kidney transplantation.
- The concomitant use of antiretroviral agents and immunosuppressive medications creates the potential for drug-drug interactions that may substantially alter blood levels of drugs and require appropriate monitoring and adjustments in dosing (Frassetto et al., 2007).
- Some of the antiretroviral agents, particularly protease inhibitors, are potent inhibitors of P-450 (e.g., ritonavir is the most potent inhibitor of P-450 that is clinically available, and when used alone or in combination [kaletra-retonavir/lopinavir], very small doses of calcineurin inhibitor [e.g., 1 mg/week of tacrolimus] may maintain adequate drug levels (Abbott et al., 2004)

Tenofovir (a component of Truvada and Atrypla) is nephrotoxic and should be avoided after transplantation.

2.6.2 Outcome of kidney transplantation in recipients with HIV

Case series have documented successful outcomes of kidney transplant recipients with HIV (Gruber et al., 2008). However, these HIV patients had been carefully selected and adequately treated for HIV at the time of transplantation. Although HIV is not an absolute contraindication to kidney transplantation, the presence of HIV has major implications in the management of patients following transplantation (4). A major issue of concern in the management of HIV patients is the need to be aware of potential drug-drug interactions among antiretroviral therapy and other medications, including immunosuppressants (Frassetto et al., 2007).

Care must be taken to identify and select those HIV-infected patients who are most likely to benefit from kidney transplantation without an unacceptably high risk of opportunistic infections.

Evidence from a National Institutes of Health (NIH)-sponsored study of organ transplantation in HIV patients has demonstrated both the effectiveness of transplantation as well as the complexity of management of kidney transplant recipients with HIV (Roland et al., 2008). Data accrued from this study has identified specific drug combinations that are associated with drug–drug interactions in these patients. Accordingly, attention must be paid and caution must be used in these patients to account for the potential impact of these interactions (Roland et al., 2008).

Although the data from the NIH study demonstrate the feasibility of transplantation for HIV-infected kidney transplant recipients, the limited number of HIV patients with CKD stage 5 undergoing kidney transplantation to date suggests the need to continue performing this procedure under research protocols and in selected centers with appropriate expertise.

Between November 2003 and June 2009 a prospective, nonrandomized trial was following a total of 150 HIV patients underwent kidney transplantation; survivors were followed for a median period of 1.7 years. In this cohort of carefully selected HIV-infected patients, both patient- and graft survival rates were high at 1 and 3 years, with no increases in complications associated with HIV infection. But there were unexpectedly high rejection rates which indicate the need for better immunotherapy (Stock et al., 2010).

Finally, it is worth noting that review of experience to date suggests that there may be an increased risk for the development of acute cellular rejection in patients with HIV undergoing organ transplantation (KDIGO, 2009).

2.7 BK virus

2.7.1 Introduction

Polyomaviruses:

Polyomaviruses have been identified in transplant recipients in association with nephropathy and ureteral obstruction (BK virus), and in association with demyelinating disease of the brain (JC virus) similar to that in AIDS (Fishman, 2002; Hirsch et al., 2006). Adult levels of seroprevalence are 65% to 90%. BK virus seems to achieve latency in renal tubular epithelial cells. JC virus also has been isolated from renal tissues but seems to have preferred tropism for neural tissues. Reactivation occurs with immunodeficiency and immunosuppression and tissue injury (e.g., ischemia-reperfusion) (Hirsch et al., 2002).

2.7.2 BK nephropathy

BK virus causes latent infection of the kidney; with reactivation during immune suppression.

BK virus is associated with a range of clinical syndromes in immunocompromised hosts, including viruria and viremia, tubulointerstitial nephritis, ureteral ulceration and stenosis, and hemorrhagic cystitis (Fishman, 2002; Hirsch et al., 2002). Active infection of renal allografts has been associated with progressive loss of graft function ("BK nephropathy") in approximately 4% of renal transplant recipients; this is referred to as polyomavirus-associated nephropathy (PVAN). The clinical presentation of disease is usually as sterile pyuria, reflecting shedding of infected tubular and ureteric epithelial cells. These cells contain sheets of virus and are detected by urine cytology as "decoy cells." In some cases, the patient presents with diminished renal allograft function or with ureteric stenosis and obstruction (Fishman, 2002).

2.7.3 Incidence

- Fifty percent of patients who develop BK viremia do so by 3 months after kidney transplantation.
- Ninety-five percent of BKV nephropathy occurs in the first 2 years after kidney transplantation (Randhawa & Brennan, 2005).

2.7.4 Risk factors

Studies have implicated donor seropositivity, high-dose immunosuppression (particularly tacrolimus and mycophenolate mofetil), pulse-dose steroids, severe ischemia-reperfusion injury, exposure to antilymphocyte therapy, increased number of HLA mismatches between donor and recipient, deceased donor renal transplants, allograft rejection and presence and degree of viremia in the pathogenesis of disease (Fishman, 2002).
The role of specific immunosuppressive agents has not been confirmed.

2.7.5 Diagnosis

The use of urine cytology to detect the presence of infected decoy cells in the urine has approximately 100% sensitivity for BK virus infection but a low (29%) predictive value (Fishman, 2002; Hirsch et al., 2002).
It is a useful screening tool but cannot establish a firm diagnosis.
Monitoring for BK virus in the plasma by DNA PCR is more specific for diagnosis of BK nephropathy than is detection with urine specimens. However, the detection of BK virus DNA in urine specimens may provide the first evidence of polyomavirus infection in the patient (Ramos et al., 2002, 2003).
Given the presence of viremia in renal allograft recipients, it is crucial to reduce immunosuppression whenever possible.
Definitive diagnosis requires a renal biopsy. Renal biopsy specimens initially show cytopathic changes in renal epithelial cells with the gradual evolution of cellular infiltration consistent with the diagnosis of interstitial nephritis. Fibrosis is often prominent occasionally with calcification. Immunostaining for cross-reacting SV40 virus shows patchy staining of viral particles within tubular cells (Fishman & Davis, 2008).

2.7.6 Screening

Whether to screen KTRs with NAT of plasma or urine has been controversial. A negative urine NAT for BKV has almost a 100% negative predictive value (Hirsch et al., 2005). By testing urine, one can avoid performing BKV testing of blood on those patients with negative urine studies. Based on this, some experts recommend screening of urine as the definitive site for BKV surveillance (Hirsch et al., 2005). However, the presence of a positive NAT for BKV in urine, in the absence of an elevated BKV load in the plasma, is not associated with an increased risk for BKV disease (Hirsch et al., 2005). Hence, the use of urine screening requires performance of NAT on the blood of those patients whose level of BK viruria exceeds established thresholds. This requires patients to return to the clinic for the additional test. Accordingly, it is suggested that NAT be performed on plasma, and not the urine of KTRs.
When NAT is not available, microscopic evaluation of the urine for the presence of decoy cells is an acceptable, albeit nonspecific, alternative screening method for BKV disease and

the risk for BKV nephropathy. A negative screening test rules out BKV nephropathy in most cases (high negative predictive value). However, a positive screening test has a very low positive predictive value for BKV nephropathy (Hirsch et al., 2005; Randhawa & Brennan, 2005). Thus, many patients with urine decoy cells will not develop BKV nephropathy. It may be inappropriate to change therapy in such patients based on the presence of urine decoy cells alone.

Emerging data suggest that BKV nephropathy can be prevented if immunosuppressive medications are reduced in patients with BKV detected by a high viral load in plasma (determined by NAT) (Brennan et al., 2005).

2.7.7 Treatment of biopsy-proven BKV nephropathy

The treatment of BKV nephropathy is unsatisfactory.

The risk of BKV nephropathy appears to be correlated with the intensity of immunosuppression, and reduction of immunosuppression can result in a decrease in BKV load and a concomitant reduction of risk of development of BKV nephropathy (Almeras et al., 2008).

Although there are some centers that would use antiviral therapy (including cidofovir, leflunomide and/or ciprofloxacin) as treatment, to date there are no definitive data confirming their effectiveness (Hirsch et al., 2005; Randhawa & Brennan, 2005). However, reduction of immunosuppression does appear to have some impact on BKV nephropathy, though variable rates of graft loss attributable to BKV nephropathy have been reported even when reduction of immunosuppression has been employed. A common practice of immunosuppressive dose reduction is withdrawal of antimetabolite (azathioprine or Mycophenolate Mofetil {MMF}) and reduction in calcineurin inhibitors (CNIs) dosage by 50%. Switching from the antimetabolite MMF to leflunomide (an immunosuppressive agent with antiviral activity and lacking nephrotoxicity) in a maintenance dose of 20 to 40 mg daily has been associated with declining BKV load in blood and improving histology (Williams et al., 2005). Some centers advocate the use of cidofovir for BK nephropathy in low doses (0.25 to 1 mg/kg every 2 weeks) (Andrei et al., 1997; Vats et al., 2003). Significant renal toxicity may be observed with this agent, and may add little to reduction in immunosuppression alone.

2.8 JC virus

JC is the agent responsible for progressive multifocal leukoencephalopathy (PML). This infection of the central nervous system by JC polyomavirus has been observed uncommonly in renal allograft recipients. This infection generally manifests with focal neurologic deficits or seizures and may progress to death after extensive demyelination (Baksh et al., 2001).

2.9 Herpes Simplex Virus (HSV)

2.9.1 Superficial HSV infection

Superficial herpes simplex virus (HSV) infection is defined as disease limited to the skin or mucosal surfaces without evidence of dissemination to visceral organs.

Serologic evidence of HSV1 and HSV2 is common in the general population. Although periodic reactivation of HSV1 and HSV2 infection occurs, these episodes tend to be self-limited in immunocompetent individuals. However, episodes of invasive or disseminated HSV may occur in KTRs receiving immunosuppressive medications, and indeed the

incidence of invasive HSV is higher in KTRs than in the general population (Koneru et al., 1988; Wertheim et al., 1985).
The highest incidence of HSV reactivation occurs early after transplantation, with the greatest risk occurring during the first month following transplantation (3). While presentation later after transplant is associated with a lower risk of dissemination, treatment of superficial infection with oral acyclovir, valacyclovir or famciclovir is still recommended, given the safety and efficacy of these medications (3).
To prevent dissemination, it seems prudent to continue treatment until there are no new, active lesions.

2.9.2 Systemic HSV infection

In contrast to superficial HSV infection, systemic HSV infection involving the lungs, liver, central nervous system or other visceral organs represents a potentially life-threatening complication. Because systemic HSV is life-threatening, hospitalization and treatment with intravenous acyclovir is warranted (3). If possible, immunosuppressive medications should be reduced or withdrawn until the infection has resolved.
Intravenous acyclovir should be continued until there is demonstrative evidence of clinical improvement as measured by resolution of fever, hypoxia and signs or symptoms of hepatitis. For treatment of HSV encephalitis, a higher dosage is given by slow infusion to prevent crystallization within the renal tubules.
Once the patient has reached this level of improvement, completion of therapy may be carried out using oral acyclovir or valacyclovir (3).

2.10 Herpes Zoster Virus (HZV)

2.10.1 Uncomplicated herpes zoster

Uncomplicated zoster is a clinical syndrome characterized by cutaneous clustering of vesicular lesions in a dermatomal distribution of one or more adjacent sensory nerves. In immunocompromised hosts, patients are at risk not only of postherpetic neuralgia but also of severe local dermatomal infection (Rubin & Tolkoff-Rubin, 1983). Similarly, immunosuppressed patients are at increased risk for the development of disseminated cutaneous zoster and visceral dissemination. The higher the level of immunosuppression, the greater the risk of dissemination.
Accordingly, prompt initiation of antiviral therapy with close follow-up is warranted for these patients, even if they have only superficial skin infection (3).

2.10.2 Disseminated or invasive herpes zoster

Patients with only skin disease, but who have lesions involving more than three dermatomes, are considered to have disseminated cutaneous zoster. Similarly, patients with visceral involvement (pneumonia, encephalitis, disseminated intravascular coagulation, or graft dysfunction) in addition to skin disease are considered to have disseminated zoster (3).
Treatment with intravenous acyclovir and temporary reduction in the amount of immunosuppressive medication is efficacious (3, Fehr et al., 2002). Although specific evidence is not available to guide which immunosuppressive agent should be reduced, it would seem logical, whenever possible, to reduce the dosage of CNIs as well as steroids. In the absence of any evidence of intercurrent rejection, an effort should be made to maintain

the reduced level of immunosuppression for a minimum of 3-5 days and until there is evidence of clinical improvement (KDIGO, 2009).

2.10.3 Pzevention of primary varicella zoster infection

The use of varicella zoster immunoglobulin has been demonstrated to prevent or modify varicella in immunosuppressed individuals exposed to varicella (3; 12; Boeckh, 2006).
If varicella zoster immunoglobulin is not available, or if >96 h have passed since the exposure, some experts recommend prophylaxis with a 7-day course of oral acyclovir (80 mg/kg/day administered in four divided doses with a maximum of 800 mg per dose) beginning on day 7-10 after varicella exposure (12; Boeckh, 2006).
The use of varicella vaccine is not recommended as a postexposure prophylactic strategy in KTRs.

2.11 Parvovirus

In the transplant population, infection with parvovirus B19 can be presented with refractory severe anemia, pancytopenia, thrombotic microangiopathy, fibrosing cholestatic hepatitis, encephalitis, and graft dysfunction. Parvovirus infection commonly occurs within the first 3 months of transplantation with reported donor transmission and can be diagnosed with bone marrow examination that reveals typical giant proerythroblasts, and the diagnosis should be confirmed by detection of B19 virus DNA in serum by PCR assay. Treatment consists of high-dose IVIG (0.5 mg/kg per day for 5 to 10 days), reduction of immunosuppression, and, if possible, discontinuation of tacrolimus therapy for recurrent or persistent disease (Pegues et al., 2010).

3. Fungal infections

3.1 Introduction

Fungal infections remain a significant cause of morbidity and mortality in renal transplant recipients, despite ongoing refinements in immunosuppressive therapy, graft preservation, and surgical techniques. The mortality from fungal infections remains high, although the incidence of fungal infections in renal transplant recipients is less than that reported for other solid organ transplant recipients, and is related to the pathogenicity of the organisms, site of infection, impaired host inflammatory response, potential for rapid clinical progression, failure to recognize a high-risk patient, and comorbidities, such as renal failure and diabetes mellitus (Pegues et al., 2010).

3.2 Antifungal prophylaxis

3.2.1 Introduction

The incidence of invasive fungal infections following solid organ transplantation ranges from 5 to 42 percent and varies with the organ being transplanted. Candida and Aspergillus species are the leading causative agents, and the majority of these infections occur within the first month after transplantation. These infections are associated with high overall mortality rates (Paya, 1993; Singh, 2000).

3.2.2 Patient selection

Patients who should be considered for antifungal prophylaxis include those with:

- Renal and hepatic dysfunction.

- Large blood transfusion requirements.
- Prolonged ICU stays.
- Additional surgery posttransplant including laparotomy and retransplantation.
- Known fungal colonization pretransplantation.
- Prior (broad-spectrum) antimicrobial use.

None of the currently available antifungal agents is ideal for all of the indications for posttransplant prophylaxis.

3.2.3 Fluconazole

Fluconazole appears to be safe and has not been associated with hepatotoxicity following liver transplantation; it can be used as prophylaxis against susceptible Candida species and reduces invasive infections in such patients (Playford et al., 2004).

Fluconazole does not have activity against filamentous fungi. In addition, some Candida species have relative resistance (high minimum inhibitory concentrations [MICs]) to the drug. Drug interactions with calcineurin inhibitors are variable but will increase these drug levels in most patients. Similarly, serum calcineurin inhibitor levels will fall when prophylaxis is discontinued; dose readjustment is essential to prevent graft rejection.

3.2.4 Itraconazole

Itraconazole capsules have poor oral bioavailability and should not be relied upon in the critically ill patient after transplantation. The itraconazole suspension has better oral bioavailability, but trials to date have failed to demonstrate the efficacy of the oral solution for the prevention of invasive aspergillosis (Menichetti et al., 1999).

Efficacy of the intravenous formulation as prophylaxis waits testing in clinical trials. Significant drug interactions with calcineurin inhibitors result in levels increased two to four fold over baseline.

3.2.5 Voriconazole

Voriconazole was approved by the FDA for the treatment of aspergillosis, scedosporiosis, and fusariosis in 2002. This azole offers broader filamentous mold activity than either fluconazole or itraconazole, but has no activity against the zygomycetes. In addition, it has excellent oral bioavailability. However, no prophylactic trials have been performed to date. In addition, as with the other azoles, voriconazole is a significant inhibitor of the cytochrome P450 enzymes. Of particular note, co-administration of voriconazole and sirolimus is contraindicated due to these interactions (11). Significant drug interactions with calcineurin inhibitors result in levels 3-5 fold over baseline in most patients.

3.2.6 Amphotericin B

Amphotericin B (both regular and lipid formulations) are used in a number of centers for the prevention of fungal infections. Several studies have demonstrated the failure of low-dose regimens as prophylaxis for invasive aspergillosis (Lorf et al., 1999; Perfect et al., 1992), and such therapies should be used with caution.

3.2.7 Echinocandins

There are multiple FDA-approved echinocandins with similar spectra of antifungal activity including caspofungin, micafungin, and anidulafungin. No trials of prophylaxis in solid organ transplantation have been performed to date. These agents are not inducers or inhibitors of the cytochrome P450 enzymes. However, cyclosporine moderately increases the area under the curve (AUC) of caspofungin and elevations in hepatic transaminases were noted in healthy subjects when the drugs were administered concomitantly. These drugs are available in IV formulations only (Mora-Duarte et al., 2002).

3.3 Candida

The most common fungal pathogen in transplant patients is Candida, with more than 50% being of non-albicans strains.

Candida infections occur most commonly during the first month following transplantation and are usually associated with transplant surgical technical complications, early rejection, and enhanced immunosuppression (Fishman, 2007).

Candida infection is most commonly associated with an endogenous source of colonization, but inadequate health care worker hand hygiene may contribute to acquisition from an exogenous source. C. albicans is the most common species, followed by C. glabrata, C. tropicalis, and C. parapsilosis. Speciation is clinically useful because nonalbicans Candida species vary in in-vitro susceptibility to amphotericin B and azoles (10).

Mucocutaneous candidal infection (e.g., oral thrush, esophageal infection, cutaneous infection at intertriginous sites, candidal vaginitis) is most common in diabetics, with high-dose steroid therapy, and during broad-spectrum antibacterial therapy. These infections are usually treatable through correction of the underlying metabolic abnormality and topical therapy with clotrimazole or nystatin without associated risks that may be present for systemically absorbed antifungal agents. However, a recent report suggested a potential drug–drug interaction between clotrimazole and tacrolimus (Vasquez et al., 2001). It is important to note that there are drug–drug interactions between fluconazole and calcineurin inhibitors.

Although data regarding the appropriate duration of prophylaxis for these agents are not available for kidney transplant recipients, the risk is greatest early after transplantation when patients are receiving their highest levels of immunosuppression, and are more likely to be exposed to antibacterial agents that increase the risk for Candida infections. Accordingly, these agents can likely be discontinued once the patient is on maintenance immunosuppression, particularly when steroid doses are stable and low (10).

Thrush also may complicate viral (HSV, CMV) or toxic (drugs including mycophenolate mofetil) esophagitis.

Other sites of Candida infection include wound infections; cystitis, pyelonephritis, and ureteral obstruction by Candida elements or "fungal ball"; intra-abdominal infections, including infected perigraft fluid collections or peritonitis; and intravascular device-associated fungemia (10).

Optimal management of candidal infection occurring in association with the presence of vascular access catheters, surgical drains, genitourinary tract stents, and bladder catheters requires removal of the foreign body and systemic antifungal therapy with fluconazole or echinocandin.

Renal parenchymal infection most often results from candidemia and hematogenous spread, although ascending infection from the bladder can occur (10).

Candiduria is a special problem in renal transplant recipients, even if the patient is asymptomatic. Particularly in individuals with poor bladder function, obstructing fungal balls can develop at the ureteropelvic junction, resulting in obstructive uropathy, ascending pyelonephritis, and the possibility of systemic dissemination. A single positive blood culture result for Candida species necessitates systemic antifungal therapy; this finding carries a risk of visceral invasion of greater than 50% in this population (Fishman & Davis, 2008).

3.4 Aspergillus

Patients at risk for aspergillosis include those receiving repeated courses of enhanced immunosuppression for rejection and those with chronic graft dysfunction, diabetes, comorbid medical illnesses, or CMV infection.

The clinical spectra of aspergillosis include: pneumonia and other tissue-invasive forms, including genitourinary, central nervous system, rhinocerebral, gastrointestinal, skin, wound, and musculoskeletal disease (Pegues et al., 2010).

Invasive aspergillosis is a medical emergency in the transplant recipient, with the portal of entry being the lungs and sinuses in more than 90% of patients and the skin in most of those remaining.

The pathological hallmark of invasive aspergillosis is blood vessel invasion, which accounts for the three clinical characteristics of this infection—tissue infarction, hemorrhage, and systemic dissemination with metastatic invasion. Early in the course of transplantation, central nervous system involvement with fungal infection is most often due to Aspergillus; 1 year or later after transplantation, other fungi (Zygomycetes, dematiaceous fungi) become more prominent (Fishman & Davis, 2008).

Diagnosis of aspergillus infection depends on a high clinical suspicion, isolation of Aspergillus species from a sterile body site or repeated isolation from the respiratory tract, and typical radiographic findings.

Radiologic appearances of pulmonary aspergillosis in kidney transplant recipients include nodules, diffuse or wedge-shaped opacities, empyema, or cavitary forms. Serial measurement of aspergillus galactomannan in the serum may aid in the early diagnosis of invasive aspergillosis in the high-risk setting (Pegues et al., 2010).

Voriconazole is the drug of choice for documented Aspergillus infection, despite its significant interactions with calcineurin inhibitors and rapamycin (Herbrecht et al., 2002).

Liposomal amphotericin is an equally effective alternative, and combination therapies are under study. Surgical debridement is usually essential for successful clearance of such invasive infections.

3.5 Pneumocystosis

3.5.1 Introduction

Pneumocystis jirovecii (formally known as Pneumocystis carinii) is an opportunistic fungal pathogen known to cause life-threatening pneumonia in immunocompromised patients, including kidney transplant recipients.

The risk of infection with Pneumocystis is greatest in the first 2-6 months after transplantation and during periods of increased immunosuppression (Fishman & Rubin, 1998; Fishman, 2001).

Most transplant centers report an incidence of Pneumocystis pneumonia of approximately 10% in the first 6 months after transplantation in patients not receiving trimethoprim/sulfamethoxazole (or alternative drugs) as prophylaxis. There is a continued risk of infection in cases of: recipients who require over immunosuppression for prolonged periods because of poor allograft function or chronic rejection, recipients with chronic CMV infection, and recipients undergoing treatments that increase the level of immunodeficiency, such as cancer chemotherapy or neutropenia secondary to drug toxicity (Fishman & Davis, 2008).

3.5.2 Clinical presentation

P. jirovecii pneumonia (PCP) is defined as the presence of lower respiratory-tract infection due to P. jirovecii.

It typically presents with fever, dyspnea, nonproductive cough, marked hypoxemia with arterial-alveolar mismatching, and diffuse interstitial infiltration or focal air space consolidation on chest radiograph. Unusual presentations are possible in renal transplant recipients, including pulmonary mass lesions.

In the transplant recipient, Pneumocystis pneumonia is generally acute to subacute in development. Atypical Pneumocystis infection (radiographically or clinically) may be seen in patients who have coexisting pulmonary infections or who develop disease while receiving prophylaxis with second-choice agents (e.g., pentamidine or atovaquone).

Significant extrapulmonary disease is uncommon in the transplant recipient (Fishman, 2001).

3.5.3 Diagnosis

The characteristic hypoxemia of Pneumocystis pneumonia produces a broad alveolar-arterial partial pressure of oxygen gradient. The level of serum lactate dehydrogenase is elevated in most patients with Pneumocystis pneumonia (>300 IU/mL).

There is no diagnostic pattern exists for Pneumocystis pneumonia on routine chest radiograph that may be entirely normal or develop the classic pattern of perihilar and interstitial ground-glass infiltrates. Chest CT scans are more sensitive to the diffuse interstitial and nodular pattern than routine radiographs.

The manifestations of P. carinii (jiroveci) pneumonia -both clinically and radiologically- are virtually identical to the manifestations of CMV and it is very difficult to determine whether both pathogens are present (Fishman & Davis, 2008).

A definitive diagnosis of PCP is made by demonstration of organisms in lung tissue or lower respiratory tract secretions. Because no specific diagnostic pattern exists on any given imaging test, it is imperative that the diagnosis of PCP be confirmed by lung biopsy or bronchoalveolar lavage (KDIGO, 2009).

3.5.4 Prophylaxis

The importance of preventing Pneumocystis infection cannot be overemphasized and although PCP is potentially a life-threatening complication of kidney transplant recipients, the use of chemoprophylaxis has been shown to be extremely effective in preventing the development of clinical disease attributable to this pathogen.

Prophylaxis against disease should be reinstituted following augmentation of immunosuppression, such as steroid bolus for acute rejection.

Prophylactic agents, in order of efficacy, include trimethoprim–sulfamethoxazole (TMP-SMX), monthly intravenous or aerosolized pentamidine, daily dapsone, daily atovaquone, and the combination of clindamycin and pyrimethamine.

Indications for the use of alternative preventive agents include the development of allergic reactions and/or drug-induced neutropenia from TMP-SMX (KDIGO, 2009).

Low-dose TMP-SMX is well tolerated and should be used in the absence of concrete data showing true allergy or interstitial nephritis.

TMP-SMX is the most effective agent for prevention of infection caused by P.carinii (jiroveci). The advantages of TMP-SMX include increased efficacy; lower cost; availability of oral preparations; and possible protection against other organisms, including T. gondii, Isospora belli, Cyclospora cayetanensis, Nocardia asteroides, and common urinary, respiratory, and gastrointestinal bacterial pathogens (Fishman & Davis, 2008). None of the alternative regimens is as good as daily TMP-SMX and none provides the antibacterial protection of that agent (Rodriguez & Fishman, 2004). Thus, another agent (daily fluoroquinolone) must be added for antibacterial activity. This may be of greatest importance in renal and lung transplant recipients where the early incidence of postoperative bacterial infections is high.

There was no difference in efficacy for PCP when TMP-SMX was given daily or three times per week (Hughes et al., 1987). However, in kidney transplant recipients, the use of daily TMP-SMX may be associated with a decreased risk of bacterial infection and may be easier for patient adherence (Fox et al., 1990).

Although definitive evidence for the duration of PCP prophylaxis is not available, most experts agree that it should be continued for at least 6 months (and perhaps as long as 1 year) following transplantation (5). Because most kidney transplant recipients will remain on immunosuppression for the rest of their lives, some experts recommend a more prolonged and perhaps even indefinite use of PCP prophylaxis.

3.5.5 Treatment

Prior to the use of TMP-SMX, mortality from PCP in kidney transplant recipients was very high (Hennequin et al., 1995; Sterling et al., 1984).

The treatment of PCP includes both the use of intravenous TMP-SMX as well as corticosteroids for kidney transplant recipients with significant hypoxemia and reduction of immunosuppressive medications (5). RCTs have demonstrated that the use of corticosteroids in the first 72 hours of PCP in HIV patients with moderate to severe PCP resulted in improved outcome, including morbidity, mortality and avoidance of intubation (5). The usual duration of treatment is 2–3 weeks.

First-line treatment is with TMP-SMX 15 mg/kg for 21 days. Treatment of severe disease should include adjunctive steroids as for HIV-infected persons with PCP (60 mg/day initially, then taper).

Second-line agents include intravenous pentamidine isethionate (4 mg/kg per day, used in patients with proven TMP-SMX allergy), dapsone-trimethoprim (100 mg dapsone daily with trimethoprim 100 mg twice daily), or clindamycin plus primaquine (600 mg 4 times daily clindamycin with 30 mg base daily primaquine).

Adverse effects of trimethoprim include nephrotoxicity, pancreatitis, and bone marrow suppression. Dapsone is associated with hemolytic anemia in patients with glucose-6-phosphate dehydrogenase deficiency.

Mild to moderate P. jiroveci pneumonia can be treated with atovaquone (750 mg orally twice daily for 21 days) in patients allergic to TMP-SMX (Pegues et al., 2010).

3.6 Cryptococcus

3.6.1 Clinical presentation after transplantation

Cryptococcal infection is rarely seen in the transplant recipient until more than 6 months after transplantation. The most common presentation of cryptococcal infection in the relatively intact transplant recipient is that of an asymptomatic pulmonary nodule, often with active organisms present, while in the chronic patient, pneumonia and meningitis are common, with skin involvement at sites of tissue injury (catheters) and in prostate or bone (Fishman & Davis, 2008).

3.6.2 Diagnosis and treatment

Cryptococcosis should be suspected in transplant recipients who present - more than 6 months after transplantation - with unexplained headaches (especially when accompanied by fevers), decreased state of consciousness, failure to thrive, or unexplained focal skin lesion (which requires biopsy for culture and pathological evaluation).
Diagnosis requires detection of serum cryptococcal antigen, but all such patients should have lumbar puncture for cell counts and cryptococcal antigen studies. Liposomal amphotericin and flucytosine (after obtaining serum levels) are probably the best initial treatment followed by high-dose fluconazole until the cryptococcal antigen is cleared from blood and cerebrospinal fluid. Scarring and hydrocephalus may be observed (Fishman & Davis, 2008).

3.7 Treatment of fungal infection

3.7.1 Amphotericin B deoxycholate (AmB)

AmB was used for treatment of invasive candidiasis, cryptococcosis, coccidioidomycosis, histoplasmosis, and aspergillosis but owing to inherent toxicities and intolerance, newer agents have increasingly been used in renal transplant recipients. Its lipid formulations are all associated with lower risks for nephrotoxicity, metabolic derangements, and infusion-associated side effects than is AmB.

3.7.2 Voriconazole

Voriconazole is superior to conventional AmB for the treatment of invasive aspergillosis and also has in vitro activity against a wider range of organisms (Herbrecht et al., 2002).

3.7.3 Itraconazole

Despite its good in vitro activity against Aspergillus species; Itraconazole use is generally reserved for treatment of less-severe aspergillosis (Menichetti et al., 1999) or maintenance therapy following initial response to lipid amphotericin or voriconazole and for treatment of endemic mycoses. All of the azoles impair calcineurin inhibitor metabolism and increase calcineurin blood levels.

3.7.4 Fluconazole

Fluconazole is the first-line agent of the treatment or prevention of reactivation coccidioidomycosis in renal transplant recipients. The development of fungal resistance or tolerance can result from the long-term use of fluconazole that also may increase the risk for fungal superinfection with C. glabrata, C. krusei, or C. tropicalis (Playford et al., 2004). Fluconazole and 5-flucytosine can be used for cryptococcal disease.

3.7.5 Echinocandins

Echinocardins including caspofungin, anidulafungin, and micafungin are fungicidal for Candida species, including fluconazole-resistant species. These agents are effective, well

tolerated, and have few drug-drug interactions. So, they increasingly are being used to treat serious infections associated with nonalbicans Candida species in transplant recipients (Mora-Duarte et al., 2002). Echinocandins are available only as intravenous formulations.
Finally, the development of any serious fungal infection in a transplant recipient mandates a critical evaluation of the immunosuppressive regimen with minimizing the corticosteroid dose, keeping the blood levels of CNIs in the low therapeutic range, and discontinuation of other immunosuppressive agents temporarily. In case of life-threatening fungal infection with clinical treatment failure despite appropriate antifungal therapy, discontinuation of immunosuppression at the cost of graft loss may be warranted.

4. Bacterial infections

4.1 Introduction

In the early post-transplantation period, the bacterial pathogens are similar to those causing health care-associated infections in the non-transplant surgical population with Enterobacteriaceae, and Staphylococcus and Pseudomonas species are the most commonly isolated health care pathogens and increasingly are multidrug resistant (Fishman, 2007).
Aerobic gram-negative bacilli, including Enterobacteriaceae and P. aeruginosa, are the most common organisms causing pneumonia and UTIs in kidney transplant recipients. Klebsiella pneumoniae and E. coli strains with resistance to extended-spectrum cephalosporins are increasingly associated with nosocomial urinary tract infections (Green et al., 2004).

4.2 Urinary Tract Infection (UTI)

A urinary tract infection (UTI) is an infection causing signs and symptoms of cystitis or pyelonephritis (including the presence of signs of systemic inflammation), which is documented to be caused by an infectious agent. Kidney allograft pyelonephritis is an infection of the kidney allograft that is usually accompanied by characteristic signs and symptoms of systemic inflammation and a positive urine and/or blood culture. Occasionally, pyelonephritis is diagnosed by allograft biopsy. Antibiotic prophylaxis is the use of an antimicrobial agent (or agents) to prevent the development of a UTI (KDIGO, 2009).
Observational studies have documented a high incidence of UTI in KTRs (Schmaldienst et al., 2002). Pyelonephritis of the kidney allograft is a common complication in KTRs (Schmaldienst et al., 2002). It may cause graft failure, sepsis and death. The use of antibiotic prophylaxis with trimethoprim–sulfamethoxazole has been demonstrated to decrease the frequency of bacterial infections, including UTI in KTRs (Fox et al., 1990). The use of trimethoprim–sulfamethoxazole for the first 9 months following kidney transplant was associated with statistically significant decreases in number of any bacterial infection, overall number of UTI and number of noncatheter UTI.
Although the use of ciproflaxicin also appeared effective in the prevention of UTI after KTRs, patients treated with this regimen were at risk for, and developed Pneumocystis jirovecii pneumonia (PCP) (Hibberd et al., 1992b). Accordingly, the use of TMP-SMX is preferred over ciprofloxacin at least during the first 6 months after transplantation.
Evidence suggests that late UTIs tend to be benign, without associated bacteremia, metastatic foci or effect on long-term graft function (Munoz, 2001).
For this reason, it is recommended to provide prophylaxis for a minimum of 6 months. For patients who are allergic to TMP-SMX, the recommended alternative agent would be

nitrofurantoin, which is widely recommended as an alternative to TMP-SMX, is chosen over ciprofloxacin (despite demonstrated effectiveness in KTRs) in an effort to limit the likelihood of emergence of antibacterial resistance.
Kidney allograft pyelonephritis may be associated with bacteremia, metastatic spread, impaired graft function and even death. Accordingly, KTRs with clinical and laboratory evidence suggestive of kidney allograft pyelonephritis should be hospitalized and be treated with intravenous antibiotics for at least the initial course of therapy. This is particularly true in early infections (first 4-6 months following kidney transplantation) (KDIGO, 2009). Recognition of the morbidity and mortality associated with allograft pyelonephritis led to recommendations in the 1980s to treat UTIs with as long as a 6-week course of antimicrobials for early UTI following transplantation. More recently, UTI after kidney transplantation has been associated with considerably lower morbidity and mortality (Munoz, 2001). Accordingly, a less-prolonged course may be required, although patients experiencing relapsing infection should be considered for a more prolonged therapeutic course.
Because of the potential for serious complications, KTRs with kidney allograft pyelonephritis should be hospitalized and treated with intravenous antibiotics, at least initially.

4.3 Mycobacterial infection

Tuberculosis (TB) and nontuberculous mycobacteria (NTM) are potential causes of serious infection in renal allograft recipients that may present as early as the first post-transplantation month.

4.3.1 Tuberculosis (TB)

4.3.1.1 Natural course and diagnosis after transplantation

The incidence of active tuberculosis is estimated to be 1% to 4% following renal transplantation and is higher in those who resided in or traveled to a country with a high prevalence of TB infection.
The most frequent source of TB infections in KTRs is reactivation of quiescent foci of Mycobacterium tuberculosis that persist after initial asymptomatic infection (Drobniewski & Ferguson, 1996). Accordingly, screening and identification of individuals with evidence of prior latent infection with TB should allow treatment prior to development of clinical disease, resulting in improved outcome.
Atypical presentations of M. tuberculosis and NTM disease may delay diagnosis and contribute to morbidity in the transplant population. Reactivation tuberculosis warrants special vigilance, especially among transplant recipients with a prior history of mycobacterial infection, with old granulomatous disease on chest radiograph, or from countries with high TB prevalence. Up to 40% of renal transplant recipients with reactivation tuberculosis will present with disseminated infection, with involvement of the skin, skeleton (bone and joint), or central nervous system and disseminated disease should be suggested with finding granuloma in biopsy specimens from extrapulmonary sites (9).
Interferon-gamma release assays such as T-SPOT.TB and QuantiFERON are an alternative to the tuberculin skin test for detecting latent TB infection (Triverio et al., 2009). Their sensitivity and specificity, however, have not been systematically evaluated in KTRs.
The use of BCG vaccine is especially common in regions where the prevalence of TB is high. In these regions, it is therefore difficult to distinguish purified-protein derivative (PPD) skin

tests that are positive due to BCG from those that are positive due to prior infection with M. tuberculosis. Accordingly, it is recommended that the history of BCG vaccination should be ignored and that a 9-month course of prophylactic isoniazid should be used (6).

The use of prophylactic isoniazid in patients with a past or current positive PPD skin test, and/or a history of TB without adequate documented treatment, has been previously recommended by the European Best Practice Guidelines for Renal Transplantation (6) and the American Society of Transplantation Guidelines for the Prevention and Management of Infectious Complications of Solid Organ Transplantation (8).

If, according to these guidelines, vaccination with BCG can give a 'false-positive' PPD skin test, then some patients may be treated unnecessarily. Most believe that the effect of BCG should not persist for more than 10 years (9).

4.3.1.2 Therapy

Because of the increase in multidrug-resistant (MDR) strains, appropriate therapy should include four agents: isoniazid (INH), rifampin (RIF), pyrazinamide (PZA), and ethambutol (EMB) or intramuscular streptomycin (SM) for 2 months or until susceptibility tests results are available followed by up to 10 months of INH and RIF (7).

Both INH and RIF affect the cytochrome P-450 enzyme system. INH increases CNIs and mTOR inhibitors levels, and RIF decreases these drug levels, increasing the risk for rejection. These interactions are usually predictable and may occur within 1 to 3 days of initiating antituberculous therapy. Appropriate dosage adjustments and monitoring are required (8).

One potential alternative is to substitute rifabutin for rifampin. Rifabutin has activity against M. tuberculosis that is similar to rifampin, but rifabutin is not as strong an inducer of CYP3A4 as rifampin (Vachharajani et al., 2002).

However, there is little published experience with rifabutin in KTRs.

4.3.2 Non-Tuberculous Mycobacteria (NTM)

Infection with NTM, including M. kansasii, M. fortuitum, M. chelonei, M. xenopi, M. marinum, and M. abscessus, has been reported in renal transplant recipients. These NTM can be isolated from sputum, lung tissue, skin, bone, and other disseminated sites. Many of the NTM are intrinsically resistant to standard antituberculous agents, and susceptibility testing should be performed against standard antituberculous agents, quinolones, macrolides, cephalosporins, and linezolid. Typical treatment includes combinations of agents for prolonged durations exceeding 12 months (Roy & Weisdorf, 1998).

4.4 Listeriosis

In renal transplant recipients, infection with L. monocytogenes typically occurs 6 or more months after transplantation and presents as meningoencephalitis or septicemia and in some cases, febrile gastroenteritis may occur. Bacteremia should be treated with intravenous ampicillin (2 gm every 4 hours for 2 weeks.), while meningitis should be treated with high-dose ampicillin and gentamicin for 3 weeks with performing repeat lumbar puncture to document cure (Pegues et al., 2010).

4.5 Legionellosis

Legionella species infections have been reported in kidney transplant recipients. Risk factors include repeated corticosteroid boluses, prolonged mechanical ventilation, and exposure to Legionella-contaminated hospital water supplies. L. micdadei and L. pneumophila commonly cause pneumonia presents with a nonproductive cough, a temperature-pulse dissociation, elevated hepatic enzymes, diarrhea, hyponatremia, myalgias, and altered mental status but extrapulmonary involvement, including culture-negative endocarditis and renal, hepatic, and central nervous system infection, have been reported. Chest x-ray findings include alveolar or interstitial infiltrates, cavities, pleural effusions, or lobar consolidation. Diagnosis can be confirmed by culture on special media or direct-fluorescent antibody testing of sputum, tissue, or bronchoalveolar fluid. In addition, a urinary antigen test should be performed for L. pneumophila serogroup 1. Empiric treatment should be administered immediately in suspected cases as delayed treatment is associated with increased mortality. In organ transplants, optimal treatment should include azithromycin and a quinolone for 14 to 21 days, depending on severity of illness (Pegues et al., 2010).

5. Parasites

5.1 Introduction

Acquisition of infection, clinical severity, and outcome of a parasitic disease depend on innate and acquired host immunity as well as the parasite's own immune response against the host when infection is established. Organ transplant recipients may acquire significant parasitic disease in 3 ways: transmission with the graft, de novo infection, or activation of dormant infection as a consequence of immunosuppression. Malaria, Trypanosoma, Toxoplasma, and Leishmania are the principal parasites that may be transmitted with bone marrow, kidney, or liver homografts, and microsporidia with xenotransplants. De novo infection with malaria and kala-azar may occur in immunocompromised travelers visiting in endemic areas, while immunocompromised natives are subject to superinfection with different strains of endemic parasites, reinfection with schistosomiasis, or rarely, with primary infections such as acanthamoeba. The list of parasites that may be reactivated in the immunocompromised host includes giardiasis, balantidiasis, strongyloidiasis, capillariasis, malaria, Chagas' disease, and kalaazar. The broad clinical syndromes of parasitic infection in transplant recipients include prolonged pyrexia, lower gastrointestinal symptoms, bronchopneumonia, and meningoencephalitis. Specific syndromes include the hematologic manifestations of malaria, myocarditis in Chagas' disease, acute renal failure in malaria and leishmaniasis, and the typical skin lesions of Chagas' and cutaneous leishmaniasis. Many antiparasitic drugs have the potential for gastrointestinal, hepatic, renal, and hematologic toxicity, and may interact with the metabolism of immunosuppressive agents. It is recommended that transplant clinicians have a high index of suspicion of parasitic infections as an important transmission threat, as well as a potential cause of significant posttransplant morbidity (Barsoum, 2004).

5.2 Malaria

Transmission of the disease has been reported with many organ transplants, as kidney (Holzer et al., 1985), bone marrow (Abdelkefi et al., 2004), and multiorgan (Chiche et al., 2003). Malarial antibodies also have been detected in a recipient of a heart transplant who received his graft from an infected donor (Fischer et al., 1999). Transmission of malaria has been traced to infected blood transfused to a kidney transplant recipient (Moran et al., 2004).

Primary or reinfection is a distinct risk in exposed transplant recipients. For this reason, chemoprophylaxis has been strongly advocated for travelers visiting endemic areas (Anteyi et al., 2003; Boggild et al., 2004). Unfortunately, infection can still be acquired in nonendemic locations including European or American airports (Giacomini, 1998) or indigenous malarial foci as those in New York (Iftikhar & Roistacher, 1995) or Georgia (MacArthur et al., 2001) in the United States.

The clinical picture of malaria in transplant recipients is usually severe, owing to the impaired immune response. It is characterized by pyrexia, which may lack the typical periodicity or rigors. Anemia is severe, being typically hemolytic and occasionally hemophagocytic (Abdelkefi et al., 2004). It is often associated with thrombocytopenia (MacArthur et al., 2001). Acute graft dysfunction may occur as a consequence of the hemodynamic consequences of falciparum infection (Barsoum, 2000). Whether the immune response to malarial infection has an impact on subsequent rejection is unknown (Barsoum, 2004).

5.3 Babesiosis

The causative organisms are protozoa closely similar to plasmodia. Babesiosis, attributed to transfusion with contaminated blood, has been reported in KTRs (Perdrizet et al., 2000). Fever, hemolytic anemia, and impaired graft function dominate the clinical picture. A hemophagosytic syndrome has been reported in an asplenic renal transplant recipient (Slovut et al., 1996). Treatment is by a combination of clindamycin and quinine, with therapeutic apheresis in severe cases (Evenson et al., 1998).

5.4 Schistosomiasis

The association between renal transplantation and schistosomiasis is frequently seen in endemic schistosomal regions and among immigrants living in western countries. The recipient, the donor or both may have active schistosomiasis or have a history of schistosomal infection, with permanent changes in the urinary or gastrointestinal tracts (Evenson et al., 1998).

KTRs may be exposed to new or reinfection of Schistosomal infection if they resume their usual habits of exposure to contaminated water. This has been reported in Egypt (Shokeir, 2001), where 23% of recipients at high risk were reinfected. The clinical profile in those cases was not significantly different from natural infection in immunocompetent individuals.

Recrudescence of schistosomal glomerulopathy has been reported in an endemic area in South America, where mesangioproliferative glomerulonephritis with schistosomal antigen deposits developed in a recent kidney transplant recipient who originally had been infected with S. mansoni (Sobh et al., 2001). Accordingly, it has been suggested to prophylactically treat patients with such infection before undergoing transplantation, since adult worms often live silently in an infected host for decades and are able to induce glomerular lesions through immune-complex deposits containing schistosomal gut antigens (Deelder et al., 1980).

5.5 Toxoplasmosis

Posttransplant toxoplasmosis has been reported most frequently with heart transplants (Hermanns et al., 2001). It also has been reported with bone marrow (Ortonne., 2001), stem cell (Lopez-Duarte et al., 2003), liver (Barcan et al., 2002), kidney (Sukthana et al., 2001), simultaneous liver-pancreas, and liver-kidney-pancreas (Hommann et al., 2002) transplants. Transmission of the disease can occur with either blood transfusion or transplanted organs. A study of 31 patients with posttransplant toxoplasmosis has shown that transmission occurred in 10, recrudescence in 2, and the mode of infection remained unknown in 19 (Renoult et al., 1997). The disease is characterized by pyrexia, lymphadenopathy, and multiorgan involvement. Anemia is common, and a hemophagocytic syndrome has been reported in several cases (Karras et al., 2004). Encephalitis is a serious and frequent complication (Lopez-Duarte et al., 2003). Peripheral neuropathy is common, taking a Guillain-Barré pattern in a recently reported case (Gonzalez et al., 2000). Chorioretinitis, similar to that seen in CMV infection, is frequently seen (Moshfeghi et al., 2004). Pulmonary infiltrates, with pleural involvement may occur (Barcan et al., 2002). Pyrimethamine is the treatment of choice.

5.6 Cryptosporidiosis

Cryptosporidium is an intestinal protozoan, which is often a benign commensal in the human intestine that can cause clinical disease in the immunocompromised patient. It is a notorious infection in intestinal transplants (Moshfeghi et al., 2004) but has also been reported as a recrudescence disease in recipients of liver (Campos et al., 2000), kidney (Minz et al., 2004), and bone marrow (Muller et al., 2004) transplants.

It may cause a diarrheal illness that can lead to significant fluid and electrolyte depletion and may be fatal. It can also persist, leading to chronic diarrhea with hepatobiliary involvement (Ferreira & Borges, 2002). There is no specific treatment, but the most widely used therapy is paromomycin.

5.7 Microsporidiasis

Microsporidia are intracellular spore-forming protozoa that are ubiquitous in the environment and may live in the intestine of insects, birds, and mammals. Human infection has been described most commonly with Enterocytozoon bieneusi in patients with HIV disease and only rarely in those with other forms of immunosuppression. Microsporidiosis have been reported in KTRs (Carlson et al., 2004; Mohindra et al., 2002).

Infection usually begins with diarrhea and cholangitis. Disseminated microsporidiosis is dominated by a febrile systemic inflammatory response, with rapid development of pneumonia and encephalitis, which is often fatal. The treatment of choice is albendazole (Anane & Attouchi, 2010).

6. References

Abbott, KC.; Swanson, SJ.; Agodoa, LY.& Kimmel, PL. (2004). Human immunodeficiency virus infection and kidney transplantation in the era of highly active antiretroviral therapy and modern immunosuppression, *J Am Soc Nephrol,* Vol., 15; pp.1633-1639.

Abdelkefi, A.; Ben Othman, T.; Torjman, L.; Ladeb, S.; Lakhal, A.; Belhadj, S. et al. (2004). Plasmodium falciparum causing hemophagocytic syndrome after allogeneic blood stem cell transplantation. *Hematol J*, Vol., 5; pp. 449-450.

Almeras, C.; Foulongne, V.; Garrigue, V.; Szwarc, I.; Vetromile, F.; Segondy, M., et al. (2008). Does reduction in immunosuppression in viremic patients prevent BK virus nephropathy in de novo renal transplant recipients? A prospective study. *Transplantation*, Vol., 85; pp. 1099–1104.

Anane, S. & Attouchi, H. (2010). Microsporidiosis: epidemiology, clinical data and therapy. *Gastroenterol Clin Biol*, Vol., 34; pp. 450-464.

Andrei, G.; Snoeck, R.; Vandeputte, M. & De Clercq, E.(1997). Activities of various compounds against murine and primate polyomaviruses. *Antimicrob Agents Chemother*, Vol., 41; pp. 587-593.

Anteyi, EA.; Liman, HM.; & Gbaji, A. (2003). Malaria prophylaxis in post renal transplant recipients in the tropics: is it necessary? *Cent Afr J Med*, Vol., 49; pp. 63-66.

Aroldi, A.; Lampertico, P.; Montagnino, G.; Passerini, P.; Villa, M.; Campise, MR, et al. (2005). Natural history of hepatitis B and C in renal allograft recipients. *Transplantation*, Vol., 79; pp. 1132–1136.

Asberg, A.; Humar, A.; Rollaq, H.; Jardine, AG.; Mouas, H.; Pescovitz, MD, et al. (2007). Oral valganciclovir is non inferior to intravenous ganciclovir for the treatment of cytomegalovirus disease in solid organ transplant recipients. *Am J Transplant*, Vol., 7; pp. 2106-2113.

Baksh, FK.; Finkelstein, SD.; Swalsky, PA.; Stoner, GL.; Ryschkewitsch, CF. & Randhawa, P. (2001). Molecular genotyping of BK and JC viruses in human polyomavirus-associated interstitial nephritis after renal transplantation. *Am J Kidney Dis*, Vol., 38; pp. 354-365.

Barcan, LA.; Dallurzo, ML.; Clara, LO.; Valledor, A.; Macias, S.; Zorkin, E., et al. (2002). Toxoplasmagondii pneumonia in liver transplantation: survival after a severe case of reactivation. *Transpl Infect Dis*, Vol., 4; pp. 93-96.

Barsoum, RS. (2000). Malarial acute renal failure. *J Am Soc Nephrol*, Vol., 11; pp. 2147-2154.

Barsoum, RS. (2004). Parasitic infections in organ transplantation. *Exp Clin Transplant*, vol, 2 ; pp. 258-2567.

Bloom, RD.; Rao, V.; Weng, F.; Grossman, RA.; Cohen, D. & Mange, KC. (2002). Association of hepatitis with posttransplant diabetes in renal transplant patients on tacrolimus. *J Am Soc Nephrol*, Vol., 13; pp. 1374-1380.

Boeckh, M. (2006). Prevention of VZV infection in immunosuppressed patients using antiviral agents. *Herpes*, Vol., 13; pp. 60–65.

Boggild, AK.; Sano, M.; Humar, A.; Salit, I.; Gilman, M. & Kain, KC. (2004). Travel patterns and risk behavior in solid organ transplant recipients. *J Travel Med*, Vol., 11; pp. 37-43.

Breinig, MK.; Zitelli, B.; Starzl, TE. & Ho, M. (1987). Epstein-Barr virus, cytomegalovirus, and other viral infections in children after liver transplantation. *J Infect Dis* Vol., 156; pp. 273–279.

Brennan, DC.; Agha, I.; Bohl, DL.; Schnitzler, MA.; Hardinger, KL.; Lockwood, M, et al. (2005). Incidence of BK with tacrolimus versus cyclosporine and impact of preemptive immunosuppression reduction. *Am J Transplant*, Vol., 5; pp. 582–594.

Caillard, S.; Lelong, C.; Pessione, F.; Moulin, B. & French PTLD Working Group. (2006). Post-transplant lymphoproliferative disorders occurring after renal transplantation in adults: Report of 230 cases from the French Registry. *Am J Transplant*, Vol., 6; pp. 2735–2742.

Caliendo, AM.; St George, K.; Kao, SY.; Allega, J.; Tan, BH.; La Fontaine, R., et al. (2000). Comparison of quantitative cytomegalovirus (CMV) PCR in plasma and CMV antigenemia assay: clinical utility of the prototype Amplicor CMV Monitor test in transplant recipients. *J Clin Microbiol*, Vol., 38; pp. 2122-2127.

Campos, M.; Jouzdani, E.; Sempoux, C.; Buts, JP.; Reding, R.; Otte, JB. & Sokal, EM. (2000). Sclerosing cholangitis associated to cryptosporidiosis in liver-transplanted children. *Eur J Pediatr*, Vol., 159; pp. 113-115.

Carlson, JR.; Li, L.; Helton, CL.; Munn, RJ.; Wasson, K.; Perez, RV., et al. (2004). Disseminated microsporidiosis in a pancreas/kidney transplant recipient. *Arch Pathol Lab Med*, Vol., 128; pp. e41-e43.

Chan, TM.; Fang, GX.; Tang, CS.; Cheng, IK.; Lai, KN. & Ho, SK. (2002). Preemptive lamivudine therapy based on HBV DNA level in HBsAg-positive kidney allograft recipients. *Hepatology*, Vol., 36; pp. 1246-1252.

Chang, TT.; Gish, RG.; de Man, R.; Gadano, A.; Sollano, J.; Chao, YC., et al. (2006). A comparison of entecavir and lamivudine for HBeAg-positive chronic hepatitis B. *N Engl J Med*, Vol., 354; pp.1001-1010.

Chiche, L.; Lesage, A.; Duhamel, C.; Salame, E.; Malet, M.; Samba, D, et al. (2003). Posttransplant malaria: first case of transmission of Plasmodium falciparum from a white multiorgan donor to four recipients. *Transplantation*, Vol., 75; pp. 166-168.

Cockfield, SM.; Preiksaitis, JK.; Jewell, LD. & Parfrey, NA. (1993). Post-transplant lymphoproliferative disorder in renal allograft recipients. Clinical experience and risk factor analysis in a single center. *Transplantation*, Vol., 56; pp. 88–96.

Cruzado, JM.; Carrera, M.; Torras, J. & Grinyó, JM. (2001). Hepatitis C virus infection and de novo glomerular lesions in renal allografts. *Am J Transplant*, Vol., 1; pp. 171-178.

Cruzado, JM.; Casanovas-Taltavull, T.; Torras, J.; Baliellas, C.; Gil-Vernet, S. & Grinyó, JM. (2003). Pretransplant interferon prevents hepatitis C virus-associated glomerulonephritis in renal allografts by HCV-RNA clearance. *Am J Transplant*, Vol., 3; pp. 357-360.

Deelder, AM.; Kornelis, D.; Van Marck, EA.; Eveleigh, PC. & Van Egmond, JG. (1980). Schistosoma mansoni: characterization of two circulating polysaccharide antigens and the immunological response to these antigens in mouse, hamster, and human infections. *Exp Parasitol*, Vol., 50; pp. 16-32.

Delladetsima, I.; Psichogiou, M.; Sypsa, V.; Psimenou, E.; Kostakis, A.; Hatzakis, A., et al. (2006). The course of hepatitis C virus infection in pretransplantation anti-hepatitis C virus-negative renal transplant recipients: a retrospective follow-up study. *Am J Kidney Dis*, Vol., 47; pp. 309-316.

Dharnidharka, VR. & Harmon, WE. (2001a). Management of pediatric postrenal transplantation infections. *Semin Nephrol*, Vol., 21; pp. 521–531.

Dharnidharka, VR.; Sullivan, EK.; Stablein, DM.; Tejani, AH.; Harmon, WE & North American Pediatric Renal Transplant Cooperative Study (NAPRTCS). (2001b).Risk factors for posttransplant lymphoproliferative disorder (PTLD) in pediatric kidney transplantation: A report of the North American Pediatric Renal Transplant Cooperative Study (NAPRTCS). *Transplantation*, Vol., 71; pp. 1065–1068.

Drobniewski, FA. & Ferguson, J. (1996) Tuberculosis in renal transplant units. *Nephrol Dial Transplant*, Vol., 11; pp. 768–770.

Evenson, DA.; Perry, E.; Kloster, B.; Hurley, R. & Stroncek, DF. (1998). Therapeutic apheresis for babesiosis. *J Clin Apheresis*, Vol., 13; pp. 32-36.

Fabrizi, F.; Dulai, G.; Dixit, V.; Bunnapradist, S. & Martin, P. (2004a). Lamivudine for the treatment of hepatitis B virus-related liver disease after renal transplantation: meta-analysis of clinical trials. *Transplantation*, Vol., 77; pp. 859-864.

Fabrizi, F.; Martin, P. & Bunnapradist, S. (2004b). Treatment of chronic viral hepatitis in patients with renal disease. *Gastroenterol Clin North Am*, Vol., 33; pp. 655-670.

Fabrizi, F.; Martin, P.; Dixit, V.; Bunnapradist, S.; Kanwal, F. & Dulai, G. (2005). Post-transplant diabetes mellitus and HCV seropositive status after renal transplantation: meta-analysis of clinical studies. *Am J Transplant*, Vol., 5; pp. 2433-2440.

Fehr, T.; Bossart, W.; Wahl, C. & Binswanger, U. (2002). Disseminated varicella infection in adult renal allograft recipients: Four cases and a review of the literature. *Transplantation*, Vol., 73; pp. 608–611.

Ferreira, MS. & Borges, AS. (2002). Some aspects of protozoan infections in immunocompromised patients- a review. *Mem Inst Oswaldo Cruz*, Vol., 97; pp. 443-457.

Filik, L.; Karakayali, H.; Moray, G.; Dalgiç, A.; Emiroğlu, R.; Ozdemir, N., et al. (2006). Lamivudine therapy in kidney allograft recipients who are seropositive for hepatitis B surface antigen. *Transplant Proc*, Vol., 38; pp. 496–498.

Fischer, L.; Sterneck, M.; Claus, M.; Costard-Jackle, A.; Fleischer, B.; Herbst, H., et al. (1999). Transmission of malaria tertiana by multi-organ donation. *Clin Transplan*, Vol., 13; pp. 491-495.

Fishman, JA. (1995). Pneumocystis carinii and parasitic infections in transplantation. *Infect Dis Clin North Am*, Vol., 9; pp. 1005-1044.

Fishman, JA. & Rubin, RH. (1998). Infection in organ-transplant recipients. *N Engl J Med*, Vol., 338; pp. 1741-1751.

Fishman, JA. (2001). Prevention of infection caused by Pneumocystis carinii in transplant recipients. *Clin Infect Dis*, Vol., 33; pp. 1397-1405.

Fishman, JA. (2002). BK virus nephropathy—polyomavirus adding insult to injury. *N Engl J Med*, Vol., 347; pp. 527-530.

Fishman, JA. (2007). Infections in organ-transplant recipients. *N Engl J Med*, Vol., 357; pp. 2601-2614.

Fishman, JA. & Davis, JA. (2008). Infections in renal transplant recipients. In: Sir Peter J.Morris, Stuart J. Knechtle. (eds). *KIDNEY TRANSPLANTATION: PRINCIPLES AND PRACTICE*, 6th ed. Elsevier, pp. 492-507. ISBN: 978-1-4160-3343-1. Philadelphia.

Fox, BC.; Sollinger, HW.; Belzer, FO. & Maki, DG. (1990). A prospective, randomized, double-blind study of trimethoprim-sulfamethoxazole for prophylaxis of infection in renal transplantation: Clinical efficacy, absorption of trimethoprim-sulfamethoxazole, effects on the microflora, and the cost-benefit of prophylaxis. *Am J Med*, Vol., 89; pp. 255–274.

Frassetto, LA.; Browne, M.; Cheng, A.; Wolfe, AR.; Roland, ME.; Stock, PG., et al. (2007). Immunosuppressant pharmacokinetics and dosing modifications in HIV-1 infected liver and kidney transplant recipients. *Am J Transplant*, Vol., 7; pp. 2816–2820.

Gane, E. & Pilmore, H. (2002). Management of chronic viral hepatitis before and after renal transplantation. *Transplantation*, Vol., 74; pp. 427–437.

Giacomini, T. (1998). Malaria in airports and their neighborhoods. *Rev Prat*, Vol, 48; pp. 264-267.

Gonzalez, MI.; Caballero, D.; Lopez, C.; Alburquerque, T.; Hernandez, R.; de la Loma, A., et al. (2000). Cerebral toxoplasmosis and Guillain-Barré syndrome after allogeneic peripheral stem cell transplantation. *Transpl Infect Dis*, Vol., 2; pp 145-149.

Green, M.; Avery, R. & Preiksaitis, J. (2004). Guidelines for the prevention and management of infectious complications of solid organ transplantation. *Am J Transplant*, Vol., 4 (Suppl 10); pp. 6-165.

Green, M.; Michaels, MG.; Katz, BZ.; Burroughs, M.; Gerber, D.; Shneider, BL., et al. (2006). CMV-IVIG for prevention of Epstein Barr virus disease and posttransplant lymphoproliferative disease in pediatric liver transplant recipients. *Am J Transplant*, Vol., 6; pp. 1906–1912.

Gruber, SA.; Doshi, MD.; Cincotta, E.; Brown, KL.; Singh, A.; Morawski, K., et al. (2008). Preliminary experience with renal transplantation in HIV+recipients: Low acute rejection and infection rates. *Transplantation*, Vol., 86; pp. 269–274.

Han, DJ.; Kim, TH.; Park, SK.; Lee, SK.; Kim, SB.; Yang, WS., et al. (2001). Results on preemptive or prophylactic treatment of lamivudine in HBsAg (+) renal allograft recipients: Comparison with salvage treatment after hepatic dysfunction with HBV recurrence. *Transplantation*, Vol., 71; pp. 387–394.

Hanafusa, T.; Ichikawa, Y.; Kishikawa, H.; Kyo, M.; Fukunishi, T.; Kokado., Y, et al. (1998). Retrospective study on the impact of hepatitis C virus infection on kidney transplant patients over 20 years. *Transplantation*, Vol., 66; pp 471-476.

Haque, T.; Wilkie, GM.; Taylor, C.; Amlot, PL.; Murad, P.; Iley, A., et al. (2002). Treatment of Epstein-Barr-viruspositive post-transplantation lymphoproliferative disease with partly HLA-matched allogeneic cytotoxic T cells. *Lancet*, Vol., 360; pp. 436-442.

Hartmann, A.; Sagedal, S. & Hjelmesaeth, J. (2006). The natural course of cytomegalovirus infection and disease in renal transplant recipients. *Transplantation*, Vol., 82; S15-S17.

Hennequin, C.; Page, B.; Roux, P.; Legendre, C. & Kreis, H. (1995). Outbreak of Pneumocystis carinii pneumonia in a renal transplant unit. *Eur J Clin Microbiol Infect Dis*, Vol., 14; pp. 122–126.

Herbrecht, R.; Denning, DW.; Patterson, TF.; Bennett, JE.; Greene, RE.; Oestmann, JW., et al. (2002). Voriconazole versus amphotericin B for primary therapy of invasive aspergillosis. *N Engl J Med*, Vol., 347; pp. 408-415.

Hermanns, B.; Brunn, A.; Schwarz, ER.; Sachweh, JS.; Seipelt, I.; Schroder, JM., et al. (2001). Fulminant toxoplasmosis in a heart transplant recipient. *Pathol Res Pract*, Vol., 197; pp.: 211-215.

Hibberd, PL.; Tolkoff-Rubin, NE.; Cosimi, AB.; Schooley, RT.; Isaacson, D.; Doran, M., et al. (1992a). Symptomatic cytomegalovirus disease in the cytomegalovirus antibody seropositive renal transplant recipient treated with OKT3. *Transplantation*, Vol., 53; pp. 68–72.

Hibberd, PL.; Tolkoff-Rubin, NE.; Doran, M.; Delvecchio, A.; Cosimi, AB.; Delmonico, FL., et al. (1992b). Trimethoprim-sulfamethoxazole compared with ciprofloxacin for the prevention of urinary tract infection in renal transplant recipients. A double-blind, randomized controlled trial. *Online J Curr Clin Trials*, Doc No 15.

Hibberd, PL.; Tolkoff-Rubin, NE.; Conti, D.; Stuart, F.; Thistlethwaite, JR.; Neylan, JF., et al. (1995). Preemptive ganciclovir therapy to prevent cytomegalovirus disease in cytomegalovirus antibody-positive renal transplant recipients. A randomized controlled trial. *Ann Intern Med*, Vol., 123; pp. 18–26.

Hirsch, HH.; Knowles, W.; Dickenmann, M.; Passweg, J.; Klimkait, T.; Mihatsch, MJ., et al. (2002). Prospective study of polyomavirus type BK replication and nephropathy in renal-transplant recipients. *N Engl J Med*, Vol., 347; pp. 488-496.

Hirsch, HH.; Brennan, DC.; Drachenberg, CB.; Ginevri, F.; Gordon, J.; Limaye, AP., et al. (2005). Polyomavirus associated nephropathy in renal transplantation: Interdisciplinary analyses and recommendations. *Transplantation*, Vol., 79; pp. 1277–1286.

Hirsch, HH.; Drachenberg, CB.; Steiger, J. & Ramos, E. (2006). Polyomavirus-associated nephropathy in renal transplantation: critical issues of screening and management. *Adv Exp Med Biol*, Vol., 577; pp. 160-173.

Hodson, EM.; Barclay, PG.; Craig, JC.; Jones, C.; Kable, K.; Strippoli, GF., et al. (2005). Antiviral medications for preventing cytomegalovirus disease in solid organ transplant recipients. *Cochrane Database Syst Rev*, CD003774.

Hodson, EM.; Jones, CA.; Strippoli, GF.; Webster, AC. & Craig, JC. (2007). Immunoglobulins, vaccines or interferon for preventing cytomegalovirus disease in solid organ transplant recipients. *Cochrane Database Syst Rev*, CD005129.

Holzer, BR.; Gluck, Z.; Zambelli, D. & Fey, M. (1985). Transmission of malaria by renal transplantation. *Transplantation*. Vol., 39; pp. 315-316.

Hommann, M.; Schotte, U.; Voigt, R.; Glutig, H.; Grube, T.; Kupper, B., et al. (2002). Cerebral toxoplasmosis after combined liver-pancreas-kidney and liver-pancreas transplantation. *Transplant Proc*, Vol., 34; pp. 2294-2295.

Hughes, WT.; Rivera, GK.; Schell, MJ.; Thornton, D. & Lott, L. (1987). Successful intermittent chemoprophylaxis for Pneumocystis carinii pneumonitis. *N Engl J Med*, Vol., 316; pp. 1627-1632.

Humar, A.; Kumar, D.; Boivin, G. & Caliendo, AM. (2002). Cytomegalovirus (CMV) virus load kinetics to predict recurrent disease in solid-organ transplant patients with CMV disease. *J Infect Dis*, Vol., 186; pp. 829–833.

Huraib, S.; Iqbal, A.; Tanimu, D. & Abdullah, A. (2001). Sustained virological and histological response with pretransplant interferon therapy in renal transplant patients with chronic viral hepatitis C. *Am J Nephrol*, Vol., 21; pp. 435-440. Iftikhar, SA. & Roistacher, K. (1995). Indigenous Plasmodium falciparum malaria in Queens, NY. *Arch Intern Med*, Vol., 155 pp. 1099-1101.

Kalil, AC.; Levitsky, J.; Lyden, E.; Stoner, J. & Freifeld, AG. (2005). Meta-analysis: the efficacy of strategies to prevent organ disease by cytomegalovirus in solid organ transplant recipients. *Ann Intern Med*, Vol., 143; pp. 870-880.

Kamar, N.; Sandres-Saune, K.; Selves, J.; Ribes, D.; Cointault, O.; Durand, D., et al. (2003a). Long-term ribavirin therapy in hepatitis C virus-positive renal transplant patients: effects on renal function and liver histology. *Am J Kidney Dis*, Vol., 42; pp. 184-192.

Kamar, N.; Toupance, O.; Buchler, M.; Sandres-Saune, K.; Izopet, J.; Durand, D., et al. (2003b). Evidence that clearance of hepatitis C virus RNA after alpha-interferon therapy in dialysis patients is sustained after renal transplantation. *J Am Soc Nephrol*, Vol., 14; pp. 2092-2098.

Karras, A.; Thervet, E.; Legendre, C. & Groupe Cooperatif de transplantation d'Ile de France. (2004). Hemophagocytic syndrome in renal transplant recipients: report of 17 cases and review of literature. *Transplantation*, Vol., 77; pp. 238-243.

KDIGO: Kidney Disease: Improving Global Outcomes (KDIGO) Transplant Work Group. KDIGO clinical practice guideline for the care of kidney transplant recipients. (2009) *Am J Transplant*, Vol., 9(Suppl 3): S1–S157.

Kletzmayr, J.; Watschinger, B.; Müller, C.; Demetriou, D.; Puchhammer-Stöckl, E.; Ferenci, P., et al. (2000). Twelve months of lamivudine treatment for chronic hepatitis B virus infection in renal transplant recipients. *Transplantation*, Vol., 70; pp. 1404-1407.

Koneru, B.; Tzakis, AG.; DePuydt, LE.; Demetris, AJ.; Armstrong, JA.; Dummer, JS., et al. (1988). Transmission of fatal herpes simplex infection through renal transplantation. *Transplantation*, Vol., 45; pp. 653–656.

Lapinski, TW.; Flisiak, R.; Jaroszewicz, J.; Michalewicz, M. & Kowalczuk, O. (2005). Efficiency and safety of lamivudine therapy in patients with chronic HBV infection, dialysis or after kidney transplantation. *World J Gastroenterol*, Vol., 11; pp. 400–402.

Lau, JY.; Davis, GL.; Brunson, ME.; Qian, KP.; Lin, HJ.; Quan, S., et al. (1993). Hepatitis C virus infection in kidney transplant recipients. *Hepatology*, Vol., 18; pp. 1027-1031.

Lee, WC.; Shu, KH.; Cheng, CH.; Wu, MJ.; Chen, CH. & Lian, JC. (2001). Long-term impact of hepatitis B, C virus infection on renal transplantation. *Am J Nephrol*, Vol., 21; pp. 300-306.

Legendre, C.; Garrigue, V.; Le Bihan, C.; Mamzer-Bruneel, MF.; Chaix, ML.; Landais, P., et al. (1998). Harmful long-term impact of hepatitis C virus infection in kidney transplant recipients. *Transplantation*, Vol., 65; pp. 667-670.

Liaw, YF.; Chien, RN.; Yeh, CT.; Tsai, SL. & Chu, CM. (1999). Acute exacerbation and hepatitis B virus clearance after emergence of YMDD motif mutation during lamivudine therapy. *Hepatology*, Vol., 30; pp. 567-572.

Lopez-Duarte, M.; Insunza, A.; Conde, E.; Iriondo, A.; Mazorra, F. & Zubizarreta, A. (2003). Cerebral toxoplasmosis after autologous peripheral blood stem cell transplantation. *Eur J Clin Microbiol Infect Dis*, Vol., 22; pp. 548-550.

Lorf, T.; Braun, F.; Rüchel, R.; Müller, A.; Sattler, B. & Ringe, B. (1999). Systemic mycoses during prophylactical use of liposomal amphotericin B (Ambisome) after liver transplantation. *Mycoses*, Vol., 42; pp. 47-53.

MacArthur, JR.; Holtz, TH.; Jenkins, J.; Newell, JP.; Koehler, JE.; Parise, ME. & Kachur, SP. (2001). Probable locally acquired mosquito-transmitted malaria in Georgia, 1999. *Clin Infect Dis*, Vol., 32; pp. E124-E128.

Marcellin, P.; Heathcote, EJ.; Buti, M.; Gane, E.; de Man, RA.; Krastev, Z., et al. (2008). Tenofovir disoproxil fumarate versus adefovir dipivoxil for chronic hepatitis B. *N Engl J Med*, Vol., 359; pp. 2442–2455.

Mahmoud, IM.; Elhabashi, AF.; Elsawy, E.; El-Husseini, AA.; Sheha, GE. & Sobh, MA. (2004). The impact of hepatitis C virus viremia on renal graft and patient survival: a 9-year prospective study. *Am J Kidney Dis*, Vol., 43; pp. 131-139.

Martin, P. & Fabrizi, F. (2008). Hepatitis C virus and kidney disease. *J Hepatol*, Vol., 49; pp. 613-624.

McDonald, RA.; Smith, JM.; Ho, M.; Lindblad, R.; Ikle, D.; Grimm, P., et al. (2008). Incidence of PTLD in pediatric renal transplant recipients receiving basiliximab, calcineurin inhibitor, sirolimus and steroids. *Am J Transplant*, Vol., 8; pp. 984–989.

Menichetti, F.; Del Favero, A.; Martino, P.; Bucaneve, G.; Micozzi, A.; Girmenia, C., et al. (1999). Itraconazole oral solution as prophylaxis for fungal infections in neutropenic patients with hematologic malignancies: A randomized, placebo-controlled, double-blind, multicenter trial. GIMEMA Infection Program. Gruppo Italiano Malattie Ematologiche dell' Adulto. *Clin Infect Dis*, Vol., 28; pp. 250-255.

Meyers, CM.; Seeff, LB.; Stehman-Breen, CO. & Hoofnagle, JH. (2003). Hepatitis C and renal disease: an update. *Am J Kidney Dis*, Vol., 42; pp. 631-657.

Minz, M.; Udgiri, NK.; Heer, MK.; Kashyap, R. & Malla, N. (2004). Cryptosporidiasis in live related renal transplant recipients: a single center experience. *Transplantation*, Vol., 77; pp. 1916-1917.

Mohindra, AR.; Lee, MW.; Visvesvara, G.; Moura, H.; Parasuraman, R.; Leitch, GJ., et al. (2002). Disseminated microsporidiosis in a renal transplant recipient. *Transpl Infect Dis*, Vol., 4; pp. 102-107.

Mora-Duarte, J.; Betts, R.; Rotstein, C.; Colombo, AL.; Thompson-Moya, L.; Smietana, J., et al. (2002). Comparison of caspofungin and amphotericin B for invasive candidiasis. *N Engl J Med*, Vol., 347; pp. 2020-2029.

Moran, E.; Collins, L.; Clayton, S.; Peto, T. & Bowler ,IC. (2004). Case of cryptic malaria. *Common Dis Public Health*, Vol., 7; pp. 142-144.

Moshfeghi, DM.; Dodds, EM.; Couto, CA.; Santos, CI.; Nicholson, DH.; Lowder, CY. & Davis, JL. (2004). Diagnostic approaches to severe, atypical toxoplasmosis mimicking acute retinal necrosis. *Ophthalmology*, Vol., 111; pp. 716-725.

Muller, CI.; Zeiser, R.; Grullich, C.; Finke, J.; Bertz, H.; Schmitt-Graff, A. & Kreisel, W. (2004) Intestinal cryptosporidiosis mimicking acute graft-versus-host disease following matched unrelated hematopoietic stem cell transplantation. *Transplantation*. Vol., 77; pp. 1478-1479.

Munoz, P. (2001). Management of urinary tract infections and lymphocele in renal transplant recipients.*Clin Infect Dis*, Vol., 33 (Suppl 1): S53–57.

Mylonakis, E.; Kallas, WM. & Fishman, JA. (2002). Combination antiviral therapy for ganciclovir-resistant cytomegalovirus infection in solid-organ transplant recipients. *Clin Infect Dis*, Vol., 34; pp. 1337-1341.

Nalesnik, M. (2001). The diverse pathology of posttransplant lymphoproliferative disorders: importance of a standardized approach. *Transpl Infect Dis*, Vol., 3; pp. 88-96.

Opelz, G. & Dohler, B. (2004). Lymphomas after solid organ transplantation: A collaborative transplant study report. *Am J Transplant*, Vol., 4; pp. 222–230.

Orloff ,SL.; Stempel, CA.; Wright, TL.; Tomlanovich, SJ.; Amend, WJ.; Stock, PG., et al. (1995). Long-term outcome in kidney transplant patients with hepatitis C (HCV) infection. *Clin Transplant*, Vol., 9; pp. 119-124.

Ortonne, N.; Ribaud, P.; Meignin, V.; Sarfati, C.; Esperou, H.; Devergie, A., et al. (2001). Toxoplasmic pneumonitis leading to fatal acute respiratory distress syndrome after engraftment in three bone marrow transplant recipients. *Transplantation*, Vol., 72; pp. 1838-1840.

Paya, CV. (1993). Fungal infections in solid-organ transplantation. *Clin Infect Dis*, Vol., 16; pp. 677-688.

Paya, C.; Fung, JJ.; Nalesnik, MA.; Kieff, E.; Green, M.; Gores, G., et al. (1999). Epstein-Barr virus-induced posttransplant lymphoproliferative disorders. *Transplantation*, Vol., 68; pp. 1517-1525.

Paya, C. & Razonable, R. (2003). Cytomegalovirus infection after organ transplantation. In: Bowden R, Ljungman P, Paya C (eds). *Transplant infections*, 2nd ed. Lippincott, Williams and Wilkins, pp 298–325.

Paya, C.; Humar, A.; Dominguez, E.; Washburn, K.; Blumberg, E.; Alexander, B., et al. (2004). Efficacy and safety of valganciclovir vs. oral ganciclovir for prevention of cytomegalovirus disease in solid organ transplant recipients. *Am J Transplant*, Vol., 4; pp. 611-620.

Pegues, DA.; Kubak, BM.; Maree, CL. & Gregson, AL. (2010). Infections in Kidney Transplantation. In: Gabriel M. Danovitch (ed). *Handbook of Kidney Transplantation* , 5th Edition. Lippincott, Williams and Wilkins, pp 252–279. ISBN-13: 978-0-7817-9374-2.

Perdrizet, GA.; Olson, NH.; Krause, PJ.; Banever, GT.; Spielman, A. & Cable, RG. (2000). Babesiosis in a renal transplant recipient acquired through blood transfusion. *Transplantation*, Vol., 70; pp. 205-208.

Perfect, JR.; Klotman, ME.; Gilbert, CC.; Crawford, DD.; Rosner, GL.; Wright, KA., et al. (1992). Prophylactic intravenous amphotericin B in neutropenic autologous bone marrow transplant recipients. *J Infect Dis*, Vol., 165; pp. 891-897.

Playford, EG.; Webster, AC.; Sorell, TC. & Craig, JC. (2004). Antifungal agents for preventing fungal infections in solid organ transplant recipients. *Cochrane Database Syst Rev*, CD004291.

Preiksaitis, JK. & Keay, S. (2001). Diagnosis and management of posttransplant lymphoproliferative disorder in solid-organ transplant recipients. *Clin Infect Dis*, Vol., 33(Suppl 1):S38.

Ramos, E.; Drachenberg, CB.; Papadimitriou, JC.; Hamze, O.; Fink, JC.; Klassen, DK., et al. (2002). Clinical course of polyoma virus nephropathy in 67 renal transplant patients. *J Am Soc Nephrol*, Vol., 13; pp. 2145-2151.

Ramos, E.; Drachenberg, CB.; Portocarrero, M.; Wali, R.; Klassen, DK.; Fink, JC., et al. (2003). BK virus nephropathy diagnosis and treatment: experience at the University of

Maryland Renal Transplant Program. In Cecka JM, Terasaki PI (eds): *Clinical Transplants 2002*. Los Angeles, UCLA Immunogenetics Center, pp 143-153.

Randhawa, P. & Brennan, DC. (2006). BK virus infection in transplant recipients: An overview and update. *Am J Transplant*, Vol., 6; pp. 2000–2005.

Reinke, P.; Fietze, E.; Ode-Hakim, S.; Prösch, S.; Lippert, J.; Ewert, R., et al. (1994). Late-acute renal allograft rejection and symptomless cytomegalovirus infection. *Lancet*, Vol., 344; pp. 1737-1738.

Renoult, E.; Georges, E.; Biava, MF.; Hulin, C.; Frimat, L.; Hestin, D. & Kessler, M. (1997). Toxoplasmosis in kidney transplant recipients: report of six cases and review. *Clin Infect Dis*, Vol., 24; pp. 625-634.

Rodriguez, M. & Fishman, JA. (2004). Prevention of infection due to Pneumocystis spp. in human immunodeficiency virus-negative immunocompromised patients. *Clin Microbiol Rev*, Vol., 17; pp. 770-782.

Roland, ME.; Barin, B.; Carlson, L.; Frassetto, LA.; Terrault, NA.; Hirose, R., et al. (2008). HIV-infected liver and kidney transplant recipients: 1- and 3-year outcomes. *Am J Transplant*, Vol., 8; pp. 355–365.

Rostaing, L.; Izopet, J.; Baron, E.; Duffaut, M.; Puel, J. & Durand, D. (1995). Treatment of chronic hepatitis C with recombinant interferon alpha in kidney transplant recipients. *Transplantation*, Vol., 59; pp. 1426-1431.

Rostaing, L.; Henry, S.; Cisterne, JM.; Duffaut, M.; Icart, J. & Durand, D. (1997). Efficacy and safety of lamivudine on replication of recurrent hepatitis B after cadaveric renal transplantation. *Transplantation*, Vol., 64; pp. 1624-1627.

Rowe, DT.; Webber, S.; Schauer, EM.; Reyes, J. & Green, M. (2001). Epstein-Barr virus load monitoring: Its role in the prevention and management of posttransplant lymphoproliferative disease. *Transpl Infect Dis*, Vol., 3; pp. 79–87.

Roy, V. & Weisdorf, D. (1998). Typical and atypical mycobacterium. In Bowden RA, Ljungman P, Paya CV (eds): *Transplant Infections*. Lippincott Raven, Philadelphia.

Rubin, RH. & Tolkoff-Rubin, NE. (1983). Viral infection in the renal transplant patient. *Proc Eur Dial Transplant Assoc*, Vol., 19; pp. 513–526.

Russo, MW.; Ghalib, R.; Sigal, S. & Joshi, V. (2006). Randomized trial of pegylated interferon alpha-2b monotherapy in aemodialysis patients with chronic hepatitis C. *Nephrol Dial Transplant*, Vol., 21; pp. 437-443.

Said, A.; Safdar, N.; Wells, J. & Lucey, MR. (2008). Liver disease in renal transplant recipients. In: Sir Peter J.Morris, Stuart J. Knechtle. (eds). *KIDNEY TRANSPLANTATION: PRINCIPLES AND PRACTICE*, 6th ed. Elsevier, pp. 508-533. ISBN: 978-1-4160-3343-1. Philadelphia.

Schmaldienst, S.; Dittrich, E. & Horl, WH. (2002). Urinary tract infections after renal transplantation. *Curr Opin Urol*, Vol., 12; pp. 125-130.

Sezer, S.; Ozdemir, FN.; Akcay, A.; Arat, Z.; Boyacioglu, S. & Haberal, M. (2004). Renal transplantation offers a better survival in HCV-infected ESRD patients. *Clin Transplant*, Vol., 18; pp. 619-623.

Shokeir, AA. (2001). Renal transplantation: the impact of schistosomiasis. *BJU Int*, Vol., 88; pp. 915-920.

Sia, IG. & Patel, R. (2000). New strategies for prevention and therapy of cytomegalovirus infection and disease in solid-organ transplant recipients. *Clin Microbiol Rev*, Vol., 13; pp. 83-121.

Singh, N. (2000). Antifungal prophylaxis for solid organ transplant recipients: Seeking clarity amidst controversy. *Clin Infect Dis*, Vol., 31; pp. 545-553.

Snyder. JJ.; Israni, AK.; Peng, Y.;Zhang, L.;Simon, TA. & Kasiske BL. (2009). Rates of first infection following kidney transplantation in yhe United States. *Kidney Int*, Vol., 75; pp 317-326.

Slovut, DP.; Benedetti, E. & Matas, AJ. (1996). Babesiosis and hemophagocytic syndrome in an asplenic renal transplant recipient. *Transplantation*, Vol., 62; pp. 537-539.

Sobh, MA.; el-Agroudy, AE.; Moustafa, FE.; Shokeir, AA.; el-Shazly, A. & Ghoneim, MA. (1992). Impact of schistosomiasis on patient and graft outcome after kidney transplantation. *Nephrol Dial Transplant*, Vol., 7; pp. 858-864.

Sterling, RP.; Bradley, BB.; Khalil, KG.; Kerman, RH. & Conklin, RH. (1984). Comparison of biopsy-proven Pneumocystis carinii pneumonia in acquired immune deficiency syndrome patients and renal allograft recipients. *Ann Thorac Surg*, Vol., 38; pp. 494–499.

Stock, PG.; Barin, B.; Murphy, B.; Hanto, D.; Diego, JM.; Light, J., et al. (2010). Outcomes of kidney transplantation in HIV-infected recipients. *N Engl J Med,* Vol., 363; pp. 2004-2014.

Straathof, KC.; Savoldo, B.; Heslop, H. & Rooney, CM. (2002). Immunotherapy for posttransplant lymphoproliferative disease. Br J *Hematol*, Vol., 118; pp. 728-740.

Strippoli, GF.; Hodson, EM.; Jones, C. & Craig, JC. (2006). Preemptive treatment for cytomegalovirus viremia to prevent cytomegalovirus disease in solid organ transplant recipients. *Transplantation*, Vol., 81; pp. 139–145.

Sukthana, Y.; Chintana, T.; Damrongkitchaiporn, S. & Lekkla, A. (2001). Serological study of Toxoplasma gondii in kidney recipients. *J Med Assoc Thai*, Vol., 84; pp. 1137-1141.

Sypsa, V.; Touloumi, G.; Tassopoulos, NC.; Ketikoglou, I.; Vafiadis, I.; Hatzis, G., et al. (2004). Reconstructing and predicting the hepatitis C virus epidemic in Greece: increasing trends of cirrhosis and hepatocellular carcinoma despite the decline in incidence of HCV infection. *J Viral Hepat*, Vol., 11; pp. 366-374.

Tan, AC.; Brouwer, JT.; Glue, P.; van Leusen, R.; Kauffmann, RH.; Schalm, SW., et al. (2001). Safety of interferon and ribavirin therapy in haemodialysis patients with chronic hepatitis C: results of a pilot study. *Nephrol Dial Transplant*, Vol., 16; pp. 193-195.

Triverio, PA.; Bridevaux, PO.; Roux-Lombard, P.; Niksic, L.; Rochat, T.; Martin, PY., et al. (2009). Interferon-gamma release assays versus tuberculin skin testing for detection of latent tuberculosis in chronic haemodialysis patients. *Nephrol Dial Transplant*, Vol., 24; pp. 1952–1956.

Vachharajani, TJ.; Oza, UG.; Phadke, AG. & Kirpalani, AL. (2002). Tuberculosis in renal transplant recipients: Rifampicin sparing treatment protocol. *Int Urol Nephrol*, Vol., 34; pp. 551–553.

van Bommel, F.; Zollner, B.; Sarrazin, C.; Spengler, U.; Hüppe, D.; Möller, B., et al. (2006). Tenofovir for patients with lamivudine-resistant hepatitis B virus (HBV) infection and high HBV DNA level during adefovir therapy. *Hepatology*, Vol., 44; pp. 318-325.

van Duijnhoven, EM.; Christiaans, MH.; Boots, JM.; Nieman, FH.; Wolffenbuttel, BH. & van Hooff, JP. (2002). Glucose metabolism in the first 3 years after renal transplantation in patients receiving tacrolimus versus cyclosporine-based immunosuppression. *J Am Soc Nephrol*, Vol., 13; pp. 213-220.

Vasquez, E.; Pollak, R. & Benedetti, E. (2001). Clotrimazole increases tacrolimus blood levels: A drug interaction in kidney transplant patients. *Clin Transplant*, Vol., 15; pp. 95–99.

Vats, A.; Shapiro, R.; Singh Randhawa, P.; Scantlebury, V.; Tuzuner, A.; Saxena, M., et al. (2003). Quantitative viral load monitoring and cidofovir therapy for the management of BK virus-associated nephropathy in children and adults. *Transplantation*, Vol., 75; pp. 105-112.

Weinberg, A.; Hodges, TN.; Li, S.; Cai, G. & Zamora, MR. (2000). Comparison of PCR, antigenemia assay, and rapid blood culture for detection and prevention of cytomegalovirus disease after lung transplantation. *J Clin Microbiol*, Vol., 38; pp. 768–772.

Wertheim, P.; Slaterus, KW.; Geelen, JL.; van der Noordaa, J. & Wilmink, JM. (1985). Cytomegalo and herpes simplex virus infections in renal transplant recipients. *Scand J Urol Nephrol Suppl*, Vol., 92; pp. 5–8.

Williams, JW.; Javaid, B.; Kadambi, PV.; Gillen, D.; Harland, R.; Thistlewaite, JR., et al. (2005). Leflunomide for polyomavirus type BK nephropathy. *N Engl J Med*, Vol., 352; pp. 1157–1158.

Winston, DJ.; Young, JA.; Pullarkat, V.; Papanicolaou, GA.; Vij, R.; Vance, E., et al. (2008). Maribavir prophylaxis for prevention of cytomegalovirus infection in allogeneic stem cell transplant recipients: a multicenter, randomized, double-blind, placebo-controlled, dose-ranging study. *Blood*, Vol., 1; pp. 5403-5410.

Wirth, S. (2006). Antiviral treatment of hepatitis B following solid organ transplantation in children. *Pediatr Transplant*, Vol., 10; pp. 271–275.

[1] Cytomegalovirus. (2004). *Am J Transplant*, Vol., 4(Suppl 10); pp. 51–58.

[2] Epstein-Barr virus and lymphoproliferative disorders after transplantation. (2004). *Am J Transplant*, Vol., 4; pp. 59–65.

[3] Guidelines for the prevention and management of infectious complications of solid organ transplantation: HHV-6, HHV-7, HHV-8, HSV-1 and -2, VZV. (2004). *Am J Transplant*, Vol., 4; pp. 66–71.

[4] Solid organ transplantation in the HIV-infected patient. (2004). *Am J Transplant*, Vol., 4; pp. 83–88.

[5] Pneumocystis jiroveci (formerly Pneumocystis carinii). (2004). *Am J Transplant*, Vol., 4 (Suppl 10); pp. 135–141.

[6] European best practice guidelines for renal transplantation. Section IV: Long-term management of the transplant recipient.(2002). IV.7.2. Late infections. Tuberculosis. *Nephrol Dial Transplant*, Vol., 17(Suppl 4); pp. 39–43.

[7]. MMWR: Treatment of tuberculosis.(2003). Centers for Disease Control and Prevention. In (vol 52, RR11), Atlanta, GA, USA, American Thoracic Society, CDC, and Infectious Diseases Society of America, pp 1–77

[8] Mycobacterium tuberculosis. (2004). *Am J Transplant*, Vol., 4 (Suppl 10); pp. 37-41.

[9] Screening for tuberculosis and tuberculosis infection in high-risk populations. (1995). Recommendations of the Advisory Council for the Elimination of Tuberculosis.*MMWRRecomm Rep*, Vol., 44; pp. 19-34.
[10] Fungal infections. (2004).*Am J Transplant*, Vol., 4(Suppl 10); pp. 110-134.
[11] VFEND" Package Insert, May 2002 Pfizer Inc, NY, NY 10017.
[12] Varicella-zoster infections. In: Pickering L, Baker C, Long S, McMillan J (eds). Red book: 2006 report of the committee on infectious disease of the American Academy of Pediatrics, 27th edn. American Academy of Pediatrics: Elk Grove Village, IL, 2006, pp 711-725.

2

Handling of Fungal Infections in Patients with Chronic Immunosuppression Post Renal Transplant

Ewa Swoboda-Kopec, Irina Netsvyetayeva, Magdalena Sikora, Mariusz Jasik and Piotr Fiedor
Warsaw Medical University
Poland

1. Introduction

Invasive fungal infections (IFI) are serious diagnostics-therapeutic problem in recipients of vascularised organs. The nature of the IFI is determined by the type of the transplanted organ. Invasive candidiasis mostly occurs in liver recipients and invasive aspergilosis - in lung recipients. The greatest risk of IFI is in recipients of simultaneous lung and heart and liver transplants. Morbidity for IFI in the first year after transplantation is estimated to be in recipients of heart and lungs 8.6%, liver 4.7%, pancreas and kidneys 4% and heart 3.4%.

Incidents of IFI among kidney recipients is estimated by differed sources to lay between 0.01 - 1.5%. Although, IFI occur rarely in kidney recipients in comparison to recipients of other organs, invasive fungal infections carries a high risk of graft loss and high mortality in this population of patients. Among recipients which have developed an IFI the risk of graft loss was determined in approx. 50% of patients, and mortality in this group was approx. 15%. Yearly survival of patients after an episode of invasive aspergilosis is 59%, for mycosis caused by mould fungi from species other then *Aspergillus sp.* 61%, invasive candidosis 66%, cryptococcosis 73%. There is definitely a greater risk for recipients of kidneys collected from cadavers, compared to living donors related to the recipient, respectively 16.5% and 7.3%. Additionally in cases of a deceased donor there is a high transfer risk for yeast-like fungi colonising in the urinary tract of a terminal state patient, in result of the breakdown of the defensive mechanism and contamination of preservative fluids, to the uninfected recipient.

Mortality is determined by the virulence of the microorganism, localisation of the infection, weakened inflammatory response of the macroorganism, frequent co-occurring of renal insufficiency and diabetes and other predisposing factors. Unspecific clinical symptoms, fast progression of the disease and, what appears to be particularly important, lack of a precisely set algorithms of diagnostic procedure, contribute to the fact that IFI in kidney recipients are a diagnostics challenge and has a questionable therapeutic result.

1.1 Factors for fungal infections

Factors for fungoid infections:

- impairment of cellular resistance
- congenital genetic defects in phagocythosis, complement system

- use of immunosuppressants, cytostatics, broad spectrum antibiotics, corticosteroids
- interruption of tissue continuity (insertion of a needle into a vessel, diagnostic puncture)
- inflammatory disorders and functional in the gastrointestinal tract (favourable factors for translocation of fungi from the intestinal lumen)
- catheterization of the urinary bladder
- parenteral feeding
- dialysis therapy
- surgical procedures, particularly in the abdominal cavity
- tracheotomy, intubation, endoscopy
- blood transfusion
- tuberculosis
- metabolic disorders
- endocrinological disorders
- pregnancy
- extreme age groups
- nutritional factors (intake of food containing moulds - strains used in food production or contaminants).

Patients with final renal insufficiency qualified for the transplant procedure, despite the main illness, often have also at least a few of the risk factors described above, are part of the population particularly predisposed to developed an IFI. There is a very high risk of IFI occurrence in recipients which had consecutive kidney transplant procedures, recipients of a simultaneous pancreas and kidney transplant and highly immunised recipients, requiring induction of the immunosuppression with anti-thymocyte globulin.

1.2 The remaining infection risk factors

The remaining infection risk factors differ depending on the period after the kidney transplant.

1.2.1 Early period

Early period - 1 month after kidney transplant. Mostly infections are caused by yeast-like fungi: *Candida sp., Trichosporon sp., Saccharomyces sp.* Risk factors in this period are related to the used surgical technique, transfer of the fungal infection form the infected organ or preservative fluid or fungal colonization form a period before the transplant. Infection with mould fungi of the *Aspergillus* genus are rare and are related to the prolonged operation time or organ transport.

1.2.2 Interim period

Interim period - from 2 to 6 months. Among etiological factors, yeast-like fungi responsible for infections in the early period are predominant, as well as mixed fungoid-bacterial infections. The basic risk factor in this time is a weakened immunological response due to:

- infections and/or reactivation of immunomodulation viruses: CMV, HIV, EBV, HBV, HCV and other
- site effects of transplanted kidney rejection therapy, with high doses of corticosteroids or other cytotoxic lymphocyte inhibitors.

1.2.3 Late period

Late period - over 6 months. Relatively often occurring infection in this period is the cryptococcosis, often in scattered form. Other etiological factors for IFI are yeast-like fungi, mould fungi of the *Aspergillus* genus and others. In this period the level of basic immunosuppression is remained on a low level, which means that in cases without complications the state of the recipients immunological system is close to the state of the general population's. IFI episodes are sporadic and caused by an individual course of the post-transplantation period or individual predispositions:

- complications in previous periods in graft function - treatment of acute rejection episodes
- exceeding of drug level limits of the basic immunosuppression protocol in systemic fluids
- reactivation of infections with immunomodulation viruses
- environmental factors.

1.3 Difficulties due to lack of an effective strategy for mycological diagnostics

Difficulties due to a lack of an effective strategy for mycological diagnostics and often sparse clinical symptoms are the reason that important data for diagnosis of invasive mycosis on kidney recipients are undervalued. Statistics on mortality due to disseminated mycosis do not contain, also for reasons outlined here, all cases. Lack of specific symptoms indicating an early period of an IFI, or transition of colonization into an active infection, lack of criteria allowing differentiation of infections and colonisations and in result lack of precisely described evidence for implementation of preventive - therapeutic treatment. Also important is to decide - does every positive mycological result, obtained by classic diagnostic methods, mean an infection and the necessity to implement antimycotic therapy, and does every colonising strain cause systemic infections, also which genotype and phenotype can benefit this process.

Additionally the treatment of a developed invasive fungal infection carries a high risk for patients due to frequent interactions between antimycotics and immunosuppressants. Taking this into account, it appears to be of outmost importance to develop a diagnostics algorithm minimising the risk of IFI in kidney recipients, based on an active surveillance of particularly predisposed recipients.

2. Invasive systemic mycosis: aspergilosis

Invasive aspergilosis (IA) is an acute infection with a mortality rate of almost 70%. Mostly it occurs in recipient of allogeneic bone marrow from an unrelated recipient - 10.3%. Among organ recipients lung recipients (Lung Transplant) are at highest risk, with morbidity at 8.4%. Among heart recipients (Heart Transplant) morbidity for IA is estimated to be 6.2%, liver (Liver Transplant) -1.7%, pancreas (Pancreas Transplant) -1.3%. Morbidity in kidney recipients (Kidney Transplant) applies for 0.7% of patient population.

An etiological factor in more then 90% of cases is *Aspergillus fumigatus*. Another species of clinical importance are: *Aspergillus niger*, *Aspergillus flavus* and *Aspergillus terreus*. Different species participation is to be observed in external and middle ear aspergilosis, in most cases *Aspergillus flavus* and *Aspergillus niger* are responsible.

Aspergillus spores are now generally present in the environment. Etiology of *Aspergillus* infections are usually results of *Aspergillus* inhalation. The invasive form is the most severe form of infection. In the initial stage, spores infect the lungs (pulmonary aspergilosis), next they get into cardiovascular vessels and to other locations eg.: sinuses (nasal sinus aspergilosis), eyes, skin, kidneys, bones, central nervous system (CNS aspergilosis).

The most common clinical manifestation is lung aspergilosis - 75% of all IA cases, *rhinosinusitis* (infection of the nasal mucosa and nasal sinuses) - 5 - 10%, disseminated multiorgan - 25%, IA with an affected central nervous system makes out 10 - 40% of all cases.

IA Diagnostic: an early diagnostic is critical for an effective therapy, also to avoid the unnecessary administration of a costly and toxic antimycotic therapy.

Traditional methods: as a „golden standard" in the diagnostic of invasive aspergilosis until now, remains the cultivation of a strain from the sample clinical material and identification fungi fimbriae by histopathology.

Appropriate test materials are bronchalalveolar washings in case of pulmonary aspergilosis and sinus washings in *rhinosinusitis* with *Aspergillus* etiology. The value of a mycological rest of sputum is restricted by its low sensitivity and specificity, difficulties in obtaining enough material (lack of a productive cough in the treated patient) or a frequent lack of morphologic elements of fungi and spore. In cases when it is not possible to sample material with invasive methods, morning sputum should be sampled a few times, on consecutive days, with securing of the material from contamination.

A difficult to diagnose form of aspergilosis is the disseminated multiorgan form. In this case the probability to cultivate an etiological factor from blood is infinitesimal compared to disseminated infections caused by other microorganisms (yeast-like fungi and bacteria). In case of invasive aspergilosis with the seizure of central nervous system, cerebrospinal fluid and serum become materials of questionable significance, the only valuable diagnostically material in this case is biopsy material sampled from the lesion. Diagnostic in this case should be based on precise analysis of all available tests: exact evaluation of the interview data, subject test results, biochemical tests results, assessment of the inflammation exponents, and results of imaging tests. As supportive tests can be used: detection of galactomannan antigen and genetic fungi material in cerebrospinal fluid and in serum.

Validity of the mycological test depends on the correct performance of every stage. Material sampling should be assisted by a microbiology specialist or a specially trained physician. It is necessary to take an appropriate number of samples and to sample material on the right microbiological medium for cultivation and direct microscopic preparation. Microscopic testing of clinical material and the correct evaluation are an immensely important stage of the diagnostic, which should be taken into account at sampling: sample material with a sterile smear dampened in a sterile 0.9% NaCl solution, transport medium should not be used for this purposes.

Histopathology diagnostic value is particularly important due to a relatively short time of waiting for results, high sensitivity and possibility to obtain positive results in an ongoing antimycotic therapy and is based on detection of fungal fimbriae. This method is restricted by lack of microorganism identification possibility and antimycotics sensitivity assessment, which can be preformed only on the basis of mycological cultivation.

Microscopic tests or cultivation are a limited possibility to retain testing material, only invasive methods and is connected to long results awaiting period.

Biopsy can be dangerous in case of weakened patients.

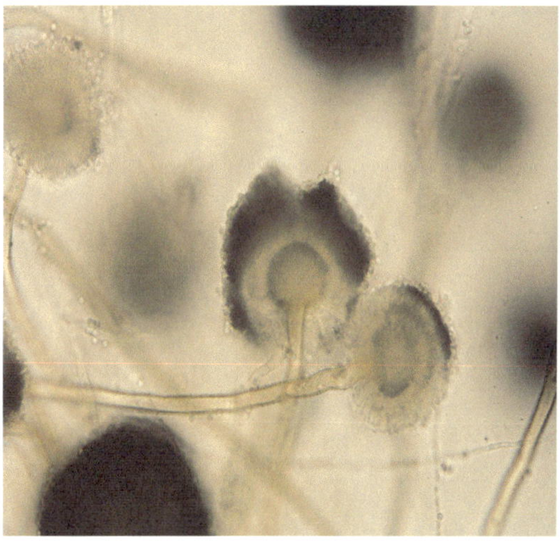
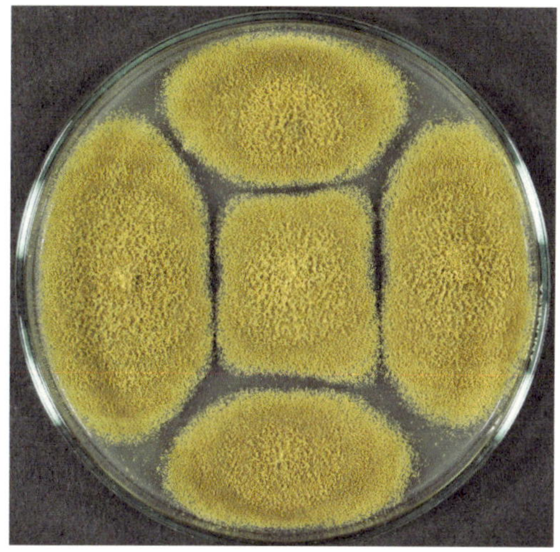

1 2

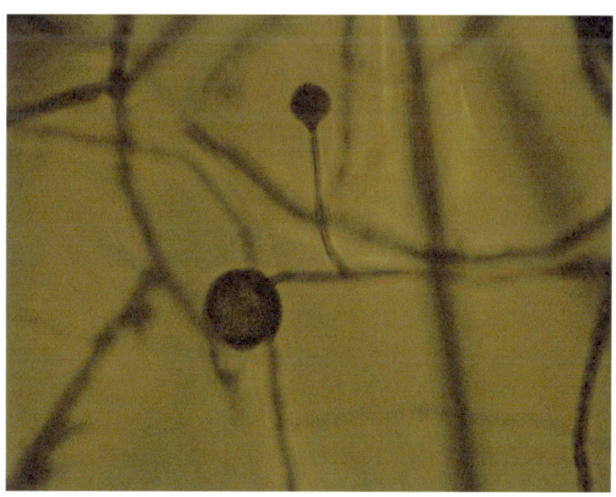

3

Fig. 1. *Aspergillus fumigatus:* **1** Microscopic slide (x400) Microscopic tests of expectoration or BAL, **2** Colonies on Sabouraud Agar. **3** *Mucor spp*. Microscopic sidle (x400).

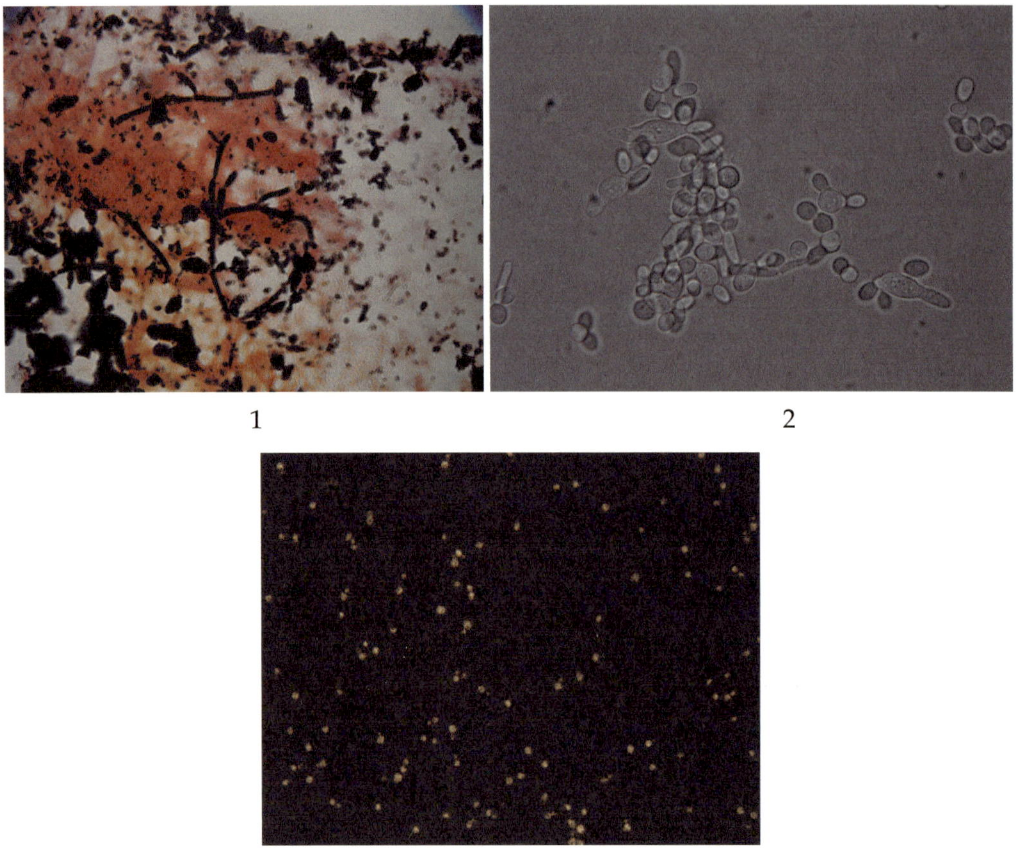

Fig. 2. **1** Invasive form of *Candida albicans* in blood (x1000), **2** *Trichosporon asahii*, microscopic slide (x400), **3** *Cryptococcus neoformans*. India Ink preparation (x400)

3. Infection with mould fungi other than Aspergillus supp. (non-Aspergillus mould infections): zygomycosis

Zygomycosis - is an invasive infection frequently with *Mucor spp., Rhizopus spp., Rhizomucor spp., Absidia spp.* fungi of the *Zygomycota* division. It has been noted in the past years that the number of zygomycosis in the general number of infections with mould fungi in a general population of recipients from 4% to 25% in the period between 2001 and 2003 has increased. Mostly the infection will have a *sinusitis* form with a tendency to quickly spread to the central nervous system - *rhinocerebral* form. Additionally the following forms can be observed: pulmonary, cutaneous and subcutaneous tissue infection, renal, gastrointestinal tract and disseminated form, often diagnosed *post-mortem.*

Most important risk factors of this type of infection are: persisting acidosis caused by a badly monitored diabetes or renal insufficiency and immunosuppressive therapy, particularly in connection with chronic nasal sinus infection. In the organ recipients population as the most important risk factor was perceived a previous exposition to voriconazole therapy of a previous infection with yeast-like fungi or *Aspergillus spp.* Often

those are „infections with breaking-point" with strains belonging to species, which do not fall in the spectrum of this drug.
Cases of zygomycosis in kidney recipients population in industrialised countries are rarely documented, but in developing countries: India, Pakistan, and Iran - they are quite common. Also the trend of „transplant tourism" observed in the last years - travelling to „third world" countries for transplants due to economic reasons and greater availability of organs, while trivialising a great risk of complications.
Rejections of transplanted organs and infection complications are serious problems, which European doctors providing post-transplant care for patient in this group may have to face. Aspergilosis with mucormycosis are most common infection complications in patients who have practised this kind of „tourism".
The death rate in this group is estimated at 59%, and further 82% suffer from graft loss, or from a disseminated form of infection with an infection of the central nervous system. The diagnostic procedure for zygomycosis is norm for all mould fungi and has been described in the chapter in aspergilosis diagnostics.

4. Invasive yest-like fungi

4.1 Invasive candidiasis (IC)

The most important exponent of the invasive candidosis is candidemia - fourth in frequency etiological factor of in hospital blood infection (BSI): 6-10% of the total positive blood culture in hospitalised patients. In patients after vascularised organ transplantation, IC makes out 53% of all IFI.
Infections with yeast-like fungi occur in 5% of kidney recipients with a death rate between 30 - 70%. Most common forms of candidosis among kidney recipients are mucosa-cutaneous and oesophagus candidosis. Heavy complications endangering the survival of the transplant are urinary tract infections: *cystitis, pielonephritis* and *ureteral obstruction by Candida elements*.
In an early period it is often conditioned by a colonisation of yeast-like fungi in the insufficient kidney in a period before the transplant and presence of urinary catheters in a post operational period, the presence of which connected with a high level of immunosuppression makes the spreading of the colonisation to the membrane and an invasive infection easier. Also a very important mechanism of developing a urinary tract infection is the pathogen translocation form the intestinal lumen. In this case it is an endeogenic infection, but with the wrong medical care and hospital hygiene it can cause spreading of the yeast-like fungi from the exogenous source.
Urinary tract infections with occurrence of additional factors can lead to candidemia, spreading of the infection and vascular complications on the transplanted kidney. Invasion of yeast-like fungi to the vascular endothelium can lead to *arteritis* or aneurysms.
Complications can lead to graft loss or patients death. Other dangerous fungal infections are suprainfections of fluid vessels forming around the transplanted kidney, peritoneum infection and catheter fungemia.
The most important factor in invasive candidosis remains the species *Candida albicans but* there is an observed growing participation of non - albicans *Candida spp*. to which belong: *C. glabrata, C. tropicalis, C. parapsilosis*. This species are characterised by being more drug resistant compared to *C. albicans*. The species *C. glabrata* shows a natural lower sensitivity to Fluconazole, and *C. parapsilosis* - to echinocandin.

One of the reasons for a larger participation of species of non - albicans *Candida* spp. possibly can be related to the wide use of prophylactic antifungal drugs. *C. parapsilosis* is characterised by a larger adhesion ability and the ability to produce a biofilm on the surface of biopolymers, including vascular catheters, which often is related to spreading of microorganisms colonised in the catheter into the system.

Widely used fluconazole prophylactic can also be one of the reasons for a larger participation of the *Trichosporon* species as a etiological factor for IFI. *Trichosporon* spp. is not the most important etiological factor for fungal infections in immunocompetent patients.

It can be a reason for an invasive mycoses in patients after vascularised organ transplant, with a high death rate. *Trichosporon* spp. is a yeast-like fungi generally occurring in nature.

Trichosporon asahii mostly is connected with surface infections such as white piedra, skin and nails mycoses in immunocompetent patients. Among the species of *Trichosporon T. asahii* is the main reason for deep invasive infections in patients treated with immunosuppressants.

The most important factor predisposing for this kind of infections are renal insufficiency, phagocytolic disability and neutropenia. Mortality in result of infections with *Trichosporon* fungi is estimated to be 80-100%, which can be related to the late diagnosis of the etiologic factor, wrong treatment and lack of correlation between the efficacy of treatment and sensitivity of the strain *in vitro*.

Additionally one of the characteristics of this species, which makes the prognosis of the course of the infection pessimistic is the variable sensitivity to amphotericin B. It can enable the strain *Trichosporon asahii* to produce biofilm.

4.2 Diagnostics of yeast-like infections

Clinical symptoms of IFI in kidney recipients are sparse and lack specificity, which makes a quick diagnosis difficult and effects efficacy of treatment and the predictions.

Classic mycological diagnostic methods: microscopic tests, culture of clinical material, identification of biochemical strain of pathogen, testing of drug resistance remain standard diagnostics. Those methods are without doubt very important in most cases and allow to implement a target treatment including a minimal inhibitory concentration of specific antifungal drugs to the etiological factor IFI.

It has to be stressed that sensitivity and specificity of the classic mycological diagnostic method are insufficient to be used as a single element for the confirmation of IFI diagnostic.

An additional problem is the often occurring mucocutaneous colonization, which causes result interpretation difficulties - not every positive result for the mycological culture allows to implement an antifungal therapy and not every negative result of the culture excludes an invasive infection.

Sparse symptoms of a systemic infection and the difficulties in a quick mycological diagnosis are reasons for delays in implementing of an appropriate antifungal therapy, which can result in the loss of the graft and even the death of the patient.

The problem to identify the participation of the infection appears interesting, also in those caused by fungi in organ rejection.

The „golden standard" in diagnostic of invasive candidosis in patients in high risk groups remains blood cultivation, which has serious restrictions. The most important are:

- low sensitivity: approx. 50% of results in patients with a confirmed or possible IC can be a false negative
- long result waiting time: in most case the waiting time is longer then 2 up to 3 days, in patients receiving antifungal drugs even 14 days.

Developed are also other criteria allowing a rather quick identification, if the active monitoring strategy of the patients state has been adjusted to the mycological diagnostic. One of this criteria is determining if the yeast-like fungi in culture of clinical material is received from one or more parts of the body.
Diagnostic of the invasive candidosis leading to the implementation of the appropriate antifungal treatment consists of clinical, radiological and microbiological tests results.

4.3 Cryptococcosis

To the *Cryptococcus* belong 37 species. The most important pathogenic species for humans is *Cryptococcus neoformans* widely spread in nature globally.
Infection vectors are birds, mostly pigeons, infection sources are also soil particles containing bird faeces contaminated with the fungi, and the most common infection mechanism is inhalation.
A specific characteristic of the yeast-like fungi from the *Cryptococcus* species, used in diagnostic routine is a lack of a polysaccharide capsule with an antiphagocytic function.
Cryptococcosis is an opportunistic infection in patients with immunological defects, it is known as an indicative illness for AIDS. The primary infection localisation are the lower airway, from which it quickly spreads to the lungs and the CNS.
The most dangerous clinical form of cryptococcosis is menigoencephalitis, other clinical forms: chronic or acute pulmonary form or disseminated in relation to the CNS, skin and other tissue and organs. After the pulmonary stage and spreading to the CNS, in the blood serum and PMR rapidly appear dissolving capsule antigens, possible to detect with enzyme immunoassay methods.
The cryptococcosis diagnostic is based on:

- microscopic determination of yeast cells with a polysaccharide capsule in cerebrospinal fluid
- microbiological cultivation of *C. neoformans* from blood or cerebrospinal fluid. The waiting time for results of this test is longer then in case of diagnostic of fungal infections with *Candida* due to a longer incubation time and can take even up to 7 days.

Detection of capsule antigens *Cryptococcus spp.* in serum or cerebrospinal fluid. Sensitivity of the method increases the parallel marking of antigens in serum and PMR.
Diagnosis of cryptococcosis can be determined only based on joined results of clinical, radiological and microbiological tests, (microbiology, histology, serology), each of those elements should be carefully considered.

4.4 Serological diagnostic

The current use of serological diagnostic is based on the detection of specific fungi species - mannoproteins, which have the role pf antigen markers. In the period of sustained systemic fungal infection, those antigens occur in the blood stream temporarily, are easily eliminated by the formed immunological complexes and by way of endocytosis through the Kupffer cells in the liver. Regular monitoring of their presence in systemic fluids has a great practical value in high risk patients.
In diagnostics of invasive aspergilosis (IA) detection of the galactomannan (GM) antigen in the blood stream is valuable (GM). GM is a polysaccharide of the vascular wall of mould fungi belonging to the *Aspergillus* species *(A. fumigatus, A. flavus, A. niger, A.terreus* and other).

A positive test result for *Aspergillus* is one of the microbiological criteria recommended by the *European Organization for Research and Treatment of Cancer* and the *Mycosis Study Group (EORTC/MSG)* to determine IA, despite negative results in classic mycological tests in patients with haematological neoplasm.
Using of similar criteria seams to be justified for diagnosis of IA in vascularised organ recipients, including kidneys. For the purpose of maximising test sensitivity it should be performed at least once a week for patients in the high risk group.
For al patients with a positive result it is recommended to repeat the test with anew blood sample.
According to the *EORTC/MSG* criteria two consecutive positive results are necessary to classify the test as a real positive.
GM detection sensitivity depends on the infection localisation. In the localised invasive pulmonary aspergilosis the sensitivity of the method is significantly lower compared to the disseminated form. Monitoring of GM levels can be useful in infection course prognosis - a drop of the levels can be connected to good prognosis.
IC serodiagnostic (invasive candidosis) is based on the detection of mannan antigen circulating in serum, which is the main component of the cellular wall of a *Candida species fungi*. Mannan is a highly immunogenic polysaccharide antigen with immunomodular characteristics. It allows to use in IC diagnostics parallel monitoring of circulating mannan and titre of antimannan antibodies.
Parallel detection of both markers allowed to increase the sensitivity to 80% and to 93% the specificity of the method. Detection of circulating *Candida spp.* antigen in serum or plasma should enhance IC diagnostic in high risk patients regarding to sensitivity and detection time of infection development. Among *Candida* antigens, mannan which is the main component oft he cellular wall of yeast-like fungi from *Candida* species, appears to be one of the most important biomarkers in the diagnostic of invasive candidosis.
Regular testing of IC high risk patients, connecting the detection of mannan antigen is helpful in diagnostic of invasive candidosis.
The usefulness of testing levels of antibodies in patients treated with immunosuppressants is controversial, but in the period of graft stability in patients without additional problems can be helpful, as long as parallel marking of mannan antigen is performed.
It should be kept in mind that the highest sensitivity is proved in IC diagnostic for *C.albicans, C.glabrata, C.tropicalis* etiology. The lowest sensitivity of mannan detection and mannan antibodies, 40-50% applies for infections with *C.krusei, C.parapsilosis, C.quilliermondii* etiology.
Beta-glucan detection methods in serum (Fungitell-Associates of Cape Cod) proposed as marker in IC diagnostic has many gaps, a positive result does not allow to determine a fungal etiological factor, allows only to differentiate between a fungal and bacterial infection. Additionally the test has a low specificity and a high cost of marking and expensive equipment means that it is rarely used in routine diagnostic.

4.5 Molecular biology methods

Development of molecular techniques, which took place in past years allowed to introduce routine microbiological diagnostic to the tests based on detection of nucleic acids of microorganisms.
In mycological diagnostic genetic methods are used for microorganism detection in material sampled from patients, as well as identification of specific species in this material. It has to

be underlines that they should be used as complimentary to the classic tests protocol or as a confirmation of its results.
Molecular methods should not be used instead of classic diagnostic techniques.
Their application with great success serve in diagnostic of infections difficult to detect with conventional cultivation methods.
Most tests are restricted to detecting of frequently occurring and consequently the most important clinically species, which are factors in general infection such as *Aspergillus fumigatus* or *Candida albicans*.
Although lately molecular identification tests are introduced for a wider group of fungal pathogens.
They have been developed for detection of some of the species *Aspergillus*: *A. flavus*, *A. niger*, *A. versicolor*, *A. terreus* and *A. nidulans* as well as etiological factors for zygomycosis isolated from clinical materials sampled from patients with a general infection.
In case of detection of ethological infections with yeast-like fungi, the newest application of molecular tests are for pathogens from the non-albicans group *Candida spp.*: *C. glabrata*, *C. tropicalis*, *C. parapsilosis*, *C. krusei*, species with an undeniable clinical expansion in recent years.
Detection methods in use are usually based on techniques which are modifications of the standard reaction PCR: real- time PCR, nested PCR, multiplex PCR to detect the ribosome gens RNA: 18s rRNA, 28s rRNA or regions ITS1 and ITS2.
Real-time reaction PCR is characterised by a fast analysis and does not require an electrophoretic test of products.
The reaction is based on the standard PCR method, allows a fast identification and quantitative assessment of the pathogen in a clinical sample. Nested PCR is a modified standard reaction in which two pairs of starters are being used: outer and inner , with different melting temperatures. The product received with outer starters becomes a live matrix for reaction with inner starters. The product received in the first stage - DNA fragment with a sequence specific for microorganisms in the second reaction stage is classified to the searched for species.
Multiplex PCR method differs from the classic method only slightly.
The reaction is performed in the same way, but with a use of more then one pair of starters with a similar melting temperature, which allows to detect more then one pathogen present in the clinical sample.
The choice of material for genetic testing is based on the localization of the infection.
In case of general infections, it is recommended to perform full blood tests on the patient, from which the DNA will be extracted in search of the pathogen.
Currently more often, particularly in mycosis diagnostics, applications are being used which do not allow for diagnostic in Rother clinical material:

- tissue biopsy,
- cerebrospinal fluid and Rother systemic fluids,
- bronchial washings (BAL),
- expectoration,
- tracheal aspiration.

Methods based on molecular techniques are characterised by higher sensitivity and specificity then classic cultivation.
It is estimated that real-time PCR sensitivity for *Candida* has 81-100% sensitivity and specificity from 97 to 86%.
While using the nested PCR method for *Candida* the reaction sensitivity can achieve 86-79%, and specificity 54%. Sensitivity in multiplex PCR is 98% with specificity of 88%.

Specificity and sensitivity in real-time PCR for *Aspergillus fumigatus* oscillates around 100% and depends on the amount of material sampled for testing.
Despite a sorter time needed for the performance of diagnostics, and in result of the waiting time for results, molecular methods hale some restrictions.
The first is the cost of testing, surely higher then in case of classic methods.
Another is a lack of possibility to determine sensitivity spectrum for antimycotics.
It is necessary to perform his test with the classic method.
It should be stressed that the possibilities of use for molecular testing is restricted to detection and identification of pathogens most frequently occurring in clinical material with the exception of the rare ones, which often cause serious infections.

5. Diagnostics algorithm for general fungal infection risk

5.1 Diagnostics algorithm for general fungal infection risk minimization in patients after kidney allotransplantation

In result of many years of observation of a 1301 kidney recipients from cadavers and/or a related donor (including 213 with diagnosed diabetes) a scheme of diagnostic procedure Has been developed, for timely diagnostic of fungal infection, differentiation from colonization with opportunistic fungi strains.
Influence of the fungal infections on an early and late function of the transplant has been analyzed and an algorithm has been developed for diagnostic procedure minimizing the risk general fungal infections in patients after a kidney allotransplantation.
For most patients a 3-drug immunosuppressive protocol has been used: Cyclosporine A (CsA) or tacrolimus (FK) with glucocorticosteroids (GS), with antiproliferative preparations: mycophenolate mofetil (MMF) or azathioprine (AZA), some of the patients received an immunosuppression induction with biological agents (ATG, OKT3).

5.2 An algorithm for an effective diagnostic procedure minimizing the risk of general fungal infections in kidney recipients

An algorithm for an effective diagnostic procedure minimizing the risk of general fungal infections in kidney recipients should include:

- strategy for a quick diagnostic of systemic mycosis in case of justified suspicion of such infection
- tactic of routine diagnostic minimizing the risk of developing a fungal infection in the general population of kidney recipients
- strict criteria for choosing of recipients from the high risk group for fungal
- programs for active monitoring of recipients from the high risk group.

5.3 Strategy for a quick diagnostic of systemic mycosis in case of justified suspicion

The diagnostic procedure should be based on all available testing methods: clinical, radiological, histological, classic microbiology diagnostic, serological methods, and molecular biology. It should be underlined that every diagnostic method has serious restrictions, the decision about the necessary implementation of a antifungal therapy should be based on the interpretation of a number of tests. The basic and crucial element of each of the schemes outlined above remains cultivation of etiological factor IFI from materials sampled from the patient: blood and other systemic fluids, biopsy materials, materials from lower airways, urine, smears from the oral cavity, throat, rectum and other parts, faeces and other materials sampled from the patient, regarding to the clinical situation at hand.

Microbiological criteria for diagnosis of general mycosis are:

- positive results for blood cultures and other physiologically sterile body cavities
- determination of fungi presence in the direct preparation from the tested material
- identification of antigens circulating by serological methods
- identification of genetic fungal material in clinical samples from usually sterile parts
- identification of specific antibodies
- determination of specific fungal enzymes in urine or other systemic fluids
- determination of morphological elements of the fungi in tissues sampled by biopsy.

Differentiation of colonization from infection:

- simultaneous cultivation of strains of the same species from different sampling locations (at least three)
- multiple cultivation of strains of the same species from one sampling location
- simultaneous occurrence of fungal antigens in serum or other naturally sterile systemic fluids
- significant (at least 4 times) of the antibodies titre in serum
- occurrence of hydrolytic enzymes specific for a species in systemic fluids.

The proposal of a procedure in cases of suspected invasive fungal infections scheme is presented in figure 3.

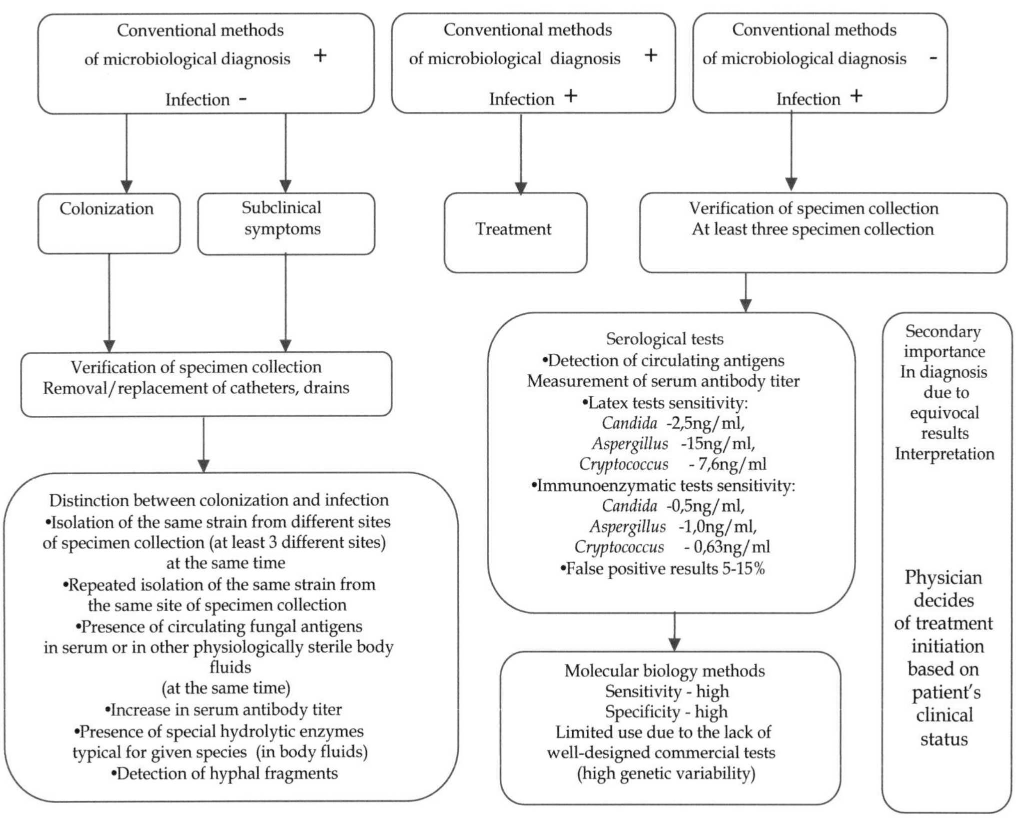

Fig. 3. Diagnostic algorithm for prevention of invasive fungal infection in solid organ transplant recipients.

5.4 Routine diagnostic tactic for minimizing risk of fungal infection in kidney recipients without risk factors disorders

Kidney recipients without additional risk factors should be monitored for a surviving skin, mucosa, urinogenital tract colonization with a classic microbiological method. Proposed is a regular cultivations for fungi in urine, oral cavity smears and qualitative diagnosis of yeast-like fungi present in the gastrointestinal tract.

Frequency of cultivations depends on the period after the Tx. In an early period it is justified to sample materials for microbiological testing not less then once every 5-7 days. In the second period once every 2-3 weeks. In the third - once every 1-2 months.

5.5 Strategy of diagnostics-prophylactic procedure minimizing the risk of a systemic fungal infection in kidney recipients with a specific predisposition

A more aggressive scheme should be applied in cases of additional risk factors for a general fungal infection.

In the early period after Tx, presence factors determined before Tx are very important:

- skin and mucosa colonization by yeast-like or mould fungi
- immunosuppression induction with biological agents in highly immunized patients
- therapy with broad-spectrum antibacterial agents
- blood transfusions
- a particularly important risk is a possibility of colonizing factor or causing a fungal infection in donor transmission from donor-recipient, especially in a diseased donor . To exclude such risk factors it is necessary to perform blood and urine cultivation for fungi
- contamination of preservative fluids with fungi
- risk factors occurring in the early period after Tx:
- skin and mucosa colonization with strains of yeast-like fungi
- bacterial infections
- another kidney transplantation
- acute insufficiency of the transplanted kidney
- repeated surgery due to early postoperative complications
- prolonged transplantation time
- treatment of acute transplant rejection with high doses of steroids or biological agents
- elevated levels of the basic immunosuppressive scheme

Risk factors in the second period after Tx:

- skin or mucosa colonization with yeast-like fungi strains
- treatment of acute transplant rejection with high doses of steroids or biological agents
- infection or reactivation of infections with immunomodulatory viruses: CMV, HHV, EBV
- leukopenia, hypogammaglobulinemia
- repeated bacterial infection
- long-term antibiotics therapy

Risk factors in the third period after Tx:

- skin or mucosa colonization with yeast-like fungi strains
- treatment of acute transplant rejection with high doses of steroids or biological agents
- infection or reactivation of infections with immunomodulatory viruses: CMV, HHV, EBV

- leukopenia, hypogammaglobulinemia
- repeated bacterial infection
- long-term antibiotics therapy
- chronic nephropathy of the transplanted kidney
- treatment of neoplastic diseases.

With the co-occurrence of two or more risk factors it a broader routine procedure, based on classic mycological diagnostic methods needs to be considered.

Together with performing cultivation of clinical samples for fungi on a regular basis, we recommend regular, weekly mannan, galactomannan and glucuronoxylomannan antigen marking, in serum with immunoenzyme method.

5.6 Therapeutic-prophylactic procedure - conclusions

Implementation of a therapeutic procedure, as far as it is possible, should each time be procedure by the identification of the etiological factor of the fungi infection species, taking into account natural resistance or a naturally lowered sensitivity to antimycotic substances.

In 7744 microbiological test of material sampled from kidney recipients, positive cultivation for fungi were received in 475 samples (6.13%). Fungi strains causing infections in his group of recipients belong mostly to the *non-albicans Candida spp.*, in which a large group are strains with a diversified sensitivity to antimycotics. *Candida albicans* was isolated only in 38.1%, where recently we domination of his species in vascularized organs recipients has been observed.

The participation of species which have replaced *C. albicans* is concerning, selected by an irrational treatment of prophylactic. Those are the strains with a restricted sensitivity to the available antimycotics, mostly from the azole group, resistant to flukonazole, namely: *C. glabrata, C. krusei, C. kefyr, C. inconspicua, Trichosporon asahi.* It has been proven that species with a natural resistance or natural sensitivity to flukonazole – *C. glabrata* and *C.krusei* make up for 40%. The acquired resistance to flukonazole has been observed in 5.27% of strains. Clinical material from which the fungi hale been cultivated, were sampled mostly from the urinary and respiratory tract, then from drainage and postoperative wounds and blood. Fungemia were caused only by strains belonging to the *non-albicans Candida spp.*

From literature and our own data appears that the popular use of flukonazole in antifungal prophylactic caused a negative selection of resistant strains. In this period it has also an increased rate of deaths due to general fungal infections with the genus *Aspergillus* has been observed.

Antifungal infection prophylactic can not be used commonly, but only in clinically justified cases, and prophylactic should be even given up, on behalf of active monitoring of recipients and progressive therapy. In this cases an implementation of drugs other then flukonazole or amphotericin B, Itrakonazole, Posaconazole should be considered. In prophylactic the toxicity of the preparations and resulting growing resistance should be considered.

Empirical therapy. In cases of suspected invasive fungal infection based on clinical evidence the appropriate drug would be amphotericin B or its liposomal forms and Itraconazole and new azoles – Voriconazole, Posaconazole as well as caspofungin. Flukonazole can be used only in large doses only in wards, where natural species resistant to flukonazole occur rarely and no prophylactic product has been used.

Treatment of diagnosed mycosis. In confirmed cases of systemic mycosis, the drug used should take into account the sensitivity to the drug of the isolated strain with a marked MIC (minimal inhibitory concentration). The dose should be calculated for each patient individually based on the MIC value. In severe cases it is possible to use a joined treatment. The length of the treatment depends on the clinical state of the patient, it usually takes a few weeks. Postoperative complications requiring a new operation bear a high risk of a fungal infection.

Due to this it appears justified to begin antimycotic treatment from the start of a repeated surgery and to perform an earlier decontamination of the gastrointestinal tract from fungal flora.

Relatively new group of antimycotic drugs are echinocandins. To this group belong: caspofungin, anidulafungin, micafungin. The mechanism of echinocandins is based on the inhibition of the polysaccharide glucan synthesis (1-3β-D-glucan), which is one of the main components of the fungi cellular wall.

Diminishing the concentration of the glucan in the cellular wall leads to changes in the permeability of the membrane and its osmotic instability, which eventually leads to cell lysis. Echinocandins can be only administered intravenously due to very low bioavailability in oral administration.

In adult patients the pharmacodynamic of those drugs is similar - all of them are used intravenously in one daily dose. They are eliminated from the organism by way of a non-enzymatic decomposition All echinocandins do not require dose modifications in case of renal insufficiency and renal replacement therapy.

Caspofungin and micafungin are metabolized in a small way in the liver, but without the cytochrome P450 superfamily enzymes. Caspofungin is the only echinocandins which requires a diminished dose in cases of moderate or severe liver insufficiency.

Echinocandins due to their mechanism are effective for fungi of the *Candida* and *Aspergillus* species similar to classic and lipid forms of amphotericin B. In a multiple site, randomised double blind a similar efficacy of caspofungin therapy with liposomal amphotericin B in treatment of fungal infection of the oesophagus in adults has been confirmed. Caspofungin has been better tolerated by the patients.

According to the IDSA 2009 guideline echinocandins are recommended as first choice drugs in fungemia treatment, particularly caused by *C. glabrata* strains in patients with neutropenia and previously treated with antimycotics from the azoles group. In the population of patients without neutropenia echinocandins are recommended as alternative therapy. Particularly justified is the use of echinocandins in case of fungemia due to their unique ability to penetrate the biofilm environment and to inhibit outer-cellular matrix composition production. This characteristics of echinocandins can have great significance in the inhibition of pathomechanisms in fungemia

Echinocandins also find use in therapy of infections with mould fungi treatment, mostly those belonging to the *Aspergillus* species, though it is restricted due to fungistatic effect of echinocandins on this type of microorganisms.

Caspofungin is recommended in treatment of invasive cadidosis and invasive aspergillosis in patients who hale previously not responded to therapy or intolerant to other antifungal drugs.

Anidulafungin approved by the FDA for treatment of esophagus candidosis, candidemia and other complications of infections with *Candida spp.* It Has been proved in clinical studies that anidulafungin has higher efficacy compared to flukonazole in patients with invasive candidosis and fungemia.

Micafungin is recommended in treatment of invasive cadidosis, for treatment of esophagus candidosis, prophylactic of infections caused by *Candida spp.* in patients with allogenic blood stem cells transplants. An important advantage of micafungin is its small potential for drug interactions. This applies for immunosuppressants: cyclosporine A, tacrolimus, mycophenolate mofetil. With a simultaneous treatment with sirolimus, Itraconazole or nifedipine with micafungin the patent should be monitored for toxic effects and if necessary the dose should be decreased. Lately reports of clinical efficacy of micafungin in treatment of infections caused by appear more frequently *non-albicans Candida species* and *Aspergillus spp.* In patients with immunological insufficiency or without.

6. Conflict of interest

The authors declare that there is no conflict of interest.

7. References

Albano, L.; Bretagne, S.; Mamzer-Bruneel, M.F.; Kacso, I.; Desnos-Ollivier, M.; Guerrini, P.; Le Luong, T.; Cassuto, E.; Dromer, F.; Lortholary, O.; French Mycosis Study Group. Evidence that graft-site candidiasis after kidney transplantation is acquired during organ recovery: a multicenter study in France. *Clin Infect Dis,* Vol.48, No.2, (January 2009), pp. 194-202, ISSN 1058-4838.

Arendrup, M.C.; Bergmann, O.J.; Larsson, L.; Nielsen, H.V.; Jarløv, J.O.; Christensson, B. (2009). Detection of candidaemia in patients with and without underlying haematological disease. *Clin Microbiol Infect,* Vol.16, No.7, (July 2010), pp. 855-862, ISSN 1198-743X.

Ascioglu, S.; Rex, J.H.; de Pauw, B.; Bennett, J.E.; Bille, J.; Crokaert, F.; Denning, D.W.; Donnelly, J.P.; Edwards, J.E.; Erjavec, Z.; Fiere, D.; Lortholary, O.; Maertens, J.; Meis, J.F.; Patterson, T.F.; Ritter, J.; Selleslag, D.; Shah, P.M.; Stevens, D.A.; Walsh, T.J. Invasive Fungal Infections Cooperative Group of the European Organization for Research and Treatment of Cancer; Mycoses Study Group of the National Institute of Allergy and Infectious Diseases. (2001). Defining opportunistic invasive fungal infections in immunocompromised patients with cancer and hematopoietic stem cell transplants: an international consensus. *Clin Infect Dis,* Vol.34, No.1, (January 2002), pp. 7-14, ISSN 1058-4838.

Badiee, P.; Kordbacheh, P.; Alborzi, A.; Zeini, F.; Mirhendy, H.; Mahmoody, M. Fungal infections in solid organ recipients. *Exp Clin Transplant,* Vol.3, No.2, (December 2005), pp. 385-389, ISSN 1304-0855.

Clancy, C.J.; Jaber, R.A.; Leather, H.L.; Wingard, J.R.; Staley, B.; Wheat, L.J.; Cline, C.L.; Rand, K.H.; Schain, D.; Baz, M.; Nguyen, M.H. (2007). Bronchoalveolar lavage galactomannan in diagnosis of invasive pulmonary aspergillosis among solid-organ transplant recipients. *J Clin Microbiol,* Vol.45, No.6, (June 2007), pp. 1759-1765, ISSN 0095-1137.

Denning, D.W, .; Kibbler, C.C.; Barnes, R.A; British Society for Medical Mycology. British Society for Medical Mycology proposed standards of care for patients with invasive fungal infections. *Lancet Infect Dis*, Vol.3, No.4, (April 2003), pp. 230-240, ISSN 1473-3099.

Erjavec, Z.; Verweij, P.E. Recent progress in the diagnosis of fungal infections in the immunocompromised host. *Drug Resist Updat,* Vol.5, No.1, (February 2002), pp. 3-10, ISSN 1368-7646.

Holzheimer, R.G.; Dralle, H. Management of mycoses in surgical patients - review of the literature. *Eur J Med Res,* Vol.7, No.5, (May 2002), pp. 200-226, ISSN 0949-2321.

Jiménez, C.; Lumbreras, C.; Aguado, J,M.; Loinaz, C.; Paseiro, G.; Andrés, A.; Morales, J.M.; Sánchez, G.; García, I.; del Palacio, A.; Moreno, E. Successful treatment of mucor infection after liver or pancreas-kidney transplantation. *Transplantation,* Vol. 73, No.3, (February 2002), pp. 476-480, ISSN 0041-1337.

Khlif, M.; Mary, C.; Sellami, H.; Sellami, A.; Dumon, H.; Ayadi, A.; Ranque, S. (2009). Evaluation of nested and real-time PCR assays in the diagnosis of candidaemia. *Clin Microbiol Infect,* Vol.15, No.7, (July 2009), pp. 656-661, ISSN 1469-0691.

Kingspor, L.; Jalal, S. Molecular detection and identification of *Candida* and *Aspergillus* spp. from clinical samples using real-time PCR. *Clin Microbiol Infect,* Vol.12, No.8, (August 2006), pp. 745-753, ISSN 1198-743X.

Magill, S.S.; Swoboda, S.M.; Shields, C.E.; Colantuoni, E.A.; Fothergill, A.W.; Merz, W.G.; Lipsett, P.A.; Hendrix, C.W. The epidemiology of Candida colonization and invasive candidiasis in a surgical intensive care unit where fluconazole prophylaxis is utilized: follow-up to a randomized clinical trial. *Ann Surg,* No.249, Vol.4, (April 2009), pp. 657-665, ISSN 0003-4932.

Matignon, M.; Botterel, F.; Audard, V.; Dunogue, B.; Dahan, K.; Lang, P.; Bretagne, S.; Grimbert, P. Outcome of renal transplantation in eight patients with Candida sp. contamination of preservation fluid. *Am J Transplant,* No.8, Vol.3, (March 2008), pp. 697-700, ISSN 1600-6135.

Netsvyetayeva, I.; Swoboda-Kopec, E.; Sikora, M.; Jaworska-Zaremba, M.; Blachnio, S.; Łuczak, M. (2008). *Trichosporon asahii* as a prospective pathogen in solid organ transplant recipients. *Mycoses,* Vol.52, No.3, (May 2009), pp. 263-265, ISSN 0933-7407.

Nucci, M.; Marr, K.A. (2005). Emerging fungal diseases. *Clin Infect Dis,* Vol.41, No.4, (August 2005), pp. 521-526, ISSN 1058-4838.

Nucci, M.; Anaissie, E. Fungal infections in hematopoietic stem cell transplantation and solid-organ transplantation--focus on aspergillosis. *Clin Chest Med,* Vol.30, No.2, (June 2009), pp. 295-306, ISSN 0272-5231.

Pappas, P.G.; Alexander, B.D.; Andes, D.R.; Hadley, S.; Kauffman, C.A.; Freifeld, A.; Anaissie, E.J.; Brumble, L.M, .; Herwaldt, L.; Ito, J.; Kontoyiannis, D.P.; Lyon, G.M.; Marr, K.A.; Morrison, V.A.; Park, B.J.; Patterson, T.F.; Perl, T.M.; Oster, R.A.; Schuster, M.G.; Walker, R.; Walsh, T.J.; Wannemuehler, K.A.; Chiller, T.M. Invasive fungal infections among organ transplant recipients: results of the Transplant-

Associated Infection Surveillance Network (TRANSNET). *Clin Infect Dis,* Vol.50, No.8, (April 2010), pp. 1101-1111, ISSN 1058-4838.

Rüping, M.J.; Vehreschild, J.J.; Cornely, O.A. Patients at high risk of invasive fungal infections: when and how to treat. *Drugs,* Vol.68, No.14, (October 2008), pp. 1941-1962, ISSN 0012-6667.

Schabereiter-Gurtner, C.; Selitsch, B.; Rotter, M.L. Hirschl, A.M.; Wilinger, B. (2007). Development of Novel Real-Time PCR Assay for Detection and Differentiation of Eleven Medically Important Aspergillus and Candida Species in Clinical Specimens *J. Clin. Microbiol,* Vol.45, No.3, (March 2007), pp. 906-914, ISSN 0095-1137.

Sendid, B.; Tabouret, M.; Poirot, J.L.; Mathieu, D.; Fruit, J.; Poulain, D. New enzyme immunoassays for sensitive detection of circulating Candida albicans mannan and antimannan antibodies: useful combined test for diagnosis of systemic candidiasis. *J Clin Microbiol,* Vol.37, No.5, (May 1999), pp. 1510-1517, ISSN 0095-1137.

Sendid, B.; Caillot, D.; Baccouch-Humbert, B.; Klingspor, L.; Grandjean, M.; Bonnin, A.; Poulain, D. (2008). Contribution of the Platelia Candida-specific antibody and antigen tests to early diagnosis of systemic Candida tropicalis infection in neutropenic adults. *J Clin Microbiol,* Vol.41, No.10, (October 2008), pp. 4551-4558, ISSN 0095-1137.

Suarez, F.; Lortholary, O.; Buland, S.; Rubio, M.T.; Ghez, D.; Mahe, V.; Quesne, G.; Poiree, S.; Buzyn, A.; Varet, B.; Berche, P.; Bougnoux, M.E. (2008). Detection of Circulating Aspergillus fumigatus DNA by Real-Time PCR Assay of Large Volumes Improves Early Diagnosis of Invasive Aspergillosis in High- Risk Adult Patients under Hematologic Surveillance. *J Cli. Microbiol,* Vol.46, No.11, (November 2008), pp. 3772-3777, ISSN 0095-1137.

Swoboda-Kopec, E.; Netsvyetayeva, I.; Paczek, L.; Dabkowska, M.; Kwiatkowski, A.; Jaworska-Zaremba, M.; Mierzwinska-Nastalska, E.; Sikora, M.; Blachnio, S.; Mlynarczyk, G.; Fiedor, P. Algorithm of clinical protocol lowering the risk of systemic mycosis infections in allografts recipients. *Transplant Proc,* Vol.41, No.8, (October 2009), pp. 3264-3266, ISSN 0041-1345.

Tortorano, A.M.; Peman, J.; Bernhardt, H.; Klingspor, L.; Kibbler, C.C.; Faure, O.; Biraghi, E.; Canton, E.; Zimmermann, K.; Seaton, S.; Grillot, R.; ECMM Working Group on Candidaemia. (2004). Epidemiology of candidaemia in Europe: results of 28-month European Confederation of Medical Mycology (ECMM) hospital-based surveillance study. *Eur J Clin Microbiol Infect Dis,* Vol.23, No.4, (April 2004), pp. 317-322, ISSN 0934-9723.

White, P.L.; Archer, A.E.; Barnes, RA. Comparison of non-culture-based methods for detection of systemic fungal infections, with an emphasis on invasive Candida infections. *J Clin Microbiol,* Vol.43, No.5, (May 2005), pp. 2181-2187. ISSN 0095-1137.

Verduyn Lunel, F.M.; Donnelly, J.P.; van der Lee, H.A.; Blijlevens, N.M.; Verweij, P.E. (2009). Circulating Candida-specific anti-mannan antibodies precede invasive candidiasis in patients undergoing myelo-ablative chemotherapy. *Clin Microbiol Infect.,* Vol.15, No.4, (April 2009), pp. 380-386, ISSN 1198-743X.

Yera, H.; Sendid, B.; Francois, N.; Camus, D.; Poulain, D. (2001). Contribution of serological tests and blood culture to the early diagnosis of systemic candidiasis. *Eur J Clin Microbiol Infect Dis.* Vol.20, No.12, (December 2001), pp. 864-870, ISSN 0934-9723.

3

CMV Infection in CMV-Seropositive Kidney Transplant Recipients

Jong Man Kim and Sung Joo Kim
Department of Surgery, Samsung Medical Center, Sungkyunkwan University School of Medicine, Republic of Korea

1. Introduction

Cytomegalovirus (CMV) infection is a major cause of morbidity in kidney transplant recipients. CMV seropositivity is common in the general population, with a reported prevalence ranging from 30 to 97% (Paya, 2001; Preiksaitis et al., 2005). After primary infection, CMV establishes life-long latency. During the past 2 decades, major advances in the management of CMV infection of transplant patients have been achieved with new diagnostic techniques and the use of antiviral agents.

Most transplant centers have protocols for the diagnosis and monitoring of CMV, while strategies for the treatment of clinically significant infections as well as prophylactic and preemptive therapy have become common practice. Such strategies address both clinically significant disease and the indirect effects of CMV infection, increased risk of allograft rejection and other infections.

Several guidelines been published within the last few years regarding the management of CMV in transplant patients, diagnostic procedures, and prevention by prophylaxis or preemptive therapy.

The following definitions are commonly used in the transplant literature and are consistent with the American Society of Transplantation (AST) and The Transplantation Society (TTS) recommendations for use in clinical trials (Humar & Michaels, 2006; Kotton et al., 2010):

- CMV infection: evidence of CMV replication regardless of symptoms
- CMV disease: evidence of CMV infection with attributable symptoms. CMV disease can be further categorized as either a viral syndrome with fever and/or malaise, leucopenia, and thrombocytopenia, or as tissue-invasive disease (e.g., pneumonitis, hepatitis, retinitis, and gastrointestinal disease).

A number of review articles on CMV-associated problems in kidney transplantation can aid the clinician working with these patients. These reviews include information on its clinical signs and symptoms, indirect effects, diagnosis, prevention, and treatment protocols. However, the manifestations of CMV infection vary among patients, in part depending on their CMV serostatus. In fact, the prevalence, clinical manifestations, and effects of CMV depend on the patient's serostatus. In this overview, we summarize the current status of CMV, focusing primarily on adult kidney transplant patients who are CMV donor positive/recipient positive (CMV D+/R+).

2. Epidemiology and pathogenesis

CMV is a widespread pathogen that causes an asymptomatic or mild mononucleosis-like primary infection, which usually occurs in early childhood or adolescence. The prevalence of CMV seropositivity ranges from 40 to 100% worldwide, with lower rates in Europe, parts of North America, and Australia, and higher rates in Africa and Asia (Ho, 1990). In regions with higher rates of CMV seropositivity, rates of CMV disease after kidney transplantation may be lower, as populations with immunity to CMV are less likely to have active disease (Kanter et al., 2009).

Like other herpes viruses, CMV can establish latency. After primary infection, the virus may persist at specific sites in the host without any detectable viral infection (Sinclair & Sissons, 2006). Sporadic reactivation events may occur, but they are generally controlled by cell-mediated immunity, cytotoxic T-cells, and NK cells. Blood leukocytes, and mononuclear cells in particular, are generally the sites of latency, but viral DNA has been detected in bone marrow hematopoietic progenitors, epithelial cells, and endothelial cells.

The latent virus can thus be easily transmitted from a transplant donor to recipient by either the leukocytes, or possibly even tissue cells, of the kidney. Transplant patients' cell-mediated immunity is impaired and cannot control the virus, resulting in reactivation of the donor virus in CMV-seronegative recipients without immunity to CMV (D+/R-), as well as in CMV-seropositive (R+). Other recipients undergo reactivation of their own latent virus. CMV is thought to be a risk factor for other viral infections, as well as invasive fungal and bacterial infections in transplant recipients (Fishman & Rubin, 1998).

Without prophylaxis, CMV infections occur in the majority of kidney transplant patients, primarily during the first 3 months, when immunosuppression is most powerful. The risk factors for CMV disease in transplant recipients include CMV seropositive donor/CMV seronegative recipient (D+/R-) and the intensity of immunosuppressive therapy. It has been reported that CMV donor positive/recipient positive status was not a risk factor for CMV replication or disease in kidney transplant recipients (Bataille et al., 2010).

3. Clinical impact of CMV infection

3.1 Direct effects

Symptoms of CMV disease are largely nonspecific, such as fever, fatigue, body aches, and myelosuppression. In some patients, CMV disease is manifested as tissue-invasive disease. The gastrointestinal tract is the most common site for tissue-invasive CMV disease, independent of the type of allograft transplant (Faure-Della Corte et al., 2010), which can cause abdominal pain and diarrhea. In severe cases, CMV ulceration of the gastrointestinal tract can lead to hemorrhage and perforation. Other organs that may manifest tissue-invasive disease include the liver, lungs, heart, pancreas, and kidneys, and may present with allograft dysfunction easily misdiagnosed as acute or chronic rejection (Couzi et al., 2010).

3.2 Indirect effects

CMV is associated with a variety of indirect effects due to the virus' ability to modulate the immune system (Couzi et al., 2010). Kidney transplant recipients with CMV infection or disease are more likely to develop opportunistic infections from other viruses (e.g., human herpesvirus [HHV]-6, HHV-7, and Epstein-Barr virus-related post-transplant lymphoprohferative disease) (Razonable & Paya, 2003; Razonable et al., 2003), bacteria (e.g.,

Nocardia spp.) (Peleg et al., 2007), and fungi (Husni et al., 1998). In addition to infections, patients with CMV infection are more likely to experience acute and chronic rejection.

CMV infection has also been described as an independent risk factor for atherosclerosis in kidney transplant recipients (Hodson et al., 2005). In addition, new-onset diabetes mellitus has been reported in patients with CMV infection or disease after kidney transplantation (Hartmann et al., 2006; Rodrigo et al., 2006). Research has shown that the development of γ-δ T cells in response to CMV is associated with a lower risk of malignancy after kidney transplantation (Couzi et al., 2010). CMV infection is associated with a higher rate of allograft failure and death in kidney transplant recipients, in part due to increased opportunistic infections as well as acute and chronic allograft rejection (Razonable & Paya, 2003; Sagedal et al., 2007). In one study, CMV persistence in the allograft was associated with reduced allograft function and survival after kidney transplantation (Helantera et al., 2006). In regard to treatment, primary antiviral prophylaxis appears to be more effective in preventing the indirect effects of CMV than pre-emptive therapy (Hodson et al., 2005; Kalil et al., 2005).

4. Diagnosis

The diagnosis of CMV infection and disease has evolved considerably. Historically, the diagnosis of CMV disease was made by histopathology, which requires an invasive procedure to obtain samples. Serologic assays appear to have limited clinical utility after transplantation, and should not be used to diagnose acute disease in kidney transplant recipients (Humar et al., 2005).

For years, culture-based methods (tissue culture and shell vial centrifugation culture) were used for CMV diagnosis. Tissue cultures can take weeks, however, and the shell vial centrifugation assay is less sensitive than molecular assays (Mazzulli et al., 1999). Nonetheless, tissue cultures are useful to grow CMV isolates in the laboratory for phenotypic antiviral resistance testing, although the latter technique has been replaced predominantly by genotypic resistance testing.

The pp65 antigenemia assay is a semi-quantitative fluorescent assay based on detection of infected cells in the peripheral blood. This assay has far higher sensitivity and specificity than culture-based methods (Mazzulli et al., 1999), and is comparable in sensitivity to CMV PCR (Caliendo et al., 2000). Though not fully quantitative, it can provide an estimate of the magnitude of viral load from the number of infected cells. Molecular diagnostic tests detect DNA or RNA, are qualitative and quantitative, and the majority are highly sensitive for CMV.

Quantitative measurement of CMV-DNA levels has become popular at many centers. Commonly used assays include PCR testing of plasma or whole blood, which is commercially available. Whole blood assays often have higher viral loads than plasma assays. In general, the highest viral loads are associated with tissue-invasive disease, while the lowest are seen with asymptomatic CMV infection (Kim et al., 2011). In addition to the absolute value of viral load, the rate of rise is also an important factor (Emery et al., 2000). Of note, it is possible for patients with tissue invasive disease (especially gastrointestinal or retinal disease) to occasionally have undetectable blood viral loads.

Both the pp65 antigenemia assay and quantitative CMV viral load testing can be utilized in preemptive protocols, to diagnose of CMV disease, and to guide management (Caliendo et al., 2000; Emery et al., 2000; Kim et al., 2011). A major problem of these assays is the lack of standardization. A recent multicenter comparison of viral load assays demonstrated up to a 1000 folds variation among them. Standardization may be achieved in the future with quantitative viral load assays (Pang et al., 2003).

5. Antiviral prophylaxis and preemptive therapy

There are very few randomized trials comparing preemptive therapy with prophylaxis in the prevention of CMV in kidney transplant recipients with CMV D+/R+ status. Reasons for this include variation among transplant programs, different end-point definitions, non-standardized testing methodologies, and different patient populations.

Two strategies are commonly used for CMV prevention: antiviral prophylaxis and preemptive therapy. Antiviral prophylaxis involves giving antiviral therapy to all 'at-risk' patients (or a specified subset) beginning in the early post transplant period for a defined duration, such as 3 to 6 months. In preemptive therapy, patients are monitored regularly by laboratory assay (often weekly) for early evidence of CMV replication. Patients with detectable replication are then treated with antiviral therapy to prevent symptomatic disease.

Each approach has advantages and disadvantages that must be considered in the context of the patient and the allograft (Table 1) (Fishman et al., 2007; Torres-Madriz & Boucher, 2008). Preemptive therapy may decrease drug costs and toxicity, but requires excellent logistic coordination in order to obtain, receive, and act on results in a timely fashion, which can be difficult if patients live far from the transplant center. In addition, due to a lack of standardized diagnostic testing, optimal threshold values for the initiation of preemptive therapy have not been defined. Antiviral prophylaxis has the theoretical advantage of preventing reactivation of other viruses such as HHV-6 and may thus be more likely to prevent the indirect effects of CMV. Meta-analyses have demonstrated that antiviral prophylaxis is associated with decreased graft loss, decreased opportunistic infections, and improved survival (Kalil et al., 2005; Small et al., 2006). Late-onset CMV disease is a potential limitation of prophylaxis.

	Prophylaxis	Preemptive therapy
Efficacy	Yes	Yes
Ease	Relatively ease to coordinate	More difficult to coordinate Test thresholds not Standardized
Late onset disease	A potential problems	Much less commonly seen
Cost	Higher drug costs	Higher laboratory costs
Toxicity	Potential for greater toxicity (myelosuppression)	Potential for less drug toxicity with shorter courses of antivirals
Indirect effects (e.g. graft loss, mortality, and opportunistic infections)	Consistent and positive impact based on meta-analyses and limited comparative trials	Very limited data that preemptive therapy affects indirect effects

Table 1. Prophylaxis versus preemptive therapy.

5.1 Antiviral prophylaxis

Drugs that have been evaluated for antiviral prophylaxis include ganciclovir, valganciclovir, acyclovir, valacyclovir, and immune globulin preparations (Table 2). All doses should be adjusted based on renal function. Ganciclovir is available in both oral and intravenous formulations. The literature contains several large, multicenter, randomized trials of prophylaxis with oral ganciclovir, valganciclovir, and valacyclovir (Hodson et al., 2008). Valganciclovir is a valine ester pro-drug of ganciclovir with better bioavailability (50-60%) than oral ganciclovir (6-9%) (Perrottet et al., 2009).

Acyclovir has less activity against CMV and is not recommended specifically for prophylaxis. The efficacy of prophylaxis with either CMV immune globulin (CMVIG) or intravenous immune globulin (IVIG) in kidney organ transplant recipients has been investigated in relatively few trials (Hodson et al., 2007), the majority of which have been randomized, but not blinded. Further research is needed to delineate the benefit of adding immune globulin to current CMV prophylaxis regimens.

Drug	Usual adult prophylaxis dose	Comments on use and major toxicity
Valganciclovir	900mg once daily	Ease on administration; leukopenia
Oral ganciclovir	1g three times daily	Low oral bioavailablility: high pill burden
IV ganciclovir	5mg/kg once daily	Intravenous access; leucopenia
Valacyclovir	2g four times daily	High pill burden; neurological effects

Table 2. Currently available drugs for CMV prophylaxis.

5.1.1 Late onset CMV disease

The major problem with CMV prophylaxis continues to be late-onset CMV disease, defined as disease occurring after discontinuation of antiviral prophylaxis. For 3-month prophylaxis regimens, this typically occurs between 3 and 6 months post transplant, but occasionally occurs later. Late onset CMV disease can be difficult to diagnose, especially in patients who live far away from their primary transplant program. Late onset CMV disease contributes to morbidity and has been associated with higher overall mortality (Limaye et al., 2004).

Potential options for dealing with late-onset CMV disease are as follows: (1) careful clinical follow-up with treatment as soon as symptoms occur, and (2) virologic monitoring after completion of prophylaxis, such as periodic measurement of antigenemia or viral load for 8 to 12 weeks. However, studies evaluating the utility of post-prophylaxis monitoring have demonstrated poor sensitivity and specificity in predicting CMV disease (Humar et al., 2004). Weekly monitoring may be required to increase sensitivity.

5.2 Preemptive therapy

Preemptive therapy involves monitoring for early evidence of CMV replication followed by early treatment to prevent symptomatic disease (Paya, 2001; Preiksaitis et al., 2005). Preemptive therapy has the potential advantage of targeting patients at higher risk, thereby decreasing drug costs and toxicity. A sound preemptive strategy includes careful selection of the patient, the optimal laboratory test, the duration of monitoring, and the type, dose, and duration of an antiviral agent.

The best laboratory test to monitor is either a viral load test or a pp65 antigenemia assay. Site-specific and assay-specific threshold values for initiation of preemptive therapy should be locally validated prior to institution of a preemptive protocol. The optimal monitoring strategy is approximately once weekly testing for 12 weeks post transplant.
Once viremia is detected, treatment should be initiated with either oral valganciclovir (900 mg twice a day) or intravenous ganciclovir (5 mg/kg twice a day). Therapy should be continued until viremia is undetectable. A randomized trial found that these agents had equal efficacy for treatment of mild to moderate CMV disease (Asberg et al., 2007). As the aim of preemptive therapy is to treat low-level asymptomatic viremia, oral valganciclovir is preferable to intravenous ganciclovir for logistical issues. Further studies are required to determine comparative efficacy of preemptive therapy versus prophylaxis, especially regarding the indirect sequelae of CMV.

5.3 Comparison of antiviral prophylaxis and preemptive therapy

Only relatively small trials have compared universal prophylaxis with preemptive therapy. In a study comparing oral ganciclovir prophylaxis with preemptive intravenous ganciclovir in kidney transplant patients, prophylaxis reduced the incidence of CMV infection over 12 months by 65% (13/73 versus 33/65 patients) and improved 4-year graft survival (Kliem et al., 2008). A trial of 98 kidney transplant patients randomly assigned to preemptive therapy or prophylaxis with valganciclovir for 100 days showed that both strategies were effective in preventing symptomatic CMV infection (Khoury et al., 2006). Another study that compared preemptive therapy with universal prophylaxis found significantly higher rates of biopsy-proven acute rejection in the preemptive therapy group (Reischig et al., 2008).
Recently, 2 studies reported directly opposed results in CMV-seropositive kidney transplant recipients receiving antiviral prophylaxis or preemptive treatment with valganciclovir. One study found no difference between groups in the incidence of CMV syndrome (4% vs. 5%; P=0.67), CMV disease (0% vs. 2%; P=0.45), or acute rejection (10% vs. 5%, P=1.00) (McGillicuddy et al., 2010). The other study found that CMV reactivation 1 year post-transplant in 67.4% and 28% of preemptive and prophylactic groups, respectively (P<0.001). In addition, the study found a significantly greater incidence of CMV disease in the preemptive group than in the prophylactic group (9.8% vs. 2.68%, P=0.021) (Weclawiak et al., 2010). Several meta-analyses found that although preemptive therapy was effective in reducing the relative risk of CMV, all-cause mortality was not altered (Hodson et al., 2005; Kalil et al., 2005; Small et al., 2006).
Guidelines regarding prophylaxis management favor the use of prophylaxis over preemptive therapy in intermediate-risk, CMV-seropositive transplant recipients, based on the available data suggesting better graft survival and clinical outcomes.(Humar & Michaels, 2006; Kotton et al., 2010) Individual transplant centers must weigh the risks and benefits of each approach, based on the frequency of CMV disease in their center, their ability to monitor recipients, cost of antiviral medications and diagnostics, local rates of late onset CMV disease, and the incidence of other opportunistic infections, graft loss, rejection, and mortality.

6. Treatment of established CMV disease

Intravenous ganciclovir has been used to successfully treat CMV disease in kidney transplant recipients in over 30 uncontrolled, non-randomized, therapeutic trials (Preiksaitis et al., 2005) and is has been considered the mainstay of therapy. The typical dose of intravenous ganciclovir is 5 mg/kg twice daily. The duration of therapy in trials varied from 2 to 4 weeks. Valganciclovir at a dose of 900 mg twice daily achieves levels similar to intravenous ganciclovir treatment. In a randomized controlled trial comparing 3 weeks of oral valganciclovir to intravenous ganciclovir for the treatment of mild to moderate CMV disease in 321 organ transplant patients, the vast majority of whom were kidney transplant recipients, both drugs had similar efficacy for the eradication of viremia 21 days post-treatment (Asberg et al., 2007). However, in the per-protocol population, a significant number of patients had persistent viremia at day 21, suggesting that longer courses of therapy are appropriate in some patients.

CMV disease should be treated for at least 2 weeks or until the following criteria are met: clinical resolution of symptoms and virologic clearance below a threshold negative value.

Intravenous ganciclovir is preferable to oral valganciclovir in patients with severe or life-threatening disease, or in patients with impaired gastrointestinal absorption (e.g., significant diarrhea). Acyclovir and oral ganciclovir are not effective in treating CMV disease in transplant recipients. While oral ganciclovir has been shown to prevent CMV disease, it is not recommended as a treatment due to concerns about emergence of ganciclovir-resistant CMV strains in the presence of CMV replication.

It is unclear whether addition of IVIG or CMVIG to existing treatment regimens has a benefit for solid organ transplant recipients, but it can be considered for patients with CMV pneumonitis or other severe disease.

Overall, molecular diagnostic tests can be used to tailor the duration of antiviral therapy based on clearance of CMV viral load or antigenemia. This risk of relapse is lower in patients who have no detectable CMV viral load at the end of therapy than for those with a detectable CMV viral load (Asberg et al., 2009; Humar et al., 2002). Therefore, patients with evidence of CMV viremia should be maintained on therapy until viremia (measured either by antigenemia or nucleic acid testing) has dropped below the negative threshold value for a given test, a value that remains poorly defined in ultra-sensitive assays. After completion of treatment, a 1 to 3 month course of secondary prophylaxis may be considered depending on the clinical situation. An alternative option is close clinical and/or virologic follow-up after discontinuation of treatment.

7. Conclusion

Although, new therapeutic procedures and the use of modern diagnostic methods have reduced the incidence of severe infections, CMV remains a common disease that negatively influences kidney transplant outcomes. In addition to viral factors and pharmacological immunosuppression, the roles of innate and adaptive immune deficiencies are now being recognized in its pathogenesis.

Prevention of CMV with antiviral prophylaxis and preemptive therapy are both effective, but have distinct disadvantages. The direct and indirect effects of CMV may be reduced by prophylaxis with antiviral agents, though late onset primary infections may complicate the post-transplant course. Furthermore, many CMV-seropositive recipients who will never develop CMV reactivation are exposed to drugs during prophylaxis. On the other hand, preemptive therapy is based on the frequent laboratory monitoring of viral load, and some patients develop a symptomatic infection before the diagnosis of CMV viremia.

Large randomized clinical trials are needed to establish a casual relationship between CMV reactivation and graft injury. In particular, they should analyze long-term graft survival and compare prophylaxis with preemptive therapy in D+/R+, with particular attention to patients receiving preemptive therapy who have no episodes of positive antigenemia and therefore are not receiving anti-CMV treatments.

8. References

Asberg, A.; Humar, A.; Jardine, A.G.; Rollag, H.; Pescovitz, M.D.; Mouas, H.; Bignamini, A.; Toz, H.; Dittmer, I.; Montejo, M. & Hartmann, A. (2009). Long-term outcomes of CMV disease treatment with valganciclovir versus IV ganciclovir in solid organ transplant recipients. American Journal of Transplantation, Vol.9, No.5, (May 2009), pp. 1205-1213, ISSN 1600-6143

Asberg, A.; Humar, A.; Rollag, H.; Jardine, A.G.; Mouas, H.; Pescovitz, M.D.; Sgarabotto, D.; Tuncer, M.; Noronha, I.L. & Hartmann, A. (2007). Oral valganciclovir is noninferior to intravenous ganciclovir for the treatment of cytomegalovirus disease in solid organ transplant recipients. American Journal of Transplantation, Vol.7, No.9, (Sep 2007), pp. 2106-2113, ISSN 1600-6135

Bataille, S.; Moal, V.; Gaudart, J.; Indreies, M.; Purgus, R.; Dussol, B.; Zandotti, C.; Berland, Y. & Vacher-Coponat, H. (2010). Cytomegalovirus risk factors in renal transplantation with modern immunosuppression. Transplant Infectious Disease, Vol.12, No.6, (Dec 2010), pp. 480-488, ISSN 1399-3062

Caliendo, A.M.; St George, K.; Kao, S.Y.; Allega, J.; Tan, B.H.; LaFontaine, R.; Bui, L. & Rinaldo, C.R. (2000). Comparison of quantitative cytomegalovirus (CMV) PCR in plasma and CMV antigenemia assay: clinical utility of the prototype AMPLICOR CMV MONITOR test in transplant recipients. Journal of Clinical Microbiology, Vol.38, No.6, (Jun 2000), pp. 2122-2127, ISSN 0095-1137

Couzi, L.; Levaillant, Y.; Jamai, A.; Pitard, V.; Lassalle, R.; Martin, K.; Garrigue, I.; Hawchar, O.; Siberchicot, F.; Moore, N.; Moreau, J.F.; Dechanet-Merville, J. & Merville, P. (2010). Cytomegalovirus-induced gammadelta T cells associate with reduced cancer risk after kidney transplantation. Journal of the American Society of Nephrology, Vol.21, No.1, (Jan 2009), pp. 181-188, ISSN 1533-3450

Emery, V.C.; Sabin, C.A.; Cope, A.V.; Gor, D.; Hassan-Walker, A.F. & Griffiths, P.D. (2000). Application of viral-load kinetics to identify patients who develop cytomegalovirus disease after transplantation. Lancet, Vol.355, No.9220, (Jun 2000), pp. 2032-2036, ISSN 0140-6736

Faure-Della Corte, M.; Samot, J.; Garrigue, I.; Magnin, N.; Reigadas, S.; Couzi, L.; Dromer, C.; Velly, J.F.; Dechanet-Merville, J.; Fleury, H.J. & Lafon, M.E. (2010). Variability and recombination of clinical human cytomegalovirus strains from transplantation recipients. Journal of Clinical Virology, Vol.47, No.2, (Feb 2009), pp. 161-169, ISSN 1873-5967

Fishman, J.A.; Emery, V.; Freeman, R.; Pascual, M.; Rostaing, L.; Schlitt, H.J.; Sgarabotto, D.; Torre-Cisneros, J. & Uknis, M.E. (2007). Cytomegalovirus in transplantation - challenging the status quo. Clinical Transplantation, Vol.21, No.2, (Mar-Apr 2007), pp. 149-158, ISSN 0902-0063

Fishman, J.A. & Rubin, R.H. (1998). Infection in organ-transplant recipients. New England Journal of Medicine, Vol.338, No.24, (Jun 1998), pp. 1741-1751, ISSN 0028-4793

Hartmann, A.; Sagedal, S. & Hjelmesaeth, J. (2006). The natural course of cytomegalovirus infection and disease in renal transplant recipients. Transplantation, Vol.82, No.2 Suppl, (Jul 2006), pp. S15-17, ISSN 0041-1337

Helantera, I.; Koskinen, P.; Finne, P.; Loginov, R.; Kyllonen, L.; Salmela, K.; Gronhagen-Riska, C. & Lautenschlager, I. (2006). Persistent cytomegalovirus infection in kidney allografts is associated with inferior graft function and survival. Transplant International, Vol.19, No.11, (Nov 2006), pp. 893-900, ISSN 0934-0874

Ho, M. (1990). Epidemiology of cytomegalovirus infections. Reviews of Infectious Diseases, Vol.12 Suppl 7, (Sep-Oct 1990), pp. S701-710, ISSN 0162-0886

Hodson, E.M.; Craig, J.C.; Strippoli, G.F. & Webster, A.C. (2008). Antiviral medications for preventing cytomegalovirus disease in solid organ transplant recipients. Cochrane Database Systematic Reviews, No.2, pp. CD003774, ISSN 1469-493X

Hodson, E.M.; Jones, C.A.; Strippoli, G.F.; Webster, A.C. & Craig, J.C. (2007). Immunoglobulins, vaccines or interferon for preventing cytomegalovirus disease in solid organ transplant recipients. Cochrane Database Systematic Reviews, No.2, pp. CD005129, ISSN 1469-493X

Hodson, E.M.; Jones, C.A.; Webster, A.C.; Strippoli, G.F.; Barclay, P.G.; Kable, K.; Vimalachandra, D. & Craig, J.C. (2005). Antiviral medications to prevent cytomegalovirus disease and early death in recipients of solid-organ transplants: a systematic review of randomised controlled trials. Lancet, Vol.365, No.9477, (Jun 2005), pp. 2105-2115, ISSN 1474-547X

Humar, A.; Kumar, D.; Boivin, G. & Caliendo, A.M. (2002). Cytomegalovirus (CMV) virus load kinetics to predict recurrent disease in solid-organ transplant patients with CMV disease. Journal of Infectious Diseases, Vol.186, No.6, (Sep 2002), pp. 829-833, ISSN 0022-1899

Humar, A.; Mazzulli, T.; Moussa, G.; Razonable, R.R.; Paya, C.V.; Pescovitz, M.D.; Covington, E. & Alecock, E. (2005). Clinical utility of cytomegalovirus (CMV) serology testing in high-risk CMV D+/R- transplant recipients. American Journal of Transplantation, Vol.5, No.5, (May 2005), pp. 1065-1070, ISSN 1600-6135

Humar, A. & Michaels, M. (2006). American Society of Transplantation recommendations for screening, monitoring and reporting of infectious complications in immunosuppression trials in recipients of organ transplantation. American Journal of Transplantation, Vol.6, No.2, (Feb 2006), pp. 262-274, ISSN 1600-6135

Humar, A.; Paya, C.; Pescovitz, M.D.; Dominguez, E.; Washburn, K.; Blumberg, E.; Alexander, B.; Freeman, R.; Heaton, N. & Mueller, B. (2004). Clinical utility of cytomegalovirus viral load testing for predicting CMV disease in D+/R- solid organ transplant recipients. American Journal of Transplantation, Vol.4, No.4, (Apr 2004), pp. 644-649, ISSN 1600-6135

Husni, R.N.; Gordon, S.M.; Longworth, D.L.; Arroliga, A.; Stillwell, P.C.; Avery, R.K.; Maurer, J.R.; Mehta, A. & Kirby, T. (1998). Cytomegalovirus infection is a risk factor for invasive aspergillosis in lung transplant recipients. Clinical Infectious Diseases, Vol.26, No.3, (Mar 1998), pp. 753-755, ISSN 1058-4838

Kalil, A.C.; Levitsky, J.; Lyden, E.; Stoner, J. & Freifeld, A.G. (2005). Meta-analysis: the efficacy of strategies to prevent organ disease by cytomegalovirus in solid organ transplant recipients. Annals of Internal Medicine, Vol.143, No.12, (Dec 2005), pp. 870-880, ISSN 1539-3704

Kanter, J.; Pallardo, L.; Gavela, E.; Escudero, V.; Beltran, S.; Morales, A.; Avila, A. & Crespo, J.F. (2009). Cytomegalovirus infection renal transplant recipients: risk factors and outcome. Transplantation Proceedings, Vol.41, No.6, (Jul-Aug 2009), pp. 2156-2158, ISSN 1873-2623

Khoury, J.A.; Storch, G.A.; Bohl, D.L.; Schuessler, R.M.; Torrence, S.M.; Lockwood, M.; Gaudreault-Keener, M.; Koch, M.J.; Miller, B.W.; Hardinger, K.L.; Schnitzler, M.A. & Brennan, D.C. (2006). Prophylactic versus preemptive oral valganciclovir for the management of cytomegalovirus infection in adult renal transplant recipients. American Journal of Transplantation, Vol.6, No.9, (Sep 2006), pp. 2134-2143, ISSN 1600-6135

Kim, J.M.; Kim, S.J.; Joh, J.W.; Kwon, C.H.; Song, S.; Shin, M.; Moon, J.I.; Kim, G.S.; Hong, S.H. & Lee, S.K. (2011). Is cytomegalovirus infection dangerous in cytomegalovirus-seropositive recipients after liver transplantation? Liver Transplantation, Vol.17, No.4, (Apr 2011), pp. 446-455, ISSN 1527-6473

Kliem, V.; Fricke, L.; Wollbrink, T.; Burg, M.; Radermacher, J. & Rohde, F. (2008). Improvement in long-term renal graft survival due to CMV prophylaxis with oral ganciclovir: results of a randomized clinical trial. American Journal of Transplantation, Vol.8, No.5, (May 2008), pp. 975-983, ISSN 1600-6143

Kotton, C.N.; Kumar, D.; Caliendo, A.M.; Asberg, A.; Chou, S.; Snydman, D.R.; Allen, U. & Humar, A. (2010). International consensus guidelines on the management of cytomegalovirus in solid organ transplantation. Transplantation, Vol.89, No.7, (Apr 2010), pp. 779-795, ISSN 1534-6080

Limaye, A.P.; Bakthavatsalam, R.; Kim, H.W.; Kuhr, C.S.; Halldorson, J.B.; Healey, P.J. & Boeckh, M. (2004). Late-onset cytomegalovirus disease in liver transplant recipients despite antiviral prophylaxis. Transplantation, Vol.78, No.9, (Nov 2004), pp. 1390-1396, ISSN 0041-1337

Mazzulli, T.; Drew, L.W.; Yen-Lieberman, B.; Jekic-McMullen, D.; Kohn, D.J.; Isada, C.; Moussa, G.; Chua, R. & Walmsley, S. (1999). Multicenter comparison of the digene hybrid capture CMV DNA assay (version 2.0), the pp65 antigenemia assay, and cell culture for detection of cytomegalovirus viremia. Journal of Clinical Microbiology, Vol.37, No.4, (Apr 1999), pp. 958-963, ISSN 0095-1137

McGillicuddy, J.W.; Weimert, N.A.; Taber, D.J.; Turner, A.; Mitchell, L.A.; Wray, D.W.; Egidi, M.F.; Kuppachi, S.; Hughes, M.G.; Baliga, P.K. & Chavin, K.D. (2010). Can preemptive cytomegalovirus monitoring be as effective as universal prophylaxis when implemented as the standard of care in patients at moderate risk? Transplantation, Vol.89, No.10, (May 2010), pp. 1218-1223, ISSN 1534-6080

Pang, X.L.; Chui, L.; Fenton, J.; LeBlanc, B. & Preiksaitis, J.K. (2003). Comparison of LightCycler-based PCR, COBAS amplicor CMV monitor, and pp65 antigenemia assays for quantitative measurement of cytomegalovirus viral load in peripheral blood specimens from patients after solid organ transplantation. Journal of Clinical Microbiology, Vol.41, No.7, (Jul 2003), pp. 3167-3174, ISSN 0095-1137

Paya, C.V. (2001). Prevention of cytomegalovirus disease in recipients of solid-organ transplants. Clinical Infectious Diseases, Vol.32, No.4, (Feb 2001), pp. 596-603, ISSN 1058-4838

Peleg, A.Y.; Husain, S.; Qureshi, Z.A.; Silveira, F.P.; Sarumi, M.; Shutt, K.A.; Kwak, E.J. & Paterson, D.L. (2007). Risk factors, clinical characteristics, and outcome of Nocardia infection in organ transplant recipients: a matched case-control study. Clinical Infectious Diseases, Vol.44, No.10, (May 2007), pp. 1307-1314, ISSN 1537-6591

Perrottet, N.; Decosterd, L.A.; Meylan, P.; Pascual, M.; Biollaz, J. & Buclin, T. (2009). Valganciclovir in adult solid organ transplant recipients: pharmacokinetic and pharmacodynamic characteristics and clinical interpretation of plasma concentration measurements. Clinical Pharmacokinetics, Vol.48, No.6, pp. 399-418, ISSN 0312-5963

Preiksaitis, J.K.; Brennan, D.C.; Fishman, J. & Allen, U. (2005). Canadian society of transplantation consensus workshop on cytomegalovirus management in solid organ transplantation final report. American Journal of Transplantation, Vol.5, No.2, (Feb 2005), pp. 218-227, ISSN 1600-6135

Razonable, R.R. & Paya, C.V. (2003). Herpesvirus infections in transplant recipients: current challenges in the clinical management of cytomegalovirus and Epstein-Barr virus infections. Herpes, Vol.10, No.3, (Dec 2004), pp. 60-65, ISSN 0969-7667

Razonable, R.R.; Rivero, A.; Brown, R.A.; Hart, G.D.; Espy, M.J.; van Cruijsen, H.; Wilson, J.; Groettum, C.; Kremers, W.; Smith, T.F. & Paya, C.V. (2003). Detection of simultaneous beta-herpesvirus infections in clinical syndromes due to defined cytomegalovirus infection. Clinical Transplantation, Vol.17, No.2, (Apr 2003), pp. 114-120, ISSN 0902-0063

Reischig, T.; Jindra, P.; Hes, O.; Svecova, M.; Klaboch, J. & Treska, V. (2008). Valacyclovir prophylaxis versus preemptive valganciclovir therapy to prevent cytomegalovirus disease after renal transplantation. American Journal of Transplantation, Vol.8, No.1, (Jan 2007), pp. 69-77, ISSN 1600-6143

Rodrigo, E.; Fernandez-Fresnedo, G.; Valero, R.; Ruiz, J.C.; Pinera, C.; Palomar, R.; Gonzalez-Cotorruelo, J.; Gomez-Alamillo, C. & Arias, M. (2006). New-onset diabetes after kidney transplantation: risk factors. Journal of the American Society of Nephrology, Vol.17, No.12 Suppl 3, (Dec 2006), pp. S291-295, ISSN 1046-6673

Sagedal, S.; Rollag, H. & Hartmann, A. (2007). Cytomegalovirus infection in renal transplant recipients is associated with impaired survival irrespective of expected mortality risk. Clinical Transplantation, Vol.21, No.3, (May-Jun 2007), pp. 309-313, ISSN 0902-0063

Sinclair, J. & Sissons, P. (2006). Latency and reactivation of human cytomegalovirus. Journal of General Virology, Vol.87, No.Pt 7, (Jul 2006), pp. 1763-1779, ISSN 0022-1317

Small, L.N.; Lau, J. & Snydman, D.R. (2006). Preventing post-organ transplantation cytomegalovirus disease with ganciclovir: a meta-analysis comparing prophylactic and preemptive therapies. Clinical Infectious Diseases, Vol.43, No.7, (Oct 2006), pp. 869-880, ISSN 1537-6591

Torres-Madriz, G. & Boucher, H.W. (2008). Immunocompromised hosts: perspectives in the treatment and prophylaxis of cytomegalovirus disease in solid-organ transplant recipients. Clinical Infectious Diseases, Vol.47, No.5, (Sep 2008), pp. 702-711, ISSN 1537-6591

Weclawiak, H.; Kamar, N.; Mengelle, C.; Esposito, L.; Mohamed, A.O.; Lavayssiere, L.; Ribes, D.; Cointault, O.; Nogier, M.B.; Cardeau-Desangles, I.; Izopet, J. & Rostaing, L. (2010). Pre-emptive intravenous ganciclovir versus valganciclovir prophylaxis for de novo cytomegalovirus-seropositive kidney-transplant recipients. Transplant International, Vol.23, No.10, (Oct 2010), pp. 1056-1064, ISSN 1432-2277

4

Posttransplant Lymphoproliferative Disorders Following Kidney Transplantation

Daan Dierickx
Department of Hematology
University Hospitals Leuven
Belgium

1. Introduction

Posttransplant lymphoproliferative disorder (PTLD) is a rare but life threatening disorder following both solid organ and hematopoietic stem cell transplantation. The disorder is characterized by an uncontrolled proliferation of lymphocytes, caused by medication induced diminished immune surveillance. From a pathological point of view PTLD has a broad and heterogeneous spectrum of appearance, ranging from a benign condition to frank lymphoma. Although not required for diagnosis of PTLD, Epstein Barr virus (EBV) plays a major role in the pathogenesis of the majority of PTLDs. Currently the gold standard in diagnosis of PTLD remains biopsy with histopathologic examination to categorize every case according to the World Health Organization 2008 classification. Similar to its heterogeneous presentation treatment options are diverse and may include preventive, preemptive, curative and palliative approaches. However, the backbone of all PTLD therapies -except maybe for real palliation- should be (partial) reconstitution of the immune system.

2. Posttransplant malignancies

Historically long term follow up of solid organ recipients was limited by low graft and patient survival, mainly due to rejection and infectious complications. However, due to improvement in care and cure of these problems, as well as permitting increased donor and recipient age, posttransplant malignancies and cardiovascular disorders have emerged as the most important long term complications. The incidence of malignancies in solid organ transplant patients is estimated to be 20% following 10 year of chronic immunosuppression.[1] Skin cancer and lymphoproliferative disorders are the two most frequent malignancies in this specific patient population. Besides these two malignancies transplant patients are vulnerable to many other neoplasms.[2] These can occur *de novo,* can be a consequence of the underlying condition leading to transplantation or –in rare cases- can be transmitted by the donor.[3] Screening, early detection and staging have become an essential part of posttransplant management, given the good prognosis associated with *in situ* or low grade malignancies. Besides classical prevention including nicotine withdrawal and ultraviolet protection is essential.[1]

3. Incidence

The incidence of PTLD varies according to the type of organ transplanted. Compared to heart, lung and intestinal transplantation, incidence of PTLD in kidney transplant recipients is relatively low and is estimated to be 1-1.5%.[4] However, due to the high kidney transplant activities, the absolute number of PTLD is probably the highest in kidney transplant recipients. Lacking large prospective trials, retrospective single center studies and registry databases have been the major source of information in collecting epidemiology, incidence, (patient, disease and treatment related) characteristics and outcome data on PTLD. The main advantage of single center retrospective analyses is the provision of more detailed information (for example EBV status, specific information on immunosuppressive regimens,…), although the number of included patients is rather small. Transplant registries on the other hand provide information on a larger number of patients, but this information is mostly very limited and depends on the goodwill and the correct registration of the physicians and transplant coordinators. Information from large population based cohort studies indicate that standardized incidence ratios (SIR), reflecting the ratio between observed and expected cases, in solid organ recipients approach 10 in non Hodgkin lymphoma and 3.5 in Hodgkin lymphoma.[5,6] Initially the highest incidence was reported in the first year following transplantation ('early onset PTLD'), although currently 'late onset PTLD' is diagnosed more frequently, probably due to the improved survival of transplant patients and to increased awareness. Because of the above described limitations of registries incidence data are best derived from small single center series. However it seems that complete and standardized nationwide prospective data registry is mandatory to permit more precise estimates on incidence of PTLD in the transplant population.

4. Risk factors

Risk factors associated with occurrence of PTLD following SOT are multiple, as shown in table 1.

EBV status at time of transplantation (donor negative/recipient positive)
Type of transplanted organ
Intensity/duration of immunosuppressive therapy
Underlying disorder
Infectious agents other than EBV (CMV?, HCV?, ...)
Age of donor and recipient
Number and severity of rejection episodes
Cytokine gene polymorphisms
HLA alleles/haplotypes/mismatches/antibodies

Table 1. Risk factors for development of PTLD

4.1 EBV mismatch

The most important independent risk factor is pre-transplantation EBV mismatch (recipient seronegative/donor seropositive), leading to a 10-75 times greater incidence of PTLD compared to EBV seropositive recipients. As EBV seroconversion positively correlates with increasing age, the higher incidence of EBV mismatch in pediatric transplant procedures may explain the higher incidence of PTLD in childhood.[7] Although transplant patients with EBV mismatch are especially prone to occurrence of early PTLD[8], EBV seronegativity remains a risk factor after one year following transplantation.[9]

4.2 Type of organ transplantation

As already mentioned before, another major risk factor comprises the type of transplanted organ. Incidence of PTLD is highest in heart-lung and multivisceral transplantation (up to 20%), followed by liver (4.5%), heart and lung (2.5%), pancreas (2%), kidney (1-1.5%) and finally matched related and unrelated hematopoietic stem cell transplantation (0.5-1%).[4] In a retrospective analysis of the Collaborative Transplant Study (CTS) database relative risk (RR) was highest in heart-lung transplantation (RR 239.5) and lowest in kidney transplant recipients (RR 12.6).[10] The reason for these differences are largely unknown. Possible hypotheses include the fact that high risk transplantations require more profound immunosuppression and contain large amounts of lymphoid tissue, leading to increased risk for EBV infection.[4]

4.3 Immunosuppressive regimen

A third important risk factor is the use of potent and prolonged immunosuppressive medication used to prevent or treat graft rejection. Taken together the risk for developing PTLD seems to be correlated with the cumulative intensity of immune suppression, leading to decreased viral and malignant surveillance. In this way repeated episodes of acute rejection increase the risk of PTLD.[2] However, measuring the cumulative immunosuppressive intensity is not easy. Firstly, transplant protocols almost always use combination therapy, making the determination of each drug separately very difficult. Secondly, registration of dose modifications/interruptions during the posttransplant period requires a major effort and consequently registration of these activities is very poor. Thirdly, besides maintenance therapy induction and repeated episodes of anti-rejection therapies might influence the risk of PTLD. Finally, no single laboratory test exists measuring the total amount of immunosuppression in a patient.[11] Due to these difficulties in determining the overall role of immunosuppression, interest has largely shifted to identification of the role of specific immunosuppressive medication.

4.3.1 Calcineurin inhibitors

Currently data on a possibly increased risk of calcineurin inhibitors (CNI) are very controversial. Although structurally unrelated to cyclosporine A, tacrolimus' mechanism of action is similar with inhibition of calcineurin and subsequent of Interleukin 2-production being the common pathway.[12] However, the immunosuppressive activity of tacrolimus seems to be stronger compared with cyclosporine A, leading to improved kidney graft survival and prevention of rejection at 1 year.[13] These stronger immunosuppressive properties seem to be translated in a higher risk for development of PTLD. In their CTS database Opelz et al found a statistical significant increased cumulative incidence of PTLD in patients receiving combination therapy with tacrolimus and mycophenolate mofetil (MMF) or azathioprine compared with patients on cyclosporin A and MMF or azathioprine.[10] This increased risk of tacrolimus compared to cyclosporin A was confirmed in a United States cohort of kidney recipients, but only in case no induction therapy was given[14], and in a Organ Procurement and Transplant Network/United Network for Organ Sharing (OPTN/UNOS) registry study, though the difference didn't reach statistical significance in this last trial.[15] On the other hand Pirsch et al didn't find a difference in PTLD incidence in a prospective randomized study comparing both CNI following kidney transplantation. However, as the follow up in this study was only one year no real conclusions can be made.[16] An important characteristic of CNI is their ability to enhance production of transforming growth factor β1 (TGFβ-1). Together with the finding that cyclosporin A can cause impaired DNA repair, a direct oncogenic effect might contribute to the occurrence of malignancies in patients treated with CNI.[17-19]

4.3.2 Antimetabolites

Azathioprine is a purine analogue which is, following metabolisation and conversion to different compounds, incorporated into replicating DNA.[20] In prevention of renal graft rejection it is largely replaced by MMF, which has been proven to be more effective than azathioprine in the prevention of allograft rejection.[21] MMF is converted in the liver to its active compound mycophenolic acid, which blocks inosine monophosphate dehydrogenase, disturbing DNA synthesis.[20] Azathioprine has well known synergism with ultraviolet radiation in carcinogenesis, leading to increased risk of skin cancers.[22] Besides the drug also induces mutagenesis due to DNA mismatch repair deficiencies, explaining also the observed increase of therapy related acute myeloid leukemia/myelodysplastic syndrome.[23] In contrast to azathioprine, several studies have shown that MMF is not associated with an increased risk[24,25] and even with a reduction in the number of PTLDs following kidney transplantation.[14,26] However, in the CTS report incidence of PTLD was similar irrespective of the use of azathioprine *versus* MMF.[10] As already discussed above combination with tacrolimus was associated with an increased risk compared to combination with cyclosporin A.[10]

4.3.3 Mammalian target of rapamycin inhibitors

Mammalian target of rapamycin (mTOR) inhibitors display their activity by blocking the serine-threonine kinase mTOR.[27] Currently two of these proliferation signaling inhibitors (PSI) are used in organ transplantation, namely sirolimus and everolimus. Apart from its immunosuppressive properties, mTOR inhibitors also possess antiproliferative characteristics, making their use very attractive especially in high risk patients and in CNI-free regimens.[28-30] However, in a recent retrospective study in kidney transplant patients maintenance therapy was associated with higher PTLD incidence.[31] In addition Mathew et al performed a multicenter analysis of renal transplant patients receiving sirolimus as base therapy or as maintenance. Although the two-year incidence of malignancies, especially skin cancer, was significantly lower, the risk of developing PTLD was increased in comparison with classical immunosuppressive therapy, especially when high dose sirolimus (5 mg/day) was given.[32]

4.3.4 Polyclonal T cell depleting antibodies

Initially used in the treatment of acute rejection following organ transplantation and of graft-versus-host disease after bone marrow transplantation, the use of anti-lymphocyte and anti-thymocyte globulins (ALG/ATG) has shifted to the prevention of both severe complications of transplantation. These antibodies bind to different antigens, not only on T cells but also on most other immunological players, although exact mechanism of action has not been fully understood yet.[33] The use of ATG was found to increase the risk for PTLD in hematopoietic stem cell transplantation[34], however its role in solid organ transplantation is less well established. In most registry studies there is a clear association between the use of ATG and the occurrence of PTLD.[10,14,31] On the other hand Hardinger et al recently published the results of a small but prospective, randomized, double-blind study in kidney transplant recipients comparing induction therapy with rabbitATG (Thymoglobulin) and horseATG (ATGAM). With 10 years follow up the composite primary endpoint of freedom from death, graft loss or acute rejection was significant higher in the Thymoglobulin-group. Importantly no patients in the Thymoglobulin group (n=48) and two in the ATGAM group (n=24) were diagnosed with PTLD.[35] In another registry study Dharnidharka et al found an increased risk in kidney transplant recipients treated with horseATG, but not with rabbitATG, although the follow up in the latter group was significantly shorter.[36]

4.3.5 Monoclonal T cell depleting and non-depleting antibodies

Muromonab CD3 (= OKT3) is a murine monoclonal antibody directed against the CD3 antigen on the surface of human T cells.[37] In their CTS study Opelz et al reported a higher incidence of early PTLD in patients receiving induction therapy with OKT3 or ATG.[10] However, other studies failed to show an association between OKT3 induction and PTLD.[37] Mainly due to xenosensitisation, pulmonary toxicity and to its relationship with malignancies, its use has been largely replaced by polyclonal or other monoclonal depleting/non-depleting antibodies.

Alemtuzumab is a humanized rat monoclonal antibody directed against the CD52 antigen. This antigen is expressed on the surface of peripheral blood lymphocytes, natural killer cells, monocytes and macrophages.[38] Because of the depletion of both B- and T-cells alemtuzumab possesses a theoretical advantage of reduced B cell mass and hence protection against (EBV related) B cell proliferation. Although data on the association between alemtuzumab induction and PTLD in kidney transplant recipients are limited, there seems to be no association.[39,40] This was confirmed in a UNOS registry study comparing no induction, depleting and non-depleting induction therapy.[31]

Based on decreased acute rejection rates anti-interleukin-2 receptor (CD25) monoclonal antibodies have emerged as an important part of immunosuppressive regimens in kidney transplant recipients due to selective depletion of activated T cells. Basiliximab is a chimeric antibody, whereas daclizumab is humanized.[41] In a study using data from the Scientific Registry of Transplant Recipients Bustami et al found a significant increased adjusted relative risk for PTLD using basiliximab or daclizumab.[42] However, other registry studies failed to find an association between anti-CD25 induction therapy and risk for PTLD, leading to the general assumption that basiliximab and daclizumab do not increase the risk for PTLD.[10] Magliocca et al retrospectively compared induction therapy with alemtuzumab and basiliximab in combined pancreas-kidney transplantation, but found no difference of PTLD occurrence in the first two years following transplantation.[43]

4.3.6 Co-stimulation blockade.

For their activation, T cells require two signals. Signal 1 represents interaction between the T cell receptor (TCR) and major histocompatibility (MHC) complex on an antigen presenting cell (APC). Co-stimulation signaling (signal 2), also achieved by interactions between APCs and T-cells, is obligatory for complete activation of the T cell. In the absence of this signal, T cells will fail to proliferate and will finally become apoptotic or anergic. Of these signal 2 interactions, those between B7 (CD80 and CD86) and CD40 [APC] and CD28 and CD40L (CD154) [T cells] respectively seem to be the most important for T cell activation. After CD28 has delivered a signal for T cell activation, CTLA4 (cytotoxic T-lymphocyte-associated antigen 4) is transiently upregulated on T cells. This molecule is a negative regulator of T-cell activation by inhibiting binding of CD28 to CD80 and CD86, due to its higher affinity compared with CD28.[44]

Inhibiting of this co-stimulation signal has become a promising approach in both autoimmune disorders and transplantation, leading to two phase III trials (BENEFIT and BENEFIT-EXTENT) comparing the selective co-stimulation blocker belatacept and cyclosporin A in kidney transplant recipients. Belatacept is a human fusion protein combining the extracellulair domain of CTLA4 with the constant-region fragment (Fc) of human IgG1. In both trials patients treated with betalacept-containing immunosuppression had an increased incidence of PTLD. Interestingly, in the BENEFIT-EXTENT study 4 of 5 PTLD cases showed central nervous system involvement. Risk factors for PTLD included EBV seronegativity pre-transplantation and the use of a more intensive regimen of belatacept.[45,46] The former finding has led to the recommendation to abandon the use of belatacept in patients with a seronegative EBV status before transplantation.[47] In another phase I/II trial with efalizumab, targeting CD11a, the alpha subunit of lymphocyte function-associated antigen-1 (LFA-1), 3 out of 38 kidney transplant recipients receiving combination therapy with high doses efalizumab and cyclosporine A were diagnosed with PTLD.[48]

In summary we can conclude that currently no firm conclusion can be made for individual contribution of these different drug classes with respect to the risk for PTLD, although use of monoclonal anti-CD3, polyclonal anti-thymocyte antibodies (ATG) and possibly some new and potent agents seem to be associated with an increased risk in most studies, whereas mycophenolate mofetil, monoclonal anti-CD52 and anti-IL2-R-antagonists probably are not. However, taking into account the increasing number of late onset PTLD, cumulative intensity seems to influence the risk mostly.

4.4 Other risk factors

Many other risk factors have been described and proposed. However their exact relationship with development of PTLD is less established in comparison to the above discussed factors.

Although the role of patient related risk factors including age, gender and race have been described, literature results are too conflicting to draw any conclusion at this moment.

Underlying immunodeficiency disorders, especially primary immune deficiency (PID) and autoimmune hepatitis leading to hematopoietic stem cell and liver transplantation respectively, seem to be associated with increased risk for development of PTLD.[49,50] The main reason for this probably is the prolonged (disease or treatment related) pretransplantation immune compromised situation. In renal transplantation no such association has been found. Whether end stage renal disease (ESRD) and subsequent need for renal replacement therapy (RRT) contribute to the PTLD risk following kidney transplantation was investigated in a large population based Australian cohort study, comparing cancer SIRs for patients with ESRD before RRT, patients on RRT and transplant patients. Because SIRs for most cancers, in particular lymphoproliferative disorders, were not increased in the ESRD and RRT groups, the risk of PTLD seems to be associated mainly by the iatrogenic immunosuppression posttransplant.[5]

About 80-85% of the PTLD cases are associated with EBV primary infection or reactivation (described in 'Pathogenesis').[4] The pathogenesis of the remaining 15-20% is less clear. These EBV negative cases have the tendency to occur late following transplantation. Possible explanations include involvement of other infectious agents or loss of EBV during PTLD evolution ('hit and run' hypothesis).[51] This hypothesis is supported by the description of Burkitt and Hodgkin lymphoma cases who seem to lack expression of EBV genes, but still have fragments of EBV DNA.[52] Different viruses have been identified as important contributors of lymphomagenesis, both in immunocompetent and immunosuppressed patients. Although Hezode et al reported on a possible higher incidence of PTLD in liver transplant patients with underlying hepatitis C cirrhosis[53], this finding could not be confirmed in a recently published large cohort study in solid organ transplant recipients.[54] Cytomegalovirus (CMV) is another virus which has been suggested as potentially PTLD-inducing virus in some single center studies, yet the number of cases are very small and currently there is no hard evidence to support its role in PTLD.[55-57]

Despite different cohorts of patients receive a similar cumulative intensity of immunosuppression, only a minority of patients will develop PTLD, pointing to a possible role of genetic susceptibility. In this way different authors have shown an increased risk for PTLD associated with cytokine gene and cytokine receptor gene polymorphisms including Tumor Necrosis Factor-α, Interferon-γ, Interleukin-10 and Transforming Growth Factor-β.[58-60] Although the use of these molecular techniques currently is not applicable in daily practice, they might become useful in predicting the risk for PTLD. However, recent data on some previously described predictive cytokine receptor gene polymorphisms were not able to confirm these findings.[61]

Given the important role of the Human Leucocyte Antigen (HLA)-system in transplantation immunology, its predictive role in development of PTLD has been suggested. Most evidence has derived from small patient populations with isolated, but not confirmed findings supporting the contribution of specific donor/patient HLA alleles, HLA haplotypes, HLA mismatches and pre-existing HLA-antibodies in the development of PTLD in transplant recipients.[62-64] Clearly, larger studies are needed to further clarify this complex association.

5. Pathogenesis

The pathogenesis and biology of PTLD is complex and multifactorial, as reflected by the large heterogeneity in time of occurrence and clinical and pathological presentation. In the majority (80-85%) of cases onset of PTLD is Epstein Barr virus (EBV) driven, leading to uncontrolled B-cell proliferation due to deficient cellular immune response. EBV is a herpesvirus, infecting more than 90% of the world population worldwide. Following primary infection, the virus persists in the host during the whole life mostly without harmful effects. However, EBV has

the capacity to transform B cells, resulting in different lymphoproliferative disorders, in particular Burkitt non Hodgkin lymphoma, Hodgkin lymphoma and PTLD.[65]
The pattern of different viral gene expression used by EBV is called the growth program. These genes encode for different functional homologues of B-cell factors involved in cell cycle regulation, inhibition of apoptosis and signal transduction.[65] In this way EBV is able to use the normal B cell program and promote proliferation and transformation of these cells.[66]
In healthy persons EBV is kept in a silent state in memory B cells without expressing any viral protein, corresponding with latency program (type 0). Based on the gene expression of different EBV-encoded genes, other growth programs can be seen (table 2). In Burkitt lymphoma the majority of EBV positive cases show a highly restricted latency I program of infection (Epstein Barr nuclear antigen-1 = EBNA-1 only program), whereas EBV positive Hodgkin lymphoma is characterized by a type II latency (default) program. Lymphoproliferative disorders occurring in immunosuppressed patients (PTLD and some HIV related lymphomas) most often express the latency III (growth) program, although other gene expression patterns have been described in PTLD.[65,67] Latency III program is critical for B cell activation and transformation, which becomes uncontrolled if not inhibited by cytotoxic T cell activity.[68] This explains why reduction of immune suppression, leading to (partial) restoration of immune control, is considered the first and most important therapeutic intervention, especially in early (EBV positive) PTLD cases.

Transcription program	EBV genes expressed	Occurrence
Type 0 (latency)	None	Peripheral blood memory B cells (healthy persons)
Type I (EBNA-1 only)	EBNA-1	Burkitt NHL
Type II (default)	EBNA-1, LMP-1, LMP-2A	Hodgkin lymphoma
Type III (growth)	EBNA-1 till -6, LMP-1, LMP-2A, LMP-2B	PTLD

Table 2. EBV transcription programs in human lymphoproliferative disorders

Another important mechanism in the pathogenesis of PTLD is situated at the graft organ level. Chronic antigen stimulation of recipient B cells by donor antigens may give rise to B cell proliferation and PTLD in case of inadequate immune surveillance. On the other hand, donor lymphoid cells (especially in organ transplantation with a high lymphoid load such as lung, bowel and liver transplantation) may be exposed to chronic recipient derived antigen stimulation, leading to donor lymphoid cell proliferation in a tolerant environment.[69] These cases of donor derived PTLD are characterized by early presentation and are often limited to the allograft, in contrast to the more frequent recipient derived PTLD occurring later and disseminated at presentation.[70]

6. Symptoms

The clinical presentation of patients with PTLD is very variable, ranging from an asymptomatic finding to fulminant general deterioration rapidly evolving into multi organ

failure. Differential diagnosis with graft rejection (in case of graft involvement) and infectious complications/sepsis (in case of symptomatic disseminated disease) may be very difficult. Children may present with painful throat, fever and adenopathies resembling an infectious mononucleosis-like picture with tonsilla and Waldeyer ring involvement. Besides classical nodal involvement with or without B symptoms, PTLD is characterized by a high incidence of extranodal invasion, including bone marrow and central nervous system (CNS) involvement.[71] Although initially a high incidence (15%) of primary and secondary CNS lymphoma was described in PTLD patients[72], recent reports show incidences between 5 and 13%.[73-75]
As already discussed above early PTLD may have a different presentation compared to late PTLD with more frequently positive EBV state and involvement of the allograft.[70,76,77]

7. Diagnosis

The gold standard in diagnosis of PTLD remains biopsy with histopathologic examination, although cytological preparations may also be useful, especially in case of effusion lymphoma. According to the current World Health Organization (WHO) PTLD is a subtype of 'Immunodeficiency associated lymphoproliferative disorders', in close correlation with other Primary Immune Deficiency (PID), Human Immunodeficiency Virus (HIV) and Methotrexate-associated lymphoproliferative disorders.[78]
In addition to morphological examination of the biopsy immunohistochemical analysis with at least CD3 and CD20 staining to differentiate between B cell and T cell origin is necessary in the evaluation of suspected PTLD. Other markers, including CD15, CD30, CD38, CD138 and MUM1 may provide additional information in case of rare subtypes. Cytogenetic and molecular analysis may provide important information on the monoclonal nature of the disorder and may help in understanding the biology of PTLD by analyzing oncogenes and tumor suppressor genes. Finally presence or absence of EBV should be demonstrated in all cases, which can be done by different techniques. EBV Early RNA (EBER) *in situ* hybridization is the preferred method as EBER transcripts are abundantly present, show relative stability and are expressed in all types of latency. Alternatives include immunoperoxidase staining for EBV Latent Membrane Protein 1 (LMP-1) or the use of Epstein Barr nuclear antigen-2 (EBNA-2) antibodies. However, LMP-1 and EBNA-2 are not expressed in all latency types, leading to false negative results.[79]
Based on morphological and immunohistochemical findings the WHO distinguishes four major categories of PTLD, ranging from polyclonal early lesions to aggressive monoclonal lymphoproliferative disorders resembling the broad spectrum of typical lymphomas occurring in immunocompetent persons (figure 1).[78]

7.1 Early lesions

Two typical early lesions have been recognized by the WHO: plasmacytic hyperplasia and infectious mononucleosis-like lesions. These abnormalities are characterized by a preservation of the underlying architecture of the tissue involved. They typically occur early (within one year) following transplantation and the large immunoblasts are infected with EBV, as shown by EBV Early RNA (EBER) *in situ hybridization* or EBV Latent Membrane Protein (LMP)-1 staining. These lesions are considered the first morphological changes in PTLD and their benign characteristics have been confirmed by the absence of oncogene or tumor suppressor gene mutations.

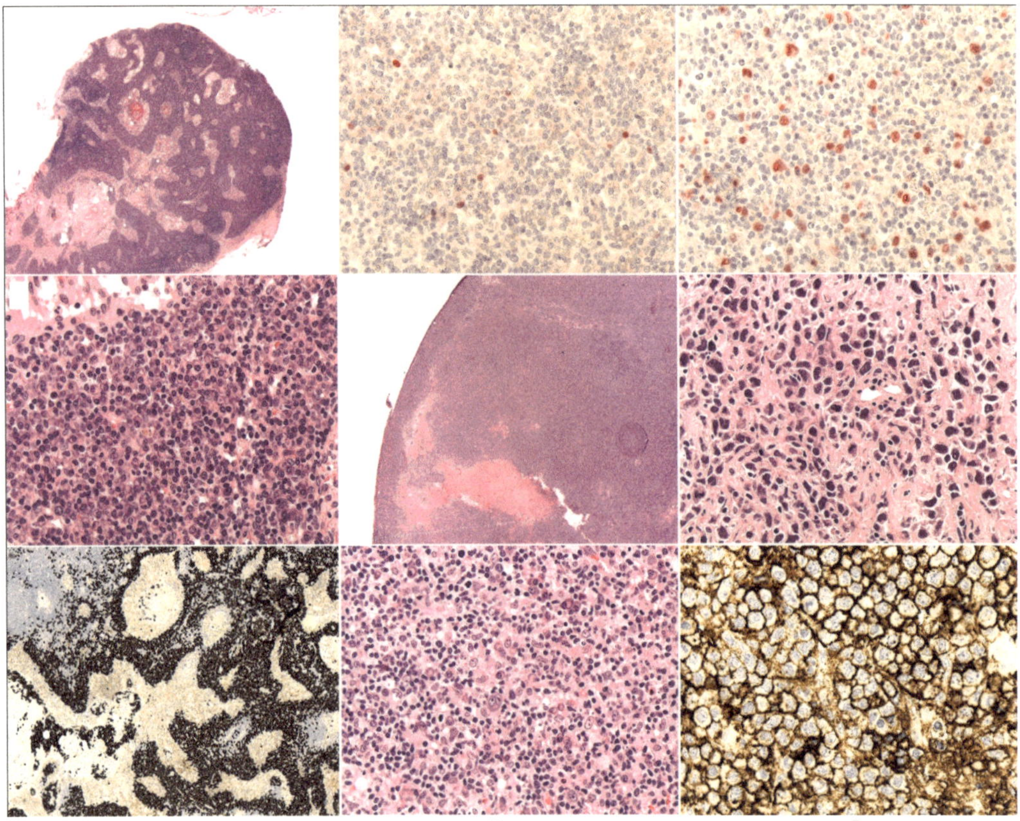

A B C
D E F
G H I

A-D. Early lesion, plasmacytic hyperplasia. A. H&E low power view. Preserved lymph node architecture. B. High power view shows numerous plasma cells. C. Plasma cells stain with CD138/syndecan. D. EBER *in situ* hybridisation shows small amount of positive cells.
E-G. Polymorphic PTLD. E. Low power view shows disturbed lymph node architecture. F. Higher power shows a polymorphic infiltrate composed of plasma cells, lymphocytes (small, medium-sized, large and Reed-Sternberg-like). G. EBER ISH shows numerous positive cells.
H-I. Monomorphic PTLD. H. Diffuse proliferation of large atypical cells. I. CD20 staining shows their B-cell origin (Courtesy to Prof Thomas Tousseyn).

Fig. 1. Morphology and immunohistochemistry of PTLD

7.2 Polymorphic PTLD

This subtype is characterized by a mixed lymphoproliferation consisting of a large spectrum of different cells like immunoblasts, mature plasma cells and intermediate sized lymphoid cells. Different specific features including atypia, necrosis and mitotic figures may be seen in the biopsy. Immunophenotyping, which has no real value in early lesions, shows a variable mixture of both B and T cells. In most cases this subtype is EBV related as well. In contrast to early lesions clonal abnormalities may be present, reflecting the transition to malignant transformation.

7.3 Monomorphic PTLD

This subtype is characterized by architectural and cytological abnormalities which can impossibly be distinguished from lymphomas occurring in immunocompetent patients. Similar to classical lymphoproliferative disorders they can be subclassified in B-, T- and NK-cell non Hodgkin lymphoma (NHL). Although not always present, most of the monomorphic PTLDs seem to be EBV driven as well. Besides the clear monoclonal appearance, additional mutations in oncogenes (N-Ras, c-Myc,...) and tumor suppressor genes (p53,...) are not uncommon.
In the majority of cases monomorphic PTLD has a B-cell phenotype, with diffuse large B cell lymphoma (DLBCL) being the prototype. Although immunoblastic, centroblastic and anaplastic DLBCL have been described, the clinical significance of these morphological subtypes is not entirely clear. However, being CD20 negative, anaplastic DLBCL may confer a poor prognosis given the fact that anti-CD20 therapy cannot be used. Other types of B-PTLD include Burkitt(-like) NHL, plasmablastic NHL and plasma cell myeloma, which can be EBV driven as well.
In contrast to B-PTLD T/NK lymphomas are rather rare following transplantation. Most T cell cases do not show positive EBV staining, although EBV positive cases have been described. Possible explanations for this last finding include expression of CD21 or other not yet identified receptors leading to EBV infection. The largest series of T- and NK-PTLD, including 130 cases, has been described by Swerdlow et al with 69% occurring after kidney transplantation. Different subtypes were identified including peripheral T cell lymphoma, unspecified (PTCL,U), hepatosplenic gamma-delta T cell lymphoma (HSGDTCL) and anaplastic large T cell lymphoma (ALCL). Most cases occurred late following transplantation and only 37% of the cases were EBV positive. The prognosis was very poor with overall survival of only 6 months, although EBV positive cases tended to have a better outcome.[80]

7.4 Hodgkin lymphoma / Hodgkin-like lymphoma

Although this subcategory constitutes only a very small proportion of PTLD, population based cohort studies have shown SIRs of 3.5 for Hodgkin lymphoma following solid organ transplantation[5,6], with the risk being even higher after bone marrow transplantation.[81] Despite most evidence is based on case reports and smaller case series HL-PTLD is mostly EBV related and is associated with a better prognosis compared to other subtypes of PTLD.[82,83] Whether there is a difference between monomorphic Hodgkin lymphoma (HL) and polymorphic Hodgkin-like lymphoma (HLL) following transplantation is not entirely clear. In an overview of the literature on this topic Semakula et al described different clinical, immunophenotypic and molecular features of both subtypes, with HLL behaving more aggressively and probably requiring a NHL-therapeutic approach, whereas real HL may be treated in the same way as classical HL.[84]
Although the WHO 2008 classification provides an important framework in correct diagnosis, some problems remain. Firstly, apart from these four categories other lymphoma subtypes have been reported following transplantation, though these have not been included in the current WHO classification. Aull et al described 16 cases of marginal zone lymphoma following solid organ transplantation. The majority of these lymphomas showed gastric localization, occurred late and were associated with Helicobacter pylori positivity (and not EBV). Treatment of most cases included reduction of immunosuppression and helicobacter pylori eradication therapy, leading to excellent disease control and prognosis.[85] It can be expected that, due to improved survival and to increasing age of transplant recipients, more

indolent lymphoproliferative disorders will occur in the transplant population. Whether these lymphomas should be considered real PTLD or only reflect an ageing population needs to be explored further.[86] Secondly it's important to stress that progression or recurrence of a lymphoproliferative disorder already existing before transplantation, does not fulfill criteria for PTLD.[87] Finally, it's clear that not all cases are easily classified in the well known lymphoma categories, reflected by the finding of several "grey zone lymphomas".

8. Staging

Once the diagnosis of PTLD has been established staging examinations need to be performed in order to exactly define the extent of involvement of lymph nodes and organs, including the allograft itself. Staging tools are comparable to those used in classical lymphomas with computed tomography (CT) scan, magnetic resonance imaging (MRI) of the brain and bone marrow examination being of great importance. The staging system most used in lymphoma is the Ann Arbor Classification (table 3).[88] However, as extranodal involvement is a frequent feature of PTLD and because CT is not able to discriminate between vital and non-vital tumor lesions, CT scan may not be the most appropriate staging tool. Besides, the use of intravenous contrast may be relatively contra-indicated in kidney transplant recipients with compromised renal function. These drawbacks have lead to emerging interest in the use of ^{18}fluorodexyglucose- positron emission tomography (FDG-PET) scan. FDG-PET is a functional imaging technique which allows characterization of metabolic active tissues by demonstration of elevated FDG-uptake in these tissues (figure 2). Last decade the use of FDG-PET has shown impressive results in detection and staging of several lymphoma subtypes, especially aggressive lymphomas. Besides FDG-PET can be used for response evaluation and follow up. However, as PET scan lacks anatomic detail due to its poor resolution, a combined approach of PET and CT has been developed for both staging and response assessment purposes. Till now, experience with PET with or without CT imaging in PTLD has been limited to rather small retrospective single center experiences. Taken together these reports reveal that PET scan may have a high sensitivity for the detection of PTLD lesions, although PET scan has shown a low accuracy in low grade lymphomas and is not the preferred examination in case of suspicion of central nervous system (CNS) localization. In the latter situation MRI of the brain and cytological examination of cerebrospinal fluid should be performed.

Stage I	**Involvement of a single lymph node region (I) <u>or</u> one extralymphatic site (IE).**
Stage II	Involvement of two or more lymph node regions, at the same side of the diaphragm (II) <u>or</u> local extralymphatic extension plus one or more lymph node regions at the same side of the diaphragm (IIE).
Stage III	Involvement of lymph node regions on both sides of diaphragm (III) which may include the spleen (IIIS) or accompanied by local extralymphatic extension (III_E) or both (IIIES).
Stage IV	Diffuse or disseminated involvement of one or more extralymphatic organs or sites, with or without associated lymphatic involvement.

Each stage number is followed by either **A** (absence of B-symptoms) or **B** (presence of B-symptoms: unexplained weight loss > 10% baseline during 6 months before, unexplained fever > 38°C, night sweats).

Table 3. Ann Arbor staging system for lymphoproliferative disorders

Fig. 2. Role of PET scan in staging and follow up

A. Heart transplant recipient diagnosed with PTLD subtype DLBCL. Pet scan shows lymphoma localisation left axilla, lung bilateral and small intestine. This scan illustrates the increased incidence of organ involvement in PTLD compared to findings in lymphoma in immunocompetent patients. B. PET scan shows a complete metabolic remission following reduction of immunosuppression and four administrations of rituximab (Courtesy to Dr Lieselot Brepoels).

9. Prevention

The often very aggressive presentation and the poor prognosis of PTLD has led to an increased interest in adequate prevention of the disorder. At this moment many centers, similar to the intensive viral monitoring following allogeneic stem cell transplantation, advocate the use of EBV viral load monitoring as a tool to initiate pre-emptive therapy in case of rapid increase of the viral load. Classical EBV serology (anti-Viral Capsid Antigen [VCA] IgM and IgG, EBV-EA and EBNA) is not reliable in patients with a dysfunctional immune system, in particular transplant recipients.[89] In this patient population viral load measurement by quantitative polymerase chain reaction (PCR) is a much more reliable test. During the last decades many authors have reported their experience with serial EBV viral load monitoring, both in adult and pediatric solid organ transplant recipients (as reviewed in ref 90 and 91).[90,91] Although these series confirm the utility of serial monitoring in prevention of PTLD, the results need to be analyzed with caution.

Firstly, most results are derived from retrospective single center studies, often mixing different populations.

Secondly, there is a huge heterogeneity in methods, cut off values and source of samples (whole blood *versus* plasma *versus* peripheral blood mononuclear cells). In a prospective single center study Tsai *et al* compared PCRs with different gene targets (EBNA, EBER and LMP) and different sample sources (plasma and lymphocytes) in lung transplant patients. Free plasma EBNA PCR showed the highest specificity and positive predictive value, making this test useful in identification and monitoring of patients with EBV-related PTLD. However, the whole PCR panel was needed to rule out the presence of EBV-related PTLD.[92] Finally, pre-emptive decisions are very variable between different centers, ranging from more intensive monitoring to reduction of immunosuppression and antiviral therapy to monoclonal anti-CD20 therapy.

In order to improve positive predictive value of EBV viremia, some authors propose to combine EBV PCR with measurements of T cell immunity like absolute lymphocyte count (<300/mm^3) or the absence of EBV-specific CD8-positive cytotoxic T cells. However, these combinations have not been validated in larger series yet.[93,94] Another approach may be the combination of EBV viral load and use of cytokine polymorphisms, as shown in a study in pediatric liver transplant recipients.[95]

In addition other, but less used, preventive tools include incorporation of cytokine measurements. Elevated Interleukin-6 (IL-6) levels have been associated with the occurrence of PTLD following solid organ transplantation, whereas a strong correlation has been found between IL-10 and EBV viral load.[96,97]

10. Treatment

As development of PTLD is the consequence of an imbalance between immunosuppression and immunosurveillance, different approaches can be made in the treatment of the disorder. These approaches include improving reconstitution of the immune system, targeting the uncontrolled proliferation of malignant B cells and decreasing (EBV) viral load.[98] Unfortunately treatment for PTLD is largely based on retrospective data with only few prospective and no randomized trials being performed till now. As a consequence formal recommendations are lacking and currently treatment is largely physician or transplant center dependent.

Taking into account that PTLD is always associated with a high degree of overimmunosuppression, the most important therapeutic intervention seems to be reduction of immunosuppression, leading to (partial) cellular (EBV specific) immunity reconstitution. However, in many cases this is insufficient and further therapy is needed. The spectrum of therapeutic options, including antiviral therapy, cytokines and chemotherapy, recently has been expanded with the use of monoclonal anti-B cell antibodies and EBV specific immunotherapy. In this chapter we will review the different currently used and future therapeutic options.

10.1 Restoration of the immune system

10.1.1 Reduction of immunosuppression

Reduction of immunosuppression (RIS) has been considered standard therapy in PTLD following kidney (and other types) transplantation allowing reconstitution of the immune system, in particular EBV-specific cytotoxic lymphocyte response.[99] Although no consensus has been reached, most transplant physicians agree to stop antimetabolites, reduce the calcineurin inhibitor dose with 50% and continue treatment with steroids.[100] It seems appropriate to re-evaluate two to four weeks following initiation of RIS, if the clinical situation doesn't oblige urgent treatment. Response rates to RIS alone in PTLD have a very wide variation ranging from almost no response to response rates exceeding 50%. This heterogeneity reflects the lack of standardization with respect to duration of RIS before re-evaluation, response criteria and reduction regimen. Reshef et al recently published their

experience with RIS alone in 67 solid organ transplant recipients diagnosed with PTLD. Overall response rate was 45%, including 37% complete responses. The authors conclude that RIS alone might be a useful therapy in low risk PTLD patients as the presence of bulky disease (> 7cm), advanced stage (Ann Arbor III-IV) and higher age (> 50 year) were independently associated with lack of response to RIS.[101] In a recent prospective trial however, examining the use of sequential RIS, interferon-α-2B and chemotherapy in 16 PTLD patients following SOT, RIS was associated with an overall response rate of 6% without any complete remission, even though acute graft rejection was seen in one third of the patients. Half of the patients showed progressive disease during the period of RIS.[102]
The main problem associated with RIS is rejection of the allograft. In contrast to heart- and lung transplantation kidney recipients can still be rescued by hemodialysis, explaining the tendency for more aggressive RIS in kidney transplantation compared to other types of organ transplantation. Whether immunosuppressive therapy can be safely reduced during chemotherapy was recently addressed in a retrospective analysis of 58 kidney transplant recipients. A significant improvement in renal function was observed in patients treated with RIS followed by CHOP chemotherapy with or without rituximab, reflecting the immunosuppressive properties of chemotherapy.[103] However, the question whether immunosuppression can be disrupted completely during chemotherapy remains unanswered. Even if immunosuppression is discontinued during chemotherapy, a reduced dose is re-initiated after termination of the chemotherapy in most centers.
Proliferation signaling inhibitors (PSI) or mammalian target of rapamycin (mTOR) inhibitors (sirolimus, everolimus) possess a unique combination of both immunosuppressive and anti-proliferative properties. From a theoretical point of view they may show superiority in the treatment of malignancies in transplant recipients, which was confirmed in small single center trials.[28,104] However, as stated before, maintenance therapy with PSI might be associated with increased risk for PTLD.[31,32]

10.1.2 Adoptive immunotherapy

The use of EBV specific cytotoxic lymphocytes (CTLs) is another attractive option to induce EBV specific cellular immune response.[65,68] This type of adoptive immunotherapy was first described in the early 1990s in patients with EBV related PTLD following hematopoietic stem cell transplantation. In contrast to PTLD following SOT, in which the disorder mostly arises in recipient lymphocytes, hematopoietic stem cell related PTLD mostly derives from donor cells. In this way donor lymphocyte infusions were given to evoke an EBV-specific response. Despite impressive response rates, a high incidence of graft versus host disease was observed.[105,106] Due to this strong alloreactive mediated complications, further attempts were made to isolate expanded EBV-specific CTLs. By infusing these CTLs, both autologous (recipient derived PTLD) and allogeneic (isolated from the donor itself or from a bank of partial HLA-matched voluntary donors), promising results were obtained in PTLD patients after SOT, recently reviewed by Merlo *et al.*[107] However, wide applicability has been limited so far because of pronounced labor-intensive procedure and by availability problems.

10.1.3 Cytokine therapy

Interferon-alpha (IFN-α) is a cytokine with well known anti-viral and anti-neoplastic properties.[108] In the late 90s several case reports and small case series have been published showing effectiveness of cytokine therapy in the treatment of PTLD. Davis *et al* treated 16 newly diagnosed patients with subcutaneous IFN-α, leading to a complete response rate of

50%. However treatment was associated with a high rate of graft rejection and was poorly tolerated.[109] However, in their recent report on the use of sequential RIS, IFN-α-2B and chemotherapy in PTLD Swinnen *et al* observed a lower overall response rate of 30% with only 15% patients with complete remission.[102]

10.2 Anti- B cell therapy

10.2.1 Cytokine therapy

Interleukin-6 (IL-6) is a cytokine produced by monocytes, fibroblasts and endothelial cells, promoting the growth of EBV-immortalized cells *in vitro*. In the early 90s Tosato *et al* demonstrated elevated serum IL-6 levels in patients with PTLD, pointing to a possible role in the pathogenesis of the disorder and providing an opportunity for new therapeutic modalities.[110] In a multicentric phase I-II trial assessing the role of anti-IL-6 monoclonal antibodies in non-responders to RIS 8 out of 12 patients responded without major side effects.[111] Although cytokine therapy clearly showed promising results in the treatment of PTLD, currently its use has been largely replaced by monoclonal anti-CD20 therapy.

10.2.2 Surgery and radiotherapy

The role of surgery and radiotherapy in the treatment of PTLD is limited to localized disease, especially in early type PTLD and mostly combined with RIS. Besides these treatment options can be used in case of local complications like bleeding, pain and compression. [71,99,112,113] In primary central nervous system (PCNSL) PTLD, radiotherapy and chemotherapy may both lead to a high response rate.[72,114,115] Although rituximab hardly crosses the blood-brain-barrier (BBB), case reports have shown promising results with the use of systemic rituximab in the treatment of PCNSL-PTLD, probably due to disruption of the BBB in patients presenting with central nervous system malignancies. However, the exact value of systemic or intrathecal rituximab needs to be determined taking into consideration the fact that in most cases anti-CD20 therapy was combined with other treatments.[116,117]

10.2.3 Chemotherapy

In most lymphoproliferative disorders in immunocompetent patients chemotherapy remains the cornerstone of therapy, often combined with lymphoma-specific immunotherapy. As a consequence chemotherapy (mostly CHOP or a CHOP-like regimen) has been considered for many years standard therapy in PTLD not responding to RIS. However, due to the immunocompromised state of the patient treatment related mortality, especially infectious, is substantially higher in this population, even though the use of broad spectrum antibiotics and G-CSF clearly has reduced the complication rate of chemotherapy.[118-120] Till now only one uncontrolled prospective trial has been published reporting the effectiveness of low dose chemotherapy in pediatric PTLD patients, leading to an overall response rate of 83% and a 2-year overall survival rate of 73%.[121] In adults all currently available evidence regarding the use of chemotherapy is based on retrospective data.[122] In an analysis of the Israel Penn International Transplant Tumor Registry outcome with different chemotherapy schedules were compared. Treatment with CHOP chemotherapy was associated with a 5 year overall survival of 24% with a PTLD-specific mortality of 34%, whereas single agent chemotherapy appeared to be inferior compared to combination chemotherapy.[118] One other approach may be sequential therapy using RIS, interferon-α and systemic chemotherapy, leading to lower tumor burden before start of

chemotherapy. This approach showed promising results in two prospective trials.[102,109] However, as described below, results and especially tolerance may be improved by substituting IFN-α by anti-CD20 monoclonal therapy.
Taken together we can conclude that, despite high initial response rates using chemotherapy after failing of RIS, toxicity and long term outcome remain problematic. However, in case of aggressive presentation of high grade lymphomas, including plasmablastic NHL, Burkitt and Burkitt-like NHL and T-cell NHL, and in case of Hodgkin or Hodgkin-like lymphoma, for which no immunotherapy is available, upfront chemotherapy needs to be considered.

10.2.4 Monoclonal anti-B cell therapy

During the last decade monoclonal anti-B-cell antibodies have emerged as a powerful treatment modality in most B-cell lymphoproliferative disorders, both indolent and aggressive. Consequently this new kind of immunotherapy was also investigated in the treatment of PTLD, most of which express CD20. Before the advent of rituximab combination of murine anti-CD21 and anti-CD24 monoclonal antibodies showed encouraging results in B-PTLD.[123] Most experience however has been obtained with rituximab, a chimeric murine/human anti-CD20 antibody, with numerous case reports, case series and larger retrospective analyses found in the international literature.[122] Besides five prospective trials have been published till now assessing the role of rituximab in PTLD, showing overall response rates ranging between 44% and 64%.[124-128] Most patients were treated with the standard rituximab dose of 375 mg/m^2/week during 4 consecutive weeks, although Gonzalez-Barca *et al* introduced the concept of risk adapted extended treatment with rituximab in case of partial response following 4 weekly admissions. With this approach the number of complete responders was upgraded from 34% after 4 admissions to 60.5% following 8 doses.[127]
Although treatment with rituximab is associated with a high response rate in PTLD, it is important to keep in mind that it does not improve (virus-specific) cellular immunity necessitating the need for simultaneous RIS.[129] Conversely, severe B-cell depletion due to treatment with rituximab was not associated with diminished EBV-specific T-cell immunity in non-transplanted patients presenting with lymphoproliferative disorders.[130]
Although toxicity of rituximab seems to be rather low in the different retrospective and prospective trials, caution is warranted based on recently described infectious complications in non-transplant related lymphoproliferatieve disorders, including progressive multifocal leucoencephalopathy and hepatitis B reactivation.[131,132]

10.3 Anti- EBV therapy

10.3.1 Antiviral therapy

As the majority of PTLD cases are associated with EBV related lymphocyte proliferation, the use of antiviral treatment was already explored almost thirty years ago.[133] The efficacy of classical antiviral drugs in the treatment of PTLD however has been very controversial. Nucleoside analogues, including aciclovir and ganciclovir, inhibiting replication of many herpes viruses, have shown *in vitro* and *in vivo* resistance against EBV related malignancies as most of these tumors do not express viral thymidine kinase (TK). Some case reports or small series have shown limited curative potential of these antiviral agents[134], which could be explained by some degree of lytic replication in PTLD although the effect of other simultaneous interventions might have influenced the responses. In the above mentioned study on the use of sequential RIS, interferon-α-2B and chemotherapy, all 16 patients received intravenous acyclovir during the period of RIS, without any response.[102] Of interest, prophylactic treatment with nucleoside analogues during three months following heart transplantation was associated with reduced PTLD risk in the Spanish registry.[135,136] This effect was also observed in a multicentric case-control study of kidney transplant recipients. The authors showed that antiviral prophylactic treatment was associated with a significant decrease in the risk of PTLD, especially in the first year posttransplant.[137] Experience with other antiviral agents like foscarnet and cidofovir, which act independently of the viral TK, is very limited. Oertel *et al* reported on their experience with foscarnet in three patients. All three patients achieved a complete remission, correlating with the expression of BZLF1/ZEBRA protein, which is an early antigen of lytic EBV activity.[138]

10.3.2 Intravenous immune globulins

The use of intravenous immune globulins (IVIG) might be another attractive therapy in PTLD, based on the presence of antibodies against EBV proteins. However, literature is limited to some isolated case reports in which IVIG is combined with different other therapies.[139] There is some more data available regarding IVIG prophylaxis following transplantation, though the results are very conflicting. Opelz *et al* examined the effect of anti-CMV prophylaxis on the occurrence of PTLD in a large registry study. The first year following kidney transplantation no case of PTLD was seen in patients who received anti-CMV IVIG compared to patients with antiviral agents or without prophylaxis. After the first year this difference disappeared. The authors conclude that anti-CMV IVIG might posses a broad range of anti-EBV activity.[140] On the other hand Green *et al* performed a randomized controlled trial in pediatric liver transplant patients, revealing no significant effect of the use of anti-CMV IVIG on occurrence of PTLD.[141] As a consequence it remains a matter of debate whether IVIG should be incorporated early in transplant programs.

10.3.3 Arginine butyrate

Recently very promising results have been described treating fifteen refractory EBV related malignancies -including 6 PTLDs- with arginine butyrate, resulting in pharmacological induction of viral TK. As this approach makes the tumor sensitive to treatment with nucleoside analogues, ganciclovir is added. With this combination therapy an overall response rate of 83% was observed in the PTLD subgroup with an acceptable toxicity profile.[142]

10.4 Retransplantation

In patients successfully treated for PTLD, but with loss of their graft due to reduced immunosuppression, retransplantation may be feasible. Birkeland *et al* reported on 5 kidney transplant recipients who underwent retransplantation without any sign of disease recurrence up to three years after transplantation.[143] In another small series Karras *et al* described six other cases without disease recurrence with a median posttransplant follow up of 30 months.[144] The largest published series was based on the OPTN/UNOS database, in which 69 patients with a history of PTLD underwent retransplantation. Time from PTLD to retransplantation ranged from < 1 year to 5-10 years. Immunosuppressive therapy was very similar to regimens used after first transplants. Patient and graft survival was very good, although outcome seemed to be better in abdominal organ retransplantation.[145]

11. Prognosis

In general the prognosis of PTLD is poor compared to 'similar' lymphoproliferative disorders in immune competent patients. In kidney transplant recipients 5 year overall survival following diagnosis of PTLD ranges from 40% to 60%, with the lowest survival rates in patients presenting with CNS involvement.[10,73]

Although several prognostic scores have been proposed by different authors, validation of this scores in different transplant populations have not been done or have shown conflicting results, partially due to heterogeneity in patient population and treatment.[74,128,146-149] However poor prognostic factors in immunocompetent lymphoma patients, including higher age, advanced disease, poor performance state and elevated lactate dehydrogenase, have also shown their value in outcome prediction of PTLD patients. Table 4 gives an

Score	Population	Number of patients	Treatment	Risk factors
International Prognostic Index (IPI)[146]	Immunocompetent patients with aggressive NHL	2031	Anthracyclin based combination chemotherapy	age, LDH, stage, performance state, number of extranodal sites
Leblond[147]	SOT	61	Heterogenous	Performance state, number of involved sites
Ghobrial[148]	SOT	107	Heterogenous	Performance state, monomorphic subtype, graft involvement
Choquet[128]	SOT	60	Heterogenous	Age, performance state, LDH
Hourighan[149]	Kidney	42	Heterogenous	LDH, B-symptoms
Evens[74]	SOT	80	Heterogenous	No rituximab therapy, CNS involvement, number of extranodal sites, albumin, bone marrow involvement

Table 4. Prognostic scores in PTLD

overview of the different proposed prognostic scores. Cesarman *et al* reported a poor response to RIS in patients showing bcl-6 mutations.[150] This finding, however, has not been examined in other studies.

New and especially validation of prognostic factors, both clinical/biochemical and molecular, may lead to better risk stratification in PTLD.

12. Future

Although we have learned a lot about all different aspects on PTLD during the last decades, even more questions remain. Further research and clinical studies are needed in this rapidly changing field with increasing transplant activities worldwide and the use of new and very potent immunosuppressive therapy.

Table 5 summarizes our current knowledge of PTLD and defines future opportunities which can only be possible by close cooperation between all departments involved in transplant patient care (transplantation unit, clinical hematology/oncology, pathology, radiology, nuclear medicine, immunology and virology) and between the different transplant centers.

Aspect	Knowledge	Future perspectives
Incidence	2%	Nationwide prospective and complete registry,…
Risk factors	Type of organ, EBV R-/D+, intensity immunosuppression	Measuring 'overall immune suppression', further search for specific role of immunosuppressive agents,…
Pathogenesis	80-85% EBV related	Role of other viruses, molecular pathways (gene expression profiling, single nucleotide polymorphism analysis, comparative genome hybridisation arrays,…),…
Diagnosis	Biopsy, WHO 2008	Non-invasive diagnosis? Role of PET/CT scan, role of magnetic resonance imaging,…
Staging	CT scan, bone marrow examination	Role of PET/CT scan, role of magnetic resonance imaging,…
Prevention	Serial monitoring EBV PCR?	Standardisation of EBV PCR, determination cut off value, role of HLA, cytokine gene polymorphisms,…
Therapy	Heterogenous	Prospective studies, international working group consensus,…
Prognosis	Poor	Identification of new (clinical and non-clinical) prognostic markers, prospective validation of prognostic scores,…

Table 5. Current knowledge and future perspectives in PTLD

13. References

[1] Buell JF, Gross TG, Woodle ES. Malignancy after transplantation. Transplantation 2005;80:S254-64.

[2] Guttierez-Dalmau A, Campistol JM. Immunosuppressive therapy and malignancy in organ transplant recipients. Drugs 2007;67:1167-98.

[3] Ajithkumar TV, Parkinson CA, Butler A, et al. Management of solid tumours in organ-transplant recipients. Lancet Oncol 2007;8:921-32.

[4] Tsao L, His ED. The clinicopathologic spectrum of posttransplantation lymphoproliferative disorders. Arch Pathol Lab Med 2007;131:1209-1218.

[5] Vajdic CM, McDonald SP, McCredie MR, et al. Cancer incidence before and after kidney transplantation. JAMA 2006;296:2823-31.

[6] Villeneuve PJ, Schaubel DE, Fenton SS, Shepherd FA, Jiang Y, Mao Y. Cancer incidence among Canadian kidney transplant recipients. Am J Transplant 2007;7:941-8.

[7] Shroff R, Rees L. The post-transplant lymphoproliferative disorder- a literature review. Pediatr Nephrol 2004;19:369-77.

[8] Quinlan SC, Pfeiffer RM, Morton LM, et al. Risk factors for early-onset and late-onset post-transplant lymphoproliferative disorder in kidney recipients in the United States. Am J Hematol 2011;56:206-9.

[9] Shahinian VB, Muirhead N, Jevnikar AM, et al. Epstein-Barr virus seronegativity is a risk factor for late-onset posttransplant lymphoroliferative disorder in adult renal allograft recipients. Transplantation 2003;75:851-6.

[10] Opelz G, Döhler B. Lymphomas after solid organ transplantation: a collaborative transplant study report. Am J Transplant 2004;4:222-30.

[11] Daniel V, Opelz G. Clinical relevance of immune monitoring in solid organ transplantation. Int Rev Immunol 2009;58:155-84.

[12] Scott LJ, McKeage K, Keam SJ, et al. Tacrolimus: a further update of its use in the management of organ transplantation. Drugs 2003;63:1247-97.

[13] Webster AC, Woodroffe RC, Taylor RS, et al. Tacrolimus versus ciclosporin as primary immunosuppression for kidney transplant recipients: meta-analysis and meta-regression of randomized trial data. BMJ 2005;331:810-20.

[14] Caillard S, Dharnidharka V, Agodoa L, et al. Posttransplant lymphoproliferative disorders after renal transplantation in the United States in era of modern immunosuppression. Transplantation 2005;15:1233-43.

[15] Cherikh WS, Kauffman HM, McBride MA, et al. Association of the type of induction immunosuppression with posttransplant lymphoproliferative disorder, graft survival, and patient survival after primary kidney transplantation. Transplantation 2003;15:1289-93.

[16] Pirsch JD. Cytomegalovirus infection and posttransplant lymphoproliferative disease in renal transplant recipients: results of the U.S. multicenter FK506 Kidney Transplant Study Group. Transplantation1999;68:1203-5.

[17] André N, Roquelaure B, Conrath J. Molecular effects of cyclosporine and oncogenesis: a new model. Med Hypotheses 2004;63:647-52.

[18] Hojo M, Morimoto T, Maluccio M, et al. Cyclosporine induces cancer progression by a cell-autonomous mechanism. Nature 1999;397:530-4.

[19] Maluccio M, Sharma V, Lagman M, et al. Tacrolimus enhances transforming growth factor-beta1 expression and promotes tumor progression. Transplantation 2003;76:597-602.
[20] Taylor A, Marcus R, Bradley JA. Post-transplant lymphoproliferative disorders (PTLD) after solid organ transplantation. Crit Rev Oncol Hematol 2005;56:155-67.
[21] Halloran P, Mathew T, Tomlanovich S, et al. Mycophenolate mofetil in renal allograft recipients: a pooled efficacy analysis of three randomized, double-blind, clinical studies in prevention of rejection. The International Mycophenolate Mofetil Renal Transplant Study Groups. Transplantation 1997;63:39-47.
[22] O'Donovan P, Perrett CM, Zhang X, et al. Azathioprine and UVA light generate mutagenic oxidative DNA damage. Science 2005;309:1871-4.
[23] Offman J, Opelz G, Doehler B, et al. Defective DNA mismatch repair in acute myeloid leukemia/myelodysplastic syndrome after organ transplantation. Blood 2004;104:822-8.
[24] Funch DP, Ko HH, Travasso J, et al. Posttransplant lymphoproliferative disorder among renal transplant patients in relation to the use of mycophenolate mofetil. Transplantation 2005;80:1174-80.
[25] Robson R, Cecka JM, Opelz G, et al. Prospective registry-based observational cohort study of the long-term risk of malignancies in renal transplant patients treated with mycophenolate mofetil. Am J Transplant 2005;5:2954-60.
[26] Birkeland SA, Hamilton-Dutoit S. Is posttransplant lymphoproliferative disorder (PTLD) caused by any specific immunosuppressive drug or by the transplantation per se? Transplantation 2003;76:984-8.
[27] Weir MR, Diekmann F, Flechner SM, et al. mTOR inhibition: the learning curve in kidney transplantation. Transpl Int 2010;23:447-60.
[28] Kahan BD, Yakupoglu YK, Schoenberg L, et al. Low incidence of malignancy among sirolimus/cyclosporine-treated renal transplant recipients. Transplantation 2005;80:749-58.
[29] Campistol JM, Eris J, Oberbauer R, et al. Sirolimus therapy after early cyclosporine withdrawal reduces the risk for cancer in adult renal transplantation. J Am Soc Nephrol 2006;17:581-9.
[30] Kauffman HM, Cherikh WS, Cheng Y, et al. Maintenance immunosuppression with target-of-rapamycin inhibitors is associated with a reduced incidence of de novo malignancies. Transplantation 2005;80:883-9.
[31] Kirk AD, Cherikh WS, Ring M, et al. Dissociation of posttransplant lymphoproliferative disease in kidney recipients treated with alemtuzumab. Am J Transplant 2007;7:2619-25.
[32] Mathew T, Kreis H, Friend P. Two-year incidence of malignancy in sirolimus-treated renal transplant recipients: results from five multicenter studies. Clin Transplant 2004;18:446-9.
[33] Mohty M. Mechanisms of action of antithymocyte globulin: T-cell depletion and beyond. Leukemia. 2007 Jul;21(7):1387-94.
[34] Landgren O, Gilbert ES, Rizzo JD, et al. Risk factors for lymphoproliferative disorders after allogeneic hematopoietic cell transplantation. Blood 2009;113:4992-5001.

[35] Hardinger KL, Rhee S, Buchanan P, et al. A prospective, randomized, double-blinded comparison of thymoglobulin versus Atgam for induction immunosuppressive therapy: 10-year results. Transplantation 2008;86:947-52.

[36] Dharnidharka VR, Stevens G. Risk for post-transplant lymphoproliferative disorder after polyclonal antibody induction in kidney transplantation. Pediatr Transplant 2005;9:622-6.

[37] Benfield MR, Tejani A, Harmon WE, A randomized multicenter trial of OKT3 mAbs induction compared with intravenous cyclosporine in pediatric renal transplantation. Pediatr Transplant 2005;9:282-92.

[38] Magliocca JF, Knechtle SJ. The evolving role of alemtuzumab (Campath-1H) for immunosuppressive therapy in organ transplantation. Transpl Int 2006;19:705-14.

[39] Watson CJ, Bradley JA, Friend PJ, et al. Alemtuzumab (CAMPATH 1H) induction therapy in cadaveric kidney transplantation--efficacy and safety at five years. Am J Transplant 2005;5:1347-53.

[40] Ciancio G, Burke GW, Gaynor JJ, A randomized trial of three renal transplant induction antibodies: early comparison of tacrolimus, mycophenolate mofetil, and steroid dosing, and newer immune-monitoring. Transplantation 2005;80:457-65.

[41] Campara M, Tzvetanov IG, Oberholzer J. Interleukin-2 receptor blockade with humanized monoclonal antibody for solid organ transplantation. Expert Opin Biol Ther 2010;10:959-69.

[42] Bustami RT, Ojo AO, Wolfe RA, et al. Immunosuppression and the risk of post-transplant malignancy among cadaveric first kidney transplant recipients. Am J Transplant 2004;4:87-93.

[43] Magliocca JF, Odorico JS, Pirsch JD, et al. A comparison of alemtuzumab with basiliximab induction in simultaneous pancreas-kidney transplantation. Am J Transplant 2008;8:1702-10.

[44] Snanoudj R, Zuber J, Legendre C. Co-stimulation blockade as a new strategy in kidney transplantation: benefits and limits. Drugs 2010;70:2121-31.

[45] Vincenti F, Charpentier B, Vanrenterghem Y, et al. A phase III study of belatacept-based immunosuppression regimens versus cyclosporine in renal transplant recipients (BENEFIT study). Am J Transplant 2010;10:535-546.

[46] Durrbach A, Pestana JM, Pearson T, et al. A phase III study of belatacept versus cyclosporine in kidney transplants from extended criteria donors (BENEFIT-EXT study). Am J Transplant 2010;10:547-557.

[47] Grinyó J, Charpentier B, Pestana JM, et al. An integrated safety profile analysis of belatacept in kidney transplant recipients. Transplantation 2010;90:1521-7.

[48] Vincenti F, Mendez R, Pescovitz M, et al. A phase I/II randomized open-label multicenter trial of efalizumab, a humanized anti-CD11a, anti-LFA-1 in renal transplantation. Am J Transplant 2007;7:1770-1777.

[49] Curtis RE, Travis LB, Rowlings PA, et al. Risk of lymphoproliferative disorders after bone marrow transplantation: a multi-institutional study. Blood 1999;94:2208-16.

[50] Zimmermann T, Hoppe-Lotichius M, Tripkovic V, et al. Liver transplanted patients with preoperative autoimmune hepatitis and immunological disorders are at increased risk for Post-Transplant Lymphoproliferative Disease (PTLD). Eur J Intern Med 2010;21:208-15.

[51] Gao Y, Lu YJ, Xue SA, et al. Hypothesis: a novel route for immortalization of epithelial cells by Epstein-Barr virus. Oncogene 2002;21:825-35.
[52] Küppers R. B cells under influence: transformation of B cells by Epstein-Barr virus. Nat Rev Immunol 2003;3:801-12.
[53] Hézode C, Duvoux C, Germanidis G, et al. Role of hepatitis C virus in lymphoproliferative disorders after liver transplantation. Hepatology 1999;30:775-8.
[54] Mortin LM, Landgren O, Chatterjee N, et al. Hepatitis C virus infection and risk of posttransplantation lymphoproliferative disorder among solid organ transplant recipients. Blood 2007;110:4599-605.
[55] Walker RC, Marshall WF, Strickler JG, et al. Pretransplantation assessment of the risk of lymphoproliferative disorder. Clin Infect Dis 1995;20:1346-53.
[56] Manez R, Breinig MC, Linden P, Wilson J, Torre-Cisneros J, Kusne S, et al. Posttransplant lymphoproliferative disease in primary Epstein-Barr virus infection after liver Transplantation: the rol of cytomegalovirus disease. J Infect Dis 1999;176:1462-7.
[57] Mattila PS, Aalto SM, Heikkilä L, et al. Malignancies after heart transplantation: presence of Epstein-Barr virus and cytomegalovirus. Clin Transplant 201;15:337-42.
[58] Dierksheide JE, Baiocchi RA, Ferketich AK, et al. IFN-gamma gene polymorphisms associate with development of EBV+ lymphoproliferative disease in hu PBL-SCID mice. Blood 2005;105:1558-65.
[59] Babel N, Vergopoulos A, Trappe RU, et al. Evidence for genetic susceptibility towards development of posttransplant lymphoproliferative disorder in solid organ recipients. Transplantation 2007;84:378-91.
[60] McAulay KA, Haque T, Crawford DH. Tumour necrosis factor gene polymorphism: a predictive factor for the development of post-transplant lymphoproliferative disease. Br J Cancer 2009;101:1019-27.
[61] Stern M, Opelz G, Döhler B, et al. Natural killer-cell receptor polymorphisms and posttransplantation non-Hodgkin lymphoma. Blood 2010;115:3960-5.
[62] Subklewe M, Marquis R, Choquet S, et al. Association of human leukocyte antigen haplotypes with posttransplant lymphoproliferative disease after solid organ transplantation. Transplantation 2006;82:1093-100.
[63] Pourfarziani V, Einollahi B, Taheri S, et al. Associations of Human Leukocyte Antigen (HLA) haplotypes with risk of developing lymphoproliferative disorders after renal transplantation. Ann Transplant 200712:16-22.
[64] Bakker NA, van Imhoff GW, Verschuuren EA, et al. HLA antigens and post renal transplant lymphoproliferative disease: HLA-B matching is critical. Transplantation 2005;80:595-9.
[65] Thorley-Lawson DA, Gross A, Persistence of the Epstein-Barr virus and the origins of associated lymphomas. N Engl J Med 2004;350:1328-37.
[66] Klein G, Klein E, Kashuba E. Interaction of Epstein-Barr virus (EBV) with human B-lymphocytes. Biochem Biophys Res Commun 2010;396:67-73.
[67] Brink AA, Dukers DF, van den Brule AJ, et al. Presence of Epstein-Barr virus latency type III at the single cell level in post-transplantation lymphoproliferative disorders and AIDS related lymphomas. J Clin Pathol 1997;50:911-8.Kutok JL, Wang F.

Spectrum of Epstein-Barr virus-associated diseases. Annu Rev Pathol 2006;1:375-404.
[68] Kutok JL, Wang F. Spectrum of Epstein-Barr virus-associated diseases. Annu Rev Pathol 2006;1:375-404.
[69] Leblond V, Choquet S. Lymphoproliferative disorder after liver transplantation. J Hepatol 2004;40:728-735.
[70] Petit B, Le Meur Y, Jaccard A, et al. Influence of host-recipient origin on clinical aspects of posttransplantation lymphoproliferative disorders in kidney transplantation. Transplantation 2002;27;73:265-71.
[71] LaCasce AS. Post-transplant lymphoproliferative disorders. Oncologist 2006;11:674 80.
[72] Buell JF, Gross TG, Hanaway MJ, et al. Posttransplant lymphoproliferative disorder: significance of central nervous system involvement. Transplant Proc 2005;37:954-5.
[73] Caillard S, Lelong C, Pessione F, et al. Post-transplant lymphoproliferative disorders occurring after renal transplantation in adults: report of 230 cases from the French Registry. Am J Transplant 2006;6:2735-42.
[74] Evens AM, David KA, Helenowski I, et al. Multicenter analysis of 80 solid organ transplantation recipients with post-transplantation lymphoproliferative disease: outcomes and prognostic factors in the modern era. J Clin Oncol 2010;28:1038-46.
[75] Dierickx D, Delforge M, Verhoef G. Prognostic factors and scores in post-transplantation lymphoproliferative disorders after solid organ transplantation. J Clin Oncol 2010;28:e366.
[76] Ghobrial IM, Habermann TM, Macon WR, et al. Differences between early and late posttransplant lymphoproliferative disorders in solid organ transplant patients: are they two different diseases? Transplantation 2005;79:244-7.
[77] Bakker NA, van Imhoff GW, Verschuuren EA, et al. Early onset post-transplant lymphoproliferative disease is associated with allograft localization. Clin Transplant 2005;19:327-34.
[78] Swerdlow SH, Webber SA, Chadburn A, Ferry JA. Post-transplant lymphoproliferative disorders. In: Swerdlow SH, Campo E, Harris NL, Jaffe ES, Pileri SA, Stein H, et al (eds). WHO classification of Tumours of Haematopoietic and Lymphoid Tissues. Lyon, France: IARC Press; 2008:343-9.
[79] Baumforth KR, Young LS, Flavell KJ, et al. The Epstein-Barr virus and its association with human cancers. Mol Pathol 1999;52:307-22.
[80] Swerdlow SH. T-cell and NK-cell posttransplantation lymphoproliferative disorders. Am J Clin Pathol 2007;127:887-95.
[81] RowlingS PA, Curtis RE, Passweg JR, et al. Increased incidence of Hodgkin's disease after allogeneic bone marrow transplantation. J Clin Oncol 1999;17:3122-7.
[82] Caillard S, Agodoa LY, Bohen EM, et al. Myeloma, Hodgkin disease, and lymphoid leukemia after renal transplantation: characteristics, risk factors and prognosis. Transplantation 2006;81:888-95.
[83] Quinlan SC, Landgren O, Morton LM, et al. Hodgkin lymphoma among US solid organ transplant recipients. Transplantation 2010;90:1011-5.
[84] Semakula B, Rittenbach JV, Wang J. Hodgkin lymphoma-like posttransplantation lymphoproliferative disorder. Arch Pathol Lab Med. 2006;130:558-60.
[85] Aull MJ, Buell JF, Peddi VR, et al. Maltoma: a helicobacter pylori-associated malignancy in transplant patients. Transplantation 2006;75:225-8.

[86] Quinlan SC, Morton LM, Pfeiffer RM, et al. Increased risk for lymphoid and myeloid neoplasms in elderly solid-organ transplant recipients. Cancer Epidemiol Biomarkers Prev 2010;19:1229-37.
[87] Dierickx D, De Rycke A, Vandenberghe P, et al. Recipient-derived chronic lymphocytic leukaemia diagnosed shortly after kidney transplantation on protocol biopsy. Nephrol Dial Transplant 2009;24:3886-90.
[88] Moormeier JA, Williams SF, Golomb HM. The staging of non-Hodgkin's lymphomas. Semin Oncol 1990;17:43-50.
[89] Gulley M, Tang W. Laboratory assays for Epstein-Barr virus-related disease. J Mol Diagn 2008;10:279-92.
[90] Gärtner B, Preiksaitis JK. EBV viral load detection in clinical virology. J Clin Virol 2010;48:82-90.
[91] Gulley ML, Tang W. Using Epstein-Barr viral load assays to diagnose, monitor, and prevent posttransplant lymphoproliferative disorder. Clin Microbiol Rev 2010;23:350-66.
[92] Tsai DE, Douglas L, Andreadis C, et al. EBV PCR in the diagnosis and monitoring of posttransplant lymphoproliferative disorder: results of a two-arm prospective trial. Am J Transplant 2008;8:1016-24.
[93] Cohen J, Gandhi M, Naik P, et al. Increased incidence of EBV-related disease following paediatric stem cell transplantation with reduced-intensity conditioning. Br J Haematol 2005;129:229-39.
[94] Meij P, van Esser JW, Niesters HG, et al. Impaired recovery of Epstein-Barr virus (EBV)--specific CD8+ T lymphocytes after partially T-depleted allogeneic stem cell transplantation may identify patients at very high risk for progressive EBV reactivation and lymphoproliferative disease. Blood 2003;101:4290-7.
[95] Lee TC, Savoldo B, Barshes NR, et al. Use of cytokine polymorphisms and Epstein-Barr virus viral load to predict development of post-transplant lymphoproliferative disorder in paediatric liver transplant recipients. Clin Transplant 2006;20:389-93.
[96] Baiocchi OC, Colleoni GW, Caballero OL, et al. Epstein-Barr viral load, interleukin-6 and interleukin-10 levels in post-transplant lymphoproliferative disease: a nested case-control study in a renal transplant cohort. Leuk Lymphoma 2005;46:533-9.
[97] Muti G, Mancini V, Ravelli E, et al. Significance of Epstein-Barr virus (EBV) load and interleukin-10 in post-transplant lymphoproliferative disorders. Leuk Lymphoma 2005;46:1397-407
[98] Gottschalk S, Rooney CM, Heslop HE. Post-transplant lymphoproliferative disorders. Annu Rev Med 2005;56:29-44.
[99] Starzl TE, Nalesnik MA, Porter KA, et al. Reversibility of lymphomas and lymphoproliferative lesions developing under cyclosporin-steroid therapy. Lancet 1984;1:583-587.
[100] Tsai D, Hardy C, Tomaszewski JE, et al. Reduction in immunosuppression as initial therapy for posttransplant lymphoproliferative disorder: analysis of prognostic variables and long-term follow-up of 42 adult patients. Transplantation 2001;71:1076-1088.
[101] Reshef R, Vardhanabhuti S, Luskin MR, et al. Reduction of immunosuppression as initial therapy for posttransplantation lymphoproliferative disorder. Am J Transplant 2011;11:336-47.

[102] Swinnen LJ, LeBlanc M, Grogan TM, et al. Prospective study of sequential reduction in immunosuppression, interferon alpha-2B, and chemotherapy for posttransplantation lymphoproliferative diosorder. Transplantation 2008;86:215-22.
[103] Trappe R, Hinrichs C, Appel U, et al. Treatment of PTLD with CHOP and rituximab reduces the risk of renal graft impairment after reduction of immunosuppression. Am J Transplant 2009;9:2331-7.
[104] Boratynska M, Watorek E, Smolska D, et al. Anticancer effect of sirolimus in renal allograft recipients with de novo malignancies. Transplant Proc 2007;39:2736-9.
[105] Papadopoulos EB, Ladanyi M, Emanuel D, et al. Infusion of donor leucocytes to treat Epstein-Barr virus-associated lymphoproliferative disorders after allogeneic bone marrow transplantation. N Engl J Med 1994;330:1185-91.
[106] O'Reilly RJ, Small TN, Papadopoulos E, et al. Adoptive immunotherapy for Epstein-Barr virus-associated lymphoproliferative disorders complicating marrow allografts. Springer Semin Immunopathology 1998;20:455-91.
[107] Merlo A, Turrini R, Dolcetti R, et al. The interplay between Epstein-Barr virus and the immune system: a rationale for adoptive cell therapy of EBV-related disorders. Haematologica 2010;95:1769-77.
[108] Faro A. Interferon-alpha and its effects on post-transplant lymphoproliferative disorders. Springer Semin Immunopathol 1998;20:425-36.
[109] Davis CL, Wood B, Sabath DE, et al. Interferon-alpha treatment of posttransplant lymphoproliferative disorder in recipients of solid organ transplants. Transplantation 1998;66:1770-9.
[110] Tosato G, Jones K, Breinig MK, et al. Interleukin-6 production in posttransplant lymphoproliferative disease. J Clin Invest 1993;91:2806-14.
[111] Haddad E, Paczesny S, Leblond V, et al. Treatment of B-lymphoproliferative disorder with a monoclonal anti-interleukin-6 antibody in 12 patients: a multicenter phase 1-2 clinical trial. Blood 2001;97:1590-7.
[112] Hauke R, Smir B, Greiner T, et al. Clinical and pathological features of posttransplant lymphoproliferative disorders: influence on survival and response to treatment. Ann Oncol 2001;12:831-4.
[113] Dotti G, Fiocchi R, Motta T, et al. Lymphomas occurring late after solid-organ transplantation: influence of treatment on the clinical outcome. Transplantation 2002;74:1095-02.
[114] Cavaliere R, Petroni G, Lopes MB, Schiff D. Primary central nervous system post-transplantation lymphoproliferative disorder. Cancer 2010;116:863-870.
[115] Moise L, Matta C, Hanna C, et al. Methotrexate- and/or cytarabine-based chemotherapy may be effective and safe in solid-organ transplant recipients with primary central nervous system lymphomas. Leuk Lymphoma 2011;52:521-4.
[116] Traum AZ, Rodig NM, Pilichowska ME, et al. Central nervous system lymphoproliferative disorder in pediatric kidney transplant recipients. Pediatr Transplant 2006;10:505-12.
[117] van de Glind G, de Graaf S, Klein C, et al. Intrathecal rituximab treatment for pediatric post-transplant lymphoproliferative disorder of the central nervous system. Pediatr Blood Cancer 2008;50:886-8.

[118] Buell JF, Gross TG, Hanaway MJ, et al. Chemotherapy for posttransplant lymphoproliferative disorder: the Israel Penn International Transplant Tumor Registry experience. Transplant Proc 2005;37:956-7.
[119] Choquet S, Trappe R, Leblond V, et al. CHOP-21 for the treatment of post-transplant lymphoproliferative disorder s(PTLD) following solid organ transplantation. Haematologica 2007;92:273-4.
[120] Lee JJ, Lam MS, Rosenberg A. Role of chemotherapy and rituximab for treatment of posttransplant lymphoproliferative disorder in solid organ transplantation. Ann Pharmacother 2007;41:1648-59.
[121] Gross TG. Low-dose chemotherapy for children with with post-transplant lymphoproliferative disease. Recent Results Cancer Res 2002;159:96-103.
[122] Dierickx D, Tousseyn T, De Wolf-Peeters C, et al. Management of posttransplant lymphoproliferative disorders following solid organ transplant: an update. Leuk Lymphoma. 2011 Feb 21. [Epub ahead of print].
[123] Benkerrou M, Jais JP, Leblond V, et al. Anti-B-cell monoclonal antibody treatment of severe posttransplant B-lymphoproliferative disorder: prognostic factors and long term outcome. Blood 1998;9:3137-47.
[124] Oertel SH, Verschuuren E, Reinke P, et al. Effect of anti-CD 20 antibody rituximab in patients with post-transplant lymphoproliferative disorder (PTLD). Am J Transplant 2005;5:2901-6.
[125] Blaes AH, Peterson BA, Bartlett N, Dunn DL, Morrison VA. Rituximab therapy is effective for posttransplant lymphoproliferative disorders after solid organ transplantation: results of a phase II trial. Cancer 2005;104:1661-7.
[126] Choquet S, Leblond V, Herbrecht R, et al. Efficacy and safety of rituximab in B-cell post-transplantion lymphoproliferative disorders: results of a prospective multicenter phase 2 study. Blood 2006;107:3053-7.
[127] Gonzalez-Barca E, Domingo-Domenech E, Capote FJ, et al. Prospective phase II trial of extended treatment with rituximab in patients with B-cell post-transplant lymphoproliferative disease. Haematologica 2007;92:1489-94.
[128] Choquet S, Oertel S, Leblond V, et al. Rituximab in the management of post-transplantation lymphoproliferative disorder after solid organ transplantation: proceed with caution. Ann Haematol 2007;86:599-607.
[129] Savoldo B, Rooney CM, Quiros-Tejeira RE, et al. Cellular immunity to Epstein-Barr virus in liver transplant recipients treated with rituximab for post-transplant lymphoproliferative disease. Am J Transplant 2005;5:566-72.
[130] Nehring AK, Dua AU, Mollee P, et al. Epstein-Barr virus T-cell immunity despite rituximab. Br J Haematol 2007;136:628-32.
[131] Carson KR, Evens AM, Richey EA, et al. Progressive multifocal leucoencephalopathy after rituximab therapy in HIV-negative patients: a report of 57 cases from the Research on Adverse Drug Events and Reports Project. Blood 2009; 113:4834-40.
[132] Yeo W, Chan TC, Leung NW, et al. Hepatitis B virus reactivation in lymphoma patients with prior resolved hepatitis B undergoing anticancer therapy with or without rituximab. J Clin Oncol 2009;27:605-11.
[133] Hanto DW, Frizzera G, Gajl-Peczalska KJ, et al. Epstein-Barr virus-induced B-cell lymphoma after renal transplantation: acyclovir therapy and transition from polyclonal to monoclonal B-cell proliferation. N Engl J Med 1982;306:913-8.

[134] Oertel S, Riess H. Antiviral treatment of Epstein-Barr virus-associated lymphoproliferations. Recent Results Cancer Res 2002;159:89-95.
[135] Crespo-Leiro MG, Alonso-Pulpón L, Arizón JM, et al. Influence of induction therapy, immunosuppressive regimen and anti-viral prophylaxis on development of lymphomas after heart transplantation: data from the Spanish Post-Heart Transplant Tumour Registry. J Heart Lung Transplant. 2007 Nov;26(11):1105-9.
[136] Crespo-Leiro MG, Alonso-Pulpon L, Vazquez de Prada JA, et al. Malignancy after heart transplantation: incidence, prognosis and risk factors. Am J Transplant 2008;8:1031-9.
[137] Funch DP, Walker AM, Schneider G, et al. Ganciclovir and acyclovir reduce the risk of post-transplant lymphoproliferative disorder in renal transplant recipients. Am J Transplant 2005;5:2894-900.
[138] Oertel S, Anagnostopoulos I, Hummel MW, Jonas S, Riess HB. Identification of early antigen BZLF1/ZEBRA protein of Epstein-Barr virus can predict the effectiveness of antiviral treatment in patients with post-transplant lymphoproliferative disease. Br J Haematol 2002;118:1120-1123.
[139] Trappe R, Riess H, Anagnostopoulos I, et al. Efficiency of antiviral therapy plus IVIG in a case of primary EBV infection associated PTLD refractory to rituximab, chemotherapy, and antiviral therapy alone. Ann Hematol 2009;88:167-72.
[140] Opelz G, Volker D, Naujokat C, Fickenscher H, Döhler B. Effect of cytomegalovirus prophylaxis with immunoglobulin or with antiviral drugs on post-transplant non-Hodgkin lymphoma: a multicentre retrospective analysis. Lancet Oncol 2007;8:112-8.
[141] Green M, Michaels MG, Katz BZ, et al. CMV-IVIG for prevention of Epstein Barr virus disease and posttransplant lymphoproliferative disease in pediatric liver transplant recipients. Am J Transplant 2006;6:1906-12.
[142] Perrine SP, Hermine O, Small T, et al. A phase 1/2 trial of arginine butyrate and ganciclovir in patients with Epstein-Barr virus-associated lymphoid malignancies. Blood 2007;109:2571-2578.
[143] Birkeland SA, Hamilton-Dutoit S, Bendtzen K. Long-term follow-up of kidney transplant patients with posttransplant lymphoproliferative disorder: duration of posttransplant lymphoproliferative disorder-induced operational graft tolerance, interleukin-18 course, and results of retransplantation. Transplantation 2003;76:153-8.
[144] Karras A, Thervet E, Le Meur Y, et al. Successful renal retransplantation after post-transplant lymphoproliferative disease. Am J Transplant 2004;4:1904-9.
[145] Johnson SR, Cherikh WS, Kauffman HM, Pavlakis M, Hanto DW. Retransplantation after post-transplant lymphoproliferative disorders: an OPTN/UNOS database analysis. Am J Transplant 2006;6:2743-9.
[146] A predictive model for aggressive non-Hodgkin's lymphoma: The International Non-Hodgkin's lymphoma Prognostic Factors Project. N Engl J Med 1993;329:987-94.
[147] Leblond V, Dhedin N, Mamzer Bruneel MF, et al. Identification of prognostic factors in 61 patients with posttransplantation lymphoproliferative disorders. J Clin Oncol 2001;19:772-8.

[148] Ghobrial IM, Habermann TH, Maurer MJ, et al: Prognostic analysis for survival in adult solid organ transplant recipients with post-transplantation lymphoproliferative disorders. J Clin Oncol 23:7574-7582, 2005
[149] Hourigan MJ, Doecke J, Mollee PN, et al: A new prognosticator for post-transplant lymphoproliferative disorders after renal transplantation. Br J Haematol 141:904-907, 2008
[150] Cesarman E, Chadburn A, Liu YF, Migliazza A, Dalla-Favera R, Knowles DM. BCL-6 gene mutations in post-transplantation lymphoproliferative disorders predict response to therapy and clinical outcome. Blood 1998;92:2294-302.

5

Post-Trasplant Lymphoproliferative Disorders (PTLD) in Adult Kidney Trasplantated Patients

Savina Aversa, Silvia Stragliotto, Fabio Canova,
Boso Caterina and Marino Dario
Istituto Oncologico Veneto, IRCC, Padova,
Italy

1. Introduction

Post-transplant lymphoproliferative disorder is a clearly recognized and potentially life threatening complication after solid organ or bone marrow transplantation. It comprises a spectrum of diseases ranging from infectious mononucleosis and lymphoid hyperplasia to highly aggressive lymphoma.

PTLD is a relatively common malignancy after transplantation with a reported incidence ranging from 2% to 10%. It's the most common form of post-transplant malignancy after skin cancer with an overall mortality often exceeding 50% (Purtilo et al., 1980; Leblond et al., 1995). Most cases of PTLD are associated with Epstein Barr virus (EBV) that leads to uncontrolled B cell proliferation in patients with a decreased function of EBV specific T cell because of immunosuppressive drugs. PTLD is not exclusively associated with EBV infection as EBV-negative PTLD, often developing late after transplantation.

Post transplant lymphomas differ from lymphomas in general population in histopathological findings, increased extranodal involvement, a more aggressive clinical course and poorer response to conventional treatment.

Registry-based reports however usually do not provide details of treatment and outcome: the existing single institution studies are largely reports and only a few studies include a significant number of patients with PTLD. Treatment of PTLD consists always in reduction of immunosuppression as first step. The role of chemotherapy remains unclear. In the past it was reserved for patients in whom other treatment options have failed even if the increased toxicities from cytotoxic agent, the high susceptibility to life-threatening infections. Actually most authors consider new anti CD20 mAB essential for treatment or as single agent or in association with CT but there is not a definitive agreement about schedules, duration of treatment and setting of patients.

2. Epidemiology

The incidence of PTLD varies according to organ transplanted, the nature of the immunosuppressive regimen and the presence or absence of EBV infection before transplantation and the age of patients. In adults PTLD has been reported to occur in 1-2,3% of kidney transplants, 1-2,8% of liver transplants, 1-6,3% of heart transplants, 2,4-5,8% of hearth-lung transplants, 4,2-10 of lung transplants and up to 10% of small bowel transplants (Table 1).

Transplanted Organ	Incidence of PTLD
Kidney	1-2,3 %
Liver	1-2,8 %
Heart	1-6,3 %
Lung	4,2-10 %
Heart/Lung	2,4-5,8 %
Bowel	10 %

Table 1. Incidence of PTLD according to transplanted organ

The incidence is significantly higher in paediatric recipients and has been reported in 1, 2-10% of kidney transplants, 4-15% of liver transplants and 6, 4-19,5 of hearth, lung and hearth and lung transplants. The higher incidence of PTLD in paediatric transplant recipient is attributable in large part to the development of primary EBV infection after transplantation. However the true incidence of PTLD in adult and paediatric recipients is difficult to determine with accuracy (Dror et a., 1999; Libertiny et al., 2001; Opelz et al., 1993) PTLD is surprisingly uncommon (<1 %) in the setting of allogenic bone marrow transplantation in the absence of specific T-cell manipulation such as use of a monoclonal anti CD3 antibody or T cell depletion of donor marrow. Although PTLD may occur at any time after transplantation, the risk of developing PTLD is greatest within the first year and declines over time thereafter. A report by the Transplant Collaborative Study showed the incidence of PTLD to be 224/100000 in the first year, 54/100000 in the second year and 31/100000 in the sixth year following transplantation (Bastard et al., 1994; Lo Coco et al., 1994; Cesarman et al., 1998; Opelz et al., 2003)

3. Pathogenesis

PTLD is often associated with clinical or serological reactivation of Epstein Barr virus infection. Tumour tissues often contain EBV-DNA sequences and express viral protein (Purtilo et al., 1980; Young et al., 1989; Hanto et al., 1981). In normal individuals, host defence mechanism make EBV infection a self limited disease and B cell proliferation is controlled by specific T cell lymphocytes. The infection is however not eradicated but persists in clinical latent form. In transplanted patients, partial suppression of T lymphocyte to prevent graft rejection, makes EBV-driven B cell proliferation uncontrolled and predispose to development of PTLD. EBV seronegative patients had a 10-76 times greater incidence of PTLD than EBV seropositive recipients (Walker et al., 1995). Active viral replication in immunosuppressed patients results in the expression of EBV encoded genes including oncogenes as LMP1, a gene that inhibits apoptosis by up regulating the anti-apoptotic gene BCL-2 (Kulwichit et al., 1998). Others alterations are involved in some PTLD, including the accumulation of cellular genetic alteration of p53, N-ras and c-myc rearrangements. BCL-6, that encodes a transcriptional repressor gene rearranged in 35-40% of diffuse large B cell lymphoma in immunocompetent patients (Bastard et al., 1994; Lo Coco et al., 1994) presents frequent somatic mutations in PTLD representing probably a consistent step in the progression from a PTLD that can be controlled by a reconstituted immune system to one that will require more aggressive therapeutic intervention (Ceserman et al., 1998). Additional stimuli are required to promote the development of PTLD and, although these are not clearly defined, the local cytokine environment and chronic stimulation of B cell by alloantigen are thought to be important.

4. Risk factors

The most important risk factor for PTLD development is the intensity of immunosuppression. Induction and rejection treatment with anti-T cell antibodies, especially OKT3 and ATG may lead to an increased risk of PTLD, as demonstrated by the higher incidence of early PTLD in hearth and hearth/lung recipient. With longer follow-up, is now evident that antibody prophylaxis increased the risk of lymphoma primarily during the first post-transplant year, whereas in subsequent years the risk is similar to that in non antibody-treated patients. Whether IL-2 receptor blocking monoclonal antibody, which was introduced in the late 1990s, also increases the risk of lymphoma is of great interest. Analysis of the critical 12-months data showed that use of anti IL-2 receptor antibodies was not associated with an increased risk of lymphoma (Gao et al., 2004) (Figure 1). There is no conclusive evidence that development of PTLD is associated with a single immunosuppressive agent (Gao et al., 2003; Pirsch et al., 1997; Weisner et al., 1998; Younes et al., 2000). Also the effect of everolimus and sirolimus on PTLD development is not clear. These drugs may theoretically be associated with a lower risk as demonstrated in animal model but the lack of prospective randomized trial assessing these differences restrains any firm conclusion (Yakupoglu et al., 2006; Majewski et al., 2003; Kusuki et al., 2009). A special category of patient at risk (10 to 50 fold increased risk) are EBV seronegative patients receiving allograft from EBV seropositive donors, leading to primary EBV infection (Walker et al., 1995). This is also the reason for the higher incidence of early PTLD observed in paediatric transplant recipients who often are still EBV seronegative at the time of transplantation.

A high incidence of EBV related lymphoproliferative disorders has been reported in a number of congenital immunodeficiency syndromes including severe combined immunodeficiency (SCID), ataxia teleangiectasia and Wischott Aldrich syndrome (Waldmann et al., 1983). Acquired immunodeficiency due to HIV disease has become a major clinical problem in many parts of the world. An increased incidence of aggressive non Hodgkin lymphoma which shares many of the unusual characteristics of PTLD is a manifestation of AIDS. The introduction of HAART has dramatically reduced the incidence of this life threatening manifestation of HIV.

Finally, the underlying indication for transplantation may also influence the risk for PTLD. For example hepatitis C infection (Burra et al., 2006) is associated with a particularly high risk of PTLD.

5. Pathologic features

A standardized approach to the classification of PTLD is important to allow consistency of reporting and to enable comparison of different treatments. Histology is essential also in differentiation between rejection and PTLD involvement of the graft. The classification of PTLD currently used is based on the histopathological appearance of the tumour. PTLD can be divided into three distinct morphological groups, as reported by the World Health Organization classification of neoplastic disease of the haematopoietic and lymphoid tissues (Table 2).

The first group comprises diffuse B cell hyperplasia, characterized by differentiated plasma cell and preservation of the normal lymphoid architecture. This type of PTLD is most often seen in children and young adults, usually occurs within the first year following transplantation and responds well to reduction in immunosuppression (Kahan et al., 2000).

The second group comprises polymorphic PTLD characterised by nuclear atypia, tumour necrosis and destruction of underlying lymphoid architecture. Lesions in this group are highly polymorphic, usually monoclonal and include plasmacytes and blast form. Polymorphic PTLD is the most common type of PTLD in both children and adults and may occur at any time after transplantation.
The third group comprises monomorphic PTLD and includes high grade invasive lymphoma of B or T lymphocytes. This type of PTLD is often seen several years after transplantation and resembles non Hodgkin lymphoma. Monomorphic B cell PTLD can be further divided into diffuse large cell lymphoma and Burkitt or Burkitt like lymphoma. PTLD may also present with discordant lesions, in which different histological subtypes can be present in a single patient.
Although the association between EBV and PTLD is well established, the presence of EBV in tumour cell is not required for the diagnosis. So, according to the international classification, any lymphoma arising in the post-transplant patient is considered to be a PTLD.

Category	**Characteristics**
Early lesion	Polyclonal Reactive plasmacytic hyperplasia and infectious mononucleosis like presentation Partial architectural preservation of the involved tissue Younger age Regress spontaneously or after reduction of immunosuppression
Polymorphic	B-cell maturation Monoclonal Variable response to immunosuppression withdrawal
Monomorphic	Monoclonal malignant B cell lymphoma Diffuse large B cell lymphoma Burkitt or Burkitt like lymphoma Plasma cell myeloma Plasmacytoma like lesion Rarely T cell neoplasma including peripheral T cell lymphoma
Hodgkin lymphoma and Hodgkin lymphoma like PTLD	Mostly seen in allogenic bone marrow transplant recipients

Table 2. World Health Organization Classification of Post-transplantation Lymphoproliferative Disorder Pathology

At least 90% of PTLD that occur in solid organ transplant patients arise from recipient cells (Weissmann e al., 1995) and the opposite apply in the case of bone marrow transplantation. Donor derived PTLD in organ transplant patient may have a predilection for the allograft (Strazzabosco et al., 1997). Some authors have suggested that they may have a worse and some a better prognosis than recipient organ PTLD even if further studies are needed in this area (Lones et al., 1997; Howard et al., 1992).

6. Clinical presentation

The clinical presentation of PTLD is highly variable; this syndrome may occur in nodal or extranodal sites as single or multiples masses.

Most patients present with fever (seen in 50%), lymphadenopathy (seen in 30%) or non-specific symptoms such as tonsillitis (particularly children) and weight loss. Around 15% of patients present as an emergency with intestinal perforation (Kahan et al., 2000) or with fulminant PTLD characterised by disseminated systemic disease that clinically resembles septic shock (Orjuela et al., 2003)

Keeping in mind that PTLD often presents at extra nodal sites (Bakker et al., 2005) (figure 2), including the allograft and digestive tract, there may be early signs and symptoms that should at least include PTLD in the differential diagnosis. This is especially true for allograft involvement of PTLD. Kidney transplant recipients with allograft involvement of PTLD often presents with renal dysfunction, hydronephrosis because of ureteral obstruction and fever. Lung transplant recipients may present with organ dysfunction. Because the GI tract is also frequently involved, GI signs and symptoms such as diarrhoea and bleeding may also lead to a diagnosis of PTLD, headache or confusion in case of CNS involvement, nasal airway obstruction in case of sinonasal PTLD involvement, or subtle orbital symptoms in case of orbital PTLD. Skin involvement is observed in approximately 5-10% of all PTLD patients and must be differentiated by other cutaneous malignancy, given the fact that organ allograft recipients have an increased risk for the development of cutaneous malignancy such as squamous and basal cell carcinoma (Allen et al., 2001; Maecker et al., 2007; Beynet et al., 2004). Given this myriad of nonspecific clinical signs and symptoms, often masquerading PTLD as infection or adverse drug effects or reactions, or even absence of symptoms at all, methods for early detection of PTLD in transplant recipients would be extremely valuable.

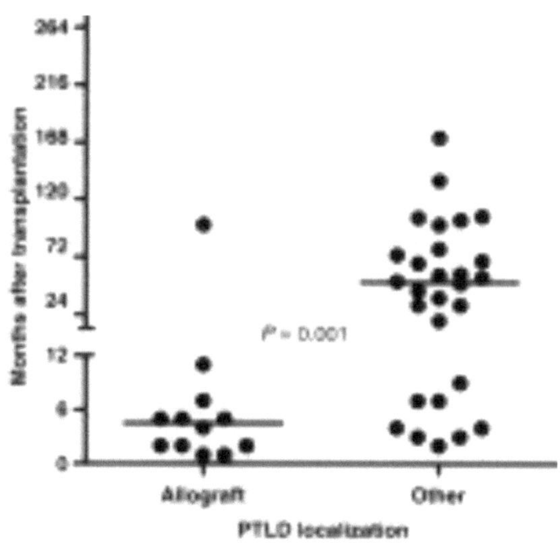

Fig. 2. Primary site of post-transplant lymphoproliferative disorder (PTLD) presentation and time after transplantation in kidney and lung transplant recipients. PTLD localized in the allograft occurred significantly earlier after transplantation when compared with PTLD localized outside the allograft (median: 4.5 months, range: 1–99 months vs. median: 51 months, range: 2–172 months, P = 0.001) (adapted from ref. Bakker NA clinical transplant 2005, printed with the permission of Blackwell Publishing).

7. Diagnosis of PTLD

The diagnosis of PTLD should be based on histological examination of biopsy tissue. Excision biopsy is preferable because PTLD may contain large areas of necrosis although needle biopsy may be acceptable when obtaining larger samples is impractical. Cytological preparation are useful, particularly in the analysis of effusion (Lechapt et al., 2001) and can provide adequate diagnostic material particularly if ancillary studies such as phenotypic, clonal and viral analysis are also performed. Tissue should be subjected to standard histology, examined for the presence of EBV by immunostaining or in-situ hybridization, cellular infiltrates characterised by relevant phenotypic markers and clonality estimated. Although it would be ideal to sample each tumour in cases of multicenter PTLD, this is seldom possible. Each tumour may represent a separate clone and the histological grade may be underestimated in multicentric cases. The surgeon run also the risk, in this case, of sampling a reactive node that may contain evidence of EBV infection, while the primary lymphomatous PTLD lies elsewhere. It is also useful consider biopsy of any lesion that respond in an atypical fashion, particularly if regression is documented in other concurrent lesion. The presence of PTLD within the graft itself may sometimes be mistaken for acute rejection and if there is diagnostic doubt, in-situ hybridisation for EBV encoded RNA, and PCR for VDJ heavy-chain rearrangements to determine clonality may be helpful. Molecular analysis of oncogenes and tumour suppressor genes will undoubtedly play an increasingly important role in predicting behaviour even if, at present, these techniques are not widely available and few genes have been analyzed

There is no separate staging system for PTLD and it is currently staged using the same system as NHL in the normal population. Staging of the disease should include CT of the abdomen and thorax and bone marrow aspiration. FDG-PET scanning is increasingly used as an important tool in the visualization of malignant lymphoma, especially for the detection of extranodal localization and post-treatment evaluation and has shown to be superior over conventional diagnostic techniques to differentiate between residual masses as a result of vital tumour or scar tissue. Bakker et al. [45] (Bakker et al., 2006) reported 12 patients whit a highly avid FDG PTLD. Additional sites of extranodal localization of PTLD not visualized on CT scanning were found in 50% of all patients (figure 3).

Additional investigations should be performed as indicated, e.g. CT or magnetic resonance scan of the cranium and spinal cord or further gastrointestinal imaging.

8. EBV DNA load monitoring after transplantation

Early detection of PTLD may allow for prompt therapy and potentially decreased mortality. In addition elevation of EBV-DNA load in blood is considered to reflect aberrant EBV induced B-cell proliferation. For this reasons much effort has been put in developing methods that might identify patients at risk for developing PTLD by measuring the amount of circulating EBV-DNA in the peripheral blood.

Despite the consensus that PTLD patients have a significantly higher EBV-DNA load compared with healthy EBV-seropositive donors or non-PTLD transplant recipients, it is still unclear which threshold values are predictive for PTLD. Many different threshold values have been reported, all with different sensitivity (60–100%) and specificity (71–100%) (Lee et al., 2005; Rowe et al., 2001; Tsai et al., 2002). Another limitation of EBV-DNA load monitoring may be the observation that PTLD developing late after transplantation is not

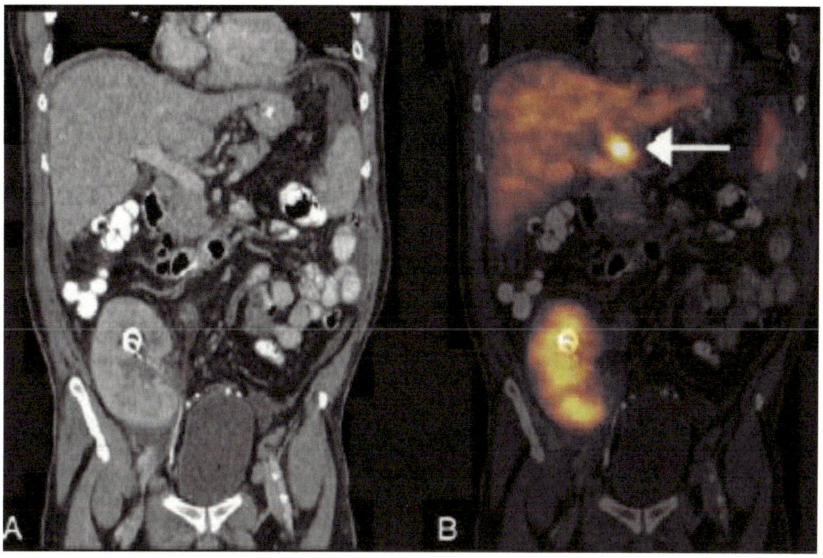

Fig. 3. Example of discordant finding. CT abdomen (A) and FDG PET fused with the same CT scan (B). Arrow indicates the histologically confirmed focal lesion with high uptake of FDG, whereas the CT scan (A) does not show any abnormalities at the site of high FDG uptake. The high uptake in the allograft, including the kidney calices and pyelum, is physiological, as is the modest uptake in liver and spleen

necessarily associated with EBV (negative staining for EBV in the tumour), and may therefore develop without a concomitant rise in EBV-DNA load. Indeed, there are studies showing EBV-negative PTLD developing late after transplantation without a rise in EBV-DNA load. These observations suggest that, although increased EBV-DNA load is generally considered to represent an increase in circulating EBV-positive tumour cells, these high EBV-DNA loads in reality may represent a separate population of proliferating B-cells that may have nothing to do with development of PTLD. Instead, these proliferating B-cells may only reflect a general state of decreased T-cell surveillance in the transplant recipient

In conclusion, because of the many variables that may influence the immune response of the individual transplant recipient, such as level of immunosuppression, time after transplantation, concomitant infections, type of organ transplanted, but also genetic factors, an exact cut-off value of EBV-DNA load critical for the development of PTLD in the individual patient cannot be defined. Therefore, rising EBV-DNA loads in the individual patient, instead of using a cut-off value, may be more appropriate to identify the individual patient at risk for the development of PTLD.

It has been suggested that concomitant combined monitoring of EBV-DNA load and EBV-specific cytotoxic T lymphocytes (CTL) responses (the absence of which may be used as a marker for possible overimmunosuppression) might better identify the individual patient at risk for PTLD development. The positive predictive value of high EBV-DNA loads as a predictor for PTLD development might be improved with this method. Smets et al. (Smets et al., 2002) showed that high EBV-DNA loads in patients who underwent primary EBV infection were indicative for PTLD development only if there was a low concomitant cellular immune response.

9. IL 10 monitoring

Some reports have suggested that levels of IL-10 might be predictive for PTLD development (Muti et al., 2003). Although the exact relationship between IL-10 and the development of PTLD has not been fully elucidated yet, IL-10 can act as an autocrine growth factor for EBV-transformed B-cells. Although this may lead to higher local levels of IL-10, it seems doubtful that this is also reflected by a higher total IL-10 load in the peripheral blood of the transplant recipient. Given the small number of studies so far and the lack of evidence regarding the exact relation between IL-10 and the development of PTLD, the relevance for identification of the patient at risk for PTLD development is not clear.

10. Clinical management

The treatment of PTLD poses a major therapeutic challenge and, although there is reasonable agreement about the overall principles of treatment no controlled studies have been undertaken and most of the recommendations result from small cohorts at single institutions. Even if no uniform approaches to the treatment have emerged, general principles are largely shared.

- Treatment must be individualised according to clinical situation and the type of organ transplanted
- Unlike non-Hodgkin lymphoma in immunocompetent patients, PTLD can be eradicated by surgical resection
- Reduction of immunosuppression is considered the first line treatment
- Antiviral agents have showed to induce regression of disease in some cases
- Chemotherapy, traditionally considered a last resort treatment, is associated with high response rate and long progression free survival
- Rituximab has emerged as treatment of choice especially in early PTLD after failure in reduce/withdrawal immunosuppression
- Radiotherapy may be appropriate for treatment of localized PTLD together with reduction in immunosuppression

10.1 Reduction of immunosuppression

Reduction of immunosuppression is the initial treatment in all patients with PTLD with the aim of increase antitumor activity. In EBV driven PTLD, this may partially restores CTL function resulting in an increase of EBV specific CTLs and elimination of virally infected lymphocytes, including those which constitute the tumour. The approach to reduce immunosuppressive drugs needs to be carefully individualised and will depend on the nature and extent of disease, the type of transplant recipient (life or no-life supporting graft) and the time from transplantation.

Steroids also are an important component of most chemotherapy regimen for PTLD and lymphoma in general.

A response to reduction in immunosuppression is usually seen within 2-4 weeks (Green et al., 1999). Reduction of immunosuppression leads to long term disease remission in 40-86% of paediatric patients and 25-63% of adults.

Features that predict response include a short interval between transplantation and PTLD and wild type BCL-6 (Ceserman et al., 1998). If PTLD develops within one year of the transplant up to 80% will respond to reducing in immunosuppression with a mortality of

40%. In contrast, after one year the response rate falls to 10% with 80% of mortality (Armitiag et al., 1991).

10.2 The role of Rituximab

PTLD is usually of B cell origin and the use of mAB to deplete B cell is a logical approach for treatment. Rituximab, a monoclonal antibody directed against CD20 antigen expressed on mature and immature B cells, results in profound and long-lasting depletion of B cell (6-8 months), together with hypogammaglobulinemia.
Rituximab is widely used in the treatment of diffuse large B cell lymphoma in immunocompetent patients with an overall survival at two years of 70% compared with 57% of patients treated with chemotherapy alone (Coiffer et al., 2002) rituximab has also recently been used in the treatment of patients with PTLD after solid organ transplantation as an adjunct to reduction of immunosuppression or chemotherapy.
The majority of the case reports describe the use of rituximab, at standard dose of 375 mg/mq once a week for four consecutive weeks, in the early onset PTLD, but it might be effective also for patients with late onset PTLD.
The patients treated with rituximab benefit from the short duration of such therapy in terms of response rate and less toxic effect. However, because of the high relapse rate observed in several studies, the combination of rituximab with cytotoxic drugs is recommended to be evaluated.

10.3 Antiviral agents

Because most PTLDs arise as a consequence of EBV infection, prophylactic measures should include avoiding over-immunosuppression of the recipient such as the use of anti-lymphocyte preparations, antiviral agents, EBV vaccination, in-vitro generated EBV specific CTL lines and avoiding, in EBV seronegative recipients, transplantation with an organ from an EBV positive donor.
Regression has been described following high dose acyclovir (Hanto et al., 1982; Morrison et al., 1994). Targeting EBV by antiviral agents has been attempted also for prophylaxis of PTLD. However, the latent EBV infected cells which carries EBV genome and express a limited number of viral proteins are not eliminated by the use of antiviral agents.
A potential approach for reducing the high risk of PTLD in EBV seronegative paediatric patients is to expose them to the EBV virus prior to transplantation to induce seroconversion and a vaccine using a viral membrane protein from EBV, gp350 (Gusy et al., 1995).

10.4 Cytokine based therapy

Agents that alter the cytokine environment of the tumour to favour remission, notably interferon-α and anti-IL-6 have been tried as adjuvant along with reduction of immunosuppression, but at present there is insufficient evidence to recommend their routine use. Interferon-α enhances T-lymphocyte cytotoxicity and has been used as an adjunct to chemotherapy to treat B cell malignancies in non-transplanted patients and in the maintenance of remission in such patients. Caution is needed when using interferon-α because of its toxicity and because it may initiate acute rejection by promoting CD8 T cell activity.
IL-6 may play a role in the development of PTLD by promoting the growth of EBV-infected B cells and increasing tumour development in EBV-immortalised cells. Serum levels of IL-6

are raised in the majority of patients with PTLD. Anti-IL-6 mAb has been used in a phase 1-2 multi-centre clinical trial (Hadda et al., 2000).

10.5 Rapamycine

Rapamycine is increasingly used as an immunosuppressive agent for solid organ transplantation. In addition to its immunosuppressive effects, it also displays anti-angiogenic and anti-tumour properties, and this make it a potentially attractive agent for patients in remission from PTLD, particularly those who develop chronic allograft rejection as a consequence of a reduction of immunosuppression. Rapamycin inhibits the growth of EBV-transformed B lymphocyte lines in-vitro by arresting the cell cycle in the G1 phase (Vaysberg et al., 2007). There are as yet no prospective studies addressing the use of rapamycin in the treatment or prevention of PTLD.

10.6 Adoptive T cell therapy

Adoptive T cell therapy using EBV-specific cytotoxic T lymphocytes (CTL) lines has generated considerable interest as a treatment for PTLD. Adoptive immunotherapy was initially advocated in allogenic bone marrow transplantation to control PTLD that was donor cell in origin. Donor CTL would restore immune surveillance against EBV driven proliferation and control PTLD. A potential risk was graft versus host disease due to the donor cell infusion: this risk could be reduced by selecting donor EBV-specific T cell ex vivo prior to infusion. This approach has been used with success as prophylaxis and treatment of PTLD after stem cell transplantation using CTL lines derived from the donor and specific for EBV gene products even if it is limited by the time required to generate the CTLs (weeks to months) and the expense for dedicated facilities.

After solid organ transplantation, PTLD is usually of recipient origin and recipient derived CTLs are required for effective killing of EBV infected B cells. It is possible to generate autologous EBV-specific CTLs from recipients who were EBV seropositive prior to transplantation. However, this approach is not applicable when PTLD arises in recipients who were EBV seronegative prior to transplantation.

10.7 Chemotherapy

Conventional cytotoxic chemotherapy which has been shown to be curative for many lymphomas in non-PTLD setting, has been viewed as a treatment of last resort due to very high morbidity and mortality rates. Chemotherapy is commonly used in the treatment of PTLD when reduction in immunosuppression fails to control the disease.

Various multi-drug regimens such as CHOP or CHOP like (cyclophosphamide, doxorubicin, vincristine and prednisone) have been used in PTLD patients (Wasson et al., 2006; Elstrom et al., 2006; Trappa et al., 2007; Taylor et al., 2006; Fohrer et al., 2006; Baudi et al., 2007; Patel et al., 2007; Aversa et al., 2008) (table 4).

In spite of the high RR up to 70%, the associated toxicity is significant and includes treatment-related deaths in about 25% of patients. The high mortality of the standard chemotherapy regimens in the PTLD population might occur because of various factors including baseline pharmacologic immunosuppression, graft dysfunction, and colonization with resistant or hospital acquired infectious organisms.

Sepsis and other complication of chemotherapy have been the major problem in some centres, while others have found refractory disease to be common. Because this high toxicity, several studies are in progress to investigate the use of other agents, such as anti-B cell mAb, in combination with lower dose and therefore less toxic chemotherapy regimes.

	Number of patients who received chemotherapy	**Chemotherapy**	**response**	**Therapy-associated mortality**
Wasson et al, 2006	9 kidney transplant retrospective	4 CHOP +/- R 1 Ganciclovir 2 Decreased immunosuppression 1 Decreased immunosuppression + Rituximab 1 Other chemotherapy	n.a.	None
Trappe et al, 2009	58 kidney transplant prospective	18 Rituximab 40 CHOP +/- R	40 CR	7 sepsis
Fohrer et al, 2006	17 kidney or kidney/pancreas transplant prospective	17 ACVBP	13 CR + PR	1 Infections
Buadi et al, 2006	14 kidney or kidney/pancreas transplant retrospective	3 ProMACE CytaBOM 1 CHOP-R 1 BMT 1 Rituximab 6 Surgery 2 Decreased immunosuppression	8 CR 1 PR 2 SD 3 NE	
Aversa et al, 2008	8 prospective	7 VACOP-B 1 STANFORD V	7 CR 1 PR	2 TRM due to interstitial pneumonia

CR: complete remission; PR: partial remission DFS : disease free survival; OS : overall survival; CHOP-R cyclophosphamide, doxorubicin, vincristine, prednisone, rituximab; PMitCEBO: prednisone, mitoxantrone, cyclophosphamide, etoposide, bleomycin, vincristine; ACVBP: doxorubicin, cyclophosphamide, vindesine, bleomycin, prednisone; ProMACE CytaBOM: cyclophosphamide, doxorubicin, etoposide, prednisone, bleomycin, vincristine, cytarabine, methotrexate, leucovorin; ABVD: doxorubicin, bleomycin, vinblastine, dacarbazine; BMT: etoposide and cyclophosphamide followed by high dose melphalan and autologous stem cell transplantation; VACOP-B: etoposide, doxorubicin, cyclophosphamide, vincristine, prednisone, bleomycin; TRM: treatment related mortality.

Table 4. Studies of chemotherapeutic treatment in patients with PTLD

11. Reference

Allen U, Hébert D, Moore D, Dror Y, Wasfy S; Canadian PTLD Survey Group-1998. Epstein-Barr virus-related post-transplant lymphoproliferative disease in solid organ transplant recipients, 1988-97: a Canadian multi-centre experience. Pediatr Transplant. 2001 Jun;5(3):198-203.

Armitage JM, Kormos R, Stuart RS. Post-transplantation lymphoproliferative disease in thoracic organ transplanted patients: ten years of cyclosporine based immunosuppression. J Heart Lung Transplat. 1991; 10: 877-886.

Aversa SML, Stragliotto S, Marino D, Calabrese F, Rigotti P, Marchini F, Gambino A, Feltrin G, Boso C, Canova F, Soldà C, Mazzarotto R and Burra P. Post-Transplant Lymphoproliferative Disorders (PTLD) after heart or kidney transplantation at a single centre: presentation and response to treatment. Acta Haematol. 2008; 120(1):36-46.

Bastard C, Deweindt C, Kerckaert JP, Lenormand B, Rossi A, Pezzella F, Fruchart C, Duval C, Monconduit M, Tilly H. LAZ3 rearrangements in non-Hodgkin's lymphoma: correlation with histology, immunophenotype, karyotype, and clinical outcome in 217 patients. Blood. 1994 May 1;83(9):2423-7.

Bakker NA, van Imhoff GW, Verschuuren EA, van Son WJ, Homan van der Heide JJ, Veeger NJ, Kluin PM, Kluin-Nelemans HC. Early onset post-transplant lymphoproliferative disease is associated with allograft localization. Clin Transplant. 2005 Jun;19(3):327-34.

Bakker NA, Pruim J, de Graaf W, van Son WJ, van der Jagt EJ, van Imhoff GW. PTLD visualization by FDG-PET: improved detection of extranodal localizations. Am J Transplant. 2006 Aug;6(8):1984-5.

Beynet DP, Wee SA, Horwitz SS, Kohler S, Horning S, Hoppe R, Kim YH. Clinical and pathological features of posttransplantation lymphoproliferative disorders presenting with skin involvement in 4 patients. Arch Dermatol. 2004 Sep;140(9):1140-6.

Buadi F, Heyeman MR, Gocke C, Rapaport A, Hakimian R, Bartlett S et al. Treatment and outcome of post-transplant lymphoproliferative disease: a single institution study. Am J Hematol. 2007 Mar;82(3):208-14.

Burra P, Buda A, Livi U, Rigotti P, Zanus G, Calabrese F, Caforio A, Menin C, Canova D, Farinati F, Aversa SML. Occurrence of post-transplant lymphoproliferative disorders among over thousand adult recipients: any role for Hepatitis C infection. Eur J Gastr Hepatol.2006, 18:1065-1070.

Cesarman E, Chadburn A, Liu YF, Migliazza A, Dalla Favera R, Knowles D. BCL-6 gene mutation in post-transplantation lymphoproliferative disorders predict response to therapy and clinical outcome. Blood 1998. 92: 2294-2302.

Coiffier B, Lepage E, Briere J, Herbrecht R, Tilly H, Bouabdallah R, Morel P, Van Den Neste E, Salles G, Gaulard P, Reyes F, Lederlin P, Gisselbrecht C. CHOP chemotherapy plus rituximab compared with CHOP alone in elderly patients with diffuse large-B-cell lymphoma. N Engl J Med. 2002 Jan 24;346(4):235-42.

Gao SZ, Chaparro SV, Perloth M, Montoya J, Miller JL, Dimiceli S, Hastie T, Oyer PE, Shoroeder J. Post-transplantation Lymphoproliferative Disease in Heart and Heart-Lung Trasplant Recipient: 30 year Experience at Stanford University. J Heart Transplant 2003, 22: 505-514.

Dror Y, Greenberg M, Taylor G, Superina R, Hébert D, West L, Connolly B, Sena L, Allen U, Weitzman S. Lymphoproliferative disorders after organ transplantation in children. Transplantation. 1999 Apr 15;67(7):990-8.

Elstrom RL, Andreadis C, Aqui NA et al. Treatment of PTLD with rituximab or chemotherapy. Am J Transplant 2006 ;6 :569-576.

Fohrer C, Caillard S, Koumarianou A, Ellero B, Woehl-Jaegle ML, Meyer C. Long-term survival in post-transplant lymphoproliferative disorders with a dose-adjusted ACVBP regimen. Br J Haematol. 2006 Sep; 134(6):602-12.

Green M, Michaels MG, Webber SA, Rowe D, Reyes J. The management of Epstein-Barr virus associated post-transplant lymphoproliferative disorders in pediatric solid-organ transplant recipients. Pediatr Transplant. 1999 Nov;3(4):271-81.

Gu SY, Huang TM, Ruan L, Miao YH, Lu H, Chu CM, Motz M, Wolf H. First EBV vaccine trial in humans using recombinant vaccinia virus expressing the major membrane antigen. Dev Biol Stand. 1995;84:171-7.

Hanto DW, Frizzera G, Gajl-Peczalska J, Purtilo DT, Klein G, Simmons RL, Najarian JS. The Epstein-Barr virus (EBV) in the pathogenesis of posttransplant lymphoma. Transplant Proc. 1981 Mar 13: 756-60.

Locker J, Nalesnik M. Molecular genetic analysis of lymphoid tumors arising after organ transplantation. Am J Pathol 1989. 135:977.

Haddad E., Paczesny S, Leblond V. et al., Treatment of B-lymphoproliferative disorder with a monoclonal anti-interleukin-6 antibody in 12 patients: a multicenter phase 1–2 clinical trial, Blood 2001; 97, 1590–1597.

Hanto DW, Frizzera G, Gajl-Peczalska KJ, Sakamoto K, Purtilo DT, Balfour HH Jr, Simmons RL, Najarian JS. Epstein-Barr virus-induced B-cell lymphoma after renal transplantation: acyclovir therapy and transition from polyclonal to monoclonal B-cell proliferation. N Engl J Med. 1982 Apr 15;306(15):913-8.

Howard TK, Klintmalm GB, Stone MJ, Cofer JB, Husberg BS, Goldstein RM, Gonwa TA Lymphoproliferative disorder masquerading as rejection in liver transplant recipients--an early aggressive tumor with atypical presentation. Transplantation. 1992 May;53(5):1145-7.

Kulwichit W, Edwards RH, Davenport EM, Baskar JF, Godfrey V, Raab-Traub N. Expression of the Epstein-Barr virus latent membrane protein 1 induces B cell lymphoma in transgenic mice. Proc Natl Acad Sci U S A. 1998 Sep 29;95(20):11963-8.

Leblond V, Sutton L, Dorent R, Davi F, Bitker MO, Gabarre J, Charlotte F, Ghoussoub JJ, Fourcade C, Fischer A, et al. Lymphoproliferative disorders after organ transplantation: a report of 24 cases observed in a single center. J Clin Oncol. 1995 Apr;13(4):961-8.

Lechapt-Zalcman E, Challine D, Delfau-Larue MH, Haioun C, Desvaux D, Gaulard P. Association of primary pleural effusion lymphoma of T-cell origin and human herpesvirus 8 in a human immunodeficiency virus-seronegative man. Arch Pathol Lab Med. 2001 Sep;125(9):1246-8.

Lee TC, Savoldo B, Rooney CM, Heslop HE, Gee AP, Caldwell Y, Barshes NR, Scott JD, Bristow LJ, O'Mahony CA, Goss JA. Quantitative EBV viral loads and immunosuppression alterations can decrease PTLD incidence in pediatric liver transplant recipients. Am J Transplant. 2005 Sep;5(9):2222-8.

Libertiny G, Watson CJ, Gray DW, Welsh KI, Morris PJ. Rising incidence of post-transplant lymphoproliferative disease in kidney transplant recipients. Br J Surg. 2001 Oct;88(10):1330-4.

Lo Coco F, Ye BH, Lista F, Corradini P, Offit K, Knowles DM, Chaganti RS, Dalla-Favera R. Rearrangements of the BCL6 gene in diffuse large cell non-Hodgkin's lymphoma. Blood. 1994 Apr 1;83(7):1757-9.

Lones MA, Lopez-Terrada D, Weiss LM, Shintaku IP, Said JW. Donor origin of posttransplant lymphoproliferative disorder localized to a liver allograft: demonstration by fluorescence in situ hybridization. Arch Pathol Lab Med. 1997 Jul;121(7):701-6.

Majewski M, Korecka M, Joergensen J, Fields L, Kossev P, Schuler W, Shaw L, Wasik MA. Immunosuppressive TOR kinase inhibitor everolimus (RAD) suppresses growth of cells derived from posttransplant lymphoproliferative disorder at allograft-protecting doses. Transplantation. 2003 May 27;75(10):1710-7.

Morrison VA, Dunn DL, Manivel JC, Gajl-Peczalska KJ, Peterson BA. Clinical characteristics of post-transplant lymphoproliferative disorders. Am J Med. 1994 Jul;97(1):14-24.

Muti G, Klersy C, Baldanti F, Granata S, Oreste P, Pezzetti L, Gatti M, Gargantini L, Caramella M, Mancini V, Gerna G, Morra E; Co-operative Study Group on PTLDs. Epstein-Barr virus (EBV) load and interleukin-10 in EBV-positive and EBV-negative post-transplant lymphoproliferative disorders. Br J Haematol. 2003 Sep;122(6):927-33.

Opelz G, Henderson R. Incidence of non-Hodgkin lymphoma in kidney and heart transplant recipients. Lancet. 1993 Dec 18-25;342(8886-8887):1514-6.

Opelz G, Dohler B. Lymphoma after Solid Organ Transplantation: a collaborative Transplant Study Report. Am J Transplant 2003; 4:222-30.

Opelz G, Daniel V, Naujokat C, Fickenscher H, Dohler B. Effect of cytomegalovirus prophylaxis with immunoglobulin or with antiviral drugs on post-transplant non Hodgkin lymphoma: a multicentre retrospective analysis. Lancet Oncology 2007; 8: 212-18.

Orjuela M, Gross TG, Cheung YK, Alobeid B, Morris E, Cairo MS. A pilot study of chemoimmunotherapy (cyclophosphamide, prednisone, and rituximab) in patients with post-transplant lymphoproliferative disorder following solid organ transplantation. Clin Cancer Res. 2003 Sep 1;9(10 Pt 2):3945S-52S.

Paranjothi S, Yusen RD, Kraus MD, Lynch JP, Patterson GA, Trulock EP. Lymphoproliferative disease after lung transplantation: comparison of presentation and outcome of early and late cases. J Heart Lung Transplant. 2001 Oct;20(10):1054-63.

Patel H, Vogl DT, Aqui N, Shaked A, Olthoff K, Markmann J, Reddy R, Stadtmauer EA, Schuster S, Tsai DE. Posttransplant lymphoproliferative disorder in adult liver transplant recipients: a report of seventeen cases. Leuk Lymphoma. 2007 May;48(5):885-91.

Pirsch JD, Miller J, Deierhoi MH, Vincenti F, Filo RS. A comparison of tacrolimus (FK506) and cyclosporine for immunosuppression after cadaveric renal transplantation. FK506 Kidney Transplant Study Group. Transplantation. 1997 Apr 15;63(7):977-83.

Purtilo DT. Epstein-Barr-virus-induced oncogenesis in immune-deficient individuals. Lancet. 1980 Feb 9;1(8163):300-3.

Rowe DT, Webber S, Schauer EM, Reyes J, Green M. Epstein-Barr virus load monitoring: its role in the prevention and management of post-transplant lymphoproliferative disease. Transpl Infect Dis. 2001 Jun;3(2):79-87.

Strazzabosco M, Corneo B, Iemmolo RM, Menin C, Gerunda G, Bonaldi L, Merenda R, Neri D, Poletti A, Montagna M, Del Mistro A, Faccioli AM, D'Andrea E. Epstein-Barr virus-associated post-transplant lympho-proliferative disease of donor origin in liver transplant recipients. J Hepatol. 1997 Apr;26(4):926-34.

Taylor AL, Bowles KM, Callaghan CJ, Wimperis JZ, Grant JW, Marcus RE, Bradley JA. Anthracycline-based chemotherapy as first-line treatment in adults with malignant post transplant lymphoproliferative disorder after solid organ transplantation. Transplantation. 2006 Aug 15;82(3):375-81.

Trappe R, Hinrichs C, Appel U, Babel N, Reinke P, Neumayer HH, Budde K, Dreyling M, Dührsen U, Kliem V, Schüttrumpf S, Hauser IA, Mergenthaler HG, Schlattmann P, Anagnostopoulos I, Doerken B, Riess H. Treatment of PTLD with rituximab and CHOP reduces the risk of renal graft impairment after reduction of immunosuppression. Am J Transplant. 2009 Oct;9(10):2331-7.

Tsai DE, Nearey M, Hardy CL, Tomaszewski JE, Kotloff RM, Grossman RA, Olthoff KM, Stadtmauer EA, Porter DL, Schuster SJ, Luger SM, Hodinka RL. Use of EBV PCR for the diagnosis and monitoring of post-transplant lymphoproliferative disorder in adult solid organ transplant patients. Am J Transplant. 2002 Nov;2(10):946-54.

Vaysberg M, Balatoni CE, Nepomuceno RR, Krams SM, Martinez OM. Rapamycin inhibits proliferation of Epstein-Barr virus-positive B-cell lymphomas through modulation of cell-cycle protein expression. Transplantation. 2007 Apr 27;83(8):1114-21.

Waldmann TA, Misiti J, Nelson DL, Kraemer KH. Ataxia-telangiectasis: a multisystem hereditary disease with immunodeficiency, impaired organ maturation, x-ray hypersensitivity, and a high incidence of neoplasia. Ann Intern Med. 1983 Sep;99(3):367-79.

Walker RC, Paya CV, Marshall WF, Strickler JG, Wiesner RH, Velosa JA, Habermann TM, Daly RC, McGregor CG. Pretransplantation seronegative Epstein-Barr virus status is the primary risk factor for posttransplantation lymphoproliferative disorder in adult heart, lung, and other solid organ transplantations. J Heart Lung Transplant. 1995 Mar-Apr;14(2):214-21.

Wasson S, Zafar MN, Best J, Reddy HK. Post-transplantation lymphoproliferative disorder in heart and kidney transplant patients: a single-centre experience. J Cardiovasc Pharmacol Ther. 2006 Mar;11(1):77-83.

Weisner RH. A long term comparison of Tacrolimus (FK 506) versus cyclosporine in liver transplantation : a report of the US FK506 Study Group. Transplantation 1998; 66:493-499.

Weissmann DJ, Ferry JA, Harris NL, Louis DN, Delmonico F, Spiro I. Posttransplantation lymphoproliferative disorders in solid organ recipients are predominantly aggressive tumors of host origin. Am J Clin Pathol. 1995 Jun;103(6):748-55.

Young L, Alfieri C, Hennessy K, Evans H, O'Hara C, Anderson KC, Ritz J, Shapiro RS, Rickinson A, Kieff E, et al. Expression of Epstein-Barr virus transformation-associated genes in tissues of patients with EBV lymphoproliferative disease. N Engl J Med. 1989 Oct 19;321(16):1080-5.

Younes BS, McDiarmid SV, Martin MG, Vargas JH, Goss JA, Busuttil RW, Ament ME. The effect of immunosuppression on posttransplant lymphoproliferative disease in pediatric liver transplant patients. Transplantation. 2000 Jul 15;70(1):94-9.

Part 2

Glomerulonephritis

6

Focal Segmental Glomerulosclerosis (FSGS) Recurrence in Kidney Allograft Recipients

Oktawia Mazanowska and Dorota Kamińska
Department of Nephrology and Transplantation Medicine Wrocław Medical University, Poland

1. Introduction

Primary or idiopathic focal and segmental glomerulosclerosis (FSGS) accounts for approximately 10% and 20% of cases of idiopathic nephrotic syndrome in children and adults, respectively. The primary pathophysiologic process appears to be an injury of glomerular visceral epithelial cells, so-called podocytes, followed by an initial proliferation of mesangial, epithelial and endothelial cells with subsequent collapse of glomerular capillary loops and eventual sclerosis. The most popular pathogenetic hypothesis suggests the involvement of one or more circulating plasma factor(s), that appears to be protein between 30 and 50 kD molecular weight, altering glomerular permeability to proteins and causing proteinuria. Familial forms of FSGS occur due to mutations of several podocyte protein genes. FSGS can be a secondary process as well. Regardless of the etiology, the natural history of the disease include: peripheral edema, refractory proteinuria, hypertension, and progressive loss of renal function. FSGS frequently recurs after kidney transplantation with the recurrence rate of 30% after first transplantation, and 80% or more in the subsequent transplants. Risk factors of recurrence include a rapid progression of the primary disease to chronic kidney disease (CKD) stage 5, younger recipient age, early onset of nephrotic range proteinuria after kidney transplantation and frequent loss of the first and subsequent allografts. Considerable number of patients with recurrent FSGS respond to plasmapheresis (PP), especially if instituted early in the course of disease and before glomerulosclerosis has been established. Combined therapy with PP and cyclophosphamide may be beneficial. Other treatments consists of intravenous cyclosporine (CsA) and oral steroids. In some patients successful treatment of recurrent FSGS with the anti-CD20 monoclonal antibody, rituximab, in conjunction with PP has been reported. As a symptomatic treatment the use of ACE inhibitors should be recommended.

2. FSGS in native kidneys

Focal segmental glomerulosclerosis (FSGS) first described by Arnold Rich in 1959 (1) is a clinicopathological entity, characterized by focal and segmental occurrence of lesions with mesangial sclerosis, obliteration of glomerular capillaries with hyalinosis and intracapillary foam cells, formation of adhesions between the glomerular tuft and Bowman's capsule, and podocyte hypertrophy. Clinically FSGS is characterized by nephrotic syndrome (NS) and progressive loss of renal function. It is the most common histopathologic diagnosis associated with idiopathic steroid-resistant NS in children, and one of the most frequent in adults, but in some patients, FSGS progress to CKD stage 5 without NS. Within 10 years of initial presentation, more than 50% of patients with FSGS develop CKD requiring renal replacement therapy (2). NAPRTCS 2007 Annual Report reveals that 14,3% of patients on dialysis and 11,4% of patients with renal transplant have FSGS as their primary diagnosis.

2.1 Pathogenesis of FSGS in native kidneys

The etiology of idiopathic FSGS and its post-transplant recurrence are still unclear; however, the recent studies on circulating permeability factor(s) (PF), genomics of podocin (NPHS2) and the emerging data on costimulatory molecules suggest an interplay of factors in different subgroups of patients with FSGS (3). Currently, FSGS is known to be due to an abnormality of the visceral epithelial cells (podocytes) of the glomerulus (4; 5). The morphological hallmark of primary FSGS is diffuse effacement of podocyte foot processes (usually > 80%), involving essentially all of the glomerular capillary loops. Damage of foot processes by the release of lymphokines/cytokines from T cells, possibly Th2 cells has been postulated (6). Transforming growth factor β (TGFβ) is probably a mediator of scarring by induction of apoptosis of podocytes and adherence of the parietal epithelial cells to the naked GBM. The familial, genetic forms of FSGS result from abnormalities in gene transcription controlling assembly of slit diaphragm, actin-based cytoskeleton, and adhesion complexes, which are essential for the podocyte function in maintaining an effective filtration barrier. Some of the gene mutations in patients with FSGS include podocin (NPHS2), nephrin (NPHS1), α actinin-4 (ACTN-4), CD2-associated protein (CD2AP), WT1 transient receptor potential cation 6 (TRPC6), and phospholipase ϵ C (PLCE1/NPHS3) (7). FSGS can also be a secondary process due to underlying conditions including obesity, HIV or parvovirus B19 infection, plasma cell proliferative disease, lithium or pamindronate treatment, urinary reflux, and heroin abuse. The amount of foot processes effacement in secondary FSGS (usually < 30%) can be used as a morphological clue to distinguish primary and secondary process. A decreased ratio of podocytes to the glomerular filtration surface area appears to be the leading mechanism of secondary FSGS (8).

2.2 Role of permeability factor(s) or intrinsic podocyte defect

The pathogenesis of FSGS is not fully clarified, but injury of podocytes is crucial. Shalhoub was the first to propose the presence of a circulating mediator secreted by T cells (9), named permeability factor (PF) by Savin's group with an anionic charge and affinity for protein A and galactose and low molecular weight (10; 11). Though several studies strongly suggest the importance of the T cell origin circulating PF, this factor has not been completely identified biochemically and may not be specific for FSGS (7). A putative PF of molecular weight between 30 and 50 kDa has been isolated from sera of patients with FSGS and increased glomerular permeability to albumin (P_{alb}) *in vitro* (12). Permeability factor(s) may exert direct effects on the nephrin and podocin in the podocyte or may alter phosphorylation of cellular proteins in the podocyte, influence the activity of serine proteases or induce of integrin-like kinase activity that leads to detachment of podocyte from GBM (11;13; 14). This factor inhibits also the synthesis of nitric oxide, probably by up-regulating asymmetric dimethyloarginine (ADMA) – an endogenous inhibitor of all nitric oxide synthases, with lose of anti-fibrotic effect in mesangium (15). Recently, McCarthy et al.

have identified a peptide - cardiotrophin-like cytokine 1 (CLC-1), which may be the presumed PF (16). Patients with a very high pretransplant level of PF had nearly 100% recurrence of their disease in the transplant kidney (12). Rarely PF may be present in patients with podocin (NPHS2) mutations. High pretransplant P_{alb} was found in 5 children with autosomal recessive podocin mutations, in which FSGS recurred after transplantation in four out of five (17). Since the PF is mildly anionic, it is unlikely that the effect of this factor is to neutralize the anionic sites on the GBM. Recent studies have suggested that there may be plasma factors that inhibit the PF (18; 19; 20). Furthermore, the net effect of the increased permeability may result from the absence or loss of an inhibitor for PF (19; 20). These inhibitory serum factors may be normal serum components such as apolipoproteins E and J (20). Further studies found that urine of patients with FSGS neutralize the PF activity of the serum, suggesting loss of an inhibitor in the urine (21), that may play a central role in the process after kidney transplantation and possibly also in the original disease (17). These findings suggest the deficiency of an inhibitor to the normally occurring PF as a primary cause for proteinuria. Alterations in the integrins (α3β1) that are involved in the attachment of podocytes to the GBM might be important in some forms of FSGS (8). Novel pathway of injury in FSGS are probably CD80/86, transmembrane proteins normally expressed on the surface of B-cells and other antigen-presenting cells, that are important players of costimulation. Reiser et al. reported the novel role of CD80 in podocytes as an inducible modifier of glomerular permselectivity (22).The knockout mice lacking CD80 were protected from lipopolysaccharide (LPS)-induced NS (22). In experimental model, LPS up-regulated CD80 expression on podocytes, resulting in rapid podocyte effacement and severe proteinuria. This link between an innate immune response and gene mutations regulating a slit-diaphragm components may represent a novel scheme for understanding the pathogenesis of recurrent FSGS in some patients (22).

2.3 Role of gene mutations for proteins exclusively expressed by podocytes

Recent studies on gene mutations encoding podocin and other components of slit-diaphragm have underscored the heterogeneity of the idiopathic forms of FSGS. Alterations of the slit-diaphragm assembly can lead to changes in the selective barrier function, resulting in proteinuria. The discovery of gene mutations of the slit-diaphragm exclusive proteins in familial NS represented a breakthrough in the research of mechanisms of NS in humans. Mutations of NPHS2 gene (encoding for podocin and localized on chromosome 1q25-31), are the most common cause of familial NS and sporadic inherited FSGS. Homozygous carriers of NPHS2 mutations develop massive proteinuria in early childhood, not responding to common therapies and progressing to CKD stage 5 (23; 24; 25). So, in children seek for podocin mutations is justified to avoid a useless prolonged course of corticosteroids because of steroid resistance. As a corollary, proteinuria should not recur in patients with NPHS2 mutations because the molecular defect of podocin should be vanished. But the recurrence of the FSGS is observed also in these patients. The recurrence of proteinuria after renal transplantation in homozygous carriers of podocin mutations is associated with high values of permeability activity for albumin (P_{alb}); which suggest a role of PF also in this inherited condition. Heterozygous carriers of NPHS2 mutations (including variants) present variable clinical phenotypes with later onset of proteinuria. Tsukaguchi et al. found that the R229Q heterozygous variant of NPHS2 (which is found in FSGS patients with the same frequency as in a normal population) appeared not to cause FSGS, but rather to enhance susceptibility to

FSGS in association with a second mutant NPHS2 allele (26). In authors material two out of 10 patients with FSGS in native kidneys revealed R229Q heterozygous variant and only one of them experienced recurrence of FSGS during the first month after transplantation (27).

3. FSGS recurrence after kidney transplantation

Recurrent FSGS after renal transplantation was described by Hoyer et al. in 1972 (28). Nowadays FSGS is the most common kidney disease known to recur after kidney transplantation and only a small proportion being *de novo*. Recurrence rate of FSGS in pediatric patients is 50% and 30% in adults (29). A reliable estimate is approximately 30% to 40% at a first graft, with an exponential increment of risk (up to 80%) at subsequent renal grafts (30; 31; 32; 33). Patients with recurrent FSGS have higher incidence of delayed graft function (DGF) and five-year graft loss rates 30-50% and up to 80% over a follow-up period of 10 years (27; 31; 34; 35; 36; 37). The most popular hypothesis suggests the involvement of one or more circulating PF altering renal permeability to proteins and causing proteinuria in allograft. According to this possibility, removal of the putative PF by plasmapheresis (PP) or selective procedures with protein A column associated with a course of immunosuppression would restore a good long-term outcome of the graft. Patients with high pretransplant P_{alb} activity have a higher risk of FSGS recurrence (30). The impact of recipient age on FSGS recurrence was confirmed by Bertelli et al. in patients without mutation of podocin with early recurrence of proteinuria in 44% of younger patients and in 23% of the older ones (30). It is taken as a proof of the existence of circulating PF(s) that are also putative effectors of original proteinuria in these patients (30).

3.1 FSGS recurrence in patients with NPHS2 mutation

Patients with clearly two pathogenic NPHS2 mutations, although have early onset of NS in native kidneys, have a very low risk (about 3%) of FSGS recurrence after kidney transplantation compared with non-NPHS2 FSGS patients (recurrence rate about 34%) (25; 30; 38). On the other hand, simple heterozygous NPHS2 mutations have a similar high recurrence as the non-familial forms (29). Recurrence of proteinuria after kidney transplantation in patients with homozygous NPHS2 mutation is caused by other pathomechanism because the transplant kidney is free from podocin mutation and the one possibility is the development of autoantibodies against the unmutated protein of the transplanted kidney, however, no antipodocin antibodies were detected (38). The alternative explanation is the co-presence of circulating PF in affected patients. In these patients good effects of plasmapheresis and/or augmented immunosuppressive treatment might support the hypothesis that possibly both genetic and endogenous systemic factors play a role in recurring pathology. Heterozygous NPHS2 mutation carriers (affected with only one NPHS2 mutation) should be distinguished from patients with two pathogenic mutations of the NPHS2 gene (homozygous or compound heterozygous mutation carriers); only the latter condition fulfill the genetic criteria of autosomal recessive disease. The percentage of patients with only one NPHS2 mutation was low (2-3%) given the fact that a second mutation has not been missed (38). Some of the homozygous carriers of podocin mutations present early recurrence of proteinuria after renal transplantation in association with high values of P_{alb}, which suggest a role of PF also in this inherited condition (30). Carraro et al. revealed the high pre-transplant P_{alb} activity in 5 children with inherited FSGS due to autosomal recessive podocin mutations (17). The post-transplant outcome was complicated in two (with 413G>A mutation) by recurrence of proteinuria after 10 and 300 days with high P_{alb} levels at onset that decreased to reach normal levels in the absence of proteinuria after the 7th cycle of PP. Co-incubation of serum with homologous nephrotic urine reduced P_{alb} to 0, whereas normal urine did not determine any change, which suggest loss of inhibitors in nephrotic urine. These data indicate that P_{alb} may be high also in NPHS2 mutated patients, probably resulting from loss of inhibitors in urine and lack of correlation of P_{alb} with proteinuria suggests a selective loss of inhibitors. In fact, high P_{alb} levels are strongly predictive of post-transplant recurrence of FSGS and P_{alb} is removed with *ex vivo* techniques such as PP and immunoabsorption. Loss of inhibitors may play a central role in the process, leading to recurrence in the allograft and possibly to proteinuria also in the original disease. (17).

3.2 Clinical manifestation and risk factors

Recurrent FSGS presents clinically with proteinuria or even full-blown nephrotic syndrome. Although recurrence of FSGS negatively influence kidney allograft survival, it has also been noticed that some individuals with proteinuria have adequate kidney function for years. Recurrence may be evident within days post-transplant (as early as the first 48 to 72 h), particularly in children (29; 38). Recurrence of FSGS can also develop any time within the first two years post-transplant. Multiple risk factors have been associated with recurrence of FSGS in the allograft. Children less than 15 years of age (generally between 6 and 15 yr), especially Caucasian white have a greater risk of recurrence (up to 40%) than do adults (36; 39). An aggressive course of primary FSGS prior to transplant, with a time interval between onset of the disease and CKD stage 5 less than 3 years is associated with higher recurrence rate (36). Both male gender and high pretransplantation panel-reactive antibodies (PRA) levels were noted to be independent risk factors for graft loss from recurrent disease. Also patients with mesangial hypercellularity in most of glomeruli as well as fewer sclerotic glomeruli have an increased incidence of recurrence (40; 41). Those with collapsing histology on native kidneys biopsy, tended to recur with the same histology and the presence of collapsing variant in the native kidney biopsy is a risk factor for recurrence (33; 42). Patients with history of prior transplant loss secondary to FSGS recurrence have a very high risk of recurrence in the current allograft, with rates as high as 80% in the second transplant and > 90% in the third and subsequent transplants (36; 43). Some studies have demonstrated higher rate of recurrence in recipients of living related grafts; probably due to closer HLA matching between living versus deceased donor or the phenotypic characteristics shared by related donor-recipient pairs that may render the kidney more susceptible to humoral factors. So some centers do not use living related allografts when transplanting particularly children (43). The more recent studies do not certify these findings, but with no advantage of graft survival in living donor transplants as observed in non-FSGS patients (44). In general living donation kidney transplantation should be avoided for children with FSGS and for adults with fulminant FSGS, but in patients not at high risk for recurrent FSGS or if the first graft showed prolonged function or was free of FSGS, living donor allografting could be considered, provided the fact that donor and recipient have been informed about the risk of disease recurrence associated with possible renal graft failure (38).

3.3 Laboratory and microscopic findings

There were no significant difference in serum creatinine concentration at the time of diagnosis between patients with and without FSGS (45). Proteinuria (at nephrotic range in many cases) and lipid levels were significantly greater in patients with FSGS (45).

Renal biopsy is often needed for definitive diagnosis, but early biopsies mostly show minimal changes on light microscopy. Effacement of foot processes on electron microscopy is the initial finding on renal biopsy, appearing within one week of recurrence. Light microscopy findings develop several weeks later (46). Hence, during the early post-transplant period, the diagnosis of FSGS recurrence, while suspected, is difficult to certify. Later, biopsies may show evidence of FSGS of the same histological subclass as in native kidneys (with 81% conformity) (47). ILPelaar et al. proposed three distinct patterns of recurrence: type I with fidelity to native disease (60%), type II with fidelity to native disease after a minimal change intermediate (20%), and type III with no fidelity to native disease (20%) (47). Arteriolar hyalinosis is more common in patients with FSGS than in patients without FSGS but the degree of interstitial fibrosis and tubular atrophy (IF/TA) was not significantly different (45).

4. Treatment of FSGS in kidney allograft recipients

Treatment strategies for recurrent FSGS are designed to inhibit secretion of the putative lymphocyte-derived PF by calcineurin inhibitors and enhance removal of PF by plasmapheresis (PP) or combined therapy with PP and cyclophosphamide. Recent reports have described the efficacy of anti-CD20 monoclonal antibody, rituximab, in conjunction with PP. Other treatments consists with intravenous cyclosporine (CsA) or high dose oral steroids. As a symptomatic treatment the use of ACE inhibitors may be recommended. But pharmacologic treatment options in recurrent FSGS are limited since most renal transplant recipients are already on maintenance steroids plus CsA or Tac, the medications most effective in the treatment of idiopathic FSGS as well (48). Because of the increased risk of graft loss in renal transplant recipients with FSGS, aggressive therapy should be recommended (37). The response of patients to PP seems to be completely individual. About 50% of patients with recurrent FSGS respond to PP, especially if instituted early in the course of disease and before glomerulosclerosis has been established. Individuals who develop recurrent FSGS after transplantation usually are given a trial of PP therapy (49). Some Centers have added oral Cyclophosphamide (2 mg/kg/day for 2 months) that reduces lymphocyte numbers and alters the balance of lymphocyte subsets or mycophenolate mofetil (MMF) to the PP protocol (40; 41). Therapeutical success in these studies have been variable. The other potentially benefit treatments is immunoadsorption with protein A columns followed by IVIG (38). Anti-proteinuric and anti-hypertensive effect of agents acting on renin-angiotensin system (ACEI and ARB) in patients with various nephropathies has been demonstrated also in recurrent FSGS (50), with 48-31% reduction of proteinuria, respectively, but with concern for graft dysfunction if early used post-transplant. Statins reduce the overall all-case as well as cardio-vascular mortality in post-transplant patients (51). The lipid-reducing treatment is significantly more common in patients with FSGS, and the level of proteinuria correlated significantly with cholesterol and TG levels. The use of lipid-lowering agents correlates with better graft prognosis; probably these drugs are used more commonly in older renal transplant recipients and with lower serum creatinine levels, and these two variables correlate with better graft survival or by pleiothropic effect of HMG-CoA reductase inhibitors on arteriolar endothelium (45). Hypercoagulable state is an important modifiable risk factor in NS also in recurrent FSGS. The work-up includes measuring of protein C, protein S, and anti-thrombin III levels and evaluating for presence of lupus anti-coagulant, anti-phospholipid and anti-cardiolipin antibodies, and for factor V Leiden mutations in the blood. In the presence of evidence for thrombophilia, continuous intravenous heparin infusion with a goal to maintain an activated partial thromboplastin time (aPTT) of 1,5 times baseline is recommended for the immediate post-transplant period (52). Typically i.v. heparin can be switched to s.c. enoxaparin after 48 h post-transplant. Argatroban has been used if heparin is contraindicated because of the presence of heparin antibodies (52). Long-term anti-coagulation is need for at least one year post-transplantation and can be achieved with warfarin (53). Following transplantation patients with FSGS should be initially monitored daily, then weekly for proteinuria with either 24-h urine protein collections or with spot urine protein/creatinine ratio. The increase in spot urine protein/creatinine ratio should be confirmed by 24-h urine protein collection and followed by kidney biopsy.

4.1 Plasmapheresis and immunoadsorptive therapies

Plasmapheresis and Protein A immunoadsorptive therapy have been considered in the management of recurrent FSGS because recognizing the role of circulating PF in the pathogenesis. With the clinical and experimental evidence, PP as a therapeutic modality should be efficient but there are no controlled trials and reports are based on small series of patients. Plasmapheresis is most beneficial when used early in the course of recurrent FSGS when recurrence occurs early post-transplant (54). Pediatric patients seem to have better outcomes in response to PP, with remission rate of 60% to 80% (33; 48). The PP protocols varies with number of PP sessions and most patients need between 8 and 12 treatments to achieve remission. The good results occurred using a protocol of plasma exchange (1,5 plasma volumes) for 3 consecutive days followed by every other day for a total of 9 treatments using 5% albumin replacement. Other typical PP prescription is 1-2 times plasma volume exchanges (usually 60 ml for every 1 kg body weight per session) and about 3-4 treatments per week until remission is achieved, usually about 10 sessions. Schachter et al. found that PP resulted in complete or partial remission in 75% of those with recurrence (3/12 complete and 5/12 partial remission; partial remission was defined when proteinuria was decreased by 50%) and 25% of patients remained dependent on regular plasma exchange to prevent recurrence of proteinuria (55). Prophylactic PP with 8 single-volume treatments over 2 weeks prior to transplantation has been attempted in patients at high risk for recurrence with variable outcome, in case reports success varied from 50% (56) to less significant benefit. Living donor transplant candidates received the first treatment one week before transplantation, and deceased donor transplants received the first treatment within 24 hours of transplant. The preemptive PP, in the week before transplantation, led to significant reduction in the rate of recurrence. But in the study of Gonzales et al. the preemptive PP (1-10 sessions) did not decrease the rate of recurrence after transplantation but was beneficial in treating high-risk patients with documented recurrence, who can achieve good graft survival (57). Some centers have added cyclophosphamide and/or mycophenolate mofetil (MMF - 2 g/day in two divided doses) to the PP protocol, but with variable results (40; 41). In report by Fuentes et al. FSGS recurrence rate was 56.3% after the first and 80% in the second transplant in children (33). Plasmapheresis treatment was carried out in 7 of 9 patients, achieving remission in six of them. Recurrence of FSGS limited graft survival (first year 66% vs 85%, third year 20% vs 68%). The report shows that PP can be effective in treating FSGS recurrence in children, although its effect on long-term graft survival seems to be more limited (33). Matalon et al. in a group of 13 adult renal transplant recipients from 3 transplant centers who underwent PP for recurrent FSGS found 50% or greater decline in proteinuria in 7 of 13 patients, but 3 of them (23%) remained PP-dependent (and required PP treatments every 2-4 weeks for up to 6 years to prevent progressive increase in proteinuria) (48). Five nonresponders progressed to CKD stage 5 over a mean time of 17 months from the recurrence. The only clinical parameter of prognostic significance was a short time interval between recurrence of FSGS and initiation of PP (48). Columns coated with staphylococcal protein A are used to treat FSGS because of the circulating factor affinity. In one study, patients were treated with protein A immunoadsorption columns with significant reduction of proteinuria and the decrease of proteinuria was about 82% at the end of the cycle (58).

4.2 Immunosuppression

Calcineurin inhibitors: The use of cyclosporine A (CsA) has not reduce the incidence of recurrent FSGS, but high doses ameliorate the clinical course of affected patients. There is consistent evidence that CsA diminishes or abolishes proteinuria. The exact mechanism of CsA in inducing remission is unknown, but immunosuppressive effects of CsA primarily result from inhibition of T helper cell activation and inhibition of release of cytokines/lymphokines, increase in glomerular cAMP as well as inhibition of glomerular PF or non-immunological effect with renal vasoconstriction. High-dose therapy with a goal to maintain high trough CsA blood level (recommended 125 to 200 ng/ml) suggest some beneficial effects (59). The reason of high whole blood CsA level is to overcome the effect of high serum cholesterol level in NS, because CsA is incorporated into the peripheral lymphocytes through LDL receptors on the cell surface. High blood level of LDL increase the amount of CsA bound to LDL and reduces the cellular uptake of LDL-CsA complex (60). In report of Salomon et al. in 14 out of 17 children treated with CsA (3mg/kg/day intravenously) for 3 weeks followed by an oral dosage to maintain trough levels between 200 and 300 ng/ml remission was achieved within 28 days (61). In other report the high-dose oral CsA (initially from 6 mg/kg/day in two divided doses) was necessary for inducting remission with complete and partial remission in 81% of treated patients (62). High dose CsA has also been used in connection with PP, but also the success was variable (38; 41; 62). Some experience in the treatment of FSGS has been reported with tacrolimus (initially at dose 0,15 - 0,1 mg/kg/day in two divided doses) and adjusted to the recommended trough blood level (5-10 ng/ml).

Rituximab: Rituximab is a chimeric mouse/human monoclonal antibody, acting on CD-20 surface marker of B-lymphocytes with selective depletion of B-lymphocytes. In transplantation rituximab is used to treat antibody-mediated rejection. Results of same very small cases series of rituximab in post-transplant recurrence of FSGS are inconsistent (63; 64). The typical regimen is 2-6 doses of 375 mg/m^2/dose of rituximab given once every one to two weeks. The efficacy of rituximab in recurrent FSGS is limited. The report of Rodriguez-Ferrero et al. summarize the effect of rituximab associated with PP treatment of 3 adult renal transplant recipients with recurrent FSGS after a 4th, a second or a third renal transplantation, respectively (65). All the patients were treated with PP once a week after recurrence; the first and second patients were treated with PP also before transplantation (133 and 62 sessions) to prevent FSGS recurrence. All of the patients received rituximab (375 $mg/m^2/wk$, 4 doses) and 1 PP session before each rituximab dose. The effectiveness of therapy was demonstrated by lack of peripheral CD19 cells after therapy. None of the patients treated with rituximab achieved complete remission, but in one patient proteinuria was reduced by 26%, in the second by 44% (65). Also Yabu et al. did not observed any advantage of rituximab therapy. Authors report 4 adult patients (3 women, 1 man; three of them received kidney transplant from living-donor) with early recurrent FSGS refractory or dependent on PP who received rituximab as sole therapy (total dose 2000 - 4200 mg). None of the patients treated with rituximab achieved remission in proteinuria, and one patient experienced early graft loss (66).

Corticosteroids: There are no data or controlled trials on corticosteroid (CS) as a sole treatment in recurrent FSGS, because patients are treated with CS in combination with CsA and/or PP. The caution is necessary when diminishing CS dosage after kidney transplantation in patients with FSGS in native kidneys (67).

In summary, even though there are no well-conducted studies, aggressive therapy of recurrent FSGS using plasmapheresis is considered to be a treatment of choice for this condition, with or without high-dose CsA, cyclophosphamide and/or MMF. However, the response is completely individual and many patients do not show improvement with any of these therapies (49).

5. Prognosis

Patients with FSGS often undergo renal transplantation because they are younger and have little comorbidity, and they are considered good transplant candidates (68). Unfortunately, recurrence of FSGS in the allograft is common. Once the FSGS has recurred in the allograft, loss of the graft occurs within 1 year in 50% to 80% of patients who do not receive any extra or specific treatment (41). FSGS patients who receive renal transplants have a 2-fold higher risk of losing graft at 10 years, compared to all patients transplanted for glomerulonephritis (37; 69). In report of Fuentes et al. in pediatric patients with recurrent FSGS graft survival was lower than in those with other etiologies of CKD (first year 75% vs 91%; 5th year 44% vs 78%) (33). In Schachter's material recurrence rate was 23% of patients with biopsy proven primary FSGS (55). Sener et al. have reported that post-transplant recurrence of FSGS may be associated with bilateral nephrectomy indicated in some patients with catastrophic NS (70). These patients should be monitored closely for early recurrence and may benefit from early PP treatment (70). The type of induction therapy for post-transplant immunosuppression is suggestive to have an effect on recurrence of FSGS as well, with higher incidence with the use of anti-lymphocyte sera (ALS) or anti-thymocyte globulin (ATG) in patients with primary FSGS. The use of ALS or ATG for initial induction therapy should be avoided in these patients because of increased recurrence rate of FSGS due to induction of certain T-cell subtypes and subsequent lymphokine/cytokine release and altering the slit-diaphragm (38). Although CsA seems to have no effect on the frequency of FSGS recurrence, there is evidence that CsA reduces proteinuria and prolongs graft survival in patients with recurrence after transplantation. Sirolimus should be used with care because of the increased possibility of recurrence (59). Although FSGS previously was associated with African-American race white recipients were at greater risk of graft loss resulting from recurrent disease. The mechanism of this association in unknown and should be investigated further (37).

The outcome of recurrent FSGS in a transplant kidney is variable, dependent on multiple factors and varies from immediate graft loss to slowly progressive proteinuria with chronic allograft injury to complete remission with no long-term consequences on the graft. Incidence of graft loss in the first 5 years post-transplant, in patients with recurrent FSGS varies, and is 20% to 50% (29). The data about the follow-up and outcome are inconsistent, not only in the graft survival rates, but also in risk factors of graft failure. In the report of Cosio et al. a significantly greater number of patients with FSGS lost their graft (39%) compared with 26% of patients with chronic allograft injury but without FSGS (45). Moroni et al. described the quite good outcomes of 52 renal transplants in 47 adults with FSGS (68). FSGS recurred in 12 out of 52 grafts (23%) and led to graft failure in 7 within 10 months. In the other 5 cases, proteinuria remitted and grafts were functioning 106 months after transplantation. The second recurrence developed in 62,5% of re-transplanted patients, who lost their first graft because of recurrence, and only one graft was lost. Patients with recurrence were more frequently male subjects (83% vs 40%), younger at diagnosis of FSGS (16 yr vs 24 yr) and of younger age at transplantation (28 yr vs 36 yr). Graft loss resulting from a second recurrence was lower than expected, and treatment with PP (in nonresponsive patients), steroids, CsA plus ACE inhibitors achieved either complete or partial remission in 80% of the cases (68).

6. *De novo* FSGS after kidney transplantation

De novo FSGS occurs in patients without the diagnosis of FSGS in native kidneys and develops more than 6 months posttransplant (45). The pathogenesis for *de novo* FSGS in allografts is unknown but two potential pathogenic mechanisms seem particularly attractive: CsA toxicity and hyperfiltration, triggered by hemodynamic stress in remnant nephrons following injury to the allograft by rejection or ischemia. In fact, *de novo* FSGS has been reported with sirolimus use (71). Primarily the glomeruli in the outer cortical region are involved with occlusive vascular changes and sometimes collapsing glomerulonephritis. The histological picture differ from recurrent FSGS, where the mild obliterative arteriolopathy preferentially involves the juxtamedullary glomeruli. Clinically, *de novo* FSGS presents with proteinuria and a less aggressive course than recurrent FSGS, but is also a negative independent predictor of graft survival. *De novo* FSGS in renal allografts most often is diagnosed in association with chronic allograft nephropathy or recurrent IgA nephropathy, transplant glomerulopathy, *de novo* membranous nephropathy but also may be not associated with other pathological conditions (45).

7. As summary

Due to increase incidence of FSGS and increasing numbers of FSGS patients coming to transplantation, the role of recurrent disease is becoming an area of greater concern to nephrologists and transplant physicians. The incidence of recurrence is generally accepted to be between 20% to 30%. Risk factors for and characteristics of recurrence include a rapid progression of the primary disease to CKD stage 5, early onset of nephrotic range proteinuria after allografting, frequent loss of the allograft, a high frequency of recurrence in subsequent allografts, and children less than 15 years of age. Some investigators have identified a circulating permeability factor, called the FSGS factor, that appears to be protein between 30 and 50 kD molecular weight. Logically, the association of PF with recurrence of FSGS guided to treat patients with plasmapheresis. The response of patients to PP seems to be completely individual. Modern immunosuppression regimens including tacrolimus, mycophenolate mofetil, sirolimus do not appear to provide additional benefit over older regimens with CsA and corticosteroids in preventing recurrence of FSGS. Patients with recurrence of FSGS clearly present a worse outcome than those who do not experience recurrent disease.

8. References

[1] Rich AR.: A hitherto undescribed vulnerability of the juxtamedullary glomeruli in lipoid nephrosis. Bulletin of the Johns Hopkins Hospital 1959; 100: 173-186
[2] Kitiyakara C., Edgers P., Kopp JB et al.: Twenty-one-year trend in ESRD due to focal segmental glomerulosclerosis in the United States. Am J Kidney Dis 2004; 44: 815-825
[3] Ghiggeri GM., Carraro M., Vincenti F.: Recurrent focal glomerulosclerosis in the era of genetics of podocyte proteins: theory and therapy. Nephrol Dial Transplant 2004; 19: 1036-1040
[4] Kretzler M.: Role of podocytes in focal sclerosis: defining the point of no return. J Am Soc Nephrol 2005; 16: 2830-2832
[5] Brenchley PE.: Vascular permeability factors in steroid-sensitive nephritic syndrome and focal segmental glomerulosclerosis. Nephrol Dial Transplant 2003; 18 (Suppl 6): vi21-25
[6] Van den Berg JG., Weening JJ.: Role of the immune system in the pathogenesis of idiopathic nephritic syndrome. Clin Sci 2004; 107: 125-136
[7] Woroniecki RP, Kopp JB.: Genetics of focal segmental glomerulosclerosis. Pediatr Nephrol 2007; 22: 638-644
[8] Chen CA., Hwang JC., Guh JY., et al.: Reduced podocyte expression of alpha3beta1 integrins and podocyte depletion in patients with primary focal segmental glomerulosclerosis and chronic PAN treated rats. J Lab Clin Med 2006; 147: 74-82
[9] Shalhoub RJ.: Pathogenesis of lipoid nephrosis: a disorder of T-cell function. Lancet 1974; 2: 556-560
[10] Savin VJ., McCarthy ET., Sharma R., et al.: Galactose binds to focal segmental glomerulosclerosis permeability factor and inhibits its activity. Transpl Res 2008; 151: 288-292;
[11] Sharma M., Sharma R., McCarthy ET., et al.: The focal segmental glomerulosclerosis permeability factor: biochemical characteristics and biological effects. Exp Biol Med 2004; 229: 85 -98
[12] Savin VJ., Sharma R., Sharma M., et al.: Circulating factor associated with increased glomerular permeability to albumin in recurrent focal segmental glomerulosclerosis. N Engl J Med 1996; 334: 878-838
[13] Hattori M., Akioka Y., Chikamoto H., et al.: Increase of integrin-linked kinase activity in cultured podocytes upon stimulation with plasma from patients with recurrent FSGS. Am J Transplant 2008; 8: 1550-1556;
[14] Carraro M., Zennaro C., Artero M., et al.: The effect of proteinase inhibitors on glomerular permeability induced in vitro by serum from patients with idiopathic focal segmental glomerulosclerosis. Nephrol Dial Transplant 2004; 19: 1969-1975
[15] Trachtman H., Futterweit S., Singhal PC., et al.: Circulating factor in patients with recurrent focal segmental glomerulosclerosis postrenal transplantation inhibits expression of inducible nitric oxide synthase and nitric oxide production by cultured rat mesangial cells. J Invest Med 1999; 47: 114-120
[16] McCarthy ET., Sharma M., Savin VJ.: Circulating permeability factors in idiopathic nephrotic syndrome and focal segmental glomerulosclerosis. Clin J Am Soc Nephrol 2010; 5: 2115-2121
[17] Carraro M., Caridi G., Bruschi M., et al.: Serum glomerular permeability activity in patients with podocin mutations (NPHS2) and steroid-resistant nephrotic syndrome. J Am Soc Nephrol 2002; 13: 1946-1952

[18] McCarthy ET, Sharma M., Sharma R., et al.: Sera from patients with collapsing focal segmental glomerulosclerosis increase albumin permeability of isolated glomeruli. J Lab Clin Med 2004; 143: 225-229
[19] Sharma R., Sharma M., McCarthy ET., et al.: Components of normal serum block the focal segmental glomerulosclerosis factor activity in vitro. Kidney Int 2000; 58: 1973-1979
[20] Candiano G., Musante L., Carraro M., et al.: Apolipoproteins prevent glomerular albumin permeability induced in vitro by serum from patients with focal segmental glomerulosclerosis. J Am Soc Nephrol 2001; 12: 143-15024
[21] Carraro M., Zennaro C., Candiano G., et al. : Nephrotic urine prevents increased rat glomerular albumin permeability induced by serum from the same patient with idiopathic nephritic syndrome. Nephrol Dial Transplant 2003; 18: 689-693
[22] Reiser J., von Gersdorff G., Loos M., et al. : Induction of B7-1 in podocytes is associated with nephrotic syndrome. J Clin Invest 2004; 113: 1390-1397
[23] Caridi G., Perfumo F., Ghiggeri GM.: NPHS2 (podocin) mutations in nephrotic syndrome. Clinical spectrum and fine mechanisms. Pediatr Res 2005; 57: 54R-61R
[24] Boute N, Gribouval D., Roselli S., et al.: NPHS2 gene, encoding the glomerular protein podocin is mutated in autosomal recessive steroid-resistant nephritic syndrome. Nat Genet 2000; 24: 349-352
[25] Weber S., Gribouval O., Esquivel EL., et al.: NPHS2 mutation analysis shows genetic heterogeneity of steroid-resistant nephritic syndrome and low post-transplant recurrence. Kidney Int 2004; 66: 571-579
[26] Tsukaguchi H., Sudhakar A., Le TC., et al.: NPHS2 mutations in late-onset focal segmental glomerulosclerosis: R229Q is a common disease allele. J Clin Invest 2002; 110: 1659-1666
[27] Mazanowska O., Kamińska D., Kościelska-Kasprzak K., et al: High risk of FSGS recurrence in kidney allograft recipients independent of heterozygous NPHS2 mutation. Adv Clin Exp Med 2008; 17: 207-212
[28] Hoyer JR., Vernier RL., Najarian JS., et al: Recurrence of idiopathic nephritic syndrome after renal transplantation. Lancet 1972; 2: 343-348
[29] Vinai M., Weber P., Seikaly MG.: Recurrence of focal segmental glomerulosclerosis in renal allograft: An in-depth review. Pediatr Tranplant 2010; 14: 314-325
[30] Bertelli R., Ginevri F., Caridi G., et al.: Recurrence of segmental glomerulosclersis after renal transplantation in patients with mutations of podocin. Am J Kidney Dis 2003; 41: 1314-1321
[31] Newstead CG.: Recurrent disease in renal transplants. Nephrol Dial Transplant 2003; 18 (Suppl 6): vi68-vi74
[32] Couser W.: Recurrent glomerulonephritis in the renal allograft: an update of selected areas. A one-center study of plasma exchange effects. Exp Clin Tranplant 2005; 3: 283-288
[33] Fuentes GM., Mesaguer CG, Carrion AP., et al.: Long-term outcome of focal segmental glomerulosclerosis after pediatric renal transplantation. Pediatr Nephrol 2010: 25: 529-534
[34] Baum MA: Outcomes after renal transplantation for FSGS in children. Pediatr Transplant 2004; 8: 329-333
[35] Hickson LJ, Gera M., Amer H ., et al.: Kidney transplantation for primary focal segmental glomerulosclerosis: Outcomes and response to therapy for recurrence. Transplantation 2009; 87: 1232-1239

[36] Tejani A., Stablein DH.: Recurrence of focal segmental glomerulosclerosis posttransplantation: a special report of the North American Pediatric Renal Transplant Cooperative Study. J Am Soc Nephrol 1992; 2: (Suppl 12): S256-S263
[37] Abbott K.C., Sawyers E.S., Oliver J.D.III, et al.: Graft loss due to recurrent focal segmental glomerulosclerosis in renal transplant recipients in the United States. Am J Kid Dis 2001; 37: : 366-373
[38] Weber S., Tönshoff B.: Recurrence of focal-segmental glomerulosclerosis in children after renal transplantation: clinical and genetic aspects. Transplantation 2005; 80: S128-S134
[39] Senggutuvan P., Cameron JS., Hartley RB., et al.: Recurrence of focal segmental glomerulosclerosis in transplant kidneys: analysis of incidence and risk factors in 59 allografts. Pediatr Nephrol 1990; 4: 21-28
[40] Cheong HI., Han HW., Park HW., et al.: Early recurrent nephrotic syndrome after renal transplantation in children with focal segmental glomerulosclerosis. Nephrol Dial Transplant 2000; 15: 78-81;
[41] Nathanson S., Cochat P., Andre JL., et al.: Recurrence of nephrotic syndrome after renal transplantation: influence of increased immunosuppression. Pediatr Nephrol 2005; 20: 1801-1804
[42] Thomas DB, Franceschini N., Hogan SL., et al.: Clinical and pathologic characteristics of focal segmental glomerulosclerosis pathologic variants. Kidney Int 2006; 69: 920-926
[43] First MR.: Living-related donor transplants should be performed with caution in patients with focal segmental glomerulosclerosis. Pediatr Nephrol 1995; 9 (Suppl): S40-S42
[44] Baum MA., Stablein DM., Panzarino VM., et al.: Loss of living donor renal allograft survival advantage in children with focal segmental glomerulosclerosis. Kidney Int 2001 59: 328-333
[45] Cosio F.G., Frankel W.L., Pelletier R.P., et al.: Focal segmental glomerulosclerosis in renal allografts with chronic nephropathy: implications for graft survival. Am J Kidney Dis 1999; 34: 731-738
[46] Requiăo-Moura LR., Moscoso-Solorzano GT, Franco MF., et al.: Prognostic factors associated with poor graft outcomes in renal recipients with post-transplant glomerulonephritis. Clin Transplant 2007; 21: 363-370
[47] IJpelaar D., Farris AB., Goemaere N., et al.: Fidelity and evolution of recurrent FSGS in renal allografts. J Am Soc Nephrol 2008; 19: 2219-2224
[48] Matalon A., Markowitz G.S., Joseph R.E., et al.: Plasmapheresis treatment of recurrent FSGS in adult renal transplant recipients. Clin Nephrol 2001; 56: 271-278
[49] Crosson J.T.: Focal segmental glomerulosclerosis and renal transplantation. Transplant Proc 2007; 39: 737-743.
[50] White CT., Macpherson CF., Hurley RM., Matsell DG.: Antiproteinuric effects of enalapril and losartan: A pilot study. Pediatr Nephrol 2003; 18: 1038-1043
[51] Navaneethan SD., Pansini F., Perkovic V., et al.: HMG CoA reductase inhibitors (statins) for people with chronic kidney disease not requiring dialysis. Cochrane Database Syst Rev 2009; (2): CD007784
[52] Morrissey PE., Ramirez PJ., Gohh RY., et al.: Management of thrombophilia in renal transplant patients. Am J Transplant 2002; 2: 872-876
[53] Kusyk T., Verran D., Stewart G., et al.: Increased risk of hemorrhagic complications in renal allograft recipients receiving systemic heparin early posttransplantation. Transplant Proc 2005; 37: 1026-1028

[54] Pradhan M., Petro J., Palmer J., et al.: Early use of plasmapheresis for recurrent post-transplant FSGS. Pediatr Nephrol 2003; 18: 934-938
[55] Schachter M.E., Monahan M., Radhakrishnan J., et al.: Recurrent focal segmental glomerulosclerosis in the renal allograft: single center experience in the era of modern immunosuppression. Clin Nephrol 2010; 3: 173-181
[56] Gohh RY., Yango AF, Morrissey PE., et al.: Preemptive plasmapheresis and recurrence of FSGS in high-risk renal transplant recipients. Am J Transplant 2005; 5: 2907-2912
[57] Gonzales E., Ettenger R., Rianthavorn P., et al.: Preemptive plasmapheresis and recurrence of focal segmental glomerulosclerosis in pediatric renal transplantation. Pediatr Transplant 2011; doi: 10.1111/j. 1399-3046.2011.01478.x. [Epub ahead of print]
[58] Dantal J., Bigot E., Bogers W., et al.: Effect of plasma adsorption on protein excretion in kidney-transplant recipients with recurrent nephrotic syndrome. N Engl J Med 1994; 330: 7-14
[59] Skhiri H., Morelon N., Noël LH., et al.: Unusual post-transplantation recurrence of focal segmental glomerulosclerosis which resolved with cyclosporine but nor with sirolimus. Transplant Int 2005; 18: 458-460
[60] Hirano T., Akashi T., Oka K., et al.: Serum cholesterol levels and kidney transplantation outcome: attenuation of cyclosporine efficacy? Transplantation 2001; 71: 659-660
[61] Salomon R., Gagnadoux MF., Niaudet P.: Intravenous cyclosporine therapy in recurrent nephritic syndrome after renal transplantation in children. Transplantation 2003; 75: 810-814
[62] Raafat RH., Kalia A., Travis LB., Divens C.: High dose oral cyclosporin therapy for recurrent focal segmental glomerulosclerosis in children. Am J Kidney Dis 2004; 44: 50-56.
[63] Apeland T., Hartmann A. : Rituximab therapy in early recurrent focal segmental sclerosis after renal transplantation. Nephrol Dial Transplant 2008; 23: 2091-2094
[64] Hristea D., Hadaya K., Marangon N., et al. : Successful treatment of recurrent focal segmental glomerulosclerosis after kidney transplantation by plasmapheresis and rituximab. Transplant Int 2007; 20: 102-105
[65] Rodriguez-Ferrero M., Ampuero J., Anaya F.: Rituximab and chronic plasmapheresis therapy of nephritic syndrome in renal transplantation patients with recurrent focal segmental glomerulosclerosis. Transplant Proc 2009; 41: 2406-2408
[66] Yabu JM., Ho B., Scandling JD., Vincenti F.: Rituximab failed to improve nephrotic syndrome in renal transplant patients with recurrent focal segmental glomerulosclerosis. Am J Transplant 2008; 8: 222-227.
[67] Greenbaum LA., Hanevold CD.: Nephrotic syndrome after conversion to alternate day steroids in two children with a history of recurrent FSGS. Pediatr Transplant 2003; 7: 395-399
[68] Moroni G., Gallelli B., Quaglini S., et al.: Long-term outcome of renal transplantation in adults with focal segmental glomerulosclerosis. Transplant Int 2009; 23: 208-216
[69] Briganti E.M., Russ GR., McNeil J.J., et al.: Risk of renal allograft loss from recurrent glomerulonephritis. N Engl J Med 2002; 347: 103-109
[70] Sener A., Bella AJ., Nguan C., et al.: Focal segmental glomerular sclerosis in renal transplant recipients: predicting early disease recurrence may prolong allograft function. Clin Transplant 2009; 23: 96-100
[71] Letavernier E., Bruneval P., Mandet C., et al.: High sirolimus levels may induce focal segmental glomerulosclerosis *de novo*. Clinical J Am Soc Nephrol 2007; 2: 326-333

Therapeutic Approach to Focal and Segmental Glomerulosclerosis (FSGS) Recurrence in Kidney Transplant Recipients

Guillaume Canaud[1,2,3], Frank Martinez[1,2] and Christophe Legendre[1,2]
[1]*Université Paris Descartes, Rue de l'Ecole de Médecine, Paris,*
[2]*Service de Transplantation et Unité de soins intensifs, Hôpital Necker, Paris,*
[3]*INSERM U845, Hôpital Necker*
[4]*Service de Néphrologie Pédiatrique, Hôpital des Enfants Malades, Paris,*
France

1. Introduction

Primary focal and segmental glomerulosclerosis (FSGS) is the most frequently acquired disease leading to end stage renal disease (ESRD) in children (NAPRTCS 2004, annual report)[1-6]. The recurrence of FSGS after kidney transplantation is frequent (20-40%) and is associated with poor graft survival[7-13]. The pathophysiology of primary FSGS remains uncertain, but secretion of a circulating factor is suspected to play a key role in excessive glomerular permeability. Excepted for the recurrence of FSGS with a previous allograft, this event is almost unpredictable and characterized by early nephrotic range proteinuria. Some studies have identified risk factors for recurrent FSGS in children, including rapid progression to ESRD, young age of onset of FSGS and, of course loss of a previous graft from recurrent disease but none of these studies can clearly separate the patients who will or will not be affected by recurrence. The treatment of recurrence remains controversial, and most reports relate to use of plasma exchange (PE) in uncontrolled trials with relatively small groups of patients and conflicting results. PE and protein immunoadsorption can markedly reduce urinary protein excretion and induce complete remission in some cases, but they usually fail to achieve sustained remission[14-16]. Steroids and cyclosporine are also associated with inconstant remission and act through different ways. More recent therapeutic approach seems promising and need to be evaluated in large trials. This review summarizes the various therapeutic approaches to FSGS recurrence.

2. Pathogenesis of FSGS recurrence

To better understand the therapeutic approaches to FSGS recurrence, we might briefly comment on its pathogenesis. The pathophysiology of this disease remains largely unclear and is thought to involve at least three types of cells (T-cells, B-cells and podocyte) and a circulating factor. In 1974, to explain what would later be called idiopathic nephrotic syndrome (INS), Shalhoub proposed the hypothesis (Shalhoub hypothesis) of T-cell dysfunction resulting in the secretion of *"circulating chemical mediator toxic to an immunologically innocent glomerular basement membrane"*[17]. Although knowledge of the pathogenesis of this disease has improved in recent years, novel therapeutics have not ameliorated the rate of its recurrence. T-cell disorder is still suspected based on much evidence for Th2 cytokine bias in INS. Sahali et al. were the first to report that T-cells from INS patients are driven toward a Th2 phenotype[18]. By screening a cDNA library from T-cells of patients with relapsing INS they found that overexpression of truncated c-maf–inducing protein (Tc-mip) induced c-maf, transactivated the IL-4 gene, and downregulated IFNγ expression, characteristic of Th2 commitment[19]. These data were also supported by the observation of increased expression of cytoplasmic IL-13 mRNA in T-cells from patients with relapsing INS as compared to those in remission and control patients[20]. Furthermore, overexpression of IL-13 in Wistar rats led to minimal change disease confirming the potential role for Th2 predominance in pathophysiology of INS[21]. More recently, the expression level of soluble ST2 protein (sST2), a marker of Th2 cells that is predicted to be regulated by c-maf, was investigated in a population of patient with FSGS recurrence after transplantation[22]. The level of sST2 were increased after transplantation in patients with recurrence compared to the control group; however this protein was unable to induce podocyte injury *in vitro* suggesting that it could be a marker of recurrence but might not be implicated in the pathogenesis of recurrence. Using a humanized mouse model, Sellier-Leclerc et al showed that $CD34^+$ stem cells, unlike $CD34^-$ peripheral blood mononuclear cells, from patients with INS induced albuminuria, suggesting the involvement of immature differentiating cells rather than mature peripheral T-cells in the pathogenesis of the disease[23]. Thus, there is evidence for T-cell dysfunction in INS, but treatments targeting T-cells (calcineurin inhibitors, anti-CD3 or anti-CD52) are not completely effective in preventing or treating FSGS recurrence. Furthermore, there is recent evidence for B-cell participation from a report of remission obtained with rituximab (anti-CD20)[24]. Indeed, it is accepted that primary FSGS is the consequence of a complex interaction between T- and B-cells leading to the secretion of a circulating factor targeting podocyte. The presence of a circulating vascular permeability factor implicated in the physiopathology of this disease is highlighted by (i) the early recurrence of nephrotic syndrome after transplantation[25], (ii) the fact that serum from patients with recurrent FSGS infused in rats can induce albuminuria[26], (iii) the occurrence of a transient nephrotic syndrome in newborn infants of women with FSGS[27], and (iv) the efficiency of plasma exchange and/or immunoadsorption at inducing remission[15]. The biochemical characteristics of this factor, however, are still unknown. Its molecular weight is suspected to be between 30-100 kDa, and Dantal et al. suggested that it could be a part of a complex with immunoglobulins[28]. Recently, Savin et al. found that this circulating factor had a high affinity for galactose and that all its activity was eliminated by galactose affinity columns[29]. The third player in this complex disease is the podocyte. Podocytes are a post-mitotic cell, arrested in G2/M phase of the cell cycle, and do not proliferate. It has been postulated that the circulating factor and/or immune cells directly interact with podocytes, and could induce the redistribution of the protein of the slit diaphragm, the loss of nephrin and/or podocin and the effacement of the foot processes, a hallmark of podocyte injury[30]. It has been suggested that foot processes effacement, if reversed, can lead to the restoration of glomerular architecture, which is typically observed in steroid-sensitive minimal change disease. The failure of repair mechanisms promotes podocyte detachment, apoptosis, podocyte depletion and FSGS. A special situation is collapsing glomerulopathy, a specific variant of FSGS. Findings in human suggest that podocytes may undergo a proliferative state and phenotypic changes in collapsing glomerulopathy[31, 32]. Importantly, evidence suggests that, in addition to podocytes, parietal epithelial cells also participate in the collapsing glomerulopathy phenotype[33]. Recently, Reiser et al. described the expression of the co-stimulatory molecule B7.1 on podocytes[34]. The significance of the presence of this molecule is not clearly understood and remains speculative.

3. Treatment of FSGS recurrence

Despite the introduction of new immunosuppressive regimens, discovery of cyclosporine, and use of induction therapies, the incidence of FSGS recurrence has remained unchanged[35-37]. In the case of recurrence treatments are not standardized, and show inconstant results. Most reports concern children and involve a small number of patients[15, 38-46]. Cyclosporine (CsA) has shown some degree of efficacy in pediatric subjects[43, 44]. Indeed, intravenous CsA after FSGS recurrence was associated with a drastic decrease of proteinuria in 82% of patients, although PE was added in some resistant cases[43]. A few reports have studied the use of tacrolimus to prevent or to treat recurrence. The results of these studies are almost inconstant[47, 48]. Due to the presence of a circulating permeability factor, most transplant teams test the efficacy of PE, which substitutes the plasma of the patient with either plasma from healthy pooled donors, albumin or colloidal substance. This treatment usually induces a reduction in proteinuria and, in some cases complete remission. Determining when to begin PEs, their frequency, duration and optimal stop time are challenging to determine, and most remissions are PE-dependant. Others supporting approaches have also been used, such as anti-human immunoglobulin affinity immunoadsorption and tryptophan immunoadsorption[28, 49].

We recently conducted a non-randomized pilot trial of intensive and prolonged multiple treatment of FSGS recurrence in adult kidney transplant recipients[50]. As this complex disease involves systemic immune dysregulation targeting podocyte, we used a strategy of concomitant high dose steroids and intravenous CsA not only for their immunosuppressive properties, but also for their podocyte cytoskeleton stabilization properties, and with PE sessions. Glucocorticoid receptors are present on podocytes, have anti apoptotic properties *in vitro* [51] and could stabilize the actin cytoskeleton[52]. CsA acts directly on podocytes by blocking calcineurin-mediated dephosphorylation of synaptopodin and stabilizes actin cytoskeleton[53]. We decided to add PE sessions based on the presence of the circulating factor and an increased five-year allograft survival rate in our own experience. Indeed, from January 1994 to December 2004, we observed that the five-year allograft survival rate was 55% in cases of FSGS recurrence (R group), compared to 93% in cases without recurrence (NR group) ($p<0.01$). In the R group, patients who benefited from PE had an increased five-year allograft survival rate (91%) similar to the NR group, whereas patients not treated with PE had a five-year allograft survival rate of only 40% ($p<0.01$).

The details of our therapeutic strategy consisted of high dose of oral steroids (1 mg/kg/d) for the first 4 weeks followed by tapering according to the following sequence: 0.75 mg/kg/d for 2 weeks, 0.5 mg/kg/d for two weeks, 0.25 mg/kg/d for two weeks and 0.2 mg/kg/d or a maximal daily dose of 10 mg thereafter. We used 14 days of intravenous CsA (2 mg/kg, targeting a blood level between 200 and 400 ng/ml) followed by oral treatment, targeting C2 levels between 1,200 and 1,400 ng/ml. PEs were performed with 5% albumin replacement (three sessions per week for three weeks, followed by two sessions per week for three weeks, one session per week until month 3, two sessions per month until month 5, and once per month until month 9). Once remission was obtained, an angiotensin-converting enzyme inhibitor and/or angiotensin receptor blocker were introduced. Rescue with rituximab therapy was anticipated in case of failure. The primary endpoint was the induction of a complete (<0.3 g per 24H) and sustained (>12 months) remission of proteinuria. The treatment was started after 3 days of nephrotic-range proteinuria without spontaneous improvement. Of 286 kidney transplant procedures performed between September 2005 and March 2007 at our institution, 18 were performed in patients with primary FSGS. After transplantation these individuals were carefully monitored for proteinuria and ten (56%, eight men, two women) exhibited recurrence. The mean age at the onset of primary FSGS in native kidneys was 19.1 ± 14.8 years, leading to ESRD 8.1 ± 8.6 years later. The mean duration of hemodialysis was 2.8 ± 2.4 years. For nine of the patients, this transplant was their first; the remaining patient had received two previous kidney transplants, both of which had been quickly lost due to recurrence. After kidney transplantation, all patients received an immunosuppressive regimen including prednisone, mycophenolate mofetil, oral CsA (n=10) or tacrolimus (n=8), along with an induction of either basiliximab (n=12) or antithymocyte globulin (Thymoglobulin®, n=6). Proteinuria occurred immediately after transplantation in six patients (60%) and early post-transplant in the remaining four (range 4-55 days). Recurrence was associated with massive proteinuria (mean 12 ± 11 g/day). We began PE within the first ten days of diagnosis in all patients, while high-dose steroids and intravenous CsA were initiated at the time of diagnosis. Complete proteinuria remission was achieved in all patients at a mean of 22.9 ± 6.6 days post-diagnosis. Three months after diagnosis, all patients were still in complete remission (mean proteinuria 0.16 ± 0.09 g/day) and all but one patient remained in remission at one year (mean proteinuria 0.19 ± 0.29 g/d). In the nine patients with complete remission, PE was tapered gradually until month 9 and then stopped. During early follow-up (mean 15.8 ± 3.3 months), none of these nine patients relapsed. At one year post-transplant, mean serum creatinine was 121 ± 29μmol/l and the measured iohexol glomerular filtration rate was 68.5 ± 18ml/min. The patient who failed to obtain sustained remission of proteinuria was the individual who had undergone a third kidney transplant. In this patient, proteinuria recurred when the frequency of PE was tapered to less than once per week. Rituximab infusion was attempted, and after two doses circulating B-cells were completely depleted (CD19 < 1/mm^3). Proteinuria was maintained in the range 1-2 g/day with PE administered twice per month.

Long term follow-up (34.2 ± 6.7 months) of this cohort revealed that all these patients were still in complete remission with a mean proteinuria level of 0.11 ± 0.07 g/day and a mean serum creatinine of 122.6 ± 18 μmol/l. The patient in partial remission went into complete remission by maintaining PE (two times per month). During the follow-up, none of these patients developed diabetes, cancer or severe infectious disease. Indeed, long-term follow-up of our cohort revealed that intensive treatment of FSGS induces not only an excellent short term response but also a complete and sustained remission of proteinuria without significant immunosuppressive regimen-associated adverse effects.

We then considered whether the treatment administered in case of FSGS recurrence impacted the pathological features of FSGS during the post-transplant course. To address this question, we retrospectively studied 77 patients from January 1984 to December 2007, including both children and adults with primary FSGS who underwent renal transplantation[54]. Of these, 42 patients experienced a recurrence of nephrotic-range proteinuria. After kidney transplantation, recurrence of proteinuria occurred immediately in 32 of the 42 cases (children, n = 28; adults, n = 4), early in 9 of the 42 cases (children, n = 4; adults, n = 5) and late in 1 of the 42 case (adult, n = 1). Briefly, at time of recurrence, day 6 to day 60 days after transplantation, no glomerular lesion was observed in 32 of 33 biopsies and we considered them as minimal change disease. Only one patient had already developed a FSGS lesion. At month 3, FSGS lesions were observed in 11 of 39 cases, and at month 12, they were observed in 14 of 37 cases. Interestingly, 17 of the 42 patients went into complete and sustained remission, and none of them developed FSGS. On the other hand, patients who never achieved complete and sustained remission developed FSGS lesions. These data suggest continuing intensive treatments if no FSGS lesion are observed on transplant biopsies.

4. Other available treatments

4.1 Preemptive PE

A few studies of preemptive PE have been reported that show inconstant efficacy and lack a control group. In 2005, Gohh et al conducted a prospective study to test whether pre-transplant PE could prevent recurrence of primary FSGS in high risk patients[55]. A high risk of FSGS recurrence was defined by a rapid evolution toward ESRD (n= 4) or prior allograft loss due to recurrence (n= 6). Patients were subjected to a course of eight PE sessions over 2 weeks in the immediate peri-operative period. Recipients of living donor kidneys initiated PE treatments 1 week before transplantation and completed their course at the end of the first post-operative week. Recipients of cadaver kidneys underwent an initial PE within 24 h of implantation. FSGS recurred in 3 of 10 patients, each of whom had lost prior transplants to recurrent FSGS. Two of these progressed to ESRD and the third had significant renal dysfunction. The authors conclude that PE may decrease incidence of FSGS recurrence in this particular population (rate of recurrence expected without PE: 60%). This therapeutic approach is difficult to organize in case of deceased donors, which is the major group of donors in many countries including our own. Furthermore, PE session before or soon after transplantation, may increase the risk of major bleeding despite the finding that no adverse event were reported in the previous study. This approach would also lead to excessive treatment in 50% of patients.

4.2 Rituximab

In 2006, Pescovitz et al reported complete remission after infusion of rituximab in a young transplant recipient[24]. After kidney transplantation this child rapidly developed FSGS recurrence resistant to PE and CsA and at month 5 developed a post-transplantation lymphoproliferative disease (PTLD). After six infusions of rituximab to treat the PTLD, proteinuria disappeared suggesting a possible interaction between B- and T-cells that leads to the secretion of permeability factor. Since that report, many transplant teams have tested the ability of rituximab to treat FSGS recurrence with inconstant results[56-59]. In fact, rituximab seems to induce remission in about 50% of cases, but some questions remain unsolved. When should the infusion begin: as an induction therapy or at time of recurrence? How many infusions should be administered, given that depletion of circulating B-cells does not always correlate with lymphoid organ depletion[60]? What are the long term side effects of this treatment? To date, no consensus has emerged, and double-blind studies are needed to determine the therapeutic potential of rituximab.

4.3 Anti-CTLA4

The co-stimulation molecule B7.1 is normally expressed on antigen presenting cells and B-cells. Recently, Reiser et al found that B7.1 is also expressed on podocyte and could be upregulated in many proteinuric states[34]. Again, the significance of the presence of this molecule is not clearly understood and remains speculative. To date, no published studies have evaluated blockade of this co-stimulation pathway for the treatment of FSGS recurrence.

4.4 Anti-TNFα

TNFα mRNA was found to be upregulated in macrophages preceding the development of nephrotic syndrome in Buffalo/Mna rats[61]. Furthermore, a high level of TNFα mRNA was detected in mononuclear cells from patients with FSGS[62]. Anti-TNFα therapy was recently tested in a child with resistant FSGS recurrence[63] and induced transient complete remission, but every relapse was sensitive to anti-TNFα infusion.

4.5 Retinoic acid, Roscovitine and cyclin dependant kinase inhibitor

Collapsing glomerulopathy recurrence is a situation in which podocytes can proliferate. Using *in vitro* and *in vivo* mouse models, retinoic acids were found to be efficient at reducing podocyte proliferation and proteinuria[64]. An on going study is evaluating treatment of collapsing glomerulopathy in native kidneys using retinoic acid (NCT00098020).

4.6 Galactose

Recently, Savin et al. found that the circulating factor has a high affinity for galactose, and that its activity can be removed by use of galactose affinity columns[29]. This group and one another reported a significant reduction in proteinuria following administration of galactose along with others therapeutics[29, 65]. A clinical trial (NCT00098020) is recruiting patients to treat primary FSGS in native kidney with galactose. Galactose has an excellent safety profile and could be an interesting therapeutic candidate.

5. Conclusion

Primary FSGS remains mysterious with a poorly understood pathogenesis. Recurrence is still frequent and associated with a poor allograft prognosis. We clearly must increase our knowledge of the pathogenesis of this disease to better identify specific risk factors for recurrence and design more specific therapeutic strategies. Our pilot study, although limited by a small population size, provides very encouraging results. Combined and intensive therapy showed a markedly beneficial effect on early proteinuria recurrence in this cohort of adult kidney transplant recipients. These preliminary results require confirmation on a larger scale with extensive follow-up. We have also described patients who went into complete and sustained remission and did not develop FSGS; patients who never achieved complete and sustained remission developed FSGS lesions. New therapeutics such as rituximab, anti-TNFα, galactose and retinoic acid should be evaluated in randomized double-blind studies. A better understanding of the molecular function of podocytes give hope that new therapeutics will be available in the next future.

6. References

[1] Habib R, Levy M, Gubler MC. Clinicopathologic correlations in the nephrotic syndrome. Paediatrician 1979;8(5-6):325-48.

[2] Cameron JS. The enigma of focal segmental glomerulosclerosis. Kidney Int Suppl 1996;57:S119-31.
[3] Haas M, Meehan SM, Karrison TG, Spargo BH. Changing etiologies of unexplained adult nephrotic syndrome: a comparison of renal biopsy findings from 1976-1979 and 1995-1997. Am J Kidney Dis 1997;30(5):621-31.
[4] Braden GL, Mulhern JG, O'Shea MH, Nash SV, Ucci AA, Jr., Germain MJ. Changing incidence of glomerular diseases in adults. Am J Kidney Dis 2000;35(5):878-83.
[5] Kitiyakara C, Eggers P, Kopp JB. Twenty-one-year trend in ESRD due to focal segmental glomerulosclerosis in the United States. Am J Kidney Dis 2004;44(5):815-25.
[6] Filler G, Young E, Geier P, Carpenter B, Drukker A, Feber J. Is there really an increase in non-minimal change nephrotic syndrome in children? Am J Kidney Dis 2003;42(6):1107-13.
[7] Cameron JS, Senguttuvan P, Hartley B, et al. Focal segmental glomerulosclerosis in fifty-nine renal allografts from a single centre; analysis of risk factors for recurrence. Transplant Proc 1989;21(1 Pt 2):2117-8.
[8] Dantal J, Baatard R, Hourmant M, Cantarovich D, Buzelin F, Soulillou JP. Recurrent nephrotic syndrome following renal transplantation in patients with focal glomerulosclerosis. A one-center study of plasma exchange effects. Transplantation 1991;52(5):827-31.
[9] Ingulli E, Tejani A. Incidence, treatment, and outcome of recurrent focal segmental glomerulosclerosis posttransplantation in 42 allografts in children--a single-center experience. Transplantation 1991;51(2):401-5.
[10] Dantal J, Soulillou JP. Relapse of focal segmental glomerulosclerosis after kidney transplantation. Adv Nephrol Necker Hosp 1996;25:91-106.
[11] Tejani A, Stablein DH. Recurrence of focal segmental glomerulosclerosis posttransplantation: a special report of the North American Pediatric Renal Transplant Cooperative Study. J Am Soc Nephrol 1992;2(12 Suppl):S258-63.
[12] Artero ML, Sharma R, Savin VJ, Vincenti F. Plasmapheresis reduces proteinuria and serum capacity to injure glomeruli in patients with recurrent focal glomerulosclerosis. Am J Kidney Dis 1994;23(4):574-81.
[13] Pardon A, Audard V, Caillard S, et al. Risk factors and outcome of focal and segmental glomerulosclerosis recurrence in adult renal transplant recipients. Nephrol Dial Transplant 2006;21(4):1053-9.
[14] Savin VJ, Sharma R, Sharma M, et al. Circulating factor associated with increased glomerular permeability to albumin in recurrent focal segmental glomerulosclerosis. The New England journal of medicine 1996;334(14):878-83.
[15] Dantal J, Bigot E, Bogers W, et al. Effect of plasma protein adsorption on protein excretion in kidney-transplant recipients with recurrent nephrotic syndrome. The New England journal of medicine 1994;330(1):7-14.
[16] Artero M, Biava C, Amend W, Tomlanovich S, Vincenti F. Recurrent focal glomerulosclerosis: natural history and response to therapy. Am J Med 1992;92(4):375-83.
[17] Shalhoub RJ. Pathogenesis of lipoid nephrosis: a disorder of T-cell function. Lancet 1974;2(7880):556-60.
[18] Sahali D, Pawlak A, Valanciute A, et al. A novel approach to investigation of the pathogenesis of active minimal-change nephrotic syndrome using subtracted cDNA library screening. J Am Soc Nephrol 2002;13(5):1238-47.

[19] Grimbert P, Valanciute A, Audard V, et al. Truncation of C-mip (Tc-mip), a new proximal signaling protein, induces c-maf Th2 transcription factor and cytoskeleton reorganization. The Journal of experimental medicine 2003;198(5):797-807.
[20] Yap HK, Cheung W, Murugasu B, Sim SK, Seah CC, Jordan SC. Th1 and Th2 cytokine mRNA profiles in childhood nephrotic syndrome: evidence for increased IL-13 mRNA expression in relapse. J Am Soc Nephrol 1999;10(3):529-37.
[21] Lai KW, Wei CL, Tan LK, et al. Overexpression of interleukin-13 induces minimal-change-like nephropathy in rats. J Am Soc Nephrol 2007;18(5):1476-85.
[22] Bruneau S, Le Berre L, Herve C, et al. Potential role of soluble ST2 protein in idiopathic nephrotic syndrome recurrence following kidney transplantation. Am J Kidney Dis 2009;54(3):522-32.
[23] Sellier-Leclerc AL, Duval A, Riveron S, et al. A humanized mouse model of idiopathic nephrotic syndrome suggests a pathogenic role for immature cells. J Am Soc Nephrol 2007;18(10):2732-9.
[24] Pescovitz MD, Book BK, Sidner RA. Resolution of recurrent focal segmental glomerulosclerosis proteinuria after rituximab treatment. The New England journal of medicine 2006;354(18):1961-3.
[25] Hoyer JR, Vernier RL, Najarian JS, Raij L, Simmons RL, Michael AF. Recurrence of idiopathic nephrotic syndrome after renal transplantation. Lancet 1972;2(7773):343-8.
[26] Zimmerman SW. Increased urinary protein excretion in the rat produced by serum from a patient with recurrent focal glomerular sclerosis after renal transplantation. Clinical nephrology 1984;22(1):32-8.
[27] Lagrue G, Branellec A, Niaudet P, Heslan JM, Guillot F, Lang P. [Transmission of nephrotic syndrome to two neonates. Spontaneous regression]. Presse Med 1991;20(6):255-7.
[28] Dantal J, Godfrin Y, Koll R, et al. Antihuman immunoglobulin affinity immunoadsorption strongly decreases proteinuria in patients with relapsing nephrotic syndrome. J Am Soc Nephrol 1998;9(9):1709-15.
[29] Savin VJ, McCarthy ET, Sharma R, Charba D, Sharma M. Galactose binds to focal segmental glomerulosclerosis permeability factor and inhibits its activity. Transl Res 2008;151(6):288-92.
[30] Kim BK, Hong HK, Kim JH, Lee HS. Differential expression of nephrin in acquired human proteinuric diseases. Am J Kidney Dis 2002;40(5):964-73.
[31] Canaud G, Bruneval P, Noel LH, et al. Glomerular Collapse Associated With Subtotal Renal Infarction in Kidney Transplant Recipients With Multiple Renal Arteries. Am J Kidney Dis 2009.
[32] Bariety J, Nochy D, Mandet C, Jacquot C, Glotz D, Meyrier A. Podocytes undergo phenotypic changes and express macrophagic-associated markers in idiopathic collapsing glomerulopathy. Kidney international 1998;53(4):918-25.
[33] Dijkman HB, Weening JJ, Smeets B, et al. Proliferating cells in HIV and pamidronate-associated collapsing focal segmental glomerulosclerosis are parietal epithelial cells. Kidney international 2006;70(2):338-44.
[34] Reiser J, von Gersdorff G, Loos M, et al. Induction of B7-1 in podocytes is associated with nephrotic syndrome. The Journal of clinical investigation 2004;113(10):1390-7.
[35] Raafat R, Travis LB, Kalia A, Diven S. Role of transplant induction therapy on recurrence rate of focal segmental glomerulosclerosis. Pediatric nephrology (Berlin, Germany) 2000;14(3):189-94.

[36] Gagnadoux MF. Ask the expert. Does antibody induction therapy with daclizumab or basiliximab increase the risk of recurrence of post-transplant focal segmental glomerulosclerosis? Pediatric nephrology (Berlin, Germany) 2002;17(4):305.

[37] Hubsch H, Montane B, Abitbol C, et al. Recurrent focal glomerulosclerosis in pediatric renal allografts: the Miami experience. Pediatric nephrology (Berlin, Germany) 2005;20(2):210-6.

[38] Laufer J, Ettenger RB, Ho WG, Cohen AH, Marik JL, Fine RN. Plasma exchange for recurrent nephrotic syndrome following renal transplantation. Transplantation 1988;46(4):540-2.

[39] Ingulli E, Tejani A, Butt KM, et al. High-dose cyclosporine therapy in recurrent nephrotic syndrome following renal transplantation. Transplantation 1990;49(1):219-21.

[40] Cochat P, Kassir A, Colon S, et al. Recurrent nephrotic syndrome after transplantation: early treatment with plasmaphaeresis and cyclophosphamide. Pediatric nephrology (Berlin, Germany) 1993;7(1):50-4.

[41] Dall'Amico R, Ghiggeri G, Carraro M, et al. Prediction and treatment of recurrent focal segmental glomerulosclerosis after renal transplantation in children. Am J Kidney Dis 1999;34(6):1048-55.

[42] Cheong HI, Han HW, Park HW, et al. Early recurrent nephrotic syndrome after renal transplantation in children with focal segmental glomerulosclerosis. Nephrol Dial Transplant 2000;15(1):78-81.

[43] Salomon R, Gagnadoux MF, Niaudet P. Intravenous cyclosporine therapy in recurrent nephrotic syndrome after renal transplantation in children. Transplantation 2003;75(6):810-4.

[44] Raafat RH, Kalia A, Travis LB, Diven SC. High-dose oral cyclosporin therapy for recurrent focal segmental glomerulosclerosis in children. Am J Kidney Dis 2004;44(1):50-6.

[45] Deegens JK, Andresdottir MB, Croockewit S, Wetzels JF. Plasma exchange improves graft survival in patients with recurrent focal glomerulosclerosis after renal transplant. Transpl Int 2004;17(3):151-7.

[46] Valdivia P, Gonzalez Roncero F, Gentil MA, et al. Plasmapheresis for the prophylaxis and treatment of recurrent focal segmental glomerulosclerosis following renal transplant. Transplant Proc 2005;37(3):1473-4.

[47] McCauley J, Shapiro R, Ellis D, Igdal H, Tzakis A, Starzl TE. Pilot trial of FK 506 in the management of steroid-resistant nephrotic syndrome. Nephrol Dial Transplant 1993;8(11):1286-90.

[48] Kessler M, Champigneulles J, Hestin D, Frimat L, Renoult E. A renal allograft recipient with late recurrence of focal and segmental glomerulosclerosis after switching from cyclosporine to tacrolimus. Transplantation 1999;67(4):641-3.

[49] Bussemaker E, Passauer J, Franz T, Gross P. Tryptophan immunoadsorption strongly reduces proteinuria in recurrent nephrotic syndrome. Nephrol Dial Transplant 2001;16(6):1270-2.

[50] Canaud G, Zuber J, Sberro R, et al. Intensive and prolonged treatment of focal and segmental glomerulosclerosis recurrence in adult kidney transplant recipients: a pilot study. Am J Transplant 2009;9(5):1081-6.

[51] Wada T, Pippin JW, Marshall CB, Griffin SV, Shankland SJ. Dexamethasone prevents podocyte apoptosis induced by puromycin aminonucleoside: role of p53 and Bcl-2-related family proteins. J Am Soc Nephrol 2005;16(9):2615-25.
[52] Ransom RF, Lam NG, Hallett MA, Atkinson SJ, Smoyer WE. Glucocorticoids protect and enhance recovery of cultured murine podocytes via actin filament stabilization. Kidney international 2005;68(6):2473-83.
[53] Faul C, Donnelly M, Merscher-Gomez S, et al. The actin cytoskeleton of kidney podocytes is a direct target of the antiproteinuric effect of cyclosporine A. Nature medicine 2008.
[54] Canaud G, Dion D, Zuber J, et al. Recurrence of nephrotic syndrome after transplantation in a mixed population of children and adults: course of glomerular lesions and value of the Columbia classification of histological variants of focal and segmental glomerulosclerosis (FSGS). Nephrol Dial Transplant 2009.
[55] Gohh RY, Yango AF, Morrissey PE, et al. Preemptive plasmapheresis and recurrence of FSGS in high-risk renal transplant recipients. Am J Transplant 2005;5(12):2907-12.
[56] Gossmann J, Scheuermann EH, Porubsky S, Kachel HG, Geiger H, Hauser IA. Abrogation of nephrotic proteinuria by rituximab treatment in a renal transplant patient with relapsed focal segmental glomerulosclerosis. Transpl Int 2007;20(6):558-62.
[57] Hristea D, Hadaya K, Marangon N, et al. Successful treatment of recurrent focal segmental glomerulosclerosis after kidney transplantation by plasmapheresis and rituximab. Transpl Int 2007;20(1):102-5.
[58] Kamar N, Faguer S, Esposito L, et al. Treatment of focal segmental glomerular sclerosis with rituximab: 2 case reports. Clinical nephrology 2007;67(4):250-4.
[59] Yabu JM, Ho B, Scandling JD, Vincenti F. Rituximab failed to improve nephrotic syndrome in renal transplant patients with recurrent focal segmental glomerulosclerosis. Am J Transplant 2008;8(1):222-7.
[60] Leandro MJ, Cambridge G, Edwards JC, Ehrenstein MR, Isenberg DA. B-cell depletion in the treatment of patients with systemic lupus erythematosus: a longitudinal analysis of 24 patients. Rheumatology (Oxford, England) 2005;44(12):1542-5.
[61] Le Berre L, Herve C, Buzelin F, Usal C, Soulillou JP, Dantal J. Renal macrophage activation and Th2 polarization precedes the development of nephrotic syndrome in Buffalo/Mna rats. Kidney international 2005;68(5):2079-90.
[62] Bakr A, Shokeir M, El-Chenawi F, El-Husseni F, Abdel-Rahman A, El-Ashry R. Tumor necrosis factor-alpha production from mononuclear cells in nephrotic syndrome. Pediatric nephrology (Berlin, Germany) 2003;18(6):516-20.
[63] Leroy S, Guigonis V, Bruckner D, et al. Successful anti-TNFalpha treatment in a child with posttransplant recurrent focal segmental glomerulosclerosis. Am J Transplant 2009;9(4):858-61.
[64] He JC, Lu TC, Fleet M, et al. Retinoic acid inhibits HIV-1-induced podocyte proliferation through the cAMP pathway. J Am Soc Nephrol 2007;18(1):93-102.
[65] De Smet E, Rioux JP, Ammann H, Deziel C, Querin S. FSGS permeability factor-associated nephrotic syndrome: remission after oral galactose therapy. Nephrol Dial Transplant 2009;24(9):2938-40.

8

Post-Transplant Glomerulonephritis in Live-Donor Renal Transplant Recipients: Clinical Course and Risk Factors

Ahmed Akl, Hany Adel and Ehab Wafa
Urology and Nephrology center, Mansoura, Egypt

1. Introduction

Kidney transplantation is the treatment of choice for end-stage renal disease. It offers better quality of life and minimizes the mortality risk for patients when compared with maintenance dialysis therapy **(Chailimpamontree W, et al., 2009).** Little data are available concerning the impact of the post-transplantation glomerulonephritis (GN) on graft outcome **(Gaston R, 2006)**. The post-transplant glomerulonephritis may be *de novo* GN or recurrence of the original kidney disease. *De novo* GN appear to have poorer prognosis than the recurrent type. Different types of glomerulonephritis were reported to recur in the graft with different recurrence rates **(Briganti EM, et al., 2002).** The recurrent glomerulonephritis was reported to be important cause of impaired graft function and consequent graft loss **(Choy B. et al., 2006)**. Studies on recurrent disease are difficult since not all patients have undergone native kidney biopsy or it was non-representative. The reported incidence of recurrent GN is thus judged by clinical suspension and could be over- or under-estimates of the true incidence **(Hariharan S, 2000).** Precise diagnosis of recurrent disease in view of concomitant histological features of chronic allograft nephropathy or chronic drug nephrotoxicity by calcineurine inhibitors is often difficult to be determined **(Requião-Moura LR, et al., 2007).** There is accumulating evidence that recurrent GN is an important and clinically relevant cause of graft loss in the long-term follow-up of renal allograft recipients. It was reported that recurrent GN is considered to be the third most common cause for graft loss 10 years after kidney transplantation. The risk of graft loss from recurrence was found to be increased from 0.6% during the first year post-transplant to 8.4% after 10 year of follow up **(Briganti EM, et al., 2002)**. The introduction of newer immunosuppressive agents and induction protocols improved the graft survival. The improvement of graft survival was through the direct reduction of the incidence of acute rejection. The incidence of post-transplant glomerulonephritis whether recurrence or de novo was not influenced **(Hariharan S, et al., 2000).** The aim of our study is to focus on the incidence, risk factors of GN after kidney transplantation and their impact on the graft function & survival.
The risk for allograft loss as a result of PTGN is thus an important factor in the decision to proceed with transplantation, and an accurate understanding of the probability of PTGN is essential for the transplant team, the patient, and a potential live donor **(Choy B, et al., 2006).** There was a marked disparity in risk for PTGN according to histological type; the

most common forms were IgA nephropathy and FSGS, whereas all other forms occurred in less than 1% of patients **(Worawon Chailimpamontree, et al., 2009).** The prognosis of each of the forms depend on various factors, including the severity or type of histological lesion **(Little M, et al., 2006),** or whether the disease is recurrent or de novo **(Bela Ivanyi, 2008).** There is as yet no effective treatment for PTGN, although intensive plasma exchange or Rituximab may be of benefit in some cases of FSGS **(Gossmann J, et al., 2007).**

2. Classification of post transplantation GN (PTGN):

Recurrent and De Novo glomerular diseases can be classified according to clinical criteria **(William A. Golgert, 2008):**

1. **True recurrence**: Native kidney disease and transplant kidney disease are the same as confirmed by kidney biopsies.
2. **Transplant glomerulopathy:** Unknown primary disease. Biopsy-proven transplant kidney disease is possibly the same disease as the native kidney disease; however, the native kidney diagnosis was never documented by renal biopsy.
3. **De novo**: Biopsy-proven kidney disease that occurs in the transplant kidney is different from the native kidney disease.

Histological classification can be divided into four types, according to the type of the disease **(William A. Golgert, 2008):**

a. **Recurrence of primary GN**: Recurrent FSGS, membranoproliferative GN (MPGN), IgA nephropathy (IgAN), Henoch-Schönlein purpura, membranous nephropathy (MN).
b. **Recurrence of secondary GN**: Systemic lupus erythematosus (SLE), hemolytic uremic syndrome/thrombotic thrombocytopenic purpura (HUS-TTP), rapidly progressive-crescentic GN, anti–glomerular basement membrane (anti-GBM) disease.
c. **Recurrence of metabolic or systemic disease**: Diabetic nephropathy, oxalosis, amyloidosis, Fabry disease, scleroderma, cystinosis, fibrillary GN.
d. **De novo diseases**: Anti-GBM disease in patients with Alport syndrome, MN, FSGS.

3. Diagnosis of GN after renal transplantation

Proteinuria and hematuria remain the hallmark findings suggesting recurrence of GN. Many transplant centers do not include a urinalysis for detecting proteinuria and hematuria as part of their routine transplant surveillance or even for some patients with worsening renal function before transplant renal biopsy. In a majority of renal transplant patients who undergo renal biopsy, tissue is not routinely submitted for immunofluorescence (IF) and for electron microscopy (EM), which is essential for the diagnosis of some forms of GN. Patients with early or mild recurrence of IgAN, MN, and lupus nephritis thus easily receive a misdiagnosis. There is no unified approach for evaluating renal transplant patients for the diagnosis of recurrent GN after renal transplantation **(William A. Golgert, 2008)**. The challenges in diagnosis of post transplantation GN are numerous and include (1) misdiagnosis or mislabeling of native kidney disease, (2) lack of a unified approach in using diagnostic tools for the diagnosis of recurrent GN, and (3) difficulties in differentiating GN from drug toxicity and alloantigen-dependant chronic immunologic damage to the transplant kidney **(Hariharan S, 1999)**.

4. Recurrent glomerulonephritis post-renal transplantation

Recurrent disease is a significant cause of allograft failure estimated to affect 1-8 % grafts **(Cameron JS, 1991)**, **(Floege J, 2003)** and **(Ramos EL, et al., 1994).** Accumulating evidence indicates that recurrent glomerulonephritis is the third most important cause of renal allograft loss at 10 years after transplantation. All forms of glomerular disease can recur after transplantation, but the likelihood of recurrence differs according to type. Focal

Usually recur > 50 %	
- Adverse effects (graft loss > 5%)	• 1ry Hemolytic Uremic Syndrome (HUS). • 1ry oxalosis • Dense deposit disease • Collapsing FSGS
- Little or no adverse effects	• DM • Systemic light chain disease
Commonly recur (5- 50 %)	
Adverse effects	• FSGS • MPGN I. • Anti-Neutrophilic-CytoplasmicAntibody(ANCA) diseases (Wegner'sgranulomatosis–microscopic polyarteritis) • Progressive systemic sclerosis • Sickle cell nephropathy
Little or no adverse effects	• IgA nephropathy • Henoch-schönlein purpura • Amyloidosis
Rarely recur (< 5%)	
- Adverse effects	• Anti-GBM
- Little or no adverse effects	• SLE • Fabry's disease
Recurrence reported (too few cases)	• Thrombotic Thrombocytopenic Purpura (TTP) • Adenosine phosphoribosyl transferase deficiency • Familial fibronectin glomerulopathy • Lipoprotein glomerulopathy
Never recur 0 %	
- Unique complications	• Hereditary nephritis/Alport's syndrome (Anti-GBM disease) • Congenital nephrosis(nephrotic syndrome)
- No unique complication	• Poly Cystic Kidney Disease (PCKD). • Osteo-onchodysplasia (nail-patella) • Acquired cystic disease • 2ry HUS(infection) • 2ry focal segmental glomerulosclerosis • Familial focal segmental glomerulosclerosis • Post-infectious acute GN

Table 1. Frequency and clinical significance of recurrent renal diseases

segmental glomerulosclerosis (FSGS), membranoproliferative glomerulonephritis, IgA nephropathy and idiopathic diarrhea-negative hemolytic uremic syndrome often recur **(Bela Ivanyi, 2008).** Isografts (identical twins) have the highest recurrence rate **(Glassock RJ, et al., 1968).** Frequency and clinical significance of recurrence varies with the disease **(Peter J. Morris, et al., 2008)** as shown in table (1).

5. Risk of recurrence

The recurrence rates vary for different types of glomerulonephritis, and the risk of subsequent graft loss also differs as shown in table (2) **(Bela Ivanyi, 2008).**

Type of glomerulonephritis	Clinical recurrence rate (% of recipients)	Rate of graft loss
FSGS	20-40	20
Membranous GN	10-30	50
MPGN type I	20-33	High
MPGN type II	67-100	34-66
Anti-GBM nephritis	<5	Can occur
ANCA-positive crescentic GN	0-20	8
IgA Nephropathy	7-30	3-16
Iopathic D- HUS	33-82	90

Table 2. Risk of Recurrence and Graft Loss for Different Types Glomerulonephritis

Only 1ry focal segmental glomerulosclerosis and MPGN recur with sufficient frequency and aggressiveness to affect graft survival **(Briganti E, et al., 2002)** and **(Busch GJ, et al., 1995)**. Recurrent GN is diagnosed by exclusion of donor-transmitted disease and de novo GN. It has a negative impact on graft survival and causes 8.4% allograft losses by 10 years in recipients with renal failure from GN **(Briganti E, et al., 2002)**. The relative impact of recurrent GN increases as graft survival lengthens, or in some population in whom 1ry GN is prevalent or severe, the clinical course and severity of recurrent glomerular disease often copies that of the patient's original disease **(Chadban S, 2001),** except for patients with vasculitis and lupus nephritis; these conditions usually controlled by transplantation immunosuppression. Focal segmental glomerulosclerosis (20%-50% recurrence rate) and dense deposit disease (50%-90% recurrence rates) have the worst prognosis and together constitute 55%-60% of all recurrent GN **(Bela Ivanyi, 2008).** Membranous GN recurs in 29%-50%, MPGN type I recurs in 20%-33%, and IgA nephropathy recurs in 58%, although with limited early (but increased later) clinical impact **(Chadban S, 2001).** Diabetic glomerulopathy also may recur but with variable clinical effects, Eighty to 100 percent of diabetic transplant recipients develop histological changes of recurrent diabetic nephropathy (DN). The time of development of nephropathy may be as little as six years post-transplantation **(Bhalla V, et al., 2003).** However, the incidence of DN as a cause of graft failure is poorly studied and has been thought to be rare **(Siddqi N, et al., 2005).**

6. Minimal change glomerulonephritis

Fourteen cases of renal transplant recipients developing nephrotic syndrome with minimal glomerular abnormalities have been reported although the cases do not represent true recurrence of a disease **(Cheigh JS, et al., 1980).** The prognosis is variable and follow-up often very short but in some reports there is progression to renal failure **(Gephardt GN, et al., 1988).** It is notable that re-biopsy in two patients showed focal segmental glomerulosclerosis (FSGS) **(Hoyer JR, et al., 1972).** Not all of the reports included venography or other imaging to exclude renal vein thrombosis and drug-associated effects are impossible to rule out.

7. Focal Segmental Glomerulosclerosis (FSGS)

FSGS has the greatest clinical impact of recurrent glomerular disease because of its high recurrence rate, poor intermediate outcome, and the number of young patients with FSGS who undergo transplantation **(Briganti EM, et al., 2002)**. Graft loss from recurrent FSGS predicts recurrence in 70% of subsequent allografts, and most of these fail, possibly precluding that individual from future transplantation **(Briganti EM, et al., 2002).** Frequency of recurrence of focal segmental glomerulosclerosis and clinical progress of FSGS is an important problem in pediatric practice as it is responsible for about 10% of childhood idiopathic nephrotic syndrome **(Kibert S, et al., 1994).** The prognosis is poor with about one-third of patients progressing to end-stage renal failure within 5 years **(Kershaw DB, et al., 1994).** Recurrence of nephrotic syndrome after renal transplantation in patients with FSGS was first reported in 1972 **(Hoyer JR, 1972).** Those individuals who do experience recurrent disease are also at high risk of delayed graft function. The recurrence rate varies with different series, but a large North American experience **(Tejani A, et al., 1992)** reported 27 out of 132 patients (20.5%), and in Europe in the same year Broyer M et al reported a rate of 20% in a series collected by the Paediatric European Dialysis and Transplant Association **(Broyer M, et al., 1992).**

More recent North American experience was reported in 1998 **(Hariharan S, et al., 1998),** 1557 renal transplants performed at a single centre between 1984 and 1994 were reviewed and FSGS was discovered in 25 patients. Some individuals will have proteinuria but adequate renal function for a number of years **(Stephanian E, et al., 1992).** A retrospective analysis of a cohort of 29 paediatric patients who received 32 grafts between 1987 and 1998 in Northern Italy was published in 1999 **(Dall'Amico R, et al., 1999).** In these individuals, proteinuria of >1g/day occurred in 15 (52%) after the first transplant and in three out of three who received a second graft. The proteinuria almost always occurred early, in 14 out of 18 occasions in this report within the first month. In about 70% of cases a transplant biopsy was performed. Recurrence of proteinuria was associated with a poor outcome compared with those individuals who did not experience recurrent disease. In the latter group normal renal function after a mean follow up of 44 months was reported **(Dall'Amico R, et al., 1999).**

Recurrence of disease is not invariably associated with a dire prognosis. For five out of eight patients aged <25 years who lost primary renal transplants to recurrence FSGS, there was prolonged function of the graft of between 4 and 10.5 years **(Stephanian E, et al., 1992).** Although one review article has recommended bilateral native nephrectomy as a prophylactic measure prior to transplantation, in the text the only reference is to a paper which points out that the manoeuvre will make the diagnosis of a recurrent FSGS posttransplantation easier **(Srivasta RN, et al., 1994).** Familial focal and segmental glomerulosclerosis, although rare, is important to recognize, as it is a different syndrome to idiopathic FSGS of childhood. A recent large multinational survey identified 26 families with multigenerational involvement and 34 families with more than one individual in a single generation affected **(Conlon PJ, et al., 1999).** Patients presented on average in their third or fourth decade and, important in the context of recurrent disease post-transplantation, 41 individuals received a renal transplant and only one experienced recurrent disease; overall 10-year graft survival was 62%. A similarly good outcome after transplantation has been reported by others. Adults with 'secondary' FSGS, for example due to renal artery stenosis or some other long standing conditions that lead to renal insufficiency, would not be expected to be at risk of recurrent disease in a renal transplant.

8. Risk factors for recurrent FSGS

It is notable that certain factors, particularly age <15 years **(Cameron JS, 1991 and Ingulli E, et al., 1991),** aggressive clinical course of the original disease with time from diagnosis to end-stage renal failure of less than 3 years **(Cameron JS, 1991 and Cheong HI, et al., 2000),** and diffuse mesangial proliferation (DMP) on native biopsy **(Conlon PJ, et al., 1999 and Senguttuvan P, et al., 1990),** are considered predictive of relapse. There is no 'cut off' that separates by age those patients destined to experience recurrence and those who will not **(Dall'Amico R, et al., 1999).** Although in general age <15 years is considered to have a poor prognosis there is evidence that, within the pediatric group, those aged >6 years have a less poor prognosis. In a pediatric registry report in 1990, only 17% of children who were aged <6 years had relapse of nephrotic syndrome after transplantation compared with 40% of those aged >6 years at the time of diagnosis of the original glomerular disease **(Rizzoni G, et al. 1991).** In the Northern Italian experience **(Dall'Amico R, et al. 1999),** there was no difference in the gender distribution or age at onset of dialysis between the group with and without recurrent disease. However, the mean interval between diagnosis and end-stage renal failure was significantly shorter in the group with recurrence. Disease duration from onset to dialysis was <2 years in nine of 15 patients with recurrent FSGS and two of 14 patients with non-recurrent FSGS (P<0.014). The importance of the native glomerular histology was explored in a publication that reported on 24 children who received 37 transplants. The native renal histology that was divided into three groups: pure FSGS, FSGS with focal mesangial proliferation (FMP) and FSGS with different mesangial Proliferation (DMP) **(Striegel JE, et al., 1986).** The finding of mesangial proliferation had a sinister prognosis for subsequent graft function.

9. Laboratory tests to predict recurrent FSGS

The reported observation that sera from patients with a recurrent FSGS causes an immediate profound increase in the albumin permeability of isolated rat glomeruli clearly offers the exciting possibility that at least the risk of recurrent disease for an individual patient could be more accurately predicted **(Savin V,et al., 1996).** Subsequent experiments that have separated the sera obtained mostly during therapeutic apheresis into sub-fractions have demonstrated that the permeability factor is a protein of molecular weight between 30 and 50 kDa **(Sharma M, et al., 1999).** A Northern Italian group examined pre-transplant serum samples from 25 patients tested in an in vitro assay of glomerular permeability to albumin. FSGS recurred in 11 of 13 children who tested positive for the permeability factor and four of 12 patients with a negative test **(Dall'Amico R, et al., 1999).**

10. Membranous Nephropathy (MN)

Recurrence of membranous nephropathy (MN) in the transplant is infrequent, with most studies reporting rates between 10 and 30 percent **(Choy BY, et al., 2006 and Cosyns JP, et al., 1998).** The mean time to recurrence, which typically presents as nephrotic range proteinuria, is approximately 10 months **(Josephson MA, et al., 1994).** Affected patients appear to have more aggressive initial disease as evidenced by progression to end-stage renal failure at a mean of four years **(Josephson MA, et al., 1994).** Recurrent disease can lead to loss of the graft **(Cosyns JP, et al., 1998 and Briganti EM, et al., 2002).** Perhaps the best estimate of the incidence of graft loss due to recurrent membranous nephropathy was provided by a study of 1505 renal transplant recipients with a history of end-stage renal disease due to biopsy-proven glomerulonephritis **(Briganti EM, et al., 2002).** Among the 81 patients with membranous disease, the incidence of allograft loss at 10 years due to recurrent disease was 12.5 percent (CI of 7.3 to 21.6 percent). Initial studies suggested that patients with living-related transplants are at higher risk for recurrence **(Berger BE, et al., 1983).** Although this hypothesis remains unproven, recurrent disease may occur earlier in living-related as compared to deceased donor transplants **(Josephson MA, et al., 1994).**

11. Membrano-Proliferative GN (MPGN)

Both idiopathic type 1 (mesangial and subendothelial deposits) and the less common type 2 (dense-deposit disease) MPGN commonly recur after renal transplantation **(Denton MD, et al., 2000).** Although these disorders have different sites of electron dense deposits, they are both associated with the other classic histologic changes of MPGN: increased glomerular cellularity and a double contour appearance of the glomerular basement membrane due to mesangial cell interposition and new basement membrane formation.

11.1 Type 1 MPGN

The reported rate of recurrent disease in idiopathic type 1 MPGN has usually ranged between 20 and 30 percent **(Glicklich D, et al., 1987 and Floege J, 2003),** although the incidence in children may be somewhat higher **(Habib R, et al., 1987).** Reported recurrence rates may represent an overestimate, since similar histologic changes can occur as part of chronic transplant rejection (transplant glomerulopathy) **(Cheigh JS, et al., 1980).** Nevertheless, findings on electron microscopy (such as the absence of immune complex deposition in transplant glomerulopathy) may help distinguish between these two disorders **(Andresdottir MB, et al., 1998).** Patients with recurrent disease may remain asymptomatic, although the majority of patients with recurrent MPGN tend to present with proteinuria, hematuria and hypertension. Hypocomplementemia may be associated with recurrent disease **(McLean RH, et al., 1976),** however, disease recurrence can occur in the absence of this finding. There is no proven beneficial therapy for the treatment of recurrent idiopathic MPGN, although the combination of aspirin and dipyridamole may stabilize renal function, similar to its efficacy in primary MPGN **(Glicklich D, et al., 1987).**

11.2 Type 2 MPGN

Type 2 MPGN "dense deposit disease" tends to recur more frequently than type 1 MPGN, ranging from 50 to 100 percent in various series **(Choy BY, et al., 2006).** Affected patients typically presented within one year following transplantation with non-nephrotic range proteinuria. Graft loss due to recurrent disease is thought to occur in only 10 to 20 percent of cases, although some centers have reported rates as high as 30 to 50 percent **(Braun MC, et al., 2005 and Andresdottir MB, et al., 1999).**

11.3 Type 3 MPGN

Type 3 MPGN is an immune complex disease which is similar to type 1 but with prominent subepithelial deposits and a complex disruption of the glomerular basement membrane. Little is known concerning recurrent disease among patients with type 3 MPGN who undergo renal transplantation. A case report described a patient with end-stage renal disease due to type 3 MPGN who presented with hematuria and proteinuria 16 months after undergoing renal transplantation **(Morales JM, et al., 1997)**. Renal biopsy revealed recurrent type 3 MPGN; graft loss occurred seven years later.

12. Immunoglobulin A (IgA) nephropathy

Recurrent IgA deposition, as determined on biopsy, may result in a wide spectrum of manifestations, ranging from an incidentally noted histologic finding to mesangioproliferative glomerulonephritis associated with hematuria, proteinuria, and progressive renal dysfunction. IgA deposition may occur alone or be concurrent with other significant pathology, including chronic rejection **(Kowalewska J, et al. 2005).**

13. De Novo Glomerulonephritis

Patients without previous glomerular disease occasionally develop lesions in the allograft that resemble 1ry glomerular disease, rather than the usual chronic transplant glomerulopathy. Although some lesions may be coincidental, at least 3 are related to an alloimmune response to the allograft: membranous nephropathy, anti-GBM in Alport's syndrome and recurrent nephrotic syndrome in congenital nephrosis. A fourth common de novo GN, focal segmental glomerulosclerosis, is believed to be related to hyper filtration injury or marked compromise as a result of calcineurin inhibitor toxicity **(Meehan SM, et al., 1998 and Cosio FG, et al., 1999).**

14. Membranous Nephropathy (MN)

De novo MN is typically a late complication affecting about 1%-2% grafts. The risk factors for de novo MN include time after transplantation, de novo MN in a first graft **(Heidet L, et al., 1994)**, HCV infection **(Josep M. Cruzadoa, et al., 2001).** Light microscopy usually shows mild glomerular basement membrane changes. Mesangeal hypercellularity is found in about 33% of biopsies **(Morales JM, et al., 1997).** In most cases, MN in the transplant is a de novo disease, occurring in patients who had a different primary renal disorder **(Truong L, et al., 1989).** The cumulative incidence of this complication is approximately 1.5 to 2 percent, but the frequency rises with time, reaching 5.3 percent at eight years in one report **(Schwarz A, et al., 1994).**

15. Pathogenesis

De novo MN is thought to be related to chronic rejection, since renal biopsy reveals signs of vascular and interstitial rejection in addition to the classic findings of MN (basement membrane thickening and immune deposits in the subepithelial space). The mechanism by which de novo MN occurs is unknown **(Truong L, et al., 1989).** Rejection leads to exposure of previously unseen glomerular antigens, resulting in a secondary antibody response. Glomerular injury due to rejection makes the capillary wall more permeable, thereby facilitating the deposition of immune complexes. Circulating antibodies may be directed against HLA antigens that are expressed on the graft. Indirect evidence in support of the importance of host factors is the seemingly high incidence of recurrence (4 of 7 in one report) in a second transplant **(Heidet L, et al., 1994).** Alloimmunization against neutral endopeptidase (NEP) is a novel pathomechanism of MN that might also account for some cases of MN after renal transplantation. Other types of alloimmunization should be investigated in MN but also in other renal and nonrenal diseases, particularly those that affect the pediatric age **(Ronco P, et al., 2005).** In comparison, de novo MN seems to be rare when a second transplant is performed in patients who did not have de novo MN in the first graft **(Heidet L, et al., 1994).**

15.1 Anti-Glomerular Basement Membrane glomerulo-nephritis (Anti-GBM)

Patients with Alport's syndrome or hereditary nephritis commonly develop anti-GBM alloantibody because they genetically lack self tolerance to GBM collagen components, however GN develops in few cases only and de novo crescentic and necrotizing GN 2ry to anti-GBM post transplantation is uncommon, seen in only 5% of adult male recipients with Alport's syndrome **(Kashtan CE, 2000).** The overall 5-year graft survival is equal to that of recipients without Alport's syndrome **(Gobel J, et al., 1992).**

15.2 Transplant Glomerulopathy (TG)

Transplant glomerulopathy (TG) is a separate histologic entity. Current evidence supports the postulate that TG is a unique pathologic and pathogenic entity distinct from other forms of chronic allograft injury **(F.G. Cosio, et al., 2008)**. Evidence is accumulating that TG has a unique pathogenesis that distinguishes it from other chronic pathologic conditions of kidney allografts **(Gloor JM, et al., 2007).** Detailed electron microscopic studies have shown basement membrane abnormalities in glomerular and peri-tubular capillaries, indicating that this is a disease of the entire renal capillary network. Staining biopsies for the complement fragment, C4d, showed positivity in subgroups of TG, suggesting the participation of anti-donor antibodies **(F.G. Cosio, et al., 2008)**. Transplant Glomerulopathy is defined by the characteristic duplication of glomerular basement membrane (GBM) observed by light microscopy as recommended by the Banff working group **(Racusen LC, et al., 2002).** It is a focal lesion particularly in its early histologic phases, affecting only a few glomeruli. However, sequential biopsies show progression with increasing percentage of affected capillary loops in an increasing number of glomeruli **(Gloor JM, et al., 2007).** The incidence of TG is increased in patients with anti-donor HLA antibodies prior to the transplant. The use of surveillance biopsies has demonstrated that TG can develop during the first few months after transplantation, although it may remain clinically quiescent for several years However, TG is progressive, leading to reduced graft survival. Current therapies for TG are likely of limited value **(F.G. Cosio, et al., 2008)**. The importance of this disease is that TG is associated with very poor allograft survival and TG is perhaps the first distinct pathologic entity arising that was first called 'chronic rejection', and then 'chronic allograft nephropathy'. The distinctiveness of TG from other forms of chronic allograft pathologies is given by the coexistence of three features: (i) histologic pattern, (ii) association with the presence of anti-HLA antibodies and (iii) the absence of other conditions that may cause duplication of GBM **(F.G. Cosio, et al., 2008)**.

Transplant Glomerulopathy is associated with poor long-term graft survival; the factors associated with reduced graft survival include graft function and proteinuria at diagnosis and the severity of GBM duplication **(F.G. Cosio, et al., 2008)**. The clinical manifestations of early TG are nonspecific, consisting of progressive, unexplained loss of kidney function, minor proteinuria and mild hypertension **(Sis B, et al., 2007).** Histological classifications of kidney allograft pathology did not separate TG from 'chronic allograft nephropathy', a nonspecific term indicating the presence of interstitial fibrosis and tubular atrophy, however, recent investigations showed that TG, particularly in its early stages, might develop independently from interstitial fibrosis, tubular atrophy and/or transplant arteriopathy **(Yamamoto I,et al., 2007).** It is important to note that glomerular inflammation coexists with TG and, in fact, becomes more common and severe as the duplication of the GBM progresses, suggesting that TG and its progression is associated with persistent capillaritis **(Gloor JM, et al., 2007).** Transplant glomerulopathy must primarily be distinguished histologically from those disorders that can cause a MPGN-pattern and/or a predominant interstitial fibrosis on renal biopsy. The MPGN-pattern of transplant glomerulopathy must be distinguished from other glomerular disorders, particularly MPGN that is associated with hepatitis C virus infection or is due to recurrent or de novo disease. These disorders may appear similar on light microscopy. The distinction may be made on electron microscopy, which typically shows thickening and duplication of the glomerular basement membranes without immune deposits in transplant glomerulopathy; by comparison, there are prominent subendothelial immune deposits in HCV-associated MPGN **(Andresdottir MB, et al., 1998).** The presence of marked interstitial fibrosis due to chronic renal transplant nephropathy must be differentiated from other causes of fibrosis, particularly that induced by calcineurin inhibitors (eg, cyclosporine or tacrolimus). In this setting, histologic evidence of the characteristic glomerulopathy, or the presence of peritubular capillary basement membrane splitting and lamination are most consistent with chronic renal allograft nephropathy. By comparison, the detection of newly formed hyaline arteriolar changes is specific for cyclosporine nephrotoxicity **(Racusen LC, et al., 2002).**

15.3 Management of Transplant Glomerulopathy

Currently, there are no known effective therapies for TG. There is strong evidence that control of blood pressure and angiotensin II inhibition are effective in slowing down the progression of glomerular diseases in native kidneys **(F. G. Cosio, et al., 2008).**

15.4 Treatment of Post Transplant Glomerulonephritis (PTGN)

15.4.1 Focal Segmental Glomerulosclerosis (FSGS)

There are only anecdotal reports of therapy in recurrent focal segmental glomerulosclerosis (FSGS). Removal of a circulating toxin with protein adsorption or plasmapheresis, or the administration of cyclophosphamide or meclofenamate (an NSAID) have been tried in selected cases with variable success **(Matalon A,et al.,2001).** Protein adsorption and plasmapheresis can markedly reduce protein excretion or even induce complete remission in at least some cases if begun early after the onset of recurrent disease before hyalinosis or more severe histologic changes have occurred **(Vincenti F, 2005).** The administration of plasmapheresis plus cyclosporine prior to transplantation has been postulated to prevent recurrent disease in high-risk patients **(Hariharan S, 2000).** A retrospective study in children found that preoperative plasmapheresis (without cyclosporine) decreased the rate of recurrent disease; four of six recurred in the nonprophylactic group versus 5 of 15 in the prophylactic group; **(Ohta T, et al., 2001).** Prolonged, daily, high dose corticosteroid is routinely used for the treatment of FSGS in non-transplant patients. Although there are only limited reports of this treatment modality for recurrent FSGS, there may be a role for steroids in this setting. In one report, two children developed recurrent FSGS after they were changed to every other day steroids **(Hanevold CD, 2003),** both patients initially responded to prolonged, daily, high dose corticosteroids, but subsequently relapsed with lower dose daily steroids. Other agents, such as Rituximab, have been tried with variable success **(Yabu JM, et al., 2008).**

15.4.2 Membrano-Proliferative Glomerulonephritis (MPGN)

There is no proven beneficial therapy for the treatment of recurrent idiopathic MPGN, although the combination of aspirin and dipyridamole may stabilize renal function, similar to its efficacy in primary MPGN **(Glicklich D, et al., 1987).** In the setting of stable graft function, especially associated with non-nephrotic range proteinuria, conservative management is generally preferred. This should include blood pressure control, the use of angiotensin converting enzyme inhibitors or angiotensin receptor blockers along with a statin. The role of cyclosporine is uncertain. Some investigators have found it to be ineffective in recurrent disease, while others have suggested that the rate of recurrence fell from 30 to 10 percent after the introduction of cyclosporine **(Lien YH, et al., 2000)**. There are also case reports describing successful treatment with cyclophosphamide or plasmapheresis **(Muczynski KA, 1995).**

While no specific treatment exists for the treatment of recurrent idiopathic MPGN, aggressive treatment using plasmapheresis and adjuvant immunosuppression may be warranted in the setting of rapidly worsening graft function or histologic findings suggestive of rapidly progressive disease. The treatment of recurrent disease in the setting of active hepatitis C virus infection is somewhat controversial; however, it should be considered in appropriate candidates **(Zeman M, et al., 2006).** The use of a wide variety of treatments has been reported. In the setting of rapidly worsening graft function or histological findings suggestive of rapidly progressive disease; plasmapheresis, substitution of tacrolimus for cyclosporine, reduction in the dose or discontinuation of the calcineurin inhibitor, increase in the corticosteroid dose, or the administration of pulse methylprednisolone may be warranted **(Braun MC, et al., 2005).** Several other treatment options; Rituximab may be useful in treating MPGN in renal transplant recipients in this setting **(Basse G, et al., 2005).**

15.4.3 Membranous Nephropathy (MN)

Cyclosporine, Tacrolimus, and Mycophenolate Mofetil do not seem to protect against or change the course of recurrent disease **(Choy BY, et al., 2006);** there is no evidence that additional immunosuppressive therapy alters the course of the membranous nephropathy. The use of Cyclosporine has not changed the incidence of de novo MN, and pulse therapy with Methylprednisolone does not appear to lower protein excretion **(Schwarz A, et al., 1994).** In a case report, the administration of Rituximab was successful in treating recurrent disease **(Gallon L, et al., 2006).**

15.5 Immunoglobulin A Nephropathy (IgAN)

There is some evidence that the use of mycophenolate mofetil may decrease the risk of IgAN recurrence, although long-term data are lacking **(Kim YS, et al., 2001).** In contrast, one analysis of transplant glomerulopathy that used recurrent IgAN as a comparative control group found no difference in the incidence of recurrence with the use of mycophenolate mofetil and/or tacrolimus **(Chandrakantan A, et al., 2005).** Retrospective analysis reported that the prevalence of recurrent IgA following transplantation was significantly reduced in patients receiving antithymocyte globulin, compared to either IL-2 induction or no induction treatment **(Berthoux F, et al., 2008).** Adapted from its use in treating IgAN in native kidneys, angiotensin converting enzyme inhibitor therapy may delay progression of recurrent disease in allografts **(Courtney AE, et al., 2006).** However, it is not clear that graft survival is actually improved by initiating either an angiotensin converting enzyme inhibitor or an angiotensin receptor blocker following the detection of recurrent IgAN **(Chandrakantan A, et al., 2005).**

16. Conclusions

The incidence of Recurrent and De novo GN occur earlier than transplant Glomerulopathy and recurrent GN is the earliest glomerular lesion observed in the first 3 months post transplantation. FSGS is the most common type of PTGN and MPGN represents the second common type.

Pre-transplant glomerulonephritis, donor age 31-40 years old, and Sirolimus protocol are risk factors for developing PTGN. Difference in blood group between the donor and recipient carries a favorable significant delay in the development of PTGN. The risk factors associated with graft loss in PTGN are; recipient age between 40 and 50 years, induction therapy with polyclonal antibody (ATG), incidence and number of acute rejection episodes, and development of chronic rejection.

Significant drop of graft survival is observed in recipients who developed PTGN after the first 2 years pos-transplant. The graft survival in the recipients with Recurrent GN is significantly lower than the graft survival of recipients who developed De novo GN and Transplant glomerulopathy. De novo GN has an independent negative impact on the long term graft loss. Middle aged donor grafts, patient receive their grafts from their off springs, and different blood groups between recipients and donors have favorable significant effect on graft survival. The patient survival in the recipients with PTGN is comparable to those without PTGN in the first 5 years post transplantation. Thereafter, significant drop of patient survival is observed in the group of recipients who suffered from De novo GN and Transplant Glomerulopathy.

17. References

Andresdottir MB; Assmann KJ; Koene RA; Wetzels JF. Immunohistological and ultrastructural differences between recurrent type I membranoproliferative glomerulonephritis and chronic transplant glomerulopathy. Am J Kidney Dis 1998 Oct; 32(4):582-8.

Basse G; Ribes D; Kamar N; Mehrenberger M; Esposito L; Guitard J; Lavayssiere L; Oksman F; Durand D; Rostaing L. Rituximab therapy for de novo mixed cryoglobulinemia in renal transplant patients. Transplantation 2005 Dec 15; 80(11):1560-4.

Bela Ivanyi, A primer on recurrent and de novo glomerulonephritis in renal allografts. NATURE CLINICAL PRACTICE NEPHROLOGY august 2008; 4 (8):446-457.

Berger BE; Vincenti F; Biava C; Amend WJ Jr; Feduska N; Salvatierra O Jr. De novo and recurrent membranous glomerulopathy following kidney transplantation. Transplantation 1983 Apr; 35(4):315-9.

Berthoux F; El Deeb S; Mariat C; Diconne E; Laurent B; Thibaudin L. Antithymocyte globulin (ATG) induction therapy and disease recurrence in renal transplant recipients with primary IgA nephropathy. Transplantation. 2008 May 27; 85(10):1505-7.

Bhalla V; Nast CC; Stollenwerk N; Tran S; Barba L; Kamil ES; Danovitch G; Adler SG. Recurrent and de novo diabetic nephropathy in renal allografts. Transplantation. 2003 Jan 15; 75(1):66-71.

Branten AJ; Vervoort G; Wetzels JF. Serum creatinine is a poor marker of GFR in nephrotic syndrome. Nephrol Dial Transplant 2005 Apr; 20(4):707-11.

Braun MC; Stablein DM; Hamiwka LA; Bell L; Bartosh SM; Strife CF. Recurrence of membranoproliferative glomerulonephritis type II in renal allografts: The North American Pediatric Renal Transplant Cooperative Study experience. J Am Soc Nephrol 2005 Jul; 16(7):2225-33.

Briganti E, Russ G, McNeil J, Atkins R, Chadban S. Risk of renal allograft loss from recurrent glomerulonephritis. N Engl J Med 2002; 347:103–109.

Briggs J, Jones E: Recurrence of glomerulonephritis following renal transplantation. Scientific Advisory Board of the ERA-EDTA Registry. European Renal Association-European Dialysis and Transplant Association. Nephrol Dial Transplant 1999; 14: 564–565.

Broyer M, Selwood N, Brunner F. Recurrence of primary renal disease on kidney graft: a European pediatric experience. J Am Soc Nephrol 1992; 2 [Suppl 12]: S255–S257.

Busch GJ, Chavers BM, Gillingham KJ, et al: Chronic renal allograft rejection in the first 6 months post-transplantation. Transplantation, 1995 60:1413.

Cameron JS. Recurrent primary disease and de novo nephritis following renal transplantation. Pediatr Nephrol 1991; 5:412–421.

Chadban S: Glomerulonephritis recurrence in renal allograft. J Am Soc Nephrol 12:394-402, 2001.

Chailimpamontree W, Dmitrienko S, Li G, Balshaw R, Magil A, Shapiro RJ, Landsberg D, Gill J, Keown PA; Genome Canada Biomarkers in transplantation Group. Probability, predictors, and prognosis of posttransplantation glomerulonephritis. J Am Soc Nephrol. 2009 Apr;20(4):843-51.

Chandrakantan A; Ratanapanichkich P; Said M; Barker CV; Julian BA. Recurrent IgA nephropathy after renal transplantation despite immunosuppressive regimens with mycophenolate mofetil. Nephrol Dial Transplant 2005 Jun; 20(6):1214-21.

Cheigh JS; Mouradian J; Susin M; Stubenbord WT; Tapia L; Riggio RR; Stenzel KH; Rubin AL. Kidney transplant nephrotic syndrome: relationship between allograft histopathology and natural course. Kidney Int 1980 Sep;18(3):358-65.

Cheong HI, Han HW, Park HW. Early recurrent nephritic syndrome after renal transplantation in children with focal segmental glomeruloselerosis. Nephrol Dial Transplant 2000; 15:78–81.

Choy BY; Chan TM; Lai KN. Recurrent glomerulonephritis after kidney transplantation. Am J Transplant. 2006 Nov; 6(11):2535-42.

Conlon PJ, Lynn K, Winn MP et al. Spectrum of disease in familial focal and segmental glomerulosclerosis. Kidney Int 1999; 56: 1863–1871.

Cosio FG; Frankel WL; Pelletier RP; Pesavento TE; Henry ML; Ferguson RM. Focal segmental glomerulosclerosis in renal allografts with chronic nephropathy: implications for graft survival. Am J Kidney Dis 1999 Oct; 34(4):731-8.

Cosyns JP; Couchoud C; Pouteil-Noble C; Squifflet JP; Pirson Y. Recurrence of membranous nephropathy after renal transplantation: probability, outcome and risk factors. Clin Nephrol 1998 Sep; 50(3):144-53.

Courtney AE; McNamee PT; Nelson WE; Maxwell AP. Does angiotensin blockade influence graft outcome in renal transplant recipients with IgA nephropathy. Nephrol Dial Transplant. 2006 Dec; 21(12):3550-4.

Dall'Amico R, Ghiggeri GM, Carraro M. Prediction and treatment of recurrent focal segmental glomerulosclerosis after renal transplantation in children. Am J Kid Dis 1999; 34: 1048–1055.

Denton MD; Singh AK. Recurrent and de novo glomerulonephritis in the renal allograft. Semin Nephrol 2000 Mar;20(2):164-75.

F. G. Cosio, J. M. Gloor, S. Sethi and M. D. Stegall Transplant Glomerulopathy. *American Journal of Transplantation* 2008; 8: 492–496.

Floege J: Recurrent glomerulonephritis following renal transplantation: an update. Nephrol dial transplant, 2003 18:1260.

Gallon L; Perico N; Dimitrov BD; Winoto J; Remuzzi G; Leventhal J; Gaspari F; Kaufman D. Long-term renal allograft function on a tacrolimus-based, pred-free maintenance immunosuppression comparing sirolimus vs. MMF. Am J Transplant. 2006 Jul; 6(7):1617-23.

Gaston RS. Current and evolving immunosuppressive regimens in kidney transplantation. Am J Kidney Dis. 2006 Apr;47(4 Suppl 2):S3-21.

Gephardt GN, Tubbs RR, Braun WE et al. Nephrotic range proteinuria with 'minimal change glomerulopathy' in human renal allografts: report of four cases. Am J Kid Dis 1988; 12:51–61.

Glassock RJ, Feldman D, Reynolds ES: Human renal isografts: a clinical and pathologic analysis. Medicine (Baltimore) 1968; 47:411.

Glicklich D; Matas AJ; Sablay LB; Senitzer D; Tellis VA; Soberman R; Veith FJ. Recurrent membranoproliferative glomerulonephritis type 1 in successive renal transplants. Am J Nephrol 1987;7(2):143-9.

Gloor JM, Sethi S, Stegall MD et al. Transplant glomerulopathy: Subclinical incidence and association with alloantibody. Am J Transplant 2007; 9: 2124-2132.

Gobel J, Olbricht CJ, Offner G, et al: Kidney transplantation in Alport's syndrome: long-term outcome and allograft anti-GBM nephritis. Clin nephrol 1992; 38:299.

Gossmann J, Scheuermann EH, Porubsky S, Kachel HG, Geiger H, Hauser IA. Abrogation of nephrotic proteinuria by rituximab treatment in a renal transplant patient with relapsed focal segmental glomerulosclerosis. Transpl Int. 2007 Jun;20(6):558-62.

Habib R, Antignac C, Hinglais N, Gagnadoux M-F, Broyer M. Glomerular lesions in the transplanted kidney in children. Am J Kidney Dis 1987; 10: 198–207.

Hanevold CD, Greenbaum LA. Nephrotic syndrome after conversion to alternate day steroids in two children with a history of recurrent FSGS. Pediatr Transplant. 2003 Oct;7(5):395-9.

Hariharan S, Adams M, Brennan D, Davis C, First M, Johnson C, Ouseph R, Peddi V, Pelz C, Roza A, Vincenti F, George V: Recurrent and de novo glomerular disease after renal transplantation: A report from Renal Allograft Disease Registry (RADR). Transplantation 1999; 68:635–641.

Hariharan S, Johnson C, Bresnahan B, Taranto S, McIntosh M, StableinD: Improved graft survival after renal transplantation in the United States, 1988 to 1996. N Engl J Med 2000; 342: 605–612.

Hariharan S, Peddi VR, Savin VJ et al. Recurrent and de novo renal diseases after renal transplantation: a report from the renal allograft disease registry. Am J Kid Dis 1998; 31:928–931.

Heidet L, Gagnadoux ME, Beziau A, et al: Recurrence of de novo membranous glomerulonephritis on renal grafts. Clin nephrol 41:314, 1994.

Hoyer JR, Vernier RI, Najarian JS et al. Recurrence of idiopathic nephrotic syndrome after renal transplantation. Lancet 1972; 11: 344–448.

Ingulli E, Tejani A. Incidence, treatment, and outcome of recurrent focal segmental glomerulosclerosis post-transplantation in 42 allografts in children—a single-center experience. Transplantation 1991; 51: 401–405

Josep M. Cruzadoa, Marta Carrerab, Joan Torrasa and Josep M. Grinyo. Hepatitis C Virus Infection and de Novo Glomerular Lesions in Renal Allografts. American Journal of Transplantation 2001; 1: 171±178.

Josephson MA; Spargo B; Hollandsworth D; Thistlethwaite JR. The recurrence of recurrent membranous glomerulopathy in a renal transplant recipient: case report and literature review. Am J Kidney Dis 1994 Nov; 24(5):873-8.

Kashtan CE: Alport syndrome: Renal transplantation and donor selection. Ren fail 2000; 22:765.

Kershaw DB, Sedman AB, Kelsch RC, Bunchman TE. Recurrent focal segmental glomerulosclerosis in pediatric renal transplant recipients: successful treatment with oral cyclophosphamide. Clin Transplant 1994; 8: 546–549.

Kibert S, Schwartz MM, Lewis E. Primary focal segmental glomerulosclerosis: clinical course and response to therapy. Am J Kidney Dis 1994; 23: 773–781.

Kim YS; Moon JI; Jeong HJ; Kim MS; Kim SI; Choi KH; Lee HY; Han DS; Park K. Live donor renal allograft in end-stage renal failure patients from immunoglobulin A nephropathy. Transplantation 2001 Jan 27; 71(2):233-8.

Kowalewska J; Yuan S; Sustento-Reodica N; Nicosia RF; Smith KD; Davis CL; Alpers CE. IgA nephropathy with crescents in kidney transplant recipients. Am J Kidney Dis 2005 Jan; 45(1):167-75.

Lien YH; Scott K. Long-term cyclophosphamide treatment for recurrent type I membranoproliferative glomerulonephritis after transplantation. Am J Kidney Dis 2000 Mar; 35(3):539-43.

Little MA; Dupont P; Campbell E; Dorman A; Walshe JJ. Severity of primary MPGN determines renal survival and post-transplantation recurrence risk. Kidney Int. 2006 Feb; 69(3):504-11.

Matalon A, Markowitz GS, Joseph RE, Cohen DJ, Saal SD, Kaplan B, D'Agati VD, Appel GB. Plasmapheresis treatment of recurrent FSGS in adult renal transplant recipients. Clin Nephrol. 2001 Oct;56(4):271-8.

McLean RH; Geiger H; Burke B; Simmons R; Najarian J; Vernier RL; Michael AF. Recurrence of membranoproliferative glomerulonephritis following kidney transplantation. Serum complement component studies. Am J Med 1976 Jan; 60(1):60-72.

Meehan SM; Pascual M; Williams WW; Tolkoff-Rubin N; Delmonico FL; Cosimi AB; Colvin RB SO: De novo collapsing glomerulopathy in renal allografts. Transplantation 1998 May 15; 65 (9):1192-7.

Morales JM, Pascual-Capdevila J, Campistol JM, et al: Membranous glomerulonephritis associated with hepatitis C virus in renal transplant patients. Transplantation 63:1634, 1997.

Morales JM; Martinez MA; Munoz de Bustillo E; Munoz MA; Gota R; Usera G. Recurrent type III membranoproliferative glomerulonephritis after kidney transplantation. Transplantation 1997 Apr 27; 63(8):1186-8.

Muczynski KA. Plasmapheresis maintained renal function in an allograft with recurrent membranoproliferative glomerulonephritis type I. Am J Nephrol 1995; 15(5):446-9.

Ohta T, Kawaguchi H, Hattori M et al. Effect of pre- and postoperative plasmapheresis on posttransplant recurrence of focal segmental glomerulosclerosis in children. Transplantation 2001; 71: 628–633.

Peter J. Morris: kidney transplantation: principles and practice. 6th edition, 2008.

Racusen LC, Solez K, Colvin R. Fibrosis and atrophy in the renal allograft. Interim report and new directions. Am J Transplant 2002; 2: 203–206.

Ramos EL, Tisher CC: Recurrent diseases in the kidney transplant. Am j kidney dis, 1994 24:142.

Requião-Moura LR, Moscoso-Solorzano GT, Franco MF, Ozaki KS, Pacheco-Silva A, Kirsztajn GM, Câmara NO. Prognostic factors associated with poor graft outcomes in renal recipients with post-transplant glomerulonephritis. Clin Transplant. 2007 May-Jun;21(3):363-70.

Rizzoni G, Ehrich JHH, Bunner FP et al. Combined report on regular dialysis and transplantation of children in Europe, 1990. Nephrol Dial Transplant 1991; 6: 31–42.

Ronco P, Debiec H. Molecular pathomechanisms of membranous nephropathy: from Heymann nephritis to alloimmunization. J Am Soc Nephrol. 2005 May;16(5):1205-13.

Savin V, Sharma R, Sharma M et al. Circulating factor associated with increased glomerular permeability to albumin in recurrent focal segmental glomerulosclerosis. NEngl J Med 1996; 334: 878–883.

Schwarz A; Krause PH; Offermann G; Keller F. Impact of de novo membranous glomerulonephritis on the clinical course after kidney transplantation. Transplantation 1994 Sep 27; 58(6):650-4.

Senguttuvan P, Cameron JS, Hartley RB et al. Recurrence of focal segmental glomerulosclerosis in transplanted kidneys: analysis of incidence and risk factors in 59 allografts. Pediatr Nephrol 1990; 4: 21–28

Sharma M, Sharma R, McCarthy ET, Savin VJ. 'The FSGS Factor': enrichment and in vivo effect of activity from focal segmental glomerulosclerosis plasma. J Am Soc Nephrol 1999; 10: 552–561.

Siddqi, N, Hariharan, S, Danovitch, G. Evaluation and Preparation of Renal Transplant Candidates. Handbook of Kidney Transplantation, Fourth Ed., Lippincott Williams Wilkins, Philadelphia 2005.

Sis B, Campbell PM, Mueller T et al. Transplant glomerulopathy, late antibody-mediated rejection and the ABCD tetrad in kidney allograft biopsies for cause. Am J Transplant 2007; 7: 1743-1752.

Srivasta RN, Kalia A, Travis LB, Diven SC, Gugliuzza KK, Rajaraman S. Prompt remission of post-renal transplant nephrotic syndrome with high-dose cyclosporine. Pediatr Nephrol 1994; 8: 94–95.

Stephanian E, Matas AJ, Mauer SM. Recurrence of disease in patients retransplanted for focal segmental glomerulosclerosis. Transplantation 1992; 53: 755–757.

Striegel JE, Sibley RK, Fryd DS, Mauer M. Recurrence of focal segmental sclerosis in children following renal transplantation. Kidney Int 1986; 19: S44–S50.

Tejani A, Nicastri AD, Sen D, Chen CK, Phadke K, Adamson O, Butt KM. Long-term evaluation of children with nephritic syndrome and focal segmental glomerular sclerosis. Nephron 1983; 35: 225–231.

Truong L; Gelfand J; D'Agati V; Tomaszewski J; Appel G; Hardy M; Pirani CL. De novo membranous glomerulonephropathy in renal allografts: a report of ten cases and review of the literature. Am J Kidney Dis 1989 Aug; 14(2):131-44.

Vincenti F, Ghiggeri GM. New insights into the pathogenesis and the therapy of recurrent focal glomerulosclerosis. Am J Transplant. 2005 Jun; 5(6):1179-85.

William A. Golgert, Gerald B. Appel, and Sundaram Hariharan Recurrent Glomerulonephritis after Renal Transplantation:An Unsolved Problem. Clin J Am Soc Nephrol 2008; (3): 800-807.

Worawon Chailimpamontree, Svetlana Dmitrienko, Guiyun Li, Robert Balshaw,Alexander Magil, R. Jean Shapiro, David Landsberg, John Gill, Paul A. Keown: Probability, Predictors, and Prognosis of Posttransplantation Glomerulonephritis. J Am Soc Nephrol 2009; 20: 843–851.

Yabu JM, Ho B, Scandling JD, Vincenti F. Rituximab failed to improve nephrotic syndrome in renal transplant patients with recurrent focal segmental glomerulosclerosis. Am J Transplant. 2008 Jan; 8(1):222-7.

Yamamoto I, Horita S, Takahashi T et al. Glomerular expression of plasmalemmal vesicle-associated protein-1 in patients with transplant glomerulopathy. Am J Transplant 2007; 7: 1954-1960.

Zeman M, Campbell P, Bain VG. Hepatitis C eradication and improvement of cryoglobulinemia-associated rash and membranoproliferative glomerulonephritis with interferon and ribavirin after kidney transplantation. Can J Gastroenterol. 2006 Jun; 20(6):427-31.

Part 3

Transplant Associated Disease

9

Psychological Aspects of Kidney Transplantation

Magdalena Trzcinska[1] and Zbigniew Włodarczyk[2]
[1]*University Hospital, Psychiatry Department, Nicolaus Copernicus University Torun, Collegium Medicum in Bydgoszcz,*
[2]*Transplantology and Surgery Department, University Hospital, Nicolaus Copernicus University Torun, Collegium Medicum in Bydgoszcz, Poland*

1. Introduction

The currently promoted holistic health care model assumes a close interaction between the somatic and mental aspects (Sheridan, Radmacher, 1998). The past few years have recorded a considerable progress in the study into the psychological determinants of somatic illnesses. The domains representing the so-called behavioural sciences show, at different levels, the relationships between the physical and mental health. Such approach, in practice, assumes that there is no illness which would be unconditioned by psychological factors (Salmon, 2002).

The mental psychological factors can be the cause of the disease, they can maintain the occurrence of pathological symptoms or they can constitute the result of the pathological process. Interestingly, the psychological knowledge does not only account for the origin of the psychopathological symptoms found in somatic disorders but it also provides constantly improved and scientifically-verified methods of their treatment.

Similarly the transplantation is a treatment method connected with numerous psychological implications for the patient and the family (Kidney Transplantation, 2000). The transplantation ward patients face psychological problems, e.g. concerning the autonomy and the responsibility for the health decisions, managing the chronic disease stress, operative procedure and the uncertainty after the transplantation. These problems often overlap with changes in behaviour, emotions and cognitive functions being a result of organic changes in the central nervous system (CNS) triggered by dialyses (Griva et al. 2002; Griva et al. 2003).

For that reason the cooperation between transplant surgeons and clinical psychologists seems to be a natural consequence of the holistic understanding of the patient, taking into account the interactions between physical and mental health. The personnel of the transplantation clinics should form interdisciplinary teams of transplant surgeons, nephrologists, qualified nurse, transplant coordinator, dietician and the clinical psychologist.

The present paper is an attempt at providing characteristics of the most essential psychological problems found in patients before and after the renal transplantation. Psychological aspects of the qualification process of potential living donors are also presented.

2. Transplantation from a living donor who is a relative: psychological aspects of the potential kidney donor's qualification process. The goal of psychological assessment

The psychological evaluation is an essential component considered in the process of qualifying a person who wants to donate a kidney to a person of immediate family. The decision on donating a kidney is difficult, conditioned by many factors and, as such, it calls for thorough consideration. It should be taken with full awareness, voluntarily, having the sense of freedom and respect for the donor. With that in mind, a potential donor should be informed by the transplant surgeon of all the facts connected with potential problems and possible complications. It is noteworthy that the decision on donating a kidney is most often taken as triggered by powerful emotions, an impulse. It is extremely rarely the case that a potential donor taking the decision has been provided with all the indispensable information on the transplantation process and thus the donor's expectations from the treatment can be unrealistic (Nolan et al., 2004, Włodarczyk et al. 1997).

The basic objective of a talk with the psychologist is to determine the nature of motivation of the potential donor as it is the aspect which creates the space for the development of potential psychopathological reactions later in time.

The opinion issued by the psychologist concerns mostly the potential donor of the organ, however, frequently it is not possible to make a psychological profile of the donor without determining the conditions sand social relations the person operates in. A special attention is paid to accurate characteristics of the relationships between the donor and the kidney receiver. Initially the talk concerns mostly the kidney donor, later also the receiver; in practice, the consultation often ends up with a talk with both persons present at the same time.

The consultation aims at getting a grasp of the psychological atmosphere in which the decision on donating the kidney was finally made and excluding the presence of any kind of pressure on the donor and, as such, it refers to motivation. The research results show that despite the fact that the decision taken by most of the potential donors is independent and spontaneous, at the same time almost all the potential donors experience some kind of pressure, which can be generated by the behaviour of the receiver, other family members but also a specific system of beliefs of the donor himself. Although taking the decision on donating the kidney to a person the donor is a member of the immediate family with is mostly motivated by the sense of moral obligation and altruist aspects, from a psychological perspective, they are not sufficient to meet the requirements of the informed consent.

For the psychologist participating in the qualification process as well as for the entire transplantation team, it must be absolutely clear why the potential donor has decided to donate a kidney to a specific person. Recognizing hidden motivation behind the declared knowingly altruist motivation is the role of the psychologist. Such information is acquired applying neither standardized psychometric tests nor structured interview; therefore the basic tool here is free interview, observation data and clinical evaluation.

One shall also remember that the very qualification process also triggers emotional anxiety in the potential donor and the intensity of the anxiety depends on how close the relationship with the kidney receiver is, his or her health condition, expectations of other family members and on many other factors. Tension affects all the persons involved in the qualification process: the donor, the patient, the other family members and the people around them. It can trigger changing moods in the donor, anxiety and increased excitability.

Anxiety in the potential donor can be connected with the anxiousness of discovering real emotions about kidney donation and present but unexpressed doubts of the donor. As already mentioned, the willingness to donate the kidney is often declared as triggered by an impulse. Such declaration is often welcomed with enthusiasm and recognition by the other family members, including the receiver himself, which makes the atmosphere impossible for the potential donor to change his or her decision. Withdrawing from the initial declaration would involve the need to confront the disappointment and the feeling of being let down by the receiver as well as fear of a negative feedback from the other family members. Besides, donating a kidney to a person of immediate family triggers a lot of gratifications and rewarding in nature: it enhances the position of the potential donor in the family, it puts the donor in the centre of attention, enhances the respect towards the donor and thus the donor's self-esteem. All that can make, despite inner doubts, the donor trigger his or her defence mechanisms which will make the donor rationalise things and become sure that the decision taken is the right one, making the penetration of and thinking over the real feelings difficult. The behaviour of donors experiencing the ambivalence towards the decision they have taken up often demonstrates a discrepancy between the declared and strong desire to donate the kidney and the focus on minor health problems, presenting excessively pessimistic forecasts concerning the transplantation or a strong, sometimes even exaggerated, glorification and idealization of the recipient and their relationship, which expresses the mechanism of reactive formation, masking real but unconscious negative feelings towards the recipient or the decision being taken. The applicable literature describes cases of potential donors who, suddenly, informed of the fact of unexpected pregnancy, a necessity to take care of their own neglected health problems first or of a longer leave, giving 'reasonable' reasons.

Yet another serious factor is also the evaluation of the family dynamics, considering the distribution of family roles; who takes essential decisions, what has been the position of the donor in the family so far. It so happens that potential family donors are the people who are lonely, neglected, kept away from taking up decisions important for the entire family or the people who have not been in the centre of attention in the family. In such persons an undisclosed motivation being the springboard for the desire to donate the kidney is the desire to enhance self-esteem, self-image, strengthening the position in the family and winning the family's respect. The risk while facing this kind of motivation involves the fact that, with time, the attention of the family refocuses on the diseased (the recipient), making the disappointment and the sense of underestimation of the donor's sacrifice in the donor greater.

Another source of motivation is the sense of guilt in healthy family members towards the diseased one, where the driving force of the decision on donating the kidney is better or worse realised desire of compensation, which refers especially to women who wish to donate the kidney to their child. Mother-donors often perceive it as a form of life-giving for the second time, which, on the one hand, can enhance the emotional bond between the mother and the child yet, on the other hand, can release the mother from unconscious or unexpressed sense of guilt connected with having given birth to a diseased child, being a defected child.

Obviously, the decision on donating the kidney often reflects the real profound bond between the donor and the receiver, however, also the situation of that kind, although seemingly not triggering any doubt, should be exposed to thorough an analysis by the psychologist since the opposite is possible; a healthy family member who wishes to be the donor is the person in the centre of attention in the family, attracting all the family admiration and recognition, whereas the person's decision on donating the kidney additionally strengthens his or her position, decreasing the importance of the receiver and deepening the receiver's dependence. The receiver is 'forced' to be thankful to the donor, which helps the development of the pathological relationship, hostility and, finally, also the difficulty of he receiver himself to accept the graft. There have been recorded cases where the receiver not being able to express his or her real feelings, after the transplantation, demonstrated the passive-aggressive approach, apparently declaring his or her care for the graft and, in fact, not following the doctor's guidelines, which was the expression of the receiver's resentment, bottled-up aggression or hostility to the donor, the symbol of which was the graft.

The motivation to donate the kidney is rarely 'pure motivation' and it is mixed in nature, being a combination of a sincere desire to help, hidden motives and fears, which obviously does not make it less valuable. However, it is important that it is possible to discuss the doubts and fears of the potential donor in the presence of the psychologist since the transplantation assumes an earlier donor's consent which would be clearly expressed, voluntary and fully informed. The people who donated their kidney in the past express their definite conviction that discussing the topic of the transplantation with the psychologist made it possible for them to take a decision with the sense of complete freedom of the choice made. The reports show that a talk with the psychologist, who is perceived as 'an advocate of the donor' is the factor which facilitates an honest exploration of the donor's own motivation and emotions. Such a talk also alleviates fear from being evaluated by others. The contact with the psychologist is also important because the decision of the donor is embedded in the emotional context of chronic stress, namely an illness of a person of the immediate family. The psychological consultation is important especially when the idea of donating the kidney to the diseased person does not come directly from the potential donor. Especially in such situation the donor needs to be able to discuss the decision and to have a closer look at all its consequences. The psychologist, being a stranger, not involved in family relations, can help to see all the aspects of the situation in a way which would be possibly most neutral and objective.

During such talk it is essential to create the sense of absolute freedom of choice, to make it possible for the donor to have a real grasp of the situation the donor enters. Irrespective of the relationship with the receiver and dependence on the receiver, the donor must remember that he or she enjoys the right to change the decision. In fact, the psychologist's talk with the donor also serves the receiver since, by penetrating into the real motivation of the donor, it often helps the receiver to avoid the emotional dependence, protecting him or her from unrealistic expectations by the donor. The talk of the psychologist with patients eligible for the family transplantation is a process during which the psychologist gets to know not only the motivation and personality of the patients but also the mechanisms creating the dynamics of a given family. Here the studies of psychopathology, personality psychology, family psychology and psychotherapy are applicable.

The evaluation of the donor-receiver relationship is important. The decision on donating the organ to a member of the immediate family is a beautiful gesture; however, the role of the psychologist is to determine the nature of the basic motivation. Is it not the case, for example, that besides the altruism and selflessness declared, it is not about, for example, an attempt at involving the receiver into the dependence with no possibility to refuse, 'relegating' a person by the family to act as the donor, without considering the person's opinion, using the position of the fall-guy or manipulating him or her with the sense of guilt? Sometimes it is also the case that the donor can manipulate with his or her decision and expect different kinds of gratification from the receiver; those are the cases of emotional blackmail; how could one refuse later anything to the person who has donated the kidney?

Yet another important aspect of the talk with the psychologist is to determine the level of knowledge of the patient on the kidney transplantation (potential donors, in fact, the same way as the receivers, often have information from informal sources). It is essential since it is the patient's image of the transplantation which determines the patient's expectations from the treatment.

While evaluating to what extent the decision on donating the kidney is an informed choice, taken with realistic consideration of not only the expected benefits but also a potential risk, it is also essential to make a thorough evaluation of the mental state of the donor. In the talk one shall consider the burden of mental diseases, and in the case of stating that the donor meets the diagnostic criteria of emotional disorder, one shall study in detail the case history. In justified cases, it can be necessary to assess the intellectual fitness of the potential donor to exclude the degree of mental retardation which makes full understanding and taking an informed decision impossible. The actions taken by the psychologist should be especially careful when the potential organ donor is, at the same time, a person directly dependent on the potential receiver.

Interestingly, besides the psychological mechanisms, also psychosocial factors are essential: socioeconomic and professional status of the donor, family situation, children, if any: the number of children, their age, attitude of the entire family (especially in the case of the transplantation between the siblings) to the idea of transplantation.

3. Psychological problems of the patients before and after kidney transplantation

Organ transplantation is a specific treatment method which is connected with many implications of psychological nature (Jakubowska-Winiecka 1999, 2001; Trzcińska, 2002). Before the transplantation the biggest problem concerns the motivation connected with taking the decision to undergo transplantation. Even though the consent to kidney transplantation, being a procedure which is to enhance the quality of life of the patient, increasing the patient's independence and which aims at the normalization of the medical parameters, seems obvious and unequivocal from the medical perspective, it is not such from the psychological point of view (Rebollo et al. 2004; Griva et al. 2002; Eggeling, 2000). The decision to enter the list of patients waiting for transplantation is made by some patients exposed to the pressure of doctors and the family. Also frequently the reservations brought up by the patients do not meet with the understanding from those nearest and dearest or the attending physician, which makes the patients themselves stop talking about their fears or resentment, however, expressing them in action. Transplant surgeons as well as transplant coordinators report on the cases from their experience in which the fear, concerns or resentment to undergo the transplantation found in patients are strong enough to make them, upon receiving the call with the information on the possibility of transplantation, give various reasons which makes it impossible at the very moment to appear in the transplantation centre, being a form of rationalising more or less unaware impulses. There are many reasons of such kinds of behaviour; one is the fear of the operative procedure and of all its implications (pain, anaesthesia, etc.). In some patients what dominates is the fear of the unsuccessful treatment itself, while some fear giving up a stable lifestyle the routine of which is determined by the rhythm enforced by the dialysis dates. The cycle of hemodialyses, usually taking place three times a week is a time-burden, it limits the independence of the patient, it makes it difficult for the patient to execute many activities and excludes the patient from many domains of social operation, however, it still gives many people the sense of security and control, based on repeatability and predictability, while the decision to undergo transplantation ruins that secure reality and makes the patient take a risk and deal with the uncertainty. The justifiability of that hypothesis can, for example, be seen from the fact that many patients after their successful transplantation do not consent to arteriovenous fistula ligation. The decision on keeping the fistula active, although it can result in numerous inconveniences or complications of medical nature, for the patient it can be some kind of 'safety net' since it expresses a kind of unconscious defence mechanism. The present research demonstrates that many patients, with time following the transplantation, despite a stable concentration of creatinine, express their need to keep the arteriovenous fistula patent, which becomes, in a way, a symbol reminding that if the graft is rejected, it is still possible to come back to dialyses.

Before the operation the basic difficulty is the time spent waiting for the organ. The diseased person has no choice but to wait long, no choice but to experience uncertainty. The person must, in a way, operate all the time with mental alertness, at any moment the person can receive the information about the need to appear at the transplantation centre. The psychological mechanisms the patient undergoes are complex: on the one hand, a strong waiting-related tension and, on the other hand, the stressful urgency of the call, a stay in an often unknown centre, city, among strangers and, finally, the procedure itself. It is after the treatment that the period of the greatest tension starts; it is when it turns out whether or not the kidney has started its functions. The observation and the stay in hospital can take very long, with no guarantee of keeping the graft. Each day of the stay in hospital gets longer and longer since the only and the most important activity is waiting for the laboratory test result which indicates whether the kidney has started to work and whether it plays its functions. It should be remembered that the patient's mood depends not so much on his or her real medical state but on its subjective interpretation, namely the way the patient understands and perceives his or her own situation. Most frequently at that stage the patients are becoming extremely susceptible to different kinds of emotional disorders (most often depressive and anxiety disorders), which require work with the psychologist. Often the frustration caused by prolonging uncertainty makes them aggressive, showing a demanding attitude, or closed to cooperation with the personnel.

Some patients' fears concern the wound healing after the treatment (some patients recover quite long, in many patients there is still anxiety, and despite the encouragement from the doctors, they are afraid to leave their bed not to make the movement harm the wound), however, fears are mostly connected with the newly received kidney.

The worst tolerated psychological aspects of being the kidney receiver include a constant never-ending uncertainty about the future of the graft. The patients after the transplantation develop different types of strategies of dealing with such uncertainty. The type of such strategy depends on the patient's personality, his or her earlier ways of managing stressful situations, locus of control, high self-esteem, as well as social support and the skills of benefiting from such support.

Those who manage definitely worse are anxious patients, dependent, demonstrating incapacity for tolerating negative emotions: distrust, excessive alertness, and showing the tendency to focus on negative aspects of the situation and the tendency to somatization. As for such people the transplantation seems not to meet its basic objective, namely the enhancement of the quality of life and increased independence and dealing with the disease more effectively; just the opposite: those people live with a constant sense of threat. They subordinate their life, and often also the life of their nearest and dearest, to the dynamics of the kidney operation. They seem as if they could not break from the need to think of the graft. They keep on measuring the amount of urine produced, record the results, and make never-ending comparisons between the results recorded on respective days. They follow the recommendations of the doctors scrupulously, often deforming their contents, thus introducing an almost military regime into their lives. In fact, their life is never, even for a while, anxiety-free, and continuous focusing on the functioning of the body triggers a vicious- circle mechanism: focusing on the body symptoms makes each change in the mood, even the smallest one, intensify fear and cause depression, which, in turn, based on biofeedback, intensifies the need to monitor the functioning of the body. The tendency to aggravate the symptoms is becoming burdensome not only for the patient himself who cannot enjoy the advantages of the renal transplant but also for those nearest and dearest and the doctors.

In some patients there is observed a negative effect of surrendering to excessive emotions. Those are the people who, often already before the transplantation, demonstrated a vivid emotional expression, poor impulse control, temperament showing a little balance between nervous processes and low tolerance to negative emotions: fear, anger, etc. Such patients, when exposed to prolonging uncertainty concerning the kidney functioning can react with an outburst of strong emotions, uncontrolled crying, sometimes anxiety attacks, psychomotor agitation. A low tolerance to prolonging stay in hospital is also observed in the patients with little insight into the emotions they are experiencing and in those who cannot verbalize their emotions. In some there is reported emotional changeability, sleeplessness, loss of appetite, sometimes apathy or other depressive or anxiety symptoms. There emerges yet another mechanism of vicious circle: living with the graft triggers tension, which becomes a springboard for creating anxious interpretations, while anxiety and other emotions affect, by means of feedback, the functioning of the kidney, e.g. by constant increase in blood pressure, while every single, even the smallest, deterioration in the somatic state in the patient deteriorates zwrotnie the patient's mental mood.

Yet another factor is the need of taking immunosuppressive drugs and its consequences in a form of side effects of those drugs which can affect the mental condition of the patient. It concerns mostly the effects connected with a change in physical appearance, which mostly affects the mood and mental well-being in women: an increase in the body weight, 'the moon face', hairiness which appears on arms and legs, deteriorated facial skin condition. Those factors can seem minor but, in fact, they determine the self-image of a given patient, affecting her self-esteem as a woman. With the change in the looks, there can appear depressive states, dejection, especially in those women whose self-esteem and the sense of identity depend on their looks considerably.

A specific problem observed in the patients being prepared for the kidney transplantation is the problem of their cognitive fitness. Many reports show an occurrence of different kinds of cognitive function deficits in dialysed patients. The applicable literature also uses the term of 'the dialysis encephalopathy', describing the dementia characteristics observed in the patients after many-year dialyses. The aetiology of cognitive dysfunctions in the dialysed patients is conditioned by many factors. In the past researchers pointed to the accumulation of aluminium in the CNS structures, originated from dialysis fluids, whereas today the researchers suggest that the degradation of the cognitive fitness is an effect of uremic toxins on CNS, disturbing the operation of the sodium pump, they increase the permeability of the blood-brain barrier. Other hypotheses point to the role of GABA neurotransmission disorders, hypoxia of the brain as a result of frequent blood-pressure drops, metabolic disorders or a persisting increased level of calcium in the brain.

The results of neuropsychological studies point unequivocally to the post-transplantation improvement of cognitive functions, mostly memory and attention enhancement, which is yet another factor determining the improvement in the quality of life in patients, as well as yet another reason for which the patients before and after the kidney transplantation should undergo neuropsychological tests.

Quite often after grafting the patients' attention is focused on the issue of the origin of the kidney received; whether it belonged to a young or older person, a woman or a man, etc. For many patients it is very important to contact the person who has received the other kidney from the same donor and to observe that person's health condition, ('If her or his kidney works, it must work in me as well since they do come from the same person'). In such cases some patients say that they are 'twins'.

4. The patient in the face of the graft rejection

Unfortunately sometimes the patients' fears are justified. It is still impossible to prevent, with a hundred-percent effect, the process of the graft rejection.

From the psychological point of view, it seems that in the case of family transplantation and receiving the kidney from a related donor, the graft rejection has a slightly different significance than in the case of the transplantation from an unrelated dead donor.

In both situations there appears a feeling of disappointment, however, in the receiver of the kidney from a relative, there is an additional special kind of the sense of guilt towards the donor ('wasting' of the received organ), which can often affect also the donor himself ('there must have been something wrong with my kidney'). In many patients who were dialysed before the transplantation there appears a fear of coming back to that burdensome procedure. Frequently the struggle of the doctors with the rejection process gets so much longer and longer that the patient, mostly mentally tired, wishes any specific and final solution to the situation, even if that would mean returning to the dialyses.

With the uncertainty getting longer and longer, bad mood, and a long stay in hospital create a sense of mental exhaustion, which often calls for a frequent contact and cooperation with the psychologist. The best is the situation of the patients hospitalized on the ward where the psychologist is a permanent treatment team member, thus ensuring a possibility of establishing a therapeutic relationship; otherwise all depends on the awareness and sensitivity of the doctors to the possibility of emerging psychological complications in the patient at different stages after the organ transplantation. It is also essential that the doctors themselves can recognise such mental states which would require consulting the psychologist or the psychiatrist, especially that many transplant patients demonstrate a strong tendency to bottle up emotions and to deny negative emotional states.

The job of the psychologist is to provide the patient with support, understanding and, mostly, an opportunity of discussing their current situation fully. In the first phase of the

contact, the patient should be given comfort of talking about his or her health, heath-related fears and to be listened to, which clearly alleviates emotional tension.
At the next stage it is applicable to involve elements of supportive therapy which aims at developing a stable patient-psychologist relationship helping the patient get the sense of security. Very good effects are recorded for the techniques of cognitive therapy; here the work focuses on dysfunctional anxiety-triggering patient's convictions and rephrasing negative unrealistic expectations from the transplantation. The techniques clearly help the patients to increase the sense of control over their own emotions. They are especially useful for the clinical psychologist who is expected to be effective over a short time. Short-term cognitive therapy helps to help the patient with perceiving the feedback mechanisms which occur between focusing on the health condition, catastrophic interpretation of symptoms and the psychophysical mood. An excellent method used to alleviate the anxiety-related tension involves also relaxation techniques.
If the renal graft rejection is the fact stated by the doctors, the job of the psychologist is to prepare the patient mentally to come back to dialyses. The most difficult job is when the rejection process can neither be confirmed nor completely excluded. It is the so-called work 'in suspense'; it mostly involves teaching the patient how to deal with anxiety, tension and other emotions referred to as negative: anger, sense of guilt. In some situations, despite the contact with the psychologist, the patients are also provided with pharmacological treatment in a form of antidepressants, anxiolytics, tranquilisers or soporifics.

5. Conclusions

Transplantation is a therapeutic method which, although, at the end of the day, enhances the quality of life of the patients, triggers numerous implications which are psychological in nature. For the patients the kidney transplantation treatment is connected with long-term emotional tension, experiencing strong anxiety and with the need to confront and to deal with strong negative emotions. While transplantation decision-taking, directly after the transplantation and throughout the functioning of the graft, in the patients there can appear psychopathological symptoms, most frequently anxiety and depressive disorders. The functioning of the patients is also often affected by cognitive deficits, frequent in dialysed patients, which undergo regression after transplantation. A special attention and psychological help are required for the patients diagnosed with graft rejection. Frequently, they will require specialist psychological treatment (psychotherapy) and psychiatric treatment (pharmacological treatment). For that reason the transplant patient requires interdisciplinary care, with the psychologist also on the team.

6. References

[1] Eggeling, S. (2000). Psychosocial implications for live - related donors. *EDTNA/ERCA Journal*, XXXVI, pp. 4-6

[2] Griva K, Hansraj S, Thompson D, Jayasena D, Davenport A, Harrison M, Newman SP. (2004) *Neuropsychological performance after kidney transplantation: a comparison between transplant types and in relation to dialysis and normative data;* Nephrol Dial Transplant; , *191*, pp. 866-74

[3] Griva K, Newman SP, Harrison MJ, Hankins M, Davenport A, Hansraj S, Thompson D. (2003) Acute neuropsychological changes in hemodialysis and peritoneal dialysis patients. *Health Psychol.*, 22, pp. 570-8
[4] Griva K, Ziegelmann JP, Thompson D, Jayasena D, Davenport A, Harrison M, Newman SP. (2002). Quality of life and emotional responses in cadaver and living related renal transplant recipients. *Nephrol Dial Transplant.*;17. pp. 2204-11. Jakubowska-Winecka, A. (1999). Psychologiczne problemy transplantacji narządów z perspektywy psychologa praktyka. Niepublikowany maszynopis. *Zakład Psychologii Klinicznej IP - CZD*, Warszawa 1999.
[5] Jakubowska-Winecka, A. (2001). Psychologiczna ocena kandydatów na żywych dawców nerki. Prezentacja na V Kongresie Polskiego Towarzystwa Transplantologicznego w Mikołajkach.
[6] Kidney transplantation. (2000) In: *Clinical transplantology*. Fujisawa GmbH.
[7] Laederach-Hofmann K, Bunzel B, Freundorfer E, Schubert MT. (2002). Changes in partner relationship after organ transplantation: comparison between heart, liver, and kidney transplantation. *Psychother Psychosom Med Psychol*. pp. 52, pp. 5-15.
[8] Nolan MT, Walton-Moss B, Taylor L, Dane K. (2004). Living kidney donor decision making: state of the science and directions for future research. *Prog Transplant*. 14, p. 201
[9] Rebollo P, Baltar JM, Campistol JM, Ortega T, Ortega F. (2004). Quality of life of patients with chronic renal allograft rejection and anemia. *J Nephrol*. 17. pp. 531-6
[10] Salmon P. (2002). *Psychologia w medycynie*. Wyd. GWP, Gdańsk.
[11] Sheridan CL, Radmacher SA. (1998). *Psychologia zdrowia*. Wyd. Instytut psychologii zdrowia Polskiego Towarzystwa Psychologicznego, Warszawa 1998.
[12] Transplantation in perspective. (2000) In: *Clinical transplantology*. Fujisawa GmbH.
[13] Trzcińska M. (2002). Psychologiczne problemy pacjentów przed transplantacją i po transplantacji nerki, *Nowiny Psycholologiczne* 2, 2002, pp. 51 - 59.
[14] Włodarczyk Z., Jarmoliński T., Runowski T., Zachwieja J., Stefaniak E., Maciejewski J. Czy i kiedy należy przeszczepiać nerki od żywych dawców? *Pediat. Pol.* 1997, sup. Nr 15, p. 116.

10

Characteristics of Anaemia Management in Patients with Chronic Kidney Disease

Zvonimir Puretic
University Hospital Centre Zagreb
Croatia

1. Introduction

Erythrocyte production is narrow regulatory process. Erythropoiesis starts with differentiation of small part of pluripotent stem cells to most primitive erythroid progenitors (Colony Forming Units - CFU and Burst Forming Units – BFU). These progenitors are developing to erythroid precursors, and follow program of specific differentiation to mature erythrocytes. (Suda et al., 1984) Haematopoietic growth factors (interleukin-3, granulocyte-macrophage factor that stimulate colonies and c-kit ligand) are important for the enhancement of progenitor cells, and together with erythropoietin produce large colonies of erythroblasts. (Sieff et al., 1986, 1989) Erythropoietin is crucial for finishing the differentiation of erythroid progenitors. Erythropoietin also has influence on receptors for erythropoietin.

If renal anaemia is not treated there are: cardiac failure, cerebrovascular ishaemic events, lowered cognitive and mental function, tiredness, reactive hypertension, left ventricular hypertrophy, increased morbidity and mortality. (Lau et al., 2010; Marti, 2004; Namiuchi et al., 2005; Streja et al., 2004)

2. Anaemia of chronic kidney disease (CKD) - appearance

Anaemia in CKD in most patients is normochromic and normocytic. It is consequence of lower erythropoietin production because of diminished mass of renal parenchyma and shorter survival of erythrocytes. Anaemia could appear already at creatinine clearance or glomerular filtration rate (GFR) < 35 ml/min/1,73m^2. (Levin, 2007; Locatelli et al., 2008)

In some diseases such as nephronophtysis, medulary cystic disease, endemic or Balkan nephropathy, anaemia can be expressed even at creatinine clearance lower than 60 ml/min/1,73m^2. (Locatelli et al., 2009) Studies in children estimated mean appearance of anaemia in CKD when GFR is lower than 43 ml/min/1,73m^2. (Fadrowski et al., 2008; Yorgin et al., 2001)

2.1 Calculated creatinine clearance from 24 hours urine speciment and estimated GFR (e-GFR)

In children could be used Schwartz (Schwartz-Haycock) formula where from creatinine in serum, height and coefficient according to the age and body mass, could be estimated GFR without 24 hours specimens (Schwartz et al.; 1984, Schwartz & Gauthier, 1985).

$$GFR = k \times (\text{height - cm/creatinine in serum - } \mu mol/L) \quad (1)$$

Measured endogenous creatinine values compared with Schwartz formula showed results that anaemia starts at GFR <58 ml/min/1,73m[2]. It is overestimation when using Schwartz´s formula for GFR. (Fadrowski et al., 2008)
In adult patients for estimation of GFR simple Cockcroft-Gault formula is used. Renal function has to be in steady state.

$$GFR=140\text{-age (ys)} \times \text{lean BW(kg) / creatinine mg/dL} \times 72 \text{ in males} \quad (2)$$

During the last years mostly is used MDRD-GFR formula for patients over 18 years of age that uses creatinine with more precise method than uncompensated kinetic Jaffe´s method. It uses an enzymatic method traceable to the IDMS method and SRM 909b level and is the most preferable formula in adults also in Croatia. (Flegar-Mestric et al., 2010)
The 4-variable equation from the Modificaton of Diet in Renal Disease (MDRD Study) and 6-variable MDRD Study were compared with standardized assay of Cockcroft-Gault equations , and is found better relation to other measurements of GFR. (Cerriotti et al., 2008; Levey et al., 2006)
Values of new enzymatic method of determination of creatinine are investigated also in children and are lower than with Jaffe´s reaction. (Cerriotti et al., 2008) That will bring changes in the estimated value for the patients using Schwartz formula with real (lower) creatinine in serum and may be better determination of estimated GFR, more similar to creatinine clearance in 24 hours urine specimens: MDRD formula can not be used in children and still Schwartz formula is actual.

3. Diagnosis of anaemia

Important is to evaluated mean values of haemoglobin (Hb) and haematocrit (Htc) in normal population according to the age and gender. (Puretic, 2000; Working Party for EBPG, 1999) In children "normal" values according to the age are presented in Table 1.

Age/gender	Hb g/L	Htc %
After birth	165 ± 30	51 ± 9
1 month	140 ± 40	41 ± 6
2-6 months	115 ± 25	35 ± 7
6 mo-2 years	120 ± 15	36 ± 3
2-6 years	125 ± 10	37 ± 3
6-12 years	135 ± 20	40 ± 5
12-18 years/males	145 ± 15	43 ± 6
12-18 years/females	140 ± 20	41 ± 5

Table 1. Mean hemoglobin values (Hb) and haematocrit (Htc) in health population of children (X±SD)

[1] Legend: k (depending on muscular mass): premature children 1st year = 29, newborns 1st year = 40, children and adolescent girls = 48, adolescent boys = 61. Mean in children > 13 years =52
[2] Note: in females GFR is 0,85 of the values in males

Diagnosis and treatment of anaemia should start at values of Hb or Htc < 80% of mean values for the age. (Table 2). (Berns, 2008; Puretic, 2009) At adults evaluation of anaemia is needed at Hb < 11o g/L in females and < 120g/L at males. (Kes & Ljutic, 2008; Locatelli et al., 2004; NKF-K/DOQI, 2006, 2007)
Laboratory diagnostics includes also: Mean Cell (Erythrocyte) Volume - MCV, Mean Content of Haemoglobin in Erythrocytes (Mean Cell Haemoglobin - MCH), Mean Concentration of Haemoglobin in Erythrocytes (Mean Cell Haemoglobin Concentration - MCHC), reticulocyte number, percentage of hypochromic erythrocytes.

Age/gender	Hb g/L	Htc %
After birth	<130	<41
1 month	<110	<33
2-6 months	<90	<28
6 mo-2 years	<95	<29
2-6 years	<100	<30
6-12 years	<110	<32
12-18 years/males	<115	<35
12-18 years/females	<110	<33
Adults/males	<120	<38
Adults/ females	<110	<33

Table 2. Indications for diagnosis and treatment of anaemia (hemoglobin and haematocrit, according to the age, and gender)

Iron parameters are: iron in serum, total iron bound capacity, ferritin and transferrin saturation (TSAT).

$$TSAT\ (\%) = Fe\ x100/TIBC \tag{3}$$

Further investigations are: occult blood in stool, C- reactive protein as marker of chronic inflammation, serum albumin and prealbumin as markers of nutrition.
Additional laboratory and clinical analysis: vitamin B_{12} and folic acid levels in plasma, blood smear, intact parathormon and parameters of haemolysis (haptoglobin, free haemoglobin, methaemalbumin, lactate dehidrogenase, bilirubin, Coomb´s tests, electrophoretic pattern of plasma proteins). (Locatelli et al.; 2009)
In doubt of myelodysplasia bone marrow puncture is needed, and consultation of haematologist. In some cases bone biopsy will confirm secondary hyperparathyreoidismus or bone marrow fibrosis.When mycrocytic anaemia is present, there is probably iron deficiency and not aluminium intoxication, because reverse osmosis in water treatment is used in all dialysis centres , and aluminium based phosphate binders are not more in use. Macrocytosis could be associated with folic acid or vitamin B_{12} deficiency.

4. Goals of anaemia treatment

In anaemia of chronic kidney disease target values for adults are haemoglobin 110-120 g/L. For children recommended are values 80% for age Table 2. (Puretic, 2009)
Values of Hb over 130 mg/L are not recommended because of high risk of heart failure, and cerebrovascular events. (Lau et al., 2010; Streja et al., 2004)

4.1 Significance of iron levels

Before erythropoietin is included in therapy it is important that serum iron is adequate and tissue storages are saturated. Iron therapy has impact on leukocyte surface molecules and reactive oxygen species in haemodialysis patients (Guz et al., 2006)
In the treatment of sideropenia the use of iron sucrose or gluconate and not colloidal forms such as dextrin is recommended. (Chertow et al., 2006) Basic parameters for adequate iron reserves are: ferritin, transferrin saturation and transferrin. Ferritin initially have to be higher than 100 mg/L, TSAT >15% and transferrin in referent values. During maintenance of erythropoietin treatment ferritin should be within range 150-300mg/L (not higher than 400- especially in children and in patients with hepatic lesion). Transferrin saturaton has to be 20-40% and transferrin serum level normal.
At high erythropoietin dosage and ferritin < 100 mg/L) females and diabetics are at higher risk of mortality. (Lau et al., 2010) Iron in patients on haemodialysis is administered intravenously, and in other intravenously or per os, but intravenous iron administration is preferable, also in patients on peritoneal dialysis. (Li & Wang, 2008) In predialysed patients better is also the use of intravenous iron (Hoerl, 2008)
Percentage of hypochromic erythrocytes at start should be usually <10%, and in maintenance phase <5%.

5. Treatment of renal anaemia

Kidney is the primary organ for erythropoietin production, but at adults small quantity is produced also in liver. In the treatment of anaemia androgen drugs are abandoned, and erythrocyte transfusions have "time limited" values, and also have complications (Slonim et al., 2008; Teruya, 2008). The guidelines for assessing appropriateness of pediatric transfusions are introduced (Roseff at al., 2002). The side-effects in potential transmission of viruses are well known. (Pampilon et al., 1998)
Eryhtropoiesis Stimulating Agents (ESA) since 1987 year are present in Croatia. (Gasparovic et al., 1990) Its importance (with the first erythropoietin alfa, and later with erythropoietin beta, darberythropoietin alfa and continuous erythropoietin receptors activation) dominates in the treatment of anaemia in chronic kidney disease and especially in dialysed patients. There are experimental studies that erythropoietin attenuates renal injury in acute kidney injury. (Spandou et al., 2006)
Dosage should be individualised, and careful monitoring of erythrocytes, haemoglobin and haematocrit is necessary so as continuous correction of other possible factors that influence anaemia.
Minimal investigations before starting erythropoietin therapy are: 1) haemoglobin and haematocrit, 2) reticulocytes, 3) mean cell volume (MCV), 4) transferrin saturation (TSAT), 5) serum ferritin and 6) occult blood in stool.

5.1 Indications

Renal anaemia: in dialysed patients and chronic kidney disease in predialysis patients with creatinine clearance < 35 ml/min/1,73m^2 or in selected cases <60 ml/min/1,73m^2. (Locatelli et al., 2009) In children and adults with chronic renal failure of transplanted kidney, and saturated iron reserves, indication is Hb <100 g/L.

5.2 Administration of erythropoietin

Subcutaneous administration of alfa or beta erythropoietin have some advantage over intravenous, because half-life is 24 hours, and intravenously administered 9 hours. (Besarab et al., 2009) In comparison to intravenous administration, during subcutaneous route minimal concentrations remain higher over longer time. That implies that erythropoietin can be administered in longer periods of time if given subcutaneously. (Portoles at al., 2005) Erythropoietin beta could be better metabolically and economically used when applied subcutaneously 3x weekly or 1x weekly, even 1 x in two weeks. (Miroescu et al., 2006) Darberythropoietin alfa is administered once weekly or once in two weeks, even at four weeks. (Carrera et al., 2006; Fang & Chang, 2009) But in patients on haemodialysis erythropoietin is given predominantly intravenously in developed countries, because it has also local side effects as inflammations, haemorrhage or calciphylaxia, and also has historical risk of pure red cell aplasia.

5.3 Initial dosage

Erythropoietin alfa or beta at adults on haemodialysis is administered 1 x 4000 IU/week in slow correction (during 2 - 3 months) or 2 - 3 x 4000 IU/ week in fast correction. Mean dosage is mostly 75-100 IU/kg/week. In peritoneal dialysis doses are lower, because in this patients haemoglobin could be recovered spontaneously during first 3 months. (Puretic, 2000)

There are no exact paediatric data in European or USA guidelines for anaemia management in chronic kidney disease, but are adult data suggested also for children (75-100 IU/kg/week).

In some sporadic reports values for children are higher. In young children: 2 years of age initial dosage is 50 U/kg 3x weekly subcutaneously or rarely intravenous. In older children dosage is 50-150 IU/kg/week or higher.

In children, in randomised double blind trial with placebo control in 222 children aged 5-18 years estimated high dosage in intravenous administration of erythropoietin alfa was 600 IU/kg/week (not to exceed 40,000) and maximal 900 IU/kg/week (not to exceed 60,000U/week). In subcutaneous administration should be used lower dosage. (recommendation of the manufacturer)

With darberythropoietin alfa usual dosage is 0,45 μg/kg BW at adults and children, even at children from age 1 year. (Fang & Chang, 2009; Portoles and al., 2005)

Continuous erythrocyte receptor activator (C.E.R.A.) administration is nowadays used only for patients over 18 years old, but could be used also in postpubertal children. (Carrera et al., 2010)

5.4 Maintenance dosage

Initial dosage after 4 weeks is titrated and changed according to haemoglobin values:

a. Lower dosage for 25% if:
    - target Hb 110-120 is reached

- Hb rises >10 g/L in two weeks

b. Enlarged dosage for 25% if:
   - Hb <100 g/L
   - Hb is not rising for 10 g/L after 4 weeks of therapy

c. not administer erythropoietin for 2-4 weeks if Hb>130 g/L

The mean dosage of erythropoietin alfa or beta in adults on dialysis in maintenance phase is 125 IU/kg/week (range 50-250). In children on chronic haemodialysis mean dosage is 175 IU/kg/week (range 50-450). On peritoneal dialysis the mean dosage is 75 IU/kg /week (range 25-325), in children and adults.

5.5 Novel Erythropoietin Stimulating Agents - ESA´s

Darberythropoietin alfa with different aminoacids structure and more sialyc acid could be administered at longer intervals: 1x weekly or once in 2 weeks, even 1 x per month and is given mostly intravenously 0,45 μg/kg/week. Intravenous half life is 25 hours. Higher sialyc acid content, larger molecular weight and negative charge prolonged its half life 3 times in comparison with erythropoietin alfa and beta. It is usually used once in two weeks. (Carrera et al., 2006; Fang & Chang, 2009)

Last years was developed a novel erythropoietin which is administered once monthly (metoxy poliethylen glycol-erythropoietin beta). It reacts on erythropoietin receptors and acts as continuous erythropoietin receptor activator (C.E.R.A.), and therefore is quite different to other ESA´s.

Initial dosage is 0,6 μg/kg every two weeks, later could be given 1 x monthly intravenously or subcutaneously. (Carrera et al., 2010)

Erythropoietins are today widely used also in patients with chronic renal failure of grade III and IV, and in patients after kidney transplantation with deterioration of graft function, and Hb <100 g/L. The use is justified in adults and in children. Conversion between these drugs is shown in Table 3.

Darberythropoietin alfa (μg) IV or SC dose per week	Erythropoietin alfa or beta (IU) IV or SC dose per week	C.E.R.A. (μg) IV or SC dose per month
<40	<8000	120
40-80	8000-16,000	200
>80	>16,000	360

Table 3. Suggestions for conversion of different erytropoiesis stimulating agents

6. Erythtropoietin in surgical treatment of dialysed patients

If surgical operation is planned in patients with chronic kidney disease erythropoietin could be administered 300 IU/kg 10 days before, than the first and fourth postoperative day to maintain Hb levels 100-130 g/L. (Locatelli et al., 2008)

If patient is on erythropoietin treatment it should not be excluded or diminished. Higher dosage of usual erythropoietin dosage has no approval preoperatively, or first week after operation.

7. Erythropoietin in acute medical disorder of dialysed patients

There are some dilemmas in administration of erythropoietin at acute disorders of organs, so as inflammation, pneumonia, cerebrovascular incident, cardiac failure. There are some opinions to stop the therapy until recovery, but it will lower haemoglobin later, especially in reconvalescent phase, so it has to be maintained at adequate levels of haemoglobin 110-120 g/L.

8. Nutritional status in additional treatment of anaemia

Malnourishment could be expressed in 40-70% in patients on haemodialysis and 30-50% on peritoneal dialysis. Anaemia in this group of patient is more severely expressed weather receive or not iron and erythropoietin therapy. Anamnesis of dietary nutrients, nutritional habits, BMI, exact „dry weight"and anthropometrical measures are important parameters in the overall treatment of anaemia. (Furumatsu et al., 2008)

In children are periodically determined: BW, body hight, head circumference, upper arm circumference, cutaneous fold thickness, development and puberty. It is necessary also to determine plasma proteins: albumin, prealbumin, transferrin, ferritin, aminoacids and cholesterol, urea, creatinine. Ferritin and transferrin are also good parameters of nutrition, and not only of anaemia. (Locatelli et al., 2006)

9. Inadequate response to erythropoietin in anaemia treatment

9.1 Erythropoietin resistance

In patients who are dialysed insufficiently or non-adequately (both, haemodyalised and peritonealy dialysed patients) resistance to erythropoietin occurs. Resistance to erythropoietin treatment is seen also at presence of the chronic inflammatory response on haemodialysis. (Locatelli et al., 2006) The cause could be allergic or toxic reaction to the artificial (bioincompatible) membranes and other plastics, or inadequate water treatment - endotoxins. Also could appear, but rarely in peritoneal dialysis because of plasticizers or endotoxins produced during manufacturing of dialysis solutions - sterile peritonitis. (Geerse et al., 2011) But controversial fact is that erythropoietin therapy acts positively on peritoneal mesangial cells and reducing inflammatory response. (Vorobiev et al., 2008)

The reasons of resistance to erythropoietin could be also subclinical infections, growth hormone deficiency, myelodysplastic syndromes, occult malignomas, HIV infection and haemoglobinopathias. It has to be excluded malnourishment, bone marrow fibrosis and chronic folate and B_{12} deficiency. (Locatelli et al., 2009)

9.2 Pure Red Cell Aplasia mediated with antibodies against erythropoietin

Acquired erythrocite aplasia is very rare disorder of severe anaemia characterized with very low reticulocyte count and practically absence of erythrocite precursors in bone marrow. All

other strains in bone marrow are normal. (Fisch et al., 2000; Howman & Kulkarni,2007) Some cases are idiopathic, in others could be present disorders as: myelodysplastic syndrome, lymphoma, leucemia, autoimmune diseases, thymoma, viral infection (Parvovirus B) or drugs (phenitoin, chloramphenicol).
The incidence of anti erithropoietin antibodies nowadays is signifficantly lower, and sporadic cases are verified also with the use of erythropoietin beta and darberythropoietin. (Bennett et al., 2007)

9.3 Pure red cell aplasia – PRCA - not induced with antibodies against erythropoietin

Numerous reports from 1989- 2004 showed incidence of 1,6/10.000 patients /year with rising to 3,43, mostly with high frequency in patients treated with erythropoietin alfa- administered subcutaneously. In intravenous administration verified were only 2 cases or 0,02/10,000 patients/year which is expected appearance in long term use of human recombinant erythropoietin in population. After change of formulation with change of protection with uncoated rubber stopper syringes, and with change of polysorbate with human plasma albumin frequency is essentially diminished and is as expected in population 0,02/10,000 patients/year. So the reason was of chemical origin. (Boven et al., 2005)

10. Erythropoietin in kidney transplantation

After kidney transplantation anaemia treatment is intriguing and may complicate post transplantation course. Early and late posttransplantation anaemia should be differentiated. (Choukroun & Martinez, 2005)

10.1 Early posttransplant anaemia

Risk factors are: blood loss during or few days after surgery, inflammation, delayed graft function and induction therapy with bone marrow suppression. According to some expert opinions soon after kidney transplantation in selected patients erythropoietin alfa or beta could be used in high dosage up to 125 IU/Kg/every other day IV (up to 400 IU/Kg/week) to partially correct anaemia in the first month after transplantation. (Van Biesen at al., 2005) Rationale was: prevention of blood transfusions and help in wound healing. In the treatment of early anaemia graft function on the other side could be deteriorated. (Gouva et al., 2004) It is contraversary to experimental studies (Spandou et al., 2006) Well known is that in good graft function transplanted kidney starts with own erythropoietin production in 8-30 days, and there is no need for erythropoietin treatment early after transplantation according to controlled studies.

10.2 Late posttransplant anemia

It appears after 1 month of kidney transplantation, and is mostly seen with chronic allograft nephropathy. (Al-Khoury et al., 2006; Baltar et al., 2007) The criteria for the treatment of anaemia are the same as in chronic kidney disease of predialysis patients. (Locatelli et al., 2009) With deterioration of graft function when GFR is lower than 35 ml/min/1,73m^2 and Hb lower than 100 g/L could start anaemia treatment with erythropoietin.

11. Conclusions

Drugs called erythropoiesis stimulating agents are today widely used in patients with chronic renal failure of grade III and IV, patients on haemodialysis or peritoneal dialysis (grade V of chronic renal failure), and in patients after kidney transplantation with deterioration of graft function. Mostly are used in patients with glomerular filtration rate, or creatinine clearance below 35 $ml/min/1,73m^2$. Administration is via intravenous or subcutaneous route. Efficacy of subcutaneous administration could be 20-30% higher, but in hemodialysed patients is justified intravenous administration.

After correction of other causes of anaemia dose of erythropoietin stimulating agents depends on haemoglobin levels, and the time to achieve recommended haemoglobin levels. Their initiation starts when haemoglobin level falls below 80% of normal values for the age. In children older than 6 years erythropoietin therapy starts at haemoglobin < 100 g/L, or haematocrit < 33%. In adults are introduced when haemoglobin is < 110 g/L, and target haemoglobin is between 110-120 g/L. During maintaining erythropoietin therapy almost always iron supplementation intravenously or peroral is needed.

After kidney transplantation anaemia can occur and may complicate posttransplantation course. According to some opinions soon after kidney transplantation in selected patients erythropoietin alfa or beta could be used in high dosage up to 125 U/Kg/every other day intravenously. According to controlled studies in good graft function grafted kidney starts with own erythropoietin production in 8-30 days and there is no need for erythropoietin treatment.

For late posttransplant anaemia (after 1st month of kidney transplantation) causes are: poor graft function with lack of erythropoietin or erythropoietin resistance, and viral or recurrent bacterial infections. Patients with later poor graft function and chronic anaemia should be treated in the same way as other patients with chronic kidney disease. Introducing erythropoietin therapy according to good clinical practice of haemoglobin levels and to maintain its level as in chronic renal failure before transplantation.

Advantages of the use of erythropoietins are multiple: there is no need for erythrocyte transfusions, and therefore lowered risk for developing of panel reacting antibodies (PRA) or HLA antibodies and transfusion transmitted viruses. Transfusions of blood have to be used only with low leucocytes protocols (e.g. filtered blood) to diminish load of transfusion transmitted viruses (HBV, HCV, CMV, EBV, HIV, TTV) and to lower possible later immunological reaction.

Routine administration of transfusions in patients with chronic kidney diseases is at haemoglobin level < 65-60 g/L, except in surgical needs, or in cardyomyopathic patients.

With recommended haemoglobin levels there is improvement of cardiovascular system, less complications including left ventricular hypertrophy, ischemic heart disease, chronic heart failure, generalised atherosclerosis and stroke. Better is growth and development of child with chronic kidney disease, so as better physical and mental activity and sense of well-being.

12. Acknowledgment

I am very gratefull to my doughter in low Marijana Bosnar-Puretic, MD, PhD for experience and patience in technical preparation of the manuscript.

13. References

Al-Khoury, S.; Shah, N., Afzali, B., Covic, A., Taylor, J. & Goldsmith, D. (2006). Post-transplantation anaemia in adult and paediatric renal allograft recipients - Guy´s Hospital experience. *Nephrol Dial Transplant*, Vol.21, pp. 1974-80

Baltar, J.; Moran, N., Ortega, F. et al. 2007) Erythropoietin safety and efficacy in chronic allograft nephropathy. *Transplant Proc* 2007; Vol. 39., pp. 2245-7

Bennett, CL.; Luminari , S., Nissenson, AR. et al. (2004). Pure red-cell aplasia and erythropoietinetin therapy. *New Engl J Med, Vol.* 351, pp. 1403-8

Berns, JS. (2008). Erythropoietin for the anemia in chronic kidney disease in hemodialysis patients. *Uptodate,* Golper, TA, Post, TW., pp. 1-8, Uptodate, http://www.uptodate.com/online/content/topic.do?topicKey=dialysis/40547&selected

Besarab, A.; Reyes, CM., & Hornberger, J. (2002). Meta-analysis of subcutaneous versus intravenous erythropoietinetin in maintenance treatment of anaemia in haemodialysis patients. *Am J Kidney Dis* , Vol.40, pp. 439-46

Boven, K.; Stryker, S., Knight , J. et al. (2005). The increased incidence of pure red cell aplasia with a Eprex formulation in uncoated rubber stopper syringes. *Kindey Int*, Vol.67, pp. 2346-53

Carrera, F.; Oliveira, L., Maia, P., Mendes T., & Ferreira, C. (2006) The efficacy of intravenous darberythropoietinetin alfa administered once every 2 weeks in chronic kidney disease patients on haemodialysis. *Nephrol Dial Transplant, Vol.*21, Issue.10, (October 2006), pp. 2846-50

Carrera, F.; Charmaine, EL., de Francisco, A., Locatelli, F., Man, JFE., Canaud, B, Kerr, PG., Macdougall, IC., Besarab, A., Villa, G., Kazes, I., Van Vlem, B., Joly, S., Beyer, U., & Dougherty, FC. (2010). Maintenance treatment of renal anaemia in hemodialysis patients with methoxy polyethilene glycol-erythropoietinetin beta versus darberythropoietinetin alfa administered monthly: a randomized comparative trial. (2010) *Nephrol Dial Transplant,* Vol.25, Issue 12 , (December 2010), pp 4009-17

Ceriotti, F.; Boyd, JC., Klein, G., Henny, J., Queralto, J., Kairisto, V., & Panteghini, M,. (2008). On behalf of the IFCC Committee on reference intervals and decision limits (C-RIDL). *Clinical Chemistry* , Vol. 54, pp. 539-66

Chertow, GM.; Mason, PD., Vaage-Nilsen, O., & Ahlmen, J. (2006). Update on adverse drug events associated with parenteral iron. *Nephrol Dial Transplant,* Vol.21, Issue .2, (February 2006), pp. 378-3

Choukroun , G.; & Martinez, F. (2005). Benefits of erythropietin in renal transplantation. *Transplantation* , Vol. 79 , Issue Supplement 3, pp. S49-50

Fadrowski, JJ.; Pierce, CB., Cole, SR., Moxey-Mims, M., Warady, BA., & Furth, SL. (2008) Hemoglobine decline in children with chronic kidney disease: baseline results from the chronic kidney disease in children prospective cohort study. *Clin J Am Soc Nephr, Vol.* 3, pp. 457-62

Fang, YW.; & Chang CH. (2009). Subcutaneous administration of darberythropoietinietin alfa effectively maintains hemoglobin concentrations at extended dose intervals in peritoneal dialysis patients. *Perit Dial Int* , Vol.29, pp. 199-203

Fisch, P.; Handgretinger, R., & Schaefer, HE. (2000). Pure red cell aplasia. *Br J Haematol,* Vol. 111,: pp. 1010-22

Flegar-Meštrić, Z.; Perkov, S., Šimonović, B.,&Juretić D. (2010). Applicability of common reference intervals for serume creatinine concentrations to the Croatian population. *Clin Chem Lab Med,* Vol. 48, pp. 231-5

Furumatsu, Y.; Nagasawa, Y., Hamato, T., et al. (2008). Integrated therapies including erythropoietin decrease the incidence of dialysis: lessons from mapping the incidence ofof end-stage renal disease in Japan. *Nephrol Dial Transplant, Vol.* 23, pp. 984-90

Gasparovic. V.; Puretic, Z., Vrhovac, B., Gjurasin, M., & Puljevic, D. (1990). Znacenje primjene rekombiniranog eritropoetina na sekundarnu anemiju kod bolesnika u terminalnoj fazi bubrezne insuficijencije na hemodijalizi. *Acta Medica Iugoslavica,* Vol.44, pp. 29-135

Geerse, DA.; Rutherford ,P., Bogers, JCA., & Konings, CJAM (2011). Sterile peritonitis associated with the use of amino-acid solution in eight peritoneal dialysis patients. *Perit Dial Int, Vol.*31, pp. 90-1

Gouva, C.; Nikopoulos, I., Ioannidis, JP., & Siamopoulos, KC. (2004). Treating anemia early in renal failure patients shows the decline in renal function:A randomized controlled trial. *Kidney Int,* Vol.55, pp. 753-60

Guz, G.; Glorieux, GL., de Smet, R., Waterloos, M-A F., Vanholder, RC., & Dhondt, AW. (2006). Impact of iron sucrose therapy on leucocyte surface molecules and reactive oxygen species in haemodialysis patients. *Nephrol Dial Transplant, Vol.*21, Issue.10, (October 2006), pp. 2834-40

Hoerl, WH. (2008). Comparing the efficacy of intravenous iron and oral iron in nondialysis patients with chronic kidney disease. *Nature Clinical Practice/Nephrol,* Vol.4, Issue 10, (October 2008), pp. 530-31, www.nature.com/clinicalpractice/nephr

Howman, R.; & Kulkarni ,H. (2007). Antibody-mediated acquaried pure red cell aplasia (PRCA) after treatment with darberythropoietinetin. *Nephrol Dial Transplant,* Vol.22, pp. 1462-4

Kes, P, & Ljutic, D. (Ed(s).) December 2008. *Smjernice za liječenje anemije u bolesnika s kroničnim zatajenjem bubrega,* Croatian Society for Nephrology, Dialysis and Transplantation, ISBN 978-953-6451-53-0, Zagreb

Lau, JH.; Gangji, AS., Rabbat, CG., & Brimble, KS. (2010). Impact of haemoglobin and erythropoietin dose changes on mortality: a secondary analysis of results from a randomized anaemia management trial. *Nephrol Dial Transplant,* (Epub); cited in *Aktuelle Nephrology,* Vol.43, Issue 2, pp. 13-14

Levey, AS.; Coresh, J., Greene, T., Stevens, LA., Zhang, Yl., Hendriksen, S., Kusek, JW., & Van Lente, F. (2006). for the Chronic Kidney Disease Epidemiology Collaboration. Using standardized serum creatinine values in the modification of diet in Renal Disease Study Equation for estimating Glomerular Filtration Rate. *Annals of Internal Medicine, American College of Physicians,* Vol.145, pp. 247-54

Levin, A.; (2007). Understanding recent hemoglobin trials in CKD: methods and lesson learned from CREATE and CHOIR. *Nephrol Dial Transplant,* Vol.22, pp. 309-12

Li, H.; & Wang, SX. (2008). Intravenous iron sucrose in peritoneal dialysis patients with renal anemia. *Perit Dial Int*, Vol.28, pp. 149-54

Locatelli, F., Aljama, P., Barany, P., Canaud, B., Carrera, F., Eckhardt, K-U., Horl, WH., Macdougall, IC., Macleod, A., Wiecek, A.,&Cameron, S. (2004). Revised European Best Practices Guidelines for the management of anaemia in patients with chronic renal failure. *Nephrol Dial Transplant, Vol.*19, Issue Supplement 2, (May 2004), pp). ii 1-47, ISSN 0931-0509

Locatelli, F.; Andrulli, S., Mermoli, B., Maffei, C., Del Vechio, L., Aterini, S., De Simone, W., Mandalari, G., Brunori, G., Amato, M., Cianciaruso, B., & Zoccali, C. (2006). Nutritional-inflammation status and resistance to erythropoietin therapy in haemoldialysis patients. *Nephrol Dial Transplant,* Vol.21, Issue 4, (April 2006), pp. 991-8

Locatelli, F.; Nissenson, AR., Barret, BJ. & al. (2008). Clinical practice guidelines for anemia in chronic kidney disease: problems and solutions. A position statement from Kidney Disease Improving Global Outcomes (KDIGO). *Kidney Int,* Vol. 74, pp. 1237-40

Locatelli, F.; Covic, A.,Eckhardt, KU., Wiecek, A., & Vanholder, R. (2009) Anaemia management in patients with chronic kidney disease: a position statement by the Anaemia Working Group of European Renal Best Practice (ERBP). *Nephrol Dial Transplant* , Vol. 24, pp. 348-54

Marti, HH. (2004). Erythropoietin and the hypoxic brain. *Journal of Experimental Biology,* Vol.207, pp. 3233-42

Miroescu, G.; Garneata, L., Ciocalteu, A . et al. (2006). Once-every-2-weeks and once-weekly erythropoietinetin beta regimens; equivalency in hemodialysis patients. *Am J Kindey Dis* , Vol. 48, pp. 45-55

Namiuchi, S.; Kagaya, Y., & Ohta, J. (2005). High serum erythropoietin level is associated with smaller infarct size in patients with acute myocardial infarction who undergo successful primary percutaneous coronary intervention. *Journal of American College in Cardiology,* Vol.45, pp. 1406-12

NKF-K/DOQI Clinical Practice Guidelines for Anemia of Chronic Kidney Disease. (2006) *Am J Kidney Dis* 2 Vol. 47, Issue supplement 4, pp. S1-18

NKF-K/DOQI Clinical Practice Guidelines and Clinical Practice Recommendations for Anemia of Chronic Kidney Disease: 2007 update for hemoglobin target. (2007), *Am J Kidney Dis,* Vol.50, pp. 474 -6

Pampilon, DH.; Rider, JR., Barbara, JA., & Williamson, LM. (1998). Prevention of transfusion - transmitted cytomegalovirus infection. *Transfusion Medicine,* Vol.9, pp. 115-23

Portoles, J.; Krisper, P., Choukroun, G., & de Francisco, ALM. (2005). Exploring dosing frequency and administration routes in the treatment of anaemia in CKD patients. *Nephrol Dial Transplant,* Vol.20, Issue Supplement 8, pp. viii13-viii17

Puretić, Z. (Ed). (May 2000). Smjernice za liječenje anemije u bolesnika s kroničnim zatajenjem bubrega, *Croatian Society for Nephrology, Dialysis and Transplantation,* ISBN 953-98163-0-0, Zagreb , pp. 7-31

Puretic, Z. (2009). Posebnosti lijecenja anemije u djece s kronicnim bolestima bubrega. *Acta Medica Croatica, Vol.*63, Issue Supplement 1, (September 2009), pp. 27-32 (abstr. english) ISSN 1330-0164

Roseff , SD., Luban, NL., & Manno, CS. (2002). Guidelines for assesing appropriatness of pediatric transfusions. *Transfusion,* Vol.42, pp. 1398-413

Schwartz, GJ.; Feld, LG., & Langford, DJ. (1984). A simple estimate of glomerular filtration rate in full term infants during the first year of life. *J Pediatr* Vol.104, pp. 849-54

Schwartz, GJ.; & Gauthier, B. (1985). A simple estimate of glomerular filtration rate in adolescent boys. *J Pediatr* Vol.106, pp. 522-7

Sieff, CA.; Emerson, SG., Mufson, A., Gesner, TG., & Nathan, DG. (1986). Dependence of highly enriched human bone marrow progenitors on hematopoietic growth factors and their response to recombinant erythropoetin. *Clinical Investigation,* Vol.77, pp. 74-8

Sief ,CA.; Ekern, SC., Nathan, DG., & Anderson, JW. (1989). Combinations of recombinant colony stimulating factors are required for optimal hematopoietic differentiation in serum-deprived culture. *Blood,* Vol.73, pp. 688-93

Slonim , AD., Joseph, JG., Turenne, WM., Sharangpeni ,A., & Luban, NL. (2008).Blood transfusion in children: a multi-institution analysis of practice and complications. *Transfusion* , Vol.48, pp. 73-80

Spandou, E.; Tsouchnikas, I., Karkavelas, G., Dounousi, E., Simeonidou, C., Guiba-Tziampiri, O., &Tsakiris, D. (2006). Erythropoietin attenuates renal injury in experimental acute renal failure ischaemic/reperfusion model. *Nephrol Dial Transplant,* Vol.21, Issue 2, (February 2006), pp. 330-6

Streja, E.; Kovesdy, CP., Greenland, S., Kopple, JD., Mc Alister, CJ., Nissenson, AR., & Kalantar-Zadeh, K. (2004) Erythropoietin, iron depletion, and relative thrombocytosis: a possible explanation for hemoglobin-survival paradox in hemodialysis. *Am J Kidney Dis,* Vol. 52, pp. 727-36

Suda, T.; Suda, J., Ogawa, M., & al. (1984). Disparate differentitation in mouse hematopoietic colonie derived from paired progenitors. *Proceedings of National Academy of Science USA,* Vol. 81, pp. 2520-4

Teruya, J. (2008). Administration and complications of red cell transfusion in infants and children. Uptodate, Mahoney, DH.,Kim, MS., pp. 1-5, Uptodate, http://www.uptodate.com/online/content/topic.do?topicKey=pedi_hem/9615&selected

Van Biesen, W.; Vanholder, R., Veys, N. et al. (2005). Efficacy of erythropoietin administration in the treatment of anemia immediately after renal transplantation. *Transplantation,* Vol.79, pp. 367-8

Vorobiov, M.; Malki, M., Shnaider, A. et al. (2008). Erythropietin prevents dialysis fluid-induced appoptosis of mesangial cells. *Perit Dial Int,* Vol. 28, pp. 648-56

Working Party for European Best Practice Guidelines for the management of anaemia in patients with chronic renal failure. (1999). European Best Practice Guidelines for the management of anaemia in patients with chronic renal failure. *Nephrol Dial Transplant, Vol.*14, Issue Supplement 5, ISSN0931-0509, (1999), pp. 1-50

Yorgin, PD.; Belson, A. , Al-Uzri, AY., & Alexander, S. (2001). The clinicl efficacy of higher hematocrit levels in children with chronic insufficiency and those undergoing dialysis. *Seminar Nephrol* , Vol.21, pp. 451-62

11

Post Transplant Anaemia

Bhadran Bose and David Mudge
*Princess Alexandra Hospital, Brisbane
Australia*

1. Introduction

Anaemia, as a complication of end stage kidney disease (ESKD), is well studied (Eschbach and Adamson 1985). Reports indicate that anaemia in this patient population is associated with numerous morbidities, but predominantly cardiovascular complications such as left ventricular hypertrophy and heart failure (Wizemann, Schafer et al. 1993; Harnett, Foley et al. 1995). Contrary to the ample data available regarding anaemia in ESKD population, much less is known about the epidemiology of post-transplant anaemia (PTA), and only few studies have systematically investigated this issue (Saito, Fujiwara et al. 1998; Yorgin, Scandling et al. 2002; Mix, Kazmi et al. 2003; Vanrenterghem, Ponticelli et al. 2003).
A successful renal allograft will correct not only the excretory functions of the kidney but also the endocrine functions (through the restored synthesis of erythropoietin and vitamin D) including the correction of anaemia. However, in the majority of transplant recipients, the renal graft does not function optimally. It is well known that renal excretory functions are not restored completely, but the extent to which renal endocrine functions are restored is only recently becoming better understood. A recent European survey of ten transplant centres revealed a prevalence of PTA as high as 42% (Molnar et al, 2011).
PTA may occur at any time after renal transplantation. Early PTA (from the time of surgery until 3 months post-operatively) is most likely to be related to pre-transplant anaemia of ESKD, the surgery itself, iron deficiency, immunosuppression, inflammation or infection (Miles, Markell et al. 1997; Turkowski-Duhem, Kamar et al. 2005) or some combination of these. Later PTA is more likely to be related to consequences of long-term immunosuppression (particularly anti-metabolite medications) or a failing allograft. All the published large scale studies to date have focused mainly on late PTA (Miles, Markell et al. 1997; Vanrenterghem, Ponticelli et al. 2003; Turkowski-Duhem, Kamar et al. 2005), and there are a lack of studies looking at the management of early PTA, in particular, the optimal management of iron deficiency at the time of kidney transplantation.
The importance of PTA is that it is one of the commonest complications after kidney transplantation, that it is strongly associated with cardiovascular morbidity (the primary cause of death of kidney transplant recipients, accounting for approximately one half of such deaths), and that its optimal treatment, either with iron, erythropoietin, or other agents, has yet to be determined by large-scale randomised controlled trials.

2. Prevalence

PTA remains a common complication after kidney transplantation, with an incidence ranging from nearly 80% at day 0 to as low as 25% at 1 year (Saito, Fujiwara et al. 1998;

Yorgin, Scandling et al. 2002; Mix, Kazmi et al. 2003; Vanrenterghem, Ponticelli et al. 2003). To date, there are very few published studies of PTA, and very few presenting data on interventions for PTA.

One of the largest studies (Vanrenterghem, Ponticelli et al. 2003) was published in the *American Journal of Transplantation*, and included 4,263 kidney transplant patients from 72 centres in 16 European countries (**TR**ansplant **E**uropean **S**urvey on **A**naemia **M**anagement [TRESAM] survey). The patients were divided into four cohorts and assessed at 6 months (n=1003), 1 year (n=960), 3 years (n=1254) and 5 years (n=1046) after kidney transplantation. Recipients of multiple organs, pregnant women and children aged <10 years were excluded from the study.

Demographic data indicate that the patients included in the TRESAM survey were representative of the European transplant population. Approximately 60% of patients were male and 40% were female, and these proportions were similar in the four cohorts. The mean (SD) age of transplant recipients at transplantation was 45.5 (13.1) years, although patients who had received their transplant more recently were significantly (p=0.01) older at transplantation than patients who had received their transplant 5 years ago. The proportion of patients in this survey who had received their kidney from a living donor was relatively low (~10%). The most prevalent underlying kidney disease in the TRESAM survey was chronic glomerulonephritis (29.8-37.0% across the four cohorts). The prevalence of diabetic nephropathy was uncharacteristically low (6.5-7.5%) by contemporary standards. The most frequently occurring co-morbidities were coronary artery disease (13.0-16.1%), hepatitis B/C (9.3-10.8%) and type 2 diabetes mellitus (8.7-10.1%).

Pre-transplant haemoglobin (Hb) concentrations in one study were significantly higher in patients who had received their transplant more recently than in patients who had received their transplant 5 years earlier, suggesting progressive anaemia with time. In that study, the mean Hb concentrations were 11.9 g/dL in the 6 month cohort *vs* 10.8 g/dL in the 5 year cohort (p<0.01; Eschbach and Adamson, 1985)

Anaemia, defined as Hb concentration ≤ 13 g/dL for male patients and ≤ 12 g/dL for female patients, was present in 38.6% of patients overall in this survey, and was equally distributed between the sexes. Of these patients, 11.6% had moderate anaemia (Hb concentration >11 and ≤ 12 g/dL for male patients and >10 and ≤11g/dL for female patients), while 8.5% had severe anaemia (Hb concentrations ≤11g/dL for male patients and ≤10 g/dL for female patients). In patients with a serum creatinine levels >2 mg/dL, 60.1% were considered anaemic, whereas in patients with a serum creatinine level ≤ 2 mg/dL, only 29.0% of patients were considered anaemic (p<0.01). The findings of the TRESAM survey were in agreement with the results published by a contemporary American group (Yorgin, Scandling et al. 2002). The aforementioned 5-year follow up of the TRESAM survey (Molnar et al, 2011) reported similar rates of anaemia at 42% overall, suggesting that the problem is not improving over time despite awareness of the problem.

The group from Boston, MA undertook a retrospective longitudinal cohort study (Mix, Kazmi et al. 2003) to characterise changes in haematocrit (Hct) following kidney transplantation and to identify factors associated with those changes. The study included 240 patients who underwent kidney transplantation in Tufts-New England Medical Centre, Boston, MA. Hct levels were available for 94% of patients at 1-month follow-up and for 95-100% of patients at subsequent follow-up intervals. At the time of transplant surgery, 22% (95% CI 16%, 28%) of the cohort had Hct < 30%. The mean Hct rose from its nadir of 33% (95% CI 27%. 39%), both at the time of transplantation and at 1 month after transplantation, to a peak of 40% (95% CI 34%, 46%) 12 months after transplantation, and declined thereafter. During the first year after transplantation, the proportion of patients with Hct <36% steadily decreased from 76% (95% CI 70%, 82%) at transplantation to 21% (95% CI 15%, 27%) at 12 months after transplantation. The proportion of patients with Hct < 33% declined over a shorter time interval, from 48% (95% CI 42%, 54%) at transplantation to 7% (95% CI 3%, 11%) at 6 months after transplantation. These data closely reflect the European experience as previously described.

3. Risk factors for PTA

In the post-transplant setting anaemia may be contributed to by blood loss, iron deficiency, bone marrow suppression by anti-proliferative agents (mycophenolate, azathioprine), erythropoietin deficiency, and inflammation (Table 1). The relative contributions of these components may be difficult to ascertain in an individual patient and may often be due to a combination of these factors.

Early PTA	Late PTA
Immunosuppressive agents	↓ red cell survival
Surgical blood loss	Immunosuppressive agents
Frequent blood sampling	↓erythrocyte production
Drugs-ACEi/ARB	Low excretory +/- endocrine graft function
Iron deficiency	EPO resistance
Delayed graft function	
Persistent uraemic toxins	

ACEi=Angiotensin converting enzyme inhibitor, ARB=Angiotensin Receptor Blocker.
EPO resistance is defined as the need of ≥300IU/Kg/week.

Table 1. Common risk factors for PTA

3.1 Early PTA

A prospective study (Turkowski-Duhem, Kamar et al. 2005) published in *Transplantation* attempted to identify independent predictors of anaemia at 6 months and 12 months post-transplant. The authors studied 99 patients who had undergone kidney transplantation at Toulouse University Hospital between January 2001 and January 2002. Anaemia as defined by WHO criteria was observed in 38.6% of patients, which is a very similar rate to that found in other published studies from the same era.

Immunosuppressive treatment, particularly with antimetabolite drugs, is one of the most likely contributors to PTA. The purine synthesis inhibitors, azathioprine and mycophenolate mofetil (MMF), are known to cause anaemia (Gossmann, Kachel et al. 1993; de Sevaux, Hilbrands et al. 1998; Kuypers, Claes et al. 2004; Shipkova, Spielbauer et al. 2004). Macrocytosis was present in the majority of the patients in those studies treated with azathioprine. Mammalian target of rapamycin (mTOR) inhibitors (e.g., sirolimus) are also associated with PTA, and particularly with microcytosis even in the absence of iron deficiency (Thaunat, Beaumont et al. 2007). In that study nearly all patient received concomitant MMF and for the 42.3% who received induction therapy with rabbit antithymocyte globulin (ATG), the incidence of PTA was lower than previously reported values, at only 25% at 1 year post-transplantation. This could merely reflect selection bias.

Some recent report suggests that sirolimus-based therapy was an independent factor of PTA (Augustine, Knauss et al. 2004). For example, the prevalence of PTA was 31% with MMF-based immunosuppression and as high as 57% with sirolimus-based immunosuppression. Through mTOR inhibition, sirolimus blocks S6 kinase activity and consequently impairs cell replication in an erythroid cell line (Jaster, Bittorf et al. 1996) leading to anaemia.

One other obvious contributor to post-transplant anaemia is iron deficiency. Iron deficiency, defined by low ferritin and a low transferrin saturation, was present in 17% (Mahmud, Aziz et al. 2002) and 34.6%(Kim, Park et al. 2003) of anaemic patients in the post-transplant setting. Patients coming to kidney transplantation are known to be frequently iron deficient both in absolute and functional terms (Lorenz, Kletzmayr et al. 2002).

Many studies have demonstrated that the occurrence of PTA is related to renal allograft function, with declining function related to worsening anaemia as is seen in the chronic kidney disease (CKD) population. The results of the TRESAM survey showed a strong correlation between Hb levels and graft function expressed as serum creatinine and creatinine clearance: the majority of anaemic patients had creatinine levels > 2 mg/dL (Vanrenterghem, Ponticelli et al. 2003). Turkowski-Duhem found an effect of post-transplant renal function on haemoglobin levels at 6 months. Both delayed graft function (DGF) and renal allograft function, defined by creatinine clearance, were independent factors associated with the occurrence of anaemia at 12 months post transplantation(Turkowski-Duhem, Kamar et al. 2005). In another study it was reported that at both 6 and 12 months post transplantation higher serum creatinine values (defined as each 1 mg/dL increase in serum creatinine level) were significant independent risk factors for anaemia (Shibagaki and Shetty 2004). Similarly, in a further study (Yorgin, Scandling et al. 2002) serum CO_2, blood urea nitrogen (BUN) and creatinine correlated with anaemia at 1 year post transplantation (Yorgin, Scandling et al. 2002). These findings were explained by the decreased production of erythropoietin (Kuypers, Claes et al.) and also the increase in erythropoietin (EPO) resistance relative to the decline in renal excretory function in the early 1990's. (van Dullemen, Luykx-de Bakker et al. 1992).

In the TRESAM survey, transplant recipients who had experienced one or more rejection episodes, or who had received a second or third graft, had lower haemoglobin levels than recipients without rejection episodes or recipients with a first transplant. An analysis using DNA microarrays identified a cluster of genes related to haemoglobin synthesis and/or erythropoiesis that was altered in kidneys with renal allograft rejection compared with normal allograft kidneys (Chua, Barry et al. 2003).

Another factor relevant to early PTA is cytomegalovirus (CMV) infection. Turkowski-Durhem showed on univariate analysis that at 12 months post transplantation, the prevalence of CMV seropositivity was significantly higher in those presenting with anaemia (78%) than in those without anaemia (51%), suggesting CMV infection might be a predisposing factor to PTA. However, on multivariate analysis, CMV status was no longer a significant predictor. . Mix et al. found that positive CMV donor status and negative recipient status (CMV D+/R-) was a factor independently associated with a greater likelihood of PTA, in this case defined as a haematocrit (Hct) <36% at 6 months post transplantation (Mix, Kazmi et al. 2003). These two observations suggest that CMV infection itself, and/or the use of drugs to prevent or treat CMV infection/disease, might result in a degree of bone-marrow suppression leading to PTA.

Angiotensin converting enzyme (ACE) inhibitor therapy is known to induce anaemia (Gossmann, Kachel et al. 1993), and has been used to treat post-transplant erythrocytosis

(Rostaing, Boisseau et al. 1995). The TRESAM survey reported that the use of ACE inhibitors or angiotensin II receptor blockers (ARB's) was associated with a higher odds ratio for anaemia (OR=1.55); they also found that it increased the risk of severe anaemia. Winckelmayer et al. observed that patients taking ACE inhibitors had significantly lower Hct levels compared with patients not taking them. In addition, a significant curvilinear dose-response relationship was found between ACE inhibitor dose and Hct level.

Turkowski-Durhem also observed that the platelet count at day-7 post transplantation was an independent predictive factor for anaemia at both 6 months (OR 0.12 (0.03-0.48); P=0.002) and 12 months (OR 0.096 (0.01 -1.04); P=0.05), i.e. more anaemic patients had a significantly lower platelet count (<200X10^9/L) than non-anaemic patients (72% vs. 38% at 6 months, and 65% vs. 45% at 12 months). The significance of the association with platelet counts at day-7 post transplant, and the occurrence of PTA at 6 and 12 months, persists even after excluding patients that received induction therapy with ATG because the latter can result in thrombocytopenia. There was no explanation given for this observation, although it could just represent a different measure of overall bone marrow suppression

The other causes of early PTA have been attributed to blood loss at the time of surgery, frequent blood sampling and the persistent effect of uraemic toxins.

3.2 Late PTA

PTA that occurs late after transplantation has been attributed to decreased red blood cell survival (Najean, Rain et al. 1997), erythrocyte hypoproduction due to iron deficiency (Teruel, Lamas et al. 1989; Beshara, Birgegard et al. 1997; Miles, Markell et al. 1997), low excretory graft function (Miles, Markell et al. 1997), and immunosuppressive agents (Solheim, Albrechtsen et al. 1987; Yoshimura, Oka et al. 1989; Creemers, van Boven et al. 1993; Zazgornik 1997).

A retrospective longitudinal analysis (Yorgin, Scandling et al. 2002) of adult renal transplant recipients was published in *American Journal of Transplantation* looking at the prevalence, severity and predictors of late PTA. The study population of adults (>18 years) transplanted during 1995 at Stanford University (n=88) and University of North Carolina (n=40) were selected. Post-transplant anaemia was a common problem which affected 30% of the study population at least once during the first 5 years after transplant. Recurrence of PTA was common (50%) and the prevalence and severity of anaemia increased with time after transplantation.

Renal excretory function is strongly correlated with anaemia in adult renal transplant recipients. Yet the effect of renal excretory function on anaemia is not absolute, as a small proportion of anaemic patients have creatinine clearance values > 75 mL/min/1.73 m^2 (i.e. normal), whereas conversely, some non-anaemic patients have creatinine clearance < 50 mL/min 1.73 m^2.(Yorgin, Scandling et al. 2002). A study by van Dullemen et al. demonstrated that EPO production decreases and EPO resistance increases proportionally to the decline in renal excretory function (van Dullemen, Luykx-de Bakker et al. 1992). Other factors not related to declining renal excretory function include DGF, acute tubulointerstitial rejection (Besarab, Caro et al. 1987; Heidenreich, Tepel et al. 1995), chronic rejection (Heidenreich, Tepel et al. 1995) and possibly long-term calcineurin inhibitor toxicity (Jensen, Hansen et al. 1994) may contribute to PTA by leading to diminished EPO production.

Since renal tubular injury may be attributable to DGF, allograft rejection and calcineurin inhibitor toxicity in renal transplant recipients, and that all of these complications are frequent, another factor which has been evaluated as an important indicator of renal tubular function is serum total CO_2. In one study, Anaemic patients had lower serum total CO_2 values ($p=0.019$ at 1 year post transplant and $p<0.0001$ at 5 years post transplant) (Yorgin, Scandling et al. 2002). The authors speculate that the presence of metabolic acidosis is a surrogate indicator of renal tubular injury, diminished renal excretory function and diminished EPO production, however this hypothesis has not been tested.

Yorgin et al also found that few anaemic patients were ever treated with EPO or even iron therapy. This finding may demonstrate a need for increased awareness of anaemia and increased concern about subnormal Hct by the patient's primary nephrologists and transplant physicians.

4. Treatment of PTA

There is a paucity of good quality and large scale intervention trials for PTA in the transplant literature, although some registry studies and multi-centre surveys do shed some light on practice patterns. For example, in the TRESAM survey rates of ESA use were reported. Surprisingly, of the 3969 patients overall for whom the use of erythropoietic therapy was documented, only 207 (5.2%) had received an erythropoietin-stimulating agent (ESA) for the treatment of anaemia. Even more striking was the fact that among the group of anaemic patients (n=1539), only 10% had received an ESA or other specific therapy. Of the 343 patients with severe anaemia, 17.8% were treated with erythropoietic therapy (Fig 1).

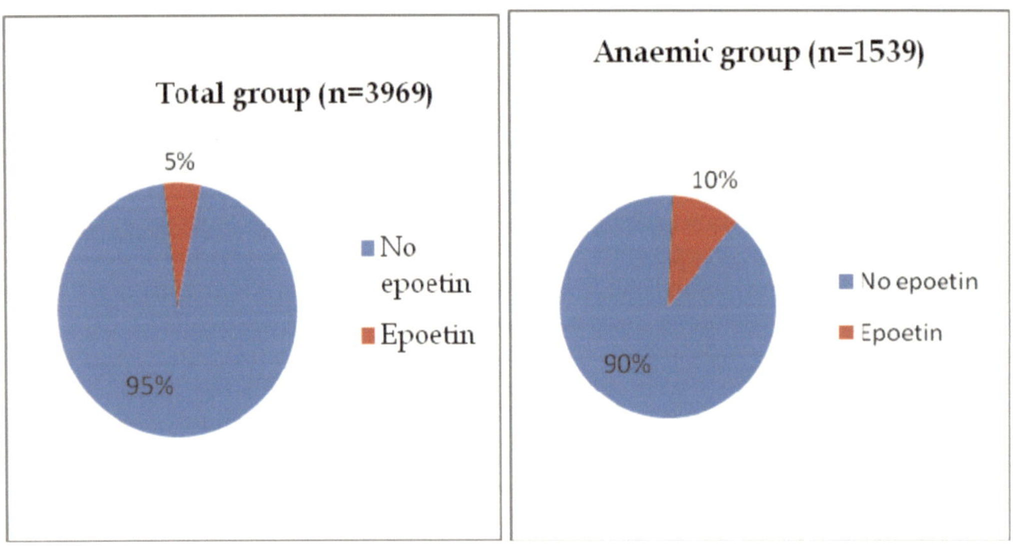

Fig. 1. Epoetin treatment in the TRESAM survey.

Possible reasons for the reluctance of nephrologists to correct anaemia in transplant patients include a relative paucity of published studies on intervention strategies for PTA, an under-recognition of the importance of the problem in terms of contribution to overall cardiovascular risk (also due to lack of specific studies demonstrating this) and finally the "psychological factor" of concerns regarding the efficacy and safety of therapy. In terms of safety of therapy, there have been concerns regarding the normalisation of Hb concentrations with ESA in the CKD population and. A few studies, involving small number of patients, have suggested that transplant recipients treated with epoetin develop hypertension, which requires treatment with anti-hypertensive drugs (Muirhead 1999; Kim, Park et al. 2003). However, to date, there have been no indications that patients treated with erythropoietic therapy after transplantation show a more rapid deterioration of their allograft function(Muirhead 1999).

4.1 Erythropoietin-stimulating agent use

Several small-scale studies suggest that ESA may be an effective treatment for post-transplant anaemia (Traindl, Barnas et al. 1994; Muirhead 1999; Kim, Park et al. 2003). The study done by *Lezaic* (Lezaic, Djukanovic et al. 1995) suggested that the response to erythropoietic therapy of patients with anaemia post-transplant is comparable with that of anaemia due to other forms of renal failure. As EPO resistance is common in these patients, they should be evaluated for secondary or tertiary hyperparathyroidism, hypothyroidism, haemolysis, and GI blood loss if a reticulocyte spike is not detected 7 days post transplantation.

Several recent studies in the CKD literature (Pfeffer et al. 2009, Drueke et al 2006) regarding haemoglobin targets have resulted in concern over the potential for increasing the risk of stroke and possibly malignancy-related death when haemoglobin targets of >13 mg/dL are aimed for. The optimum Hb target for kidney transplant recipients remains unknown. Future trials will need to assess these endpoints in the post-transplant situation in order to establish the safety of ESA in this setting.

4.2 Iron therapy

Replacement of depleted iron stores are necessary for the correction of PTA. Functional iron deficiency is a common problem in CKD populations and may also be a problem in kidney transplant recipients. The best form of iron replacement in this setting is yet to be established. Oral iron is poorly absorbed, often not tolerated, and may interfere with the absorption of immunosuppressants. Intravenous iron has been used to replenish iron stores (Macdougall 1999) in transplant recipients as it has been in CKD patients in order to get around the problems of oral iron supplements. But a study currently in press but whose protocol was recently published (Mudge, Tan et al. 2009) showed that intravenous versus oral iron was not associated with a reduction in PTA, but did lead to a non-significant reduction in gastro-intestinal side-effects, numerically fewer blood transfusions and was equally efficacious in the treatment of post-transplant anaemia.

The measurement of iron status in post-kidney transplant patients, as in CKD patients, remains problematic. Existing measurements include serum iron, ferritin, and transferrin saturation. Ferritin is elevated in the setting of inflammation and therefore may not be indicative. New measures of iron status such as hepcidin show promise for more accurate estimation of iron status in this setting, but as yet a reference range has not been elucidated.

4.3 Other treatments

Other nutritional parameters such as B vitamins (B12, folate etc) are important in the pathogenesis of anaemia, and patients who have been treated with haemodialysis prior to transplantation are at risk of B-group vitamin deficiencies due to the removal of these water soluble vitamins with long-term dialysis, and especially with extended-hours dialysis

(Coveney, 2010). Most such patients would be supplemented with B-group vitamins during their dialysis treatment however.

5. Conclusions

PTA is a common problem in kidney transplant recipients and further studies are needed to better determine the relative contributions of iron deficiency, EPO deficiency, and bone marrow suppression, with a view to better determining the optimum strategy for its correction in individual patients. Anaemia is a risk factor for cardiovascular events and may be a contributor to the high cardiovascular event rate seen in kidney transplant recipients.

6. References

Augustine, J. J., T. C. Knauss, et al. (2004). "Comparative effects of sirolimus and mycophenolate mofetil on erythropoiesis in kidney transplant patients." American journal of transplantation : official journal of the American Society of Transplantation and the American Society of Transplant Surgeons 4(12): 2001-2006.

Besarab, A., J. Caro, et al. (1987). "Dynamics of erythropoiesis following renal transplantation." Kidney international 32(4): 526-536.

Beshara, S., G. Birgegard, et al. (1997). "Assessment of erythropoiesis following renal transplantation." European journal of haematology 58(3): 167-173.

Chua, M. S., C. Barry, et al. (2003). "Molecular profiling of anemia in acute renal allograft rejection using DNA microarrays." American journal of transplantation : official journal of the American Society of Transplantation and the American Society of Transplant Surgeons 3(1): 17-22.

Coveney, N., Polkinghorne, K.R., Linehan, L. et al. (2010). "Water-soluble vitamin levels in extended hors hemodialysis." Hemodialysis International Nov 24. doi: 10.1111/j.1542-4758.2010.00505.x. [Epub ahead of print]

Creemers, G. J., W. P. van Boven, et al. (1993). "Azathioprine-associated pure red cell aplasia." Journal of internal medicine 233(1): 85-87.

de Sevaux, R. G., L. B. Hilbrands, et al. (1998). "A randomised, prospective study on the conversion from cyclosporine-prednisone to cyclosporine-azathioprine at 6 months after renal transplantation." Transplant international : official journal of the European Society for Organ Transplantation 11 Suppl 1: S322-324.

Drueke, T.B. et al (2006). "Normalization of hemoglobin level in patients with chronic kidney disease and anemia." New England Journal of Medicine 355(20): 2071-2084.

Eschbach, J. W. and J. W. Adamson (1985). "Anemia of end-stage renal disease (ESRD)." Kidney international 28(1): 1-5.

Gossmann, J., H. G. Kachel, et al. (1993). "Anemia in renal transplant recipients caused by concomitant therapy with azathioprine and angiotensin-converting enzyme inhibitors." Transplantation 56(3): 585-589.

Harnett, J. D., R. N. Foley, et al. (1995). "Congestive heart failure in dialysis patients: prevalence, incidence, prognosis and risk factors." Kidney international 47(3): 884-890.

Heidenreich, S., M. Tepel, et al. (1995). "Prognostic value of serum erythropoietin levels in late acute rejection of renal transplants." American journal of kidney diseases : the official journal of the National Kidney Foundation 25(5): 775-780.

Jaster, R., T. Bittorf, et al. (1996). "Inhibition of proliferation but not erythroid differentiation of J2E cells by rapamycin." Biochemical pharmacology 51(9): 1181-1185.

Jensen, J. D., H. E. Hansen, et al. (1994). "Increased serum erythropoietin level during azathioprine treatment in renal transplant recipients." Nephron 67(3): 297-301.

Kim, H. C., S. B. Park, et al. (2003). "Anemia following renal transplantation." Transplantation proceedings 35(1): 302-303.

Kuypers, D. R., K. Claes, et al. (2004). "Clinical efficacy and toxicity profile of tacrolimus and mycophenolic acid in relation to combined long-term pharmacokinetics in de novo renal allograft recipients." Clinical pharmacology and therapeutics 75(5): 434-447.

Lezaic, V., L. Djukanovic, et al. (1995). "Recombinant human erythropoietin treatment of anemia in renal transplant patients." Renal failure 17(6): 705-714.

Lorenz, M., J. Kletzmayr, et al. (2002). "Anemia and iron deficiencies among long-term renal transplant recipients." Journal of the American Society of Nephrology : JASN 13(3): 794-797.

Macdougall, I. C. (1999). "Strategies for iron supplementation: oral versus intravenous." Kidney international. Supplement 69: S61-66.

Mahmud, S. N., R. Aziz, et al. (2002). "Anemia characteristics after renal transplantation." Transplantation proceedings 34(6): 2428.

Miles, A. M., M. S. Markell, et al. (1997). "Anemia following renal transplantation: erythropoietin response and iron deficiency." Clinical transplantation 11(4): 313-315.

Mix, T. C., W. Kazmi, et al. (2003). "Anemia: a continuing problem following kidney transplantation." American journal of transplantation : official journal of the American Society of Transplantation and the American Society of Transplant Surgeons 3(11): 1426-1433.

Mudge, D. W., K. S. Tan, et al. (2009). "Intravenous versus oral iron supplementation for correction of post-transplant anaemia in renal transplant patients." BMC nephrology 10: 14.

Muirhead, N. (1999). "Erythropoietin and renal transplantation." Kidney international. Supplement 69: S86-92.

Najean, Y., J. D. Rain, et al. (1997). "Red cell and platelet kinetics in chronic cytopenias following transplantation." Hematology and cell therapy 39(5): 233-236.

Pfeffer, M.A., Burdmann, M.D., Chen, C.Y., et al. (2009). "A trial of darbepoetin alfa in type 2 diabetes and chronic kidney disease" New England Journal of Medicine 361(21): 2019-32

Rostaing, L., M. Boisseau, et al. (1995). "Correction of post-renal transplant erythrocytosis by enalapril." Scandinavian journal of urology and nephrology 29(4): 399-406.

Saito, S., T. Fujiwara, et al. (1998). "Anemia following renal transplantation." Transplantation proceedings 30(7): 3025-3026.

Shibagaki, Y. and A. Shetty (2004). "Anaemia is common after kidney transplantation, especially among African Americans." Nephrology, dialysis, transplantation : official publication of the European Dialysis and Transplant Association - European Renal Association 19(9): 2368-2373.

Shipkova, M., B. Spielbauer, et al. (2004). "cDNA microarray analysis reveals new candidate genes possibly linked to side effects under mycophenolate mofetil therapy." Transplantation 78(8): 1145-1152.

Solheim, B. G., D. A. Albrechtsen, et al. (1987). "Hemolytic anemia in cyclosporine-treated recipients of kidney or heart grafts from donors with minor incompatibility for ABO antigens." Transplantation proceedings 19(5): 4236-4238.
Teruel, J. L., S. Lamas, et al. (1989). "Serum ferritin levels after renal transplantation: a prospective study." Nephron 51(4): 462-465.
Thaunat, O., C. Beaumont, et al. (2007). "Late introduction of sirolimus induces anemia in renal transplant recipients." Transplantation 83(9): 1283; author reply 1284.
Traindl, O., U. Barnas, et al. (1994). "Recombinant human erythropoietin in renal transplant recipients with renal anemia." Clinical transplantation 8(1): 45-48.
Turkowski-Duhem, A., N. Kamar, et al. (2005). "Predictive factors of anemia within the first year post renal transplant." Transplantation 80(7): 903-909.
van Dullemen, H. M., S. Luykx-de Bakker, et al. (1992). "Inhibitors of recombinant human erythropoietin in chronic renal failure." The Netherlands journal of medicine 41(1-2): 56-63.
Vanrenterghem, Y., C. Ponticelli, et al. (2003). "Prevalence and management of anemia in renal transplant recipients: a European survey." American journal of transplantation : official journal of the American Society of Transplantation and the American Society of Transplant Surgeons 3(7): 835-845.
Wizemann, V., R. Schafer, et al. (1993). "Follow-up of cardiac changes induced by anemia compensation in normotensive hemodialysis patients with left-ventricular hypertrophy." Nephron 64(2): 202-206.
Yorgin, P. D., J. D. Scandling, et al. (2002). "Late post-transplant anemia in adult renal transplant recipients. An under-recognized problem?" American journal of transplantation : official journal of the American Society of Transplantation and the American Society of Transplant Surgeons 2(5): 429-435.
Yoshimura, N., T. Oka, et al. (1989). "Cyclosporine-associated microangiopathic hemolytic anemia in a renal transplant recipient." The Japanese journal of surgery 19(2): 223-228.
Zazgornik, J. (1997). "Azathioprine induced macrocytosis and red cell aplasia in renal transplant patients." Nephrology, dialysis, transplantation : official publication of the European Dialysis and Transplant Association - European Renal Association 12(3): 628.

12

New Onset Diabetes After Solid Organ Transplantation

Phuong-Thu T. Pham[1], Phuong-Mai T. Pham[2], Parikh S[1], Son V. Pham[3], Phuong-Anh T. Pham[4] and Phuong-Chi T. Pham[5]
[1]*Department of Medicine, Nephrology Division, Kidney Transplant Program, David Geffen School of Medicine at UCLA*
[2]*Department of Medicine, Greater Los Angeles VA Medical Center and David Geffen School of Medicine at UCLA*
[3]*Department of Medicine, Cardiology Division, Bay Pines VA Medical Center, Bay Pines, Florida*
[4]*Department of Medicine, Division of Cardiovascular Diseases, VA Medical Center, University of Tennessee Health Science Center, Memphis, TN*
[5]*Department of Medicine, Nephrology Division, UCLA-Olive View Medical Center and David Geffen School of Medicine*
United States of America

1. Introduction

New onset diabetes mellitus after transplantation (NODAT) is a serious and common complication following solid organ transplantation. NODAT has been reported to occur in 2% to 53% of all solid organ transplants. Kidney transplant recipients who develop NODAT have variably been reported to be at increased risk of fatal and nonfatal cardiovascular events and other adverse outcomes including infection, reduced patient survival, graft rejection, and accelerated graft loss compared with those who do not develop diabetes. Limited clinical studies in liver, heart and lung transplants similarly suggested that NODAT has an adverse impact on patient and graft outcomes. The following chapter presents an overview of the literature on the current diagnostic criteria for NODAT, its incidence after solid organ transplantation, suggested risk factors and potential pathogenic mechanisms. The impact of NODAT on patient and allograft outcomes and suggested guidelines for early identification and management of NODAT will also be discussed.

2. Definition and diagnosis of new onset diabetes after transplantation

Historically, post-transplant diabetes has been variably defined as having random glucose levels greater than 200 mg/dl fasting, glucose levels greater than 140 mg/dl, or the need for insulin or oral hypoglycemic agents in the post-transplant period. In 2003, the International Expert Panel consisting of experts from both the transplant and diabetes fields set forth the International Consensus Guidelines for the diagnosis and management of NODAT (Davidson et al., 2003; Wilkinson et al., 2005). It was recommended that the definition and diagnosis of NODAT should be based on the definition of diabetes mellitus and impaired glucose tolerance (IGT) described by the World Health Organization (WHO) (Montori et al., 2002; Wilkinson et al, 2005). The current WHO and American Diabetes Association (ADA) guidelines for the diagnosis of prediabetic states (IFG and IGT) and diabetes mellitus are provided in Table 1 (modified from Davidson et al., 2003).

Criteria for the diagnosis of diabetes mellitus

- Symptoms[1] of diabetes mellitus + casual[2] PG concentrations ≥ 200 mg/dL (11.1 mM)

or

- FPG ≥ 126 mg/dL (7.0 mM). Fasting is defined as no caloric intake for at least 8 hours

or

- 2-hr PG ≥ 200 mg/dL (11.1 mM) during an oral glucose tolerance test[3]

A confirmatory laboratory test based on measurements of venous PG must be done on another day in the absence of unequivocal hyperglycemia accompanied by acute metabolic decompensation.

Criteria for normal FPG and IFG or IGT

FPG
WHO criteria
FPG < 110 mg/dL (6.1 mM) = normal fasting glucose
FPG ≥ 110 mg/dl (6.1 mM) and < 126 mg/dl (7.0 mM) = IFG
2003 ADA updated consensus report
FPG < 100 mg/dL (5.6 mM) = normal fasting glucose
FPG ≥ 100 mg/dl (5.6 mM) and < 126 mg/dl (7.0 mM) = IFG
or
OGTT
2-hr PG < 140 mg/dl (7.8 mM) = normal glucose tolerance
2-hr PG ≥ 140 mg/dl (7.8 mM) and < 200 mg/dl (11.1 nM) = IGT

WHO: World Health Organization; PG: plasma glucose; FPG: fasting plasma glucose; IFG: impaired fasting glucose; IGT: impaired glucose tolerance; OGTT: oral glucose tolerance test
[1] Classic symptoms of diabetes include polyuria, polydipsia, and unexplained weight loss.
[2] Casual is defined as any time of day without regard to time since last meal.
[3] OGTT: the test should be performed as described by WHO, using a glucose load containing equivalent of 75 g anhydrous glucose dissolved in water.

Table 1. WHO and 2003 updated ADA criteria for the diagnosis of diabetes mellitus

3. Incidence

New onset diabetes mellitus after transplantation has been reported to occur in 4% to 25% of renal transplant recipients, 2.5% to 25% of liver transplant recipients, 4% to 40% of heart transplant recipients, and 30% to 35% of lung transplant recipients (Baid et al., 2001; Davidson et al., 2003; Knobler et al., 1998; Ye et al., 2010a). There has been scant literature on the incidence of diabetes mellitus after a successful pancreas transplant. In one-single center study persistent diabetes mellitus despite evidence of functioning pancreas allografts occurred in 19% of patients (22/144) at 39 months post-transplant (Dean et al., 2008).

The variation in the reported incidence may be due in part to the lack of a standard definition of the condition, the duration of follow-up, the presence of both modifiable and non-modifiable risks factors, and the type of organ transplants among others. In HCV-infected liver recipients, the prevalence of NODAT has been reported to range between 40% to 60% (Baid et al., 2001; Bigam et al., 2000; Knobler et al., 1998). While the prevalence of diabetes reported to the International Society of Heart Lung Transplant (ISHLT) are 19% at 1-year and 28% at 5 years for lung transplant recipients, and 15.4% at 1-year and 20% at 5-years for heart-lung transplant recipients (Trulock et al., 2007), a lower prevalence has been reported (Silverborn et al., 2005). In one single-center study consisting of 126 lung and heart-lung transplant recipients, diabetes has a reported prevalence of 6% at 1 year and 7% at 5 years. The lower prevalence of diabetes in this study was thought to be due in part to a lower frequency of cystic fibrosis patients (8.7% vs. 16.0% in the ISHLT database) and the exclusion of patients with pre-existing diabetes (Silverborn et al., 2005).

Similar to the nontransplant settings, the use of fasting plasma glucose (FPG) versus oral glucose tolerance test (OGTT) to define diabetes mellitus also changes the prevalence of NODAT. In a prospective study designed to evaluate the use of OGTT for risk-stratifying patients for NODAT, Sharif et al. demonstrated that among 122 renal transplant recipients without diabetes who had two FPG level measurements within the range of 100-125 mg/dl (5.6-6.9 mmol/l) for more than 6 months after transplantation, OGTTs revealed that 10% had overt diabetes mellitus, 9% had IGT alone, 18% had IFG alone (all defined by WHO criteria), and 14% had combined IFG and IGT (Sharif et al., 2006).

4. Risk factors for NODAT

Risk factors for the development of NODAT are categorized as non-modifiable and modifiable or potentially modifiable, the former category to facilitate the identification of high risk individuals, and the latter two categories to optimize the management of NODAT. Suggested risk factors for NODAT are summarized in Figure 1. It is noteworthy that most clinical studies evaluating the incidence and risk factors for NODAT have been performed in kidney and liver transplant recipients.

Limited studies in pancreas transplant recipients suggest that pre-transplant body mass index (BMI), high pretransplant insulin requirements and acute rejection episodes are risk factors for persistent post-transplant diabetes mellitus despite the presence of a functioning pancreas allograft (Dean et al., 2008).

Retrospective analysis of the UNOS/OPTN database demonstrated that the risk factors for NODAT after heart transplant are similar to those reported in kidney transplant recipients including older age, non-white race, higher BMI, recipient CMV positivity, tacrolimus (vs. cyclosporine) and steroid use (vs. no steroid) at discharge. Ischemic heart disease was also found to be associated with an increased incidence of NODAT (Ye et al., 2010b). In a single-center study consisting of 97 consecutive adult heart transplant recipients, a family history of diabetes and the need for insulin beyond the first 24 hours after transplantation were shown to be risk factors for the development NODAT (Depczynski et al., 2000).

4.1 Nonmodifiable risk factors

There has been ample literature suggesting that age, Hispanic and African American race and ethnicity are risks factors for NODAT (Cosio et al., 2001; Kasiske et al., 2003; P.T. Pham et al., 2007a, 2007b).

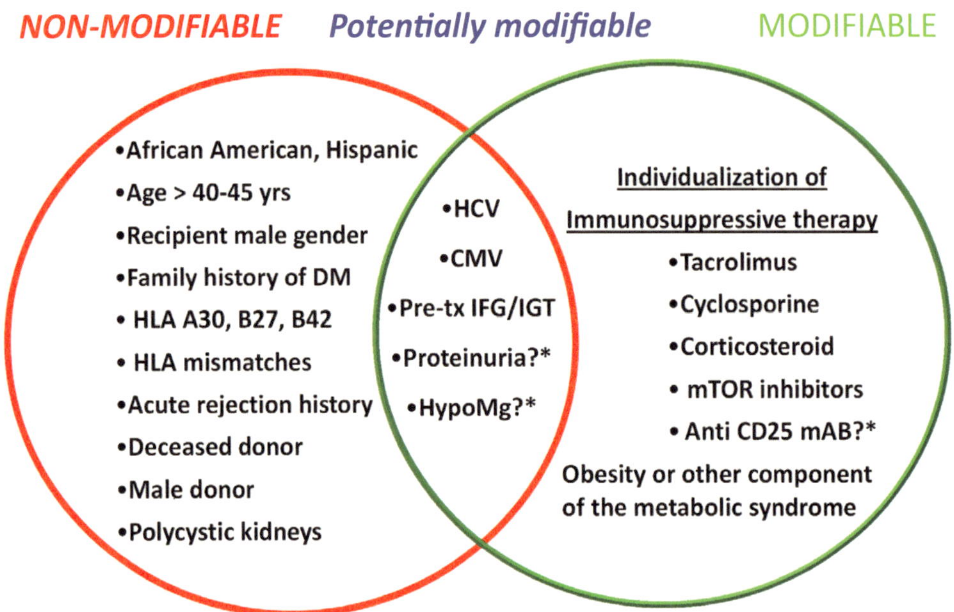

***See text**

Abbreviations: **HCV:** hepatitis C; **CMV:** cytomegalovirus; **Pre-Tx:** pre-transplant; **HypoMg:** hypomagnesemia
Anti CD25 mAb: anti CD25 monoclonal antibody

NB: Restoration of insulin metabolism by a functioning graft may unmask pre-transplant impaired glucose tolerance or diabetes & is not a risk factor *perse*

Fig. 1. Risk Factors for NODAT

Similar to type 2 diabetes in the general population, both genetic and environmental factors have been suggested to play a role in the development of NODAT. There is strong evidence suggesting that individuals with a family history of diabetes among first-degree relatives have an increased risk of developing NODAT with one study reporting a seven fold increase in the condition (Davidson et al., 2003). The increased prevalence of NODAT associated with a family history of diabetes has been documented across all types of solid organ transplantation. In a Spanish multicenter cross-sectional study consisting of 1410 recipients of kidney transplants, 489 liver transplants, 207 heart transplants, and 72 lung transplants, a positive family history of diabetes was associated with a 50% increased in the risk of developing NODAT (odds ratio of 1.51) (Martinez-Castelao et al., 2005).

Other non-modifiable risk factors include recipient male gender, the presence of certain HLA antigens such as HLA A 30, B27, B42, increasing HLA mismatches, DR mismatch, deceased donor kidneys, male donor, and acute rejection history (Depczynski et al., 2000). Adult polycystic kidney disease (ADPKD) has been suggested to confer an increased risk of developing NODAT in some studies but not in others (P.T. Pham et al., 2007b). The pathogenic mechanism of ADPKD-associated NODAT has not been studied. Of interest, ADPKD patients with normal native kidney function have been shown to have insulin resistance and compensatory hyperinsulinemia (Vareesangthip et al., 1997).

Although not a risk factor per se, increased insulin clearance after a successful kidney transplant can unmask pre-transplant impaired glucose tolerance or pre-existing diabetes mellitus that manifests clinically as NODAT.

4.2 Modifiable risk factors

4.2.1 Corticosteroid-associated NODAT

The now well-established contributory role of corticosteroid on NODAT was first described by Starlz in 1964 in renal transplant recipients. The diabetogenic effect of corticosteroids has been suggested to be dose-dependent. Single-center studies have demonstrated that oral prednisolone dose reduction to 5 mg daily significantly improves glucose tolerance during the first year after transplantation (Hjelmesaeth et al., 1997) while a 0.01 mg/kg/day increase in prednisolone dose is associated with a 5% risk of developing NODAT (Hjelmesaeth et al., 2001).

In a small study involving 57 stable renal transplant recipients, Midtvedt and colleagues found that prednisolone dose reduction from a mean of 16 mg daily (range 10 to 30) to 9 mg (range 5 to 12.5) resulted in an average increase in insulin sensitivity index of 24% (Midtvedt et al., 2004). However, complete withdrawal of 5 mg/day of prednisolone did not influence insulin sensitivity significantly. Whether complete withdrawal of chronic low dose corticosteroid therapy (prednisolone 5 mg daily) improves glucose metabolism remains to be studied. Nonetheless, in recent years several studies have suggested a potential beneficial effect of steroid-free immunosuppression on NODAT risk reduction (Luan et al., 2011).

In a retrospective analysis of the Organ Procurement Transplant Network/Scientific Registry of Transplant Recipient (OPTN/SRTR) database consisting of > 25,000 kidney transplant recipients engrafted between 1/2004 and 12/13/2006, Luan et al. demonstrated that steroid-free immunosuppression was associated with a significant reduction in the likelihood of developing NODAT compared with steroid-containing regimens (Luan et al., 2011). The cumulative incidence of NODAT within three years post-transplant were 12.3% in steroid-free vs. 17.7% in steroid-containing regimens, $p < 0.001$. Overall, steroid-containing regimens at the time of hospital discharge were associated with a 42% increased risk for NODAT. Notably, patients from programs that frequently adopted steroid-free regimens had reduced odds of NODAT compared with those from programs that commonly used steroid-contatining regimens.

The dose dependent diabetogenic effect of corticosteroid was also observed in recipients of nonrenal organ transplants. In a retrospective review involving 88 heart transplant recipients, Depczynski and colleagues found that patients who developed NODAT had received higher mean doses of prednisolone at 3 months compared with those who remained free of diabetes at a mean follow-up of 27 months (0.21 ± 0.03 vs. 0.19 ± 0.03 mg/kg/day, $p< 0.01$) (Depczynski et al., 2000).

4.2.2 Calcineurin inhibitor-associated NODAT: cyclosporine vs. tacrolimus

Although clinical trials comparing the incidence of NODAT in CSA- vs. Tac-treated patients have yielded mixed results, Tac has more consistently been shown to have a greater diabetogenic effect (Ekberg et al., 2007; P.T. Pham et al., 2007b; Woodward et al., 2003).

The DIRECT Study (Diabetes Incidence after Renal Transplantation: Neoral C2 monitoring versus Tacrolimus) was the first multi-center open label, randomized trial to assess glucose abnormalities in de novo kidney transplant patients who were randomized to cyclosporine microemulsion- (CsA-ME) or tacrolimus-based immunosuppression (Vincente et al., 2007). The incidence of NODAT or IFG (defined by WHO/ADA criteria) at 6-month post-transplant was significantly lower in CsA-ME- vs. tacrolimus- treated patients, (26% vs. 33.6%, p=0.046). Furthermore, a lower proportion of CsA-ME patients with NODAT required hypoglycemic medication or dual therapy with insulin and oral hypoglycemic agents compared with their tacrolimus-treated counterparts.

The greater diabetogenic effect of tacrolimus compared to CSA has been reported to occur across renal and nonrenal transplant groups. In a meta-analysis to evaluate the reported incidence of NODAT after solid organ transplantation, Heisel and colleagues found a higher incidence of insulin-dependent diabetes mellitus (IDDM) in Tac- vs. CSA-treated liver, heart, and lung transplant recipients (Heisel et al, 2004). In renal transplant recipients, IDDM occurred in 9.8% of Tac- vs. 2.7% of CSA-treated patients ($p<0.00001$). Similar trends were observed among recipients of non renal organ transplants (11.1% vs. 6.2%, respectively ($p<0.003$). Nonetheless, not all studies showed that Tac is more diabetogenic than cyclosporine (Meiser et al., 1998). It has been suggested that these study inconsistencies stemmed in part from the difference in the definitions of NODAT and the difference in calcineurin inhibitor dose and drug levels (Maes et al., 2001; Meiser et al., 1998). In a single-center study consisting of 139 renal transplant recipients without known pretransplant glucose abnormalities, Maes and colleagues have shown that high Tac trough levels, particularly levels greater than 15 ng/ml in the first month after transplant was a significant risk factor for persistent impaired fasting glucose or diabetes mellitus beyond the first year after transplantation (Maes et al., 2001). In a single-center study consisting of 45 OLT recipients treated with either CSA (n=9) or high- (n=15) vs. low- (n=13) dose Tac, the incidence of NODAT were 11%, 40% and 23%, respectively (Cai et al., 1998).

4.2.3 Interaction between tacrolimus and concomitant hepatitis C infection (HCV)

In a retrospective study of more than 400 kidney transplant recipients with no known pre-transplant diabetes, Bloom and colleagues have shown that among the HCV(+) cohort, NODAT occurred more often in the Tac- compared with the CSA-treated groups (57.8% vs. 7.7%, $p< 0.0001$) (Bloom et al., 2002). In contrast, among the HCV (-) cohort, the rates of NODAT were similar between the two calcineurin inhibitor (CNI) groups (Tac vs. CSA: 10% vs. 9.4%, respectively, $p= 0.521$). Whether concomitant exposure to tacrolimus and HCV plays a synergistic role in the development of NODAT remains speculative.

4.2.4 Effects of sirolimus on glucose metabolism

Early large randomized clinical trials suggested that sirolimus is devoid of diabetogenic effects either used alone or in combination therapy with CNI. However, the diabetogenicity of sirolimus has now been well-described. Teutenico et al. demonstrated that calcineurin inhibitors to sirolimus conversion therapy and tacrolimus withdrawal in a regimen consisting of tacrolimus and sirolimus were associated with a 30% increased incidence of impaired glucose tolerance (Teutenico et al., 2005). In one single-center study, tacrolimus and sirolimus combination therapy was found to be associated with a higher incidence of NODAT than tacrolimus alone immunosuppression (Sulanc et al., 2005). Subsequent large registry study also demonstrated an association between sirolimus and the development of NODAT. In an analysis of the USRDS database consisting of more than 20,000 primary kidney transplant recipients receiving sirolimus (Sir) or CNI (CsA or Tac) or both in various combination therapy with an antimetabolite (MMF or AZA), Johnston et al. demonstrated that patients treated with sirolimus in combination with a CNI (CsA or Tac) had the highest incidence of NODAT (Johnston et al., 2008). The authors further demonstrated that patients treated with (Sir + Tac) combination therapy had a hazard ratio of developing NODAT of 1.9 compared with those receiving (Tac + MMF/AZA), suggesting that sirolimus was associated with an increased risk for NODAT independent of any effect of tacrolimus.

4.2.5 Anti-CD25 monoclonal antibodies

In a single-center study consisting of 74 stable kidney transplant recipients with 3 month-follow-up, Bayes et al. demonstrated that basiliximab induction therapy is an independent risk factor for NODAT (OR: 3.28; p=0.041) (Bayes et al., 2007). Aasebo et al. similarly demonstrated that the use of basiliximab induction therapy significantly increased NODAT risk (n=264) (Aesebo et al., 2010). At 10 weeks post-transplant, NODAT, impaired glucose tolerance (IGT) or impaired fasting glucose (IFG) occurred in 51.5% in the basiliximab group compared with 36.9% in the group that did not receive basiliximab induction (p=0.017).

5. Potential pathogenic mechanisms of immunosuppressive drug--induced NODAT

5.1 Calcineurin inhibitors

Impaired insulin secretion has been suggested to contribute to the development of CNI-associated NODAT (Crutchlow & Bloom, 2007). Experimental studies have shown that CNIs impair the function of cultured β-cells by impairing insulin gene expression (Crutchlow et al., 2007; Van Hooff et al., 2004). In recipients of pancreas transplants, both calcineurin inhibitors CSA and Tac have been shown to cause reversible toxicity to islet cells. In a study of 26 pancreas allograft biopsies from 20 simultaneous kidney-pancreas transplant recipients, a significant correlation was seen between the presence of islet cell damage and serum levels of Tac and CSA, as well as with the Tac peak level (Drachenberg et al., 1999). Cytoplasmic swelling and vacuolization, and marked decrease or absence of dense-core secretory granules in β-cells were demonstrated on electron microscopy. The islet cell damage was more frequent and severe in the Tac- (10/13) compared to the CSA-treated groups (5/13). Serial biopsies from two patients with hyperglycemia and evidence of islet cell damage receiving Tac immunosuppression demonstrated reversibility of the damage upon discontinuation of tacrolimus.

5.2 Sirolimus (mTOR inhibitors)

Suggested pathogenic mechanisms of sirolimus-induced hyperglycemia include sirolimus-associated impaired insulin-mediated suppression of hepatic glucose production, ectopic triglyceride deposition leading to insulin resistance, and direct β cell toxicity (Crutchlow & Bloom, 2007). However, studies on the effects of sirolimus on insulin action and secretion have yielded variable and conflicting results. Currently existing literature suggests that the effects of sirolimus on glucose metabolism appear to be cell-species- and dose-dependent (Subramanian & Trence, 2007).

5.2.1 Anti-CD25 monoclonal antibodies

The pathogenic mechanisms of anti-CD25-induced NODAT have not been established. However, suppression of regulatory T-cells has been suggested to play a contributory role (Aasebo et al., 2010). Studies in diabetes-prone mice have shown that anti-IL2-antibody treatment trigger insulinitis and early onset diabetes through inhibition of Foxp3-expressing CD25+ CD4+ regulatory T-cells (Setoguchi et al., 2005).

Suggested pathogenic mechanisms of immunosuppressive drug-induced NODAT are summarized in table 2.

Immunosuppressive agent	Pathogenic mechanism(s)	Comments
Corticosteroids	•↓Peripheral insulin sensitivity • Inhibit pancreatic insulin production & secretion • ↑Hepatic gluconeogenesis • Promote protein degradation to free amino acids in muscle, lipolysis	•Dose-dependent •Impact of complete withdrawal of chronic low-dose steroids unclear •Potential ↓NODAT risk in steroid-free regimens
Cyclosporine	• ↓insulin secretion (CsA < Tac) • ↓insulin synthesis • ↓β-cell density	•Dose-dependent, •Diabetogenic effect ↑ with ↑ steroid dose*
Tacrolimus	• ↓insulin secretion (Tac > CsA) • ↓insulin synthesis	•Dose-dependent, •Diabetogenic effect ↑ with ↑ steroid dose*
Sirolimus	•↑Peripheral insulin resistance • Impair pancreatic β-cell response	↑Diabetogenicity when use with CNIs

Abbreviations: CNI: calcineurin inhibitors
* Demonstrated in some but not all studies

Table 2. Drug-Induced NODAT: potential pathogenic mechanism(s)

6. Obesity

Similar to the general population, obesity has been shown to be associated with the development of NODAT in most studies (Setoguchi et al., 2005). Analysis of the USRDS database revealed that obesity, defined as a BMI of $\geq$ 30 kg/m^2 is one of the strongest risk factors for NODAT (Relative risk of 1.73, $P < 0.0001$). Although some studies failed to demonstrate an association between obesity and the development of NODAT, obesity and its associated peripheral insulin resistance state is a known risk factor for type 2 diabetes. The mechanism whereby obesity induces insulin resistance is poorly understood. Nonetheless, the pattern of body fat distribution has been suggested to play a contributory role. Studies in healthy women showed that upper body or male-type obesity has a much greater association with insulin resistance and impaired glucose tolerance than lower body or female-type obesity (Kissebah et al., 1982). Similar studies in the transplant settings is lacking. It is speculated that intra-abdominal fat or waist-to-hip ratio may be more important risk factors for NODAT than total body weight or BMI (Davidson et al., 2003).

7. Hypertriglyceridemia / Hypertension

Early retrospective studies suggested that the greater the number of the metabolic syndrome components, the greater the risk for the development of NODAT (Eckel, 2007). In a recent retrospective analysis consisting of 640 nondiabetic renal transplant recipients Bayer et al. demonstrated that the prevalence of NODAT at 1-year increased with increasing number of

metabolic syndrome score 0: 0%, 1: 24%, 2: 29%, 3: 31%, 4: 35%, 5: 74%, p=0.001) (Bayer et al., 2010). Multivariate analysis incorporating the individual metabolic syndrome components as covariates demonstrated that of all the pre-transplant metabolic syndrome components, only low-density lipoprotein was independently associated with the development of NODAT.
The precise role of the metabolic syndrome or metabolic syndrome component(s) in the development of NODAT remains to be defined. Nonetheless, the overlapping metabolic risk factors for type 2 diabetes and cardiovascular disease (e.g. obesity, hyperglycemia, dyslipidemia, hypertension) warrants early identification and aggressive management of individual risk factors

8. Proteinuria

Early report from single-center study suggested an association between proteinuria on day 5 after transplantation and the development of NODAT (Kuypers et al., 2008). However, these findings have been challenged because proteinuria on day 5 may just reflect the highly concentrated urine associated with hyperglycemia-induced osmotic diuresis from the early posttransplant use of high dose corticosteroid or residual native kidney proteinuria. Furthermore, it has been shown that immediate posttransplant proteinuria generally resolves several weeks after transplantation (Myslak et al., 2006). Nonetheless, in a subsequent single-center retrospective study designed to evaluate the impact of early proteinuria (3 and 6 months after transplantation) and urinary albumin excretion (UAE) on NODAT, Roland et al. demonstrated that low-grade (<1g/day) and very low-grade (< /0.3 g/day) proteinuria were independent risk factor for NODAT (p=0.0042 and p=.00025, respectively) (Roland et al., 2008). Furthermore, there was a dose-dependent relationship across UAE categories with NODAT. NODAT-free survival was greater in patients with normoalbuminuria than in those with microalbuminuria, and greater in those with microalbuminuria than in those with macroalbuminuria (p=0.0326). The authors also demonstrated that pulse pressure was an independent risk factor for NODAT, suggesting that early low-grade proteinuria and pulse pressure may be markers of the metabolic syndrome or vascular damage or both.

9. Hypomagnesemia

In the general population, not only has hypomagnesemia been shown to be associated with type 2 diabetes, but numerous studies have also reported an inverse relationship between glycemic control and serum Mg levels (P.C. Pham et al., 2007). Similar to the nontransplant settings, hypomagenesemia has also been shown to be an independent predictor of NODAT in recipients of renal and liver transplants. In a single-center retrospective analysis consisting of 254 renal transplant recipients Van Laecke et al. demonstrated that hypomagnesemia during the first-month posttransplantation was associated with the development of NODAT independent of the immunosuppressive regimen used (van Laecke et al., 2009). While the association between the use of CNIs was strongly related to hypomagnesemia, NODAT disappeared after adjustment for Mg levels suggesting that the diabetogenic effect of CNIs is at least in part related to hypomagnesemia. Conversely, the use of mTOR inhibitors appeared to be a risk factor for NODAT after adjustment for Mg levels. The same group of authors subsequently demonstrated that both pretransplant hypomagenesemia and hypomagnesemia in the first-month posttransplantation were independent predictors of NODAT in recipients of liver transplants (Van Laecke et al., 2010). Nonetheless, not all studies demonstrated that hypomagnesemia is a risk factor for NODAT. In one small single-center study consisting of 205 non-previously diabetic patients with > 1 year graft survival, neither the mean values of Mg nor the percentage of patients with hypomagnesemia differed between NODAT and non-NODAT patients (Santos et al., 2010).

Whether Mg supplementation and correction of Mg deficiency reduce the incidence of insulin resistance or NODAT remains to be studied.

10. Potentially modifiable risk factors

10.1 Impaired glucose tolerance before transplantation

Abnormal glucose metabolism has been reported to be a risk factor for the development of NODAT in some but not all studies. In a study consisting of 490 recipients of kidney transplants, Cosio et al. demonstrated that higher pretransplant glucose is a risk factor for NODAT at one year (Cosio et al., 2005). Using patients with pretransplant FPG levels between 90 and 100 as the reference group, patients with plasma glucose < 90 mg/dL have lower risk of NODAT (OR=.46, P=0.01). In contrast, the risk of NODAT increases as the pretransplant FPG levels increases (FPG =101-109, OR=1.5; and FPG = 110-125, OR=7.6, P < 0.0001). Among patients with IFG pretransplant, 70% had hyperglycemia at one year (IFG 43% and NODAT 27%). In one single-center study Eprinchard et al demonstrated that pretransplant IGT is a risk factor for NODAT with a relative risk of developing NODAT of 2.4 (Eprinchard et al., 2011).

10.2 HCV-associated NODAT

The association between HCV infection and impaired fasting glucose or the development of overt type 2 diabetes mellitus in the general population has long been suggested. Potential mechanisms of the diabetogenic effect of HCV infection include insulin resistance, decreased hepatic glucose uptake and glycogenesis, and direct cytopathic effect of the virus on pancreatic β cells (Bloom & Lake, 2006). Similar to the non-transplant settings, the link between hepatitis C and the development of NODAT has also been recognized in solid organ transplant recipients. The pathogenesis of HCV-associated NODAT, however, remains poorly understood. Clinical studies in recipients of orthotopic liver transplant (OLT) recipients have implicated insulin resistance associated with active HCV infection as a predominant pathogenic mechanism. Independent investigators have shown a temporal relationship between recurrent allograft hepatitis and increasing viral loads and the development of NODAT (Baid et al., 2001; Delgado-Borrego et al., 2004). Furthermore, patients who responded to antiviral therapy were observed to have improvement in glycemic control (Baid et al., 2001; Delgado-Borrego et al., 2004; Simo et al., 2006). In a small cohort of 17 non-diabetic HCV (+) and 33 non-diabetic HCV (-) OLT recipients, Baid and colleagues have shown that the presence of HCV infection was independently associated with a 62% increase in insulin resistance (P=0.0005) (Baid et al., 2001). It was suggested that the virus had a direct effect on insulin resistance as no difference in β cell function or hepatic insulin extraction between the HCV (+) and (-) groups was observed.

In a small study consisting of 16 renal transplant candidates with sustained virologic response to interferon treatment given in the pre-transplant period, none developed

NODAT at a mean follow-up of 22.5 months (range, 2 to 88 months) (Kamar et al., 2003). It is conceivable that successful pre-transplant treatment of hepatitis C could potentially reduce the incidence of NODAT after kidney transplantation.

10.3 Cytomegalovirus-associated NODAT

The link between cytomegalovirus (CMV) infection and the development of NODAT was first reported in 1985 in a renal transplant recipient (Lehr et al., 1985). Limited studies suggested that both asymptomatic CMV infection and CMV disease are independent risk factors for the development of NODAT. In a study consisting of 160 consecutive non-diabetic renal transplant recipients who were prospectively monitored for CMV infection during the first three months after transplantation, Hjelmesaeth and colleagues found that asymptomatic CMV infection was associated with a four-fold increased risk of new-onset diabetes (adjusted RR= 4.00; p=0.025) (Hjelmasaeth et al., 2004). Patients with active CMV infection had a significantly lower median insulin release compared to their CMV negative counterparts, suggesting that impaired pancreatic β cell insulin release may be involved in the pathogenic mechanism of CMV-associated NODAT. It is speculated that CMV-induced release of proinflammatory cytokines may lead to apoptosis and functional disturbances of pancreatic β-cells (Hjelmasaeth et al., 2005).

11. Impact of NODAT on patient and allograft outcomes

11.1 Kidney transplants

Clinical studies evaluating the impact of NODAT on patient and allograft outcomes after solid organ transplantation have yielded variable results. Nonetheless, there has been ample literature suggesting that kidney transplant recipients who developed NODAT are at two- to three- fold increased risk of fatal and nonfatal cardiovascular disease events as compared with nondiabetic patients (Ojo, 2006; Hjelmasaeth et al., 2006). The development of NODAT has also been shown to be associated with an adverse impact on patient survival and an increased risk of graft rejection and graft loss, as well as an increased incidence of infectious complications (Ojo, 2006). Data from the United Renal Data System consisting of over 11,000 Medicare beneficiaries who received primary kidney transplants between 1996 and 2000 demonstrated that compared to "no diabetes", NODAT was associated with a 63% increased risk of graft failure (p< 0.0001), a 46% increased risk of death-censored graft failure (p< 0.0001) and an 87% increased risk of mortality (p< 0.0001) (Kasiske et al., 2003).

In contrast to earlier reports, a retrospective analysis of the UNOS/OPTN database (involving patients transplanted between 2004-2007) failed to demonstrate the negative impact of NODAT on transplant survival or CV mortality during a median follow-up of 548 days. The study consisted of >37,000 renal transplant recipients with a functioning transplant for at least 1 year. Risk stratification according to diabetes status (pre-transplant diabetes, NODAT) and acute rejection (AR) at 1 year demonstrated that pre-transplant diabetes is the major predictor of all-cause and cardiovascular mortality whereas acute rejection during the first year is the major predictor of death-censored transplant failure. In contrast, NODAT alone was not associated significantly with any study outcomes (Kuo et al., 2010). Nonetheless, the study results were regarded as inconclusive due to the wide confidence intervals and the relatively short duration of follow-up. It is noteworthy that in a large registry study consisting of more than 27,000 primary kidney transplant recipients with graft survival of at least 1 year and with longer-term follow-up, Cole et al. demonstrated that patients with NODAT had decreased survival compared with those who developed neither NODAT nor acute rejection (HR 3.85; $p < 0.0001$) (Cole et al., 2008).

11.2 Non-renal solid organ transplants

Clinical studies evaluating the impact of NODAT on patient and allograft outcomes after non-renal solid organ transplantation have yielded variable results (Baid et al., 2001; John & Thuluvath, 2002; Valentine et al., 2001).

In a study consisting of 66 heart transplant recipients, post-transplant insulin resistance or post-transplant hyperglycemia (glucose levels > 8.9 mmol/L 2 hours after a standard oral glucose tolerance test) was found to be a predictive factor for transplant coronary artery stenosis ($p \leq 0.01$) and death ($p \leq 0.005$) during a 5-year post-tarnsplant follow-up period (Valentine et al., 2001). Patients with post-transplant hyperglycemia were also found to have a higher mean coronary artery intimal thickness than those without post-transplant hyperglycemia (0.35 ± 0.05 vs. $0.20 \pm .02$, respectively; $p \leq 0.05$).

In a single-center study consisting of 435 liver transplant recipients John et al. demonstrated that cardiovascular complications, major and minor infections, neurologic and neuropsychiatric complications were twice as common in patients who developed NODAT (n= 46) compared with their age- and sex-matched counterparts without pre- or post-transplant diabetes (n=92) (John & Thuluvath, 2002). However, there was no difference in patient survival between the two groups at 1-, 2- and 5-years follow-up. In contrast, Baid et al. demonstrated that NODAT was an independent risk factor for mortality after liver transplantation (HR 3.67, $p < 0.0001$) particularly in those with hepatitis C. The cumulative mortality in HCV (+) NODAT (+) vs. HCV (+) NODAT (-) patients was 56% vs. 14%, respectively (p=0.001) (Baid et al., 2001).

12. Detection and management of diabetes mellitus in recipients of solid organ transplants

12.1 Pre-transplant baseline evaluation

Suggested guidelines for pre-transplant baseline evaluation of potential transplant candidates is shown in Figure 2. Patients with evidence of IGT or abnormal OGTT before transplantation should be counseled on lifestyle modifications including weight control, diet, and exercise. The goals for the life-style modification involved achieving and maintaining a weight reduction of at least 7 percent of initial body weight through a healthy low-calorie, low-fat diet and at least 150 minutes of physical activity per week.

Pre-transplant treatment of HCV-infected renal transplant candidates should be considered. Selection of an immunosuppressive regimen should be tailored to each individual patient, weighing the risk of developing diabetes after transplantation against the risk of acute rejection.

12.2 Early detection of NODAT after transplantation

Studies investigating the best predictive tool for identifying patients at risk for developing NODAT early after transplantation are currently lacking. While fasting plasma glucose (FPG) is readily available in clinical practice it may be normal in kidney transplant recipients with abnormal glucose homeostasis. It has been suggested that transplant patients have an atypical form of insulin resistance and their plasma glucose often peeks before lunch. Hence the use of FPG alone may preclude the accurate diagnosis of NODAT. Kuypers et al. demonstrated that a normal (vs. diabetic) OGTT on day 5 was associated with a significantly reduced risk for NODAT (odds ratio 0.03, P=0.0002) (Kuypers et al., 2008). However, it is noteworthy that while acute rejection has been suggested to increase the risk for NODAT, it usually does not occur before day 5. Obtaining OGTT and FPG at day 5, therefore, may preclude the subset of patients with higher risk of developing NODAT. Hence, it has been suggested that performing OGTT at 10-12 weeks post-transplantation might be useful as an alternative or supplementary test to day 5 OGTT (P.T. Pham & P.C. Pham, 2008).

The routine recommendation of performing an OGTT early after transplantation awaits further studies. Suggested pre-transplant baseline evaluation and post-transplant screening for NODAT is shown in Figure 2.

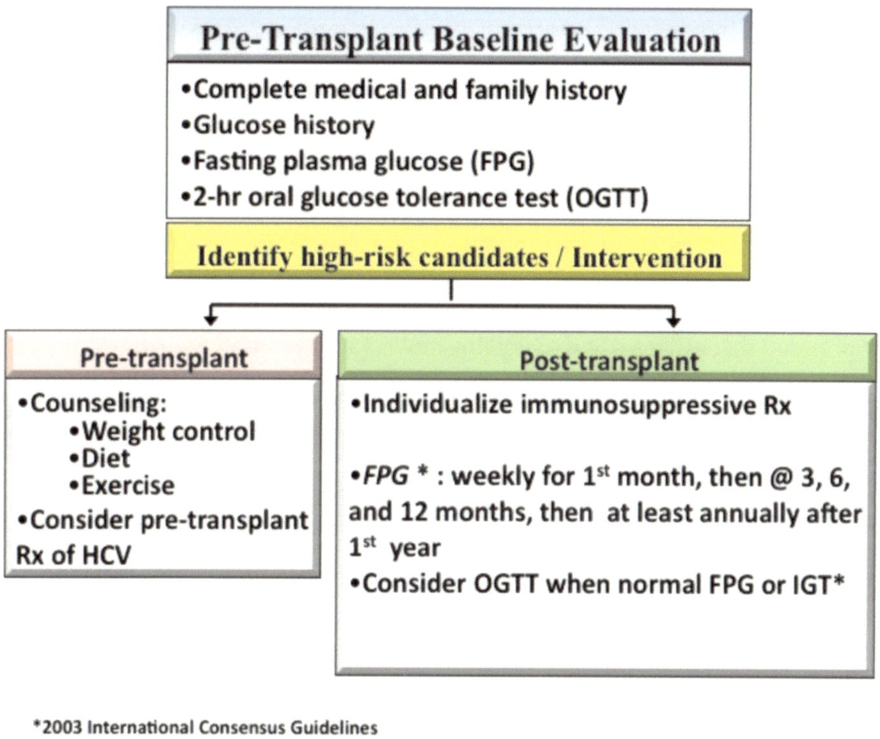

Fig. 2. Sugested guidelines for pre-transplant baseline evaluation and post-transplant screening for NODAT

12.3 Management of established NODAT

The management of NODAT should follow the conventional approach for patients with type 2 diabetes mellitus as recommended by many clinical guidelines established by well-recognized organizations including the American Diabetes Association (ADA).

Similar to the nontransplant settings, a target hemoglobin A1C level < 6.5%-7% is recommended. Fasting plasma glucose should be below 100 mg/dL (6.11 mmol/L), and a 2-hour postprandial plasma glucose should be below 140 mg/dL (7.77 mmol/L) (Mannon,

2008). Nonetheless, it should be noted that the Action to Control Cardiovascular Risk in Diabetes (ACCORD) trial was discontinued prematurely because of a satistically significant increase in all-cause mortality in the intensive- compared with the standard- glycemic treatment groups (Gerstein et al., 2008). At 1 year, stable median A_{1C} levels of 6.4% and 7.5% were achieved in the intensive-therapy and standard groups, respectively. The intensive-therapy group had a relative increase in mortality of 22% and an absolute increase of 1.0% during a follow-up period of 3.5 years. Death from cardiovascular causes were similar between the two treatment groups. It is also notable that hypoglycemia requiring assistance and weight gain of more than 10 kg were more frequent in the intensive-therapy group ($P < 0.001$). Long-term follow-up of the ACCORD study demonstrated that intensive therapy failed to reduce the risk of advanced measures of microvascular outcomes but delayed the onset of micro- and macro-albuminuria and some measures of ocular complications and peripheral neuropathy which persisted over the 5 year study period despite the transition from intensive to conventional treatment of glycemia after 3.7 years (Ismail-Beigi et al., 2010).

Study similar to that of the ACCORD study in recipients of solid organ transplantation is lacking. Nonetheless, the determination of hemoglobin A1C target levels for solid organ transplant recipients should be individualized based on hypoglycemia risks.

13. Modifiable risk factor management strategy

13.1 Dietary modification and physical activity

The Diabetes Prevention Program has demonstrated that a structured diet and physical activity program that achieves and maintains modest weight loss for overweight adults with IGT can significantly reduce the development of diabetes. Defining realistic goals such as a target weight loss of 5-10% of total body weight and patient- centered approach to education may be invaluable in achieving success. Suggested non-insulin management of NODAT is shown in table 3.

13.2 Modification of immunosuppression

Modification of immunosuppression should be considered in high-risk patients. Corticosteroid dose reduction has been shown to significantly improve glucose tolerance during the first year after transplantation (Kasiske et al., 2003). However, any dose reduction should be weighed against the risk of acute rejection. Steroid-sparing regimen or steroid avoidance protocol should be tailored to each individual patient. Tac to CSA conversion therapy in patients who fail to achieve target glycemic control or in those with difficult to control diabetes has yielded variable results. The use of CNI and mTOR inhibitor combination therapy should probably be avoided. Belatacept -- a selective T cell costimulation blocker, is a promising new immunosuppressant that has been suggested to have better cardiovascular and metabolic risk profiles compared with cyclosporine (lower blood pressure, better lipid profiles and lower NODAT incidence) (Vanrenterghem et al., 2011).

13.3 Renin-angiotensin inhibition

A meta-analysis of 10 randomized controlled trials to assess the effects of renin angiotensin inhibition [five with angiotensin-converting enzyme inhibitors (ACEIs) and five with

Agents	Action	Adverse effects / Comments
INSULIN SENSITIZERS (e.g. Metformin, Butoformin, Phenformin)	↓ hepatic glucose production, ↑ glucose uptake by skeletal muscle	• Diarrhea, dyspepsia, lactic acidosis w/ renal insufficiency • No weight gain, no hypoglycemia
INSULIN SECRETAGOGUES	↑ pancreatic insulin secretion	
Sulfonylureas (SUs) (e.g. Glipizide, Glyburide, Glimepiride)		***SUs***: weight gain, edema, hypoglycemia (esp. in renal insufficiency & elderly)
Meglitinides (e.g. Repaglinide, Nateglinide)		***Meglitinides***: weight gain, hypoglycemia (lower risk than SUs) Rapid onset & offset, hepatically excreted (use w/ renal insufficiency)
OTHERS W/ DIFFERENT ACTIONS		
Thiazolidinedione derivatives (TZD) [e.g. Pioglitazone, Rosiglitazone (the drug has been suspended in Europe since 2010, use with caution, see text)]	Bind to peroxisome proliferator-activated receptors (PPARs) & stimulate insulin sensitive genes	• Weight gain, peripheral edema (esp. w/ insulin), anemia, pulmonary edema, CHF, fractures • Slow onset of action, no hypoglycemia, no reliance on renal excretion, contraindicated in class III-IV CHF or hepatic impairment
Glucagon-like peptide-1 analogues (e.g. Exenatide, Liraglutide)	↑ pancreatic insulin secretion	Either favorable or neutral effect on weight gain (delays gastric emptying, ↑ satiety)
Dipeptidyl peptidase 4 inhibitors (e.g. Sitagliptin, Saxagliptin)	↑ Endogenous incretins	• Avoid vildagliptin in hepatic impairment & stage IV-V CKD, dose should be adjusted for renal insufficiency. • Watch for immunosuppresive drug interaction • Weight neutral, no hypoglycemia, ? β cell preservation

Table 3. Non-insulin drug therapy for NODAT

angiotensin receptor blockers (ARBs)] on the incidence of new cases of type 2 diabetes mellitus in patients with arterial hypertension and congestive heart failure demonstrated that renin-angiotensin inhibition with either ACEIs or ARBs consistently and significantly reduced the incidence of type 2 diabetes mellitus compared with placebo, or beta-blockers/diuretics or amlodipine (Scheen, 2004). This finding has not yet been validated in either transplant recipients or prospective trials in the general population (Bosch et al., 2006). Nonetheless, ACE-I and/or ARB are commonly used due to its well-established antiproteinuric, cardioprotective, and blood pressure lowering effect.

13.4 Pharmacological management

When lifestyle modification fails to achieve adequate glycemic control, medical intervention is recommended. Orally administered agents can be used either alone or in combination with other oral agents or insulin. The choice of pharmacologic therapy is based on the potential advantages and disadvantages associated with the different classes of oral agents. Table 3 summarizes the mechanisms of action and potential advantages and disadvantages of different classes of oral agents.

It is noteworthy that the results of the Dialysis Outcomes and Practice Patterns Study (DOPPS) demonstrated that in long-term hemodialysis patients rosiglitazone was associated with a significantly higher all-cause (hazard ration 1.59) and cardiovascular mortality and a 3.5 fold increase of hospitalizations due to myocardial infarction (Ramirez et al., 2009). In contrast to the DOPPS study results, in an analysis of the national cohort study consisting of more than 5,000 dialysis patients with type 2 diabetes Brunelli et al. observed a lower incidence of all-cause mortality in patients not on insulin vs. insulin requiring diabetic patients (Brunelli et al., 2009). Similar studies in the transplant settings are lacking. Nonetheless, great caution should be exercised when rosiglitazone is used in the setting of kidney transplantation because all kidney transplant recipients should be regarded as having at least stage II-IV chronic kidney disease. It should be noted that rosiglitazone has been suspended in Europe since 2010

Incretin-based therapy appears to provide an attractive treatment option for patients with NODAT owing to its favorable effect on weight reduction /weight neutrality. Data on its safety and efficacy in renal transplant recipients are currently lacking. A randomized, placebo-controlled, double-blind, prospective trial to evaluate the safety and efficacy of vildagliptin in patients with NODAT is currently underway (Haidinger et al., 2010). Caution should be exercised when these agents are used in the transplant setting, particularly with regards to drug to drug interactions. Vildagliptin should be avoided in patients with hepatic impairment and stage IV-V chronic kidney disease and the dose of sitagliptin should be adjusted for renal insufficiency.

Finally, drug to drug interactions should be carefully considered. Interested readers are referred to the following references (Cheng & Fantus, 2005; Hatorp et al., 2003; Niemi et al., 2000).

14. Summary

NODAT is a common complication after solid organ transplantation and has variably been reported to have an adverse impact on patient and allograft outcomes. Risk stratification and intervention to minimize risk should be an integral part in the management of the transplant recipients. Clinicians must be familiar with the patients' immune history prior to manipulating their immunosuppressive therapy.in an attempt to ameliorate NODAT risk. When lifestyle modification fails to achieve adequate glycemic control, medical intervention is often necessary.

The routine care of patients with NODAT should include an evaluation of hemoglobin A1C level every three months and regular screening for diabetic complications. It should be noted that hemoglobin A1C cannot be accurately interpreted within the first three months post transplantation due to various factors including possible blood transfusions in the early posttransplant period and the presence of anemia or impaired allograft function. Blood transfusions may render the test invalid until new hemoglobin is formed and the presence of anemia and kidney impairment can directly interfere with the A1C assay. An artifactual reduction in A1C level has been reported in islet cell transplant recipients taking dapsone for pneumocystis carinii (P. jiroveci) prophylaxis. The cause is yet unknown, but a reduction in red blood cell lifespan and/or hemolysis has been implicated (Froud et al., 2007).

Fasting lipid profile should be measured annually. In transplant recipients with multiple CVD risk factors, more frequent monitoring of lipid profile should be performed at the discretion of the clinicians. Statins or the HMG-CoA reductase inhibitors are the most widely used lipid lowering agents in both the nontransplant and transplant settings. Table 4 summarizes the suggested guidelines for the management of NODAT (P.T. Pham et al., 2007c; Qaseem et al., 2011).

Non-pharmacological

Dietary modification
Dietitian referral
Diabetic dyslipidemia: diet low in saturated fats and cholesterol & high in complex carbohydrates & fiber
AHA[1] guidelines: limiting cholesterol (< 200 mg/day for those with DM), < 7% calories from saturated fats, 2-3% calories from trans-fatty acids, < 2,400 mg sodium a day, > 25g/day of dietary fiber & 2 servings of fish a week

Lifestyle modification
Exercise
Weight reduction or avoidance of excessive weight gain
Smoking cessation

Modification of immunosuppressive medications[2]

Rapid steroid taper, steroid-sparing or steroid avoidance protocols
Tacrolimus to cyclosporine conversion therapy
Avoid CNI and mTOR inhibitors combination therapy

Pharmacological therapy

Acute, marked hyperglycemia (may require in-patient management)
Consider insulin drip when glucose > 400 mg/dL[3]
Chronic hyperglycemia: treat to target HbA1C < 6.5%[4]
Oral glucose-lowering agent monotherapy or combination therapy[5] and/or insulin therapy
Consider diabetologist referral if HbA1C remains > 9.0%

Monitoring of patients with NODAT

HbA1C every 3 months
Screening for microalbuminuria
Regular ophthalmologic exam
Regular foot care
Annual fasting lipid profile
Aggressive treatment of dyslipidemia nd hypertension

---

[1]AHA: American Heart Association
[2]Clinicians must be familiar with the patients'immune history prior to manipulating their immunosuppressive therapy
[3]The American College of Physicians expert panel recommends not using intensive insulin therapy to normalize blood glucose in general surgical and medical intensive care unit (SICU/MICU) patients with or without diabetes (reference 84). Studies in the transplant settings are lacking. The determination of target blood glucose for transplant recipients should be individualized at the discretion of the clinician.
[4]See text

Table 4. Management of NODAT

15. References

Aasebo, W., Midvedt, K., Valderhaugh, T.G., et al. (2010). Impaired gluose homeostasis in renal transplant recipients receiving basiliximab. *Nephrology Dialysis Transplantation*, Vol. 25, No. 4, (November 2010), pp. 1279-1286, ISSN 0931-0509

Baid, S., Cosimi, A.B., Farrell, et al. (2001). Posttransplant diabetes mellitus in liver transplant recipients: risk factors, temporal relationship with hepatitis C virus allograft hepatitis, and impact on mortality. *Transplantation*, Vol. 72, No. 6, (September 2010), pp. 1066-1072, ISSN 0041-1337

Bayer, N.D., Cochetti, P.T., Kumar, M.S.A., et al. (2010). Association of metabolic syndrome with development of New-Onset Diabetes after transplantation. *Transplantation*, Vol. 90, No. 8, (October 2010), pp. 861-866, ISSN 0041-1337

Bayes, B., Pastor, M.C., Lauzurica, R., et al. (2007). Do anti-CD25 monoclonal antibodies potentiate posttransplant diabetes mellitus? *Transplantation Proceedings*, Vol. 39, No. 7, (February 2007), pp. 2248-2250, ISSN 0041-1345

Bigam, D., Pennington, J., Carpentier, A., et al. (2000). Hepatitis-C related cirrhosis: a predictor of diabetes after liver transplantation. *Hepatology*, Vol. 32, No. 1, (July 2000), pp. 87-90, ISSN 1527-3350

Bloom, R.D., Rao, V., Weng, F., et al. (2002). Association of hepatitis C with posttransplant diabetes in renal transplant patients on tacrolimus. *Journal of American Society of Nephrology*, Vol. 13, No. 5, (May 2002), pp. 1374-1380, ISSN 1046-6673

Bloom, R.D., Lake, J.R. (2006). Emerging issues in hepatitis C virus-positive liver and kidney transplant recipients. *American Journal of Kidney Transplantation*, Vol. 6, No. 10, (October 2006), pp. 2232-2237, ISSN 1600-6135

Bosch, J., Yusuf, S., Gerstein, H.C., et al. (2006). Effect of ramipril on the incidence of diabetes. *New England Journal of Medicine*, Vol. 355, No. 15, (October 2006), pp. 1551-1562, ISSN 0028-4793

Brunelli, S.M., Thadhani, R., Ikizler, T.A., et al. (2009). Thiazolidinedione use is associated with better survival in hemodialysis patients with non-insulin dependent diabetes. *Kidney International*, Vol. 75, No. 9, (May 2009), pp. 961-968, ISSN 0085-2538

Cai, T.H., Esterl, R.M., Nichols, F., et al. (1998). Improved immunosuppression with combination tacrolimus (FK506) and mycophenolic acid in orthotopic liver transplantation. *Transplantation Proceedings*, Vol. 30, No. 4, (June 1998), pp. 1413-1414, ISSN 0041-1345

Cheng, A.Y.Y., Fantus, I.G. (2005). Oral antihyperglycemic therapy for type 2 diabetes mellitus. *Canadian Medical Association Journal*, Vol. 172, No. 2, (January 2005), pp. 213-226, ISSN 0820-3946

Cole, E.H., Johnston, O., Rose, C.L., et al. (2008). Impact of acute rejection and new-onset diabetes on long-term transplant graft and patient survival. *Clinical Journal of the American Society of Nephrology*, Vol. 3, No. 3, (May 2008), pp. 814-821, ISSN 1555-9041

Cosio, F.G., Pesavento, T.E., Osei, K., et al. (2001). Post-transplant diabetes mellitus: Increasing incidence in renal allograft recipients transplanted in recent years. *Kidney International*, Vol. 59, No. 2, (February 2001), pp. 732-737, ISSN 0085-2538

Cosio, F.G., Kudva, Y., van der Velde, M., Larson, T.S., et al. (2005). New onset hyperglycemia and diabetes mellitus are associated with increased cardiovascular risk after kidney transplantation. *Kidney International*, Vol. 67, No. 6, (June 2005), pp. 2415-2421, ISSN 0085-2538

Crutchlow, M.F., Bloom, R.D. Transplant-associated hyperglycemia: A new look at an old problem. (2007). *Clinical Journal of the American Society of Nephrology*, Vol. 2, No. 2, (March 2007), pp. 343-355, ISSN 1555-9041

Davidson, J., Wilkinson, A.H., Dantal, J., et al. (2003). New-onset diabetes after transplantation: 2003 International Consensus Guidelines. *Transplantation*, Vol. 75, No. 10, (May 2003), pp. SS3-SS24, ISSN 0041-1337

Dean, P.G., Kudva, Y.C., Larson, T.S., et al. (2008). Post transplantation diabetes after pancreas transplantation. *American Journal of Transplantation*, Vol. 8, No. 1, (January 2008), pp. 175-182, ISSN 1600-6135

Delgado-Borrego, A., Casson, D., Schoenfeld, D., et al. (2004). Hepatitis C virus is independently associated with increased insulin resistance after liver transplantation. *Transplantation*, Vol 77, No. 5, (March 2004), pp. 703-710, ISSN 0041-1337

Depczynski, B., Daly, B., Campbell, D., et al. (2000). Predicting the occurrence of diabetes mellitus in recipients of heart transplants. *Diabetic Medicine*, Vol. 17, No. 1, (January 2000), pp. 15-19, ISSN 1464-5491

Drachenberg, C.B., Klassen, D.K., Weir, M.R., et al. (1999). Islet cell damage associated with tacrolimus and cyclosporine: morphological features in pancreas allograft biopsies and clinical correlation. *Transplantation*, Vol. 68, No. 3, (August 1999), pp. 396-402, ISSN 0041-1337

Eckel, R.H. (2007). Mechanisms of the components of the metabolic syndrome that predispose to diabetes and atherosclerotic CVD. *Proceedings of the Nutrition Society*, Vol. 66, No. 1, (February 2007), pp. 82-95, ISSN 0029-6651

Eprinchard, C.S., Braun, P.P., Heibel, F., et al. (2011). Incidence and risk factors of glucose metabolism disorders in kidney transplant recipients: role of systematic screening by oral glucose tolerance test. *Transplantation*. Vol. 91, No. 7, (April 2011), ISSN 0041-1337

Ekberg, H., Tedesco-Silva, H., Demirbas, A., et al. (2007). Reduced exposure to calcineurin inhibitors in renal transplantation. *New England Journal of Medicine,* Vol. 357, (December 2007), pp. 2562-2575, ISSN 0028-4793

Froud, T., Faradji, R.N., Monroy, K., et al. (2007). Dapsone-induced artifactual A1C reduction in islet transplant recipients. *Transplantation*, Vol. 83, No. 6, (March 2007), pp. 824-825, ISSN 0041-1337

Gerstein, H.C., Miller, M.E., Byinhton, R.P., et al. (2008). Effects of intensive glucose lowering in type 2 diabetes. *New England Journal of Medicine*, Vol. 358, No. 24, (June 2008), pp. 2545-2559, ISSN 0028-4793

Haidinger, M., Werzowa, J., Voigt, H-C., et al. (2010). A randomized, placebo-controlled, double-blind, prospective trial to evaluate the effect of vildagliptin in new-onset diabetes mellitus after kidney transplantation. *Trials*, Vol. 11, No. 91, (October 2010), pp. 1-6, ISSN 1745-6215

Hatorp, V., Hansen, K.T., Thomsen, M.S. (2003). Influence of drugs interacting with CYP3A4 on the pharmacokinetics, pharmacodynamics and safety of the prandial glucose regulator repaglinide. *Journal of Clinical Pharmacology*, Vol. 43, No. 6, pp. 649-660, ISSN 0091-2700

Heisel, O., Heisel, R., Balshaw, R., et al. (2004). New onset diabetes mellitus in patients receiving calcineurin inhibitors: a systematic review and meta-analysis. *American Journal of Transplantation*, Vol. 4. No. 4, (April 2004), pp. 583-595, ISSN 1600-6135

Hjelmesaeth, J., Hartmann, A., Kofstad, J., et al. (1997). Glucose intolerance after renal transplantation depends upon prednisolone dose and recipient age. *Transplantation*, Vol. 64, No. 7, (October 1997), pp. 979-983, ISSN 0041-1337

Hjelmesaeth, J., Hartmann, A., Kofstad, J., et al. (2001). Tapering off prenisolone and cyclosporine the first year after renal transplantation: the effect on glucose tolerance. *Nephrology Dialysis Transplantation*, Vol. 16, No. 4, (April 2001), pp. 829-835, ISSN 0931-0509

Hjelmesaeth, J., Sagedal, S., Hartmannn, A. et al. (2004). Asymptomatic cytomegalovirus infection is associated with increased risk for new-onset diabetes and impaired insulin release after renal transplantation. *Diabetologia*, Vol. 47, No. 9, (September 2004), pp. 1550-1556, ISSN 0012-186X

Hjelmesaeth, J., Muller, F., Jenssen, T., et al. (2005). Is there a link between cytomegalovirus infection and new-onset posttransplant diabetes mellitus? Potential mechanisms of virus induced β-cell damage. *Nephrology Dialysis Transplantation*, Vol. 20, No. 11, (November 2005), pp. 2311-2315, ISSN 0931-0509

Hjelmesaeth, J., Hartmann, A., Leivestad, T. et al. (2006). The impact of early-diagnosed new-onset post-tarnsplantation diabetes mellitus on survival and major cardiac events. *Kidney International*, Vol. 69, No. 3, (February 2006), pp. 588-595, ISSN 0085-2538

Ismail-Beigi, F., Craven, T., Banerji, M.A., et al. Effect of intensive treatment of hyperglycemia on microvascular outcomes in type 2 diabetes: an analysis of the ACCORD randomized trial. *Lancet*, Vol. 376, No. 9739, (August 2010), pp. 419-430, ISSN 0140-6736

Kasiske, B.L., Snyder, J.J., Gilbertson, D., et al. (2003). Diabetes mellitus after kidney transplantation in the United States. *American Journal of Transplantation*, Vol. 3, No. 10, (October 2003), pp. 178-185, ISSN 1600-6135

Knobler, H., Stagnaro-Green, A., Wallenstein, S., et al. (1998). Higher incidence of diabetes in liver transplant recipients with hepatitis C. *Journal of Clinical Gastroenterology*, Vol. 26, No. 1 (January 1998), pp. 30-33, ISSN 0192-0790

Luan, F.L., Steffick, D.E., Ojo, A.O. (2011). New-Onset Diabetes Mellitus in kidney transplant recipients discharged on steroid-free immunosuppression. *Transplantation*, Vol. 91, No. 3, (February 2011), pp. 334-341, ISSN 0041-1337

John, P.R., Thuluvath, P.J. (2002). Outcomes of patients with new-onset diabetes mellitus after liver transplantation compared with those without diabetes mellitus. *Liver transplantation*, Vol. 8, No. 8, (August 2002), pp. 708-713, ISSN 1527-6465

Johnston, O., Rose, C.L., Webster, A.C., et al. (2008). Sirolimus is associated with New-Onset Diabetes in kidney transplant recipients. *Journal of American Society of Nephrology*, Vol. 19, No. 7, (July 2008), pp. 1411-1418, ISSN 1046-6673

Kamar, N., Toupance, O., Buchler, M., et al. (2003). Evidence that clearance of hepatitis C virus RNA after α-interferon therapy in dialysis patients is sustained after renal transplantation. *Journal of American Society of Nephrology*, Vol. 14, No. 8, (August 2003), pp. 2092-2098, ISSN 1046-6673

Kissebah, A.H., Vydelingum, N., Murray, R., et al. (1982). Relation of body fat distribution to metabolic complications of obesity. *Journal of Clinical Endocrinology and Metabolism*, Vol. 54, No. 2, (May 1982), pp. 254-260, ISSN 0021-972X

Kuo, H-T., Sampaio, M.S., Vincenti, F. ,et al. (2010). Associations of pretransplant diabetes mellitus, New-Onset Diabetes Mellitus after Transplant, and acute rejection with transplant outcomes: An analysis of the Organ Procurement and Transplant Network/United Network for Organ Sharing (OPTN/UNOS) database. *American Journal of Kidney Disease*, Vol. 56, No. 6, (December 2010), pp. 1127-1139, ISSN 0272-6386

Kuypers, D.R., Claes, K., Bammens, B., et al. (2008). Early clinical assessment of glucose metabolism in renal allograft recipients: Diagnosis and prediction of post-transplant diabetes mellitus. *Nephrology Dialysis Transplantation*, Vol. 23, No. 6, (June 2008), pp. 2033-2042, ISSN 0931-0509

Lehr, H., Jao, S., Waltzer, W.C., et al. (1985). Cytomegalovirus-induced diabetes mellitus in a renal transplant recipient. *Transplantation Proceedings*, Vol. 17, No. 5, (October 1985), pp. 2152-2154, ISSN 0041-1345

Maes, B.D., Kuypers, D., Messiaen, T., et al. (2001). Posttransplant diabetes mellitus in FK-506-treated renal transplant recipients: analysis of incidence and risk factors. *Transplantation*, Vol. 72, No. 10, (November 2001), pp. 1655-1661, ISSN 0041-1337

Mannon, R.B. (2008). Therapeutic management of posttransplant diabetes mellitus. *Transplantation Reviews*, Vol. 22, No. 2, (April 2008), pp. 116-124, ISSN 0955-470X

Martinez-Castelao, A., Hernandez, M.D., Pascual, J., et al. (2005). Detection and treatment of post kidney transplant hyperglycemia: A Spanish multicenter cross-sectional study. *Transplantation Proceedings*, Vol. 37, No. 9, (November 2005), pp. 3813-3816, ISSN 0041-1345

Meiser, B.M., Uberfuhr, P., Fuchs, A., et al. (1998). Single-center randomized trial comparing tacrolimus (FK506) and cyclosporine in the prevention of acute myocardial rejection. *The Journal of Heart and Lung Transplantation*, Vol. 17, No. 8(August 1998), pp. 782-788, ISSN 1053-2498

Midtvedt, K., Hjemesaeth, J., Hartmann, A., et al. (2004). Insulin resistance after renal transplantation: the effect of steroid dose reduction and withdrawal. *Journal of the American Society of Nephrology*, Vol. 15, No. 12, (December 2004), pp. 3233-3239, ISSN 1046-6673

Montori, V.M., Velosa, J.A., Basu, A. et al. (2002). Post transplantation diabetes: A systematic review of the literature. *Diabetes Care*, Vol. 25, No. 3, (March 2002), pp. 583-592, ISSN 0149-5992

Myslak, M., Amer, H., Morales, P. et al. (2006). Interpreting post-transplant proteinuria in patients with proteinuria pre-transplant. *American Journal of Transplantation*, Vol. 6, No. 7, (July 2006), pp. 1660-1665, ISSN 1600-6135

Niemi, M., Backman, J.T., Neuvonen, P.J., et al. (2000). Rifampin decreases the plasma concentrations and effects of repaglinide. *Clinical Pharmacology and Therapeutics*, Vol. 68, No. 5, (July 2000), pp. 495-500, ISSN 0009-9236

Ojo, A.O. (2006). Cardiovascular complications after renal transplantation and their prevention. *Transplantation*, Vol. 82, No. 5, (September 2006), pp. 603-611, ISSN 0041-1337

Pham, P.C., Pham, P.M., Pham, S.V. et al. (2007). Hypomagnesemia in patients with type 2 diabetes. *Clinical Journal of the American Society of Nephrology*, Vol. 2, No. 2, (March 2007), pp. 366-373, ISSN 1555-9041

Pham, P.T., Danovitch, G.M., Pham, P.C. (2007a). The medical management of the renal transplant recipient . In: *Comprehensive Clinical Nephrology, 3rd ed.*, R.J. Johnson & John Feehally, pp. 1085-1101, Mosby, ISBN 978-0-323-04602-2, Philadelphia, PA

Pham, P.T., Pham, P.C., Lipshutz, G., et al. (2007b). New onset diabetes mellitus after solid organ transplantation. *Endocrinology and Metabolism Clinics of North America,* Vol. 36, No. 4, (December 2007b), pp. 873-890, ISSN 0889-8529

Pham, P.T., Pham, P.C., Danovitch, G.M. (2007c). Posttransplant cardiovascular disease. *Seminars in Nephrology*, Vol. 27, No. 4, (July 2007c), pp. 430-444, ISSN 0270-9295

Pham, P.T., Pham, P.C. (2008). Assessing the risk of post-transplantation diabetes mellitus with an oral glucose tolerance test. *Nature Clinical Practice Nephrology*, Vol. 4, No. 11, (November 2008), pp. 600-601, ISSN 1759-5061

Qaseem, A., Humphrey, L., Chou, R., et al. (2011). Use of intensive therapy for the management of glycemic control in hospitalized patients: A clinical practice guideline from the American College of Physicians. *Annals of Internal Medicine*, Vol. 154, No. 4, (February 2011), pp. 260-267, ISSN 0003-4819

Ramirez, S.P., Albert, J.M., Blayney, M.J., et al. (2009). Rosiglitazone is associated with mortality in chronic hemodialysis patients. *Journal of the American Society of Nephrology*, Vol. 20, No. 5, (May 2009), pp. 1094-1101, ISSN 1046-6673

Roland, M., Gatault, P., Al-Naijjar, A., et al. (2008). Early pulse pressure and low-grade proteinuria as independent long-term risk factors for New-Onset Diabetes After kidney Transplantation. *American Journal of Transplantation*, Vol. 8, No. 8, (August 2008), pp. 1719-1728, ISSN 1600-6135

Santos, L., Rodrigo, E., Pinera, C., et al. (2010). Elevated serum Gamma-Glutaryltransferase and hypomagnesemia are not related with new-onset diabetes after transplantation. *Transplantation Proceedings*, Vol. 42, No. 8, (October 2010), pp. 2914-2916, ISSN 0041-1345

Scheen, A.J. Renin-angiotensin system inhibition prevents type 2 diabetes mellitus. Part 1. A meta-analysis of randomized clinical trials. *Diabetes and Metabolism*, Vol. 30, No. 6, (December 2004), pp. 487-496, ISSN 1262-3636

Setoguchi, R., Hori, S., Takahashi, T., et al. (2005). Hemoestatic maintenance of natural Fox3(+) CD25(+) CD4(+) regulatory T cells by interleukin (IL)-2 and induction of autoimmune disease by IL-2 neutralization. *The Journal of Experimental Medicine*, Vol. 201, pp. 723-735, ISSN 0022-1007

Sharif, A., Moore, R.H., Baboolal, K. (2006). The use of oral glucose tolerance tests to risk stratify for new-onset diabetes after transplantation: an underdiagnosed phenomenon. *Transplantation*, Vol. 82, No. 12, (December 2006), pp. 1667-1672, ISSN 0041-1337

Silverborn, M., Jeppsson, A., Martensson, G., & Nilsson, F. (2005). New-onset cardiovascular risk factors in lung transplant recipients. *The Journal of Heart and Lung Transplantation*, Vol. 24, No. 10, (October 2005), pp. 1536-1543, ISSN 1053-2498

Simo, R., Lecube, A., Genesca, J., et al. (2006). Sustained virological response correlates with reduction in the incidence of glucose abnormalities in patients with chronic hepatitis C virus infection. *Diabetes Care*, Vol. 29, No. 11, (November 2006), pp. 2462-2466, ISSN 0149-5992

Subramanian, S., Trence, D.L. (2007). Immunosuppression agents: effects on glucose and lipid metabolism. *Endocrinology and Metabolism Clinics of North America*, Vol. 36, No. 4, (December 2007), pp. 891-905, ISSN 0889-8529

Sulanc, E., Lane, J.T., Puumala, S.E., et al. (2005). New-onset diabetes after kidney transplantation: an application of 2003 International Guidelines. *Transplantation*, Vol. 80, No. 7, (October 2005), pp. 945-952, ISSN 0041-1337

Teutônico, A., Schena, P.F., Di Paolo, S. (2006). Glucose metabolism in renal transplant recipients: Effect of calcineurin inhibitor withdrawal and conversion to sirolimus. *Journal of American Society of Nephrology*, Vol. 16, No. 10, (October 2005), pp. 3128-3135, ISSN 1046-6673

Trulock, E.P., Christie, J.D., Edward, L.B., et al. (2007). Registry of the International society for heart and lung Transplantation: twenty-fourth official adult lung and heart-lung transplantation report. *The Journal of Heart and Lung Transplantation*, Vol. 26, No. 8, (August 2007), pp. 782-795, ISSN 1053-2498

Valentine, H., Rickenbacker, P., Kemna, M., et al. (2001). Metabolic abnormalities characteristics of dysmetabolic syndrome predict the development of transplant coronary artery disease: prospective study. *Circulation*, Vol. 103, pp. 2144-2152, ISSN 0009-7322

Van Hooff, J.P., Christiaans, M.H.L., van Duijhoven, E.M. (2004). Evaluating mechanisms of post-transplant diabetes mellitus. *Nephrology Dialysis Transplantation*, Vol. 19, Suppl. 6, (December 2004), pp. vi18-vi12, ISSN 0931-0509

Van Laecke, S., Van Biesen, W., Verbeke, F., et al. (2009). Posttransplantation hypomagnesemia and its realtion with immunosuppression as predictors of New-Onset Diabetes after Transplantation. *American Journal of Transplantation*, Vol. 9, No. 9, (September 2009), pp. 2140-2149, ISSN 1600-6135

Van Laecke, S., Desideri, F., Geerts, A., et al. (2010). Hypomagenesemia and the risk of New-Onset Diabetes after liver transplantation. *Liver Transplantation*, Vol. 16, No. 11, (November 2010), pp. 1278-1287, ISSN 1527-6465

Vanrenterghem, Y., Bresnahan, B., Campistol, J., et al. (2011). Belatacept-based regimens are associated with improved cardiovascular and metabolic risk factors compared with cyclosporine in kidney transplant recipients. (BENEFT- and BENEFITEXT Studies). *Transplantation*, (March 2011), [Epub ahead of print], ISSN 1534-0608

Vareesangthip, K., Tong, P., Wilkinson, R., et al. (1997). Insulin resistance in adult polycystic kidney disease. *Kidney International*, Vol. 52, No. 2, (August 1997), pp. 503-508, ISSN 0085-2538

Vincenti, F., Friman, S., Sceuermann, E., et al. (2007). Results of an International, randomized trial comparing glucose metabolism disorders and outcome with cyclosporine versus Tacrolimus. *American Journal of Transplantation*, Vol. 7, No. 6, (June 2007), pp. 1506-1514, ISSN 1600-6135

Wilkinson, A.H., Davidson, J., Dotta, F., et al. (2005). Guidelines for the treatment and management of new-onset diabetes after transplantation. *Clinical Transplantion*, Vol. 19, No. 3, (June 2005), pp. 291-298, ISSN 0902-0063

Woodward, R.S., Schnitzler, M.A., Baty, J., et al. (2003). Incidence and cost of new onset diabetes mellitus among U.S. wait-listed and transplanted renal allograft recipients.

American Journal of Transplantation, Vol. 3, No. 5, (May 2003), pp. 590-598, ISSN 1600-6135

Ye, X., Kuo, H-T., Sampaio, M.S., et al. (2010a). Risk factors for the development of new-onset diabetes mellitus after transplant in adult lung transplant recipients. *Clinical Transplantation,* (December 2010a), DOI:10.1111/j.1399-0012.2010.01383.x, ISSN 1399-0012

Ye, X., Kuo, H-T, Sampaio, M, et al. (2010b). Risk factors for development on New-Onset Diabetes Mellitus in adult heart transplant recipients. *Transplantation,* Vol. 89, No. 12, (June 2010b), ISSN 0041-1337

13

Sexual and Reproductive Function in Chronic Kidney Disease and Effect of Kidney Transplantation

Mahboob Lessan-Pezeshki[1] and Shirin Ghazizadeh[2]
[1]*Nephrology Research Center, Imam Khomeini Hospital, Tehran University of Medical Sciences,*
[2]*Obstetrics and Gynecology Department, Tehran University of Medical Sciences, Iran*

1. Introduction

Chronic renal failure has been known to be associated with impotence and loss of libido in men and for many women, infertility and menstrual irregularities. There have been ongoing improvements in survival and quality of life after renal transplantation. These have been accompanied by an improvement in reproductive function and reversal of the relative infertility that occurs despite maintenance hemodialysis. One of the most impressive aspects of successful renal transplantation in the young person is the ability of the male patient to father a child and the female patient to give birth to a healthy baby.

Pregnancy does not appear to have any adverse effect on the long-term survival of renal allografts. Because the outcome of pregnancy in transplantation are so different than those in chronic dialysis, it is advisable to treat end-stage renal disease patients with transplantation and wait until renal function has been stable before undertaking a planned pregnancy. Women are usually advised to wait at least 1 year after living-related kidney Transplantation, and 2 years after cadaveric kidney transplantation; however, waits of 5 years or more have been associated with impaired renal function post-partum.

All women of child-bearing age should be counseled about the possibility and risks of pregnancy after kidney transplantation. Types of immunosuppressive regimens and assessment of graft function should be considered during preconception counseling. Contraceptive counseling should be provided before transplantation surgery, because ovulatory cycles may begin within 1 to 2 months after transplantation in women with grafts that are functioning well. It is strongly advised that every sexually active transplant recipient attend a family-planning counseling session, ideally before transplantation is performed. Breastfeeding is discouraged for patients taking any immunosuppressive drugs.

In this chapter we will first have a short review on reproductive physiology in male and female and irregularities caused by end stage renal disease and then we will review the experience of women undergoing child birth after transplantation, with a focus on outcomes and suggested management strategies including contraception counseling.

2. Male reproduction

2.1 Physiology of reproduction in men

The male reproductive tract consists of the testis, epididymis, vas deference, prostate, seminal vesicles, ejaculatory duct, bulbouretral glands, and urethra. The testes contain two cell types: the Sertoli cells, which line the seminiferous tubules (the site of spermatogenesis), and the Leydig cells (the site of androgen synthesis). In the male, the pituitary gland secretes luteinizing hormone (LH) and follicle-stimulating hormone (FSH), which act on the testes. LH stimulates the synthesis and secretion of testosterone by the Leydig cells, and FSH stimulates the sertoli cells to secrete inhibin. FSH and testosterone act on the seminiferous tubules to stimulate spermatogenesis. In human it takes about 75 days for spermatogonia to develop into mature sperm cells (Berek 2002).

During ejaculation, mature spermatozoa are released from the vas deferens along with fluid from the prostate, seminal vesicle, and the bulbourethral glands. The semen released is a gelatinous mixture of spermatozoa and seminal plasma; however it thins out 20 -30 minutes after ejaculation by a process called liquefaction (Berek 2002).

Both LH and FSH play roles in normal spermatogenesis. Thus, spermatogenesis does not occur spontaneously in men who have hypogonadotropic hypogonadism of prepubertal onset. Spermatogenesis can be initiated in these men by the administration of human chorionic gonadotropin (hCG), which has potent LH effects, and an FSH preparation, such as human menopausal gonadotropin (hMG) (Finkel 1985).

2.2 Male reproduction in end stage renal disease

For many male patients with renal failure, impotence and loss of libido have been seen frequently; these problems may improve but rarely normalize with the institution of maintenance dialysis, commonly resulting in a decreased quality of life (Holdsworth 1978; Diemont 2000; Rosas 2003). By comparison, a well-functioning renal transplant is much more likely to restore sexual activity; however, some features of reproductive function may remain impaired.

The uremic milieu plays an important role in the genesis of sexual dysfunction in end stage renal disease. Psychologic and physical stresses that may contribute to disturbances in sexual function are also commonly present in patients with chronic renal failure (Holdsworth 1978; Steele 1996; Toorians, Janssen et al. 1997).

2.2.1 Gonadal function

Advanced chronic kidney disease is associated with impaired spermatogenesis and testicular damage (Holdsworth 1977; Holdsworth 1978). Semen analysis typically shows a decreased volume of ejaculate, oligo- or complete azoospermia, and a low percentage of motile sperm. Testicular histology shows reduced spermatogenic activity varying from decreased numbers of mature spermatocytes to complete aplasia of germinal elements. Other findings include damage to the seminiferous tubules, atrophy of Sertoli cells, and interstitial fibrosis and calcifications.

The factors responsible for testicular damage in uremia are not well understood. It is possible that plasticizers in dialysis tubing, such as phthalate, may play a role in patients undergoing maintenance hemodialysis.

Uremia also impairs gonadal steroidogenesis. The serum total and free testosterone concentrations are typically reduced, although the binding capacity and concentration of sex hormone-binding globulin are normal (Lim 1976; Levitan 1984; de Vries 1984). Another manifestation of diminished testosterone secretory capacity is the subnormal and delayed testosterone response to the administration of human chorionic gonadotropin (HCG), a compound with luteinizing hormone-like actions (Stewart-Bentley 1974). By comparison, although the total plasma estrogen concentration is frequently elevated, the serum estradiol concentration is typically normal (Lim 1978).

2.2.2 Pituitary function

The serum concentration of luteinizing hormone (LH) is elevated in uremic men (Lim 1978); this is due to diminished testosterone feedback.

Follicle stimulating hormone (FSH) secretion is also elevated, although to a more variable degree (Holdsworth 1978; de Vries 1984). Elevated FSH levels are probably the result of decreased testosterone and inhibin, a Sertoli cell product. The plasma FSH concentration tends to be highest in those uremic patients with the most severe damage to seminiferous tubules and presumably the lowest levels of inhibin. It has been suggested that increased FSH levels may portend a poor prognosis for recovery of spermatogenic function after renal transplantation. The gonadotropin reserve is generally intact, since the plasma level of both gonadotropins increased appropriately following administration of gonadotropin-releasing hormone (GnRH) (LeRoith 1980). The appropriate increase in FSH and LH in response to the administration of clomiphene (a nonsteroidal antiestrogen that stimulates gonadotropin secretion by blockade of estrogen mediated negative feedback on the hypothalamus) (Lim 1978), also indicates a normal gonadotropin reserve.

2.2.3 Hyperprolactinemia

The basal levels of serum prolactin are elevated in the majority of uremic patients, and the response to thyrotropin-releasing hormone (TRH) is reduced and delayed (Hagen C 1976). The mechanisms for the hyperprolactinemia in chronic renal failure are not well defined. Increased autonomous production rate of prolactin is a major mechanism for the hyperprolactinemia but decreased metabolic clearance rate may also play a role (Cowden 1981). The demonstration of resistance to stimulation or suppression of prolactin in CRF is consistent with increased autonomous production (Pece 1979). The state of secondary hyperparathyroidism of CRF may contribute to the increased production rate of prolactin, because PTH stimulates prolactin secretion (Issac 1978). The treatment of CRF patients with erythropoietin was associated with a decreased in serum prolactin levels and improvement in sexual dysfunction (Schaefer, Stanhope et al. 1989), but did not normalize rate of the response to TRH (Ramirez 1976). These observations suggest that either anemia and/or deficiency of erythropoietin per se participate in the genesis of the hyperprolactinemia of CRF.

2.2.4 Gynecomastia

Variable degrees of gynecomastia are often encountered in the male uremic patient treated with maintenance hemodialysis (Lim 1978). Gynecomastia usually develops during initial months of dialysis and regresses as dialysis continues. It may be transient or may last for periods of several months. The etiology may be related to the improvement in the nutritional status of uremic patient with dialysis theray and, as such, is similar to the mechanism of refeeding gynecomastia. It must be emphasized that in almost all cases of

Gynecomastia, there is an alteration either in the ratio between the serum level of androgen and estrogen, in favor of the latter, or in the ratio between the action of androgen and estrogen at the tissue level (Sawin 1973). Indeed, in patients with advanced CRF and those treated with hemodialysis, the ratio between the serum levels of free testosterone and estradiol is reduced because of a decreased in testosterone levels.

2.3 Erectile dysfunction in end stage renal disease:

Erectile dysfunction is defined as the inability to achieve and maintain an erection sufficient to permit satisfactory sexual intercourse. It may result from psychologic, neurologic, hormonal, arterial or cavernosal impairment or from a combination of these factors. Most of the studies in sexual dysfunctions in CRF patients have focused on impotence. Erectile dysfunction is common in patients with CRF and is observed in excess of 50% of these patients (Procci 1981). These data are based on results obtained from interviews with or by the completion of questionnaires by the patients and/or their spouses. Several factors appear to participate in the genesis of impotence in CRF patients. These include abnormalities in the neurohormonal control system of erection hormones of the hypothalamic-pituitary-gonadal axis , secondary hyperparathyroidism and, dysfunction of the corporal smooth muscle of the penis or in their response to relaxing stimuli and/or derangements in the arterial supply or the venous drainage of the penis (Schrier RW 2001). Patients with a history of abnormal erectile function prior to the onset of renal disease may have a secondary cause, such as a neuropathy or peripheral vascular disease.

The presence of a neurogenic bladder suggests an underlying neuropathy, while findings of peripheral vascular disease point toward inadequate penile blood flow. The lack of secondary sexual characteristics combined with small soft testicles suggests hypogonadism. The ingestion of a number of medications, such as beta blockers and tricyclic antidepressants, may be a cause of erectile dysfunction.

Among those without an obvious cause of impotence after an initial evaluation, consideration should be given to a psychologic difficulty, such as stress or depression. The values of Nocturnal Penile Tumescence (NPT) among a large population of uremic patients are significantly lower than normal. The administration of a nocturnal penile tumescence test may help distinguish between an organic and a psychologic disorder; the absence of an erection during sleep suggests underlying organic dysfunction. A positive test, however, does not exclude a physical cause.

2.3.1 Management

The first step in the treatment of uremic men with sexual dysfunction is increasing the delivered dose of dialysis, discontinuing medications with side effects of impotence and correcting the anemia of chronic renal disease. As an example, the administration of recombinant human erythropoietin to raise the hematocrit to 33 to 36 percent may enhance sexual function (Delano 1989).

Sildenafil has been effectively used in the treatment of erectile dysfunction in both hemodialysis and peritoneal dialysis patients and is often used for psychologic, vascular, or neurogenic causes (Ifudu 1998; Palmer 1999; Turk 2001; Seibel 2002; Rosas 2003; Grossman 2004). Concurrent use of sildenafil and nitrates in any form, regularly or intermittently, is contraindicated.

Since the elevation of serum levels of prolactin plays a role in the impotence of male uremic patient, correction of hyperprolactinemia by bromocriptin is also associated with improvement of sexual dysfunction.

Cabergoline, which causes nausea much less often than does bromocriptine and is at least as effective in treating hyperprolactinemia, should be tried first (Biller BM; Molitch ME; Vance ML; Cannistraro KB; Davis KR; Simons JA; Schoenfelder JR; Klibanski A 1996). The administration of testosterone to uremic men usually fails to restore libido or potency, despite normalized serum testosterone.

A vacuum tumescence device may be effective in restoring potency in uremic impotent males unresponsive to medical therapy. Administration of zinc is also a reasonable therapeutic option in uremic men.

2.4 Renal transplantation

Kidney transplantation is the best and most effective option that can be offered to patients with severe renal damage to restore their health and the possibility of recovering their sexual and reproductive functions.

After successful transplantation, about two thirds of male patients observe improved libido and a return of sexual function to predialysis levels. Fertility as assessed by sperm counts, improves in half patients. The sex hormone profile tends to normalize; plasma testosterone and follicle stimulating hormone levels increase; and luteinizing hormone levels which may be high in dialysis patients, decrease to normal or low levels (Danovitch GM 2005).

The factors that might cause certain difficulties for the recovery of sexual and reproductive functions in this type of patients include prolonged use of peritoneal dialysis, high follicle stimulating hormone (FSH) serum levels before the transplant, and a deficient function of the graft (De Celis and Pedron-Nuevo 1999).

A certain improvement has been reported as to semen quality in the three main parameters (number, morphology, and motility of the spermatozoa) in patients after kidney transplantation (De Celis and Pedron-Nuevo 1999).

Several studies conducted to evaluate the effects of immunosuppressive regimens suggest that some of these agents are potentially gonadotoxic since they affect testicular function and decrease fertility. This is mainly due to an indirect effect on the hypothalamus-pituitary-gonadal axis, or directly suppressant on the germinal epithelium of the testis, where the spermatogenetic process is primarily affected because of an interruption of the cycle needed for the development of an adequate amount of normal spermatozoa.

This would result in oligo/asthenozoospermia, teratozoospermia, or azoospermia. Cyclosporine (CSA) is an important therapeutic agent and a common component in multiple immunosuppressive regimens used in recipients of kidney transplants and for a growing number of autoimmune disorders. Some studies imply that CSA is a potentially gonadotoxic drug, producing adverse effects on the reproductive capability in experimental models as well as in humans. In certain animal species, such as the Sprague-Dawley strain rats, Seethalakshmi et al. showed that the administration of CSA induces a deficient intratesticular synthesis of androgens and a reduction in spermatogenesis, although this reduction was reversible after exogenous gonadotrophins were administered (Seethalakshmi 1990). On the other hand, it has also been possible to observe the adverse effect of CSA by means of testicular biopsies performed in dogs (Seethalakshmi 1988) and rats (Seethalakshmi 1990) treated with CSA for short periods, where marked abnormalities in spermatogenesis were seen. Cyclosporine (CSA) may impair testosterone biosynthesis through direct damage to leydig cells and germinal cells, an indirect impairment of the hypothalamic-pituitary-gonadal axis has also been suggested.

Computer-aided sperm analysis (CASA) in infertile renal transplant recipients showed that both sperm concentration and straight line velocity (VSL) were inversely correlated to the cyclosporine whole blood trough levels. Stabilization of the cyclosporine whole blood trough level within the target therapeutic level could improve the fertility potential in kidney transplant recipients. Duration of hemodialysis before transplantation is also important in this regard. The time spent on hemodialysis is inversely correlated with the percentage of motile spermatozoa and the amplitude of lateral head displacement (ALH) (Eid, Abdel-Hamid et al. 1996).

Azathioprine (AZA), another drug that is frequently combined with CSA, is considered to be genotoxic (Olshan 1994). However, very few studies have analyzed the effects of AZA on the reproductive function of humans. Several studies suggest that prednisone might not be involved in sperm cell damage.

Kaczmarek and coworkers found that heart transplant recipients treated with sirolimus had significantly lower free testosterone levels and significant higher levels of gonadotropic hormones luteinizing hormone and follicle-stimulating hormone compared with calcineurin inhibitor-based immunosuppression group (Kaczmarek 2004). Patients treated with sirolimus throughout the post-transplant period have a significantly reduced total sperm count compared to patients who did not receive sirolimus and a decreased proportion of motile spermatozoa. Moreover, the fathered pregnancy rate was lower in patients receiving sirolimus-based regimens (Zuber, Anglicheau et al. 2008).

There is also concern about infertility associated with Ganciclovir which is used for treatment of cytomegalovirus (CMV) infection in transplant patients (Nevins and Dunn 1992). There is no increased incidence of neonatal malformations in pregnancies fathered by transplant recipients (Danovitch GM 2005).

2.4.1 Sexual functions in renal transplant patients

Renal transplant recipients have all suffered from uremia. They have frequently spent a significant amount of time on dialysis and often have other comorbidities including hypertension and diabetes. Although a successful transplant may improve erectile function and return of libido, in many cases some degree of sexual dysfunction may persist. On the contrary a recent study showed that, erectile function worsens after RT in patients<45 yr (Mirone, Longo et al. 2009).

Hypertension is common among transplant patients; CSA can exacerbate preexisting high blood pressure and also induce hypertension in patients, who had normal blood pressure prior to the kidney transplant.

Antihypertensive medications have negative effects on male sexual functions, such as libido and erection (Matthew RW 2005). Those medications which are implicated in erectile dysfunction include beta blockers (propranolol, labetalol), Alpha blockers (prazosin), sympatholytics (clonidine), vasodilators (hydralazine), and diuretics (thiazides, spironolactone).

Other drugs which may also play a role in erectile dysfunction in transplant patients are: HMG- CoA reductase inhibitors (lovastatin, simvastatin), antidepressant (serotonin reuptake inhibitors, tricyclics, monoamine oxidase inhibitors) and H2 antagonists (cimetidine, ranitidine, famotidine).

Ketoconazole which is used in some transplant centers in order to increase cyclosporine level and reducing the cost of calcineurin inhibitors can cause erectile dysfunction because of its antiandrogenic action.
Additional factors such as smoking and alcohol intake may account for failure of male sexual function to improve after transplantation.
Cigarette smoking may induce vasoconstriction and penile venous leakage because of its contractile effect on the cavernous smooth muscle (Juenemann 1987). Alcohol in small amounts improves erection and increases libido because of its vasodilatory effect and the suppression of anxiety; however, large amounts can cause central sedation, decreased libido, and transient erectile dysfunction. Chronic alcoholism may cause hypogonadism and polyneuropathy, which may affect penile nerve function (Miller 1988).
Autonomic neuropathy may impair erectile function, and interruption of both hypogastric arteries may occasionally impair vascular supply.

2.4.2 Management of erectile dysfunction in transplant patients

Male patients should be asked about their sexual function and referred for urologic evaluation when necessary. Historically, androgens were touted as enhancing male sexual function. Today, more effective treatments are available, and testosterone therapy should be discouraged in men in whom erectile dysfunction is not associated with hypogonadism (Lue T F 2000). Sildenafil is a selective inhibitor of phosphodiesterase type 5, which inactivates cyclic GMP. Since its release in March 1998, it has become the drug of choice for most men with erectile dysfunction. When sexual stimulation releases nitric oxide into the penile smooth muscle, inhibition of phosphodiesterase type 5 by sildenafil causes a marked elevation of cyclic GMP concentrations in the glans penis, corpus cavernosum, and corpus spongiosum, resulting in increased smooth-muscle relaxation and better erection. Sildenafil has no effect on the penis in the absence of sexual stimulation, when the concentrations of nitric oxide and cyclic GMP are low (Lue T F 2000). Sildenafil has little effect on libido. Among more than 3700 men with 1631 patient years of exposure to sildenafil, most adverse events were mild to moderate and self-limited in duration (Esteban de la Rosa, Bravo Soto et al. 2003). Among men taking 25 to 100 mg of sildenafil, 16 percent reported headache, 10 percent flushing, 7 percent dyspepsia, 4 percent nasal congestion, and 3 percent abnormal vision (described as a mild and transient color tinge or increased sensitivity to light). These rates were twice as high among men taking 100 mg of sildenafil as among men who were taking lower doses. The visual effect is probably related to inhibition of phosphodiesterase type 6 in the retina. No chronic visual impairment has been reported, and the incidence of visual side effects was similar in diabetic and nondiabetic men (Price 1998). Nevertheless, because of the short duration of the clinical trials and the difficulty in detecting subtle retinal changes, the long-term safety of sildenafil treatment is still unknown. In men with retinal diseases, an ophthalmologic consultation may be warranted before sildenafil treatment is initiated. Adverse cardiovascular events (nasal congestion, headache, and flushing) were mild and transient in the majority of men. The rate of serious cardiovascular events (angina and coronary-artery disorder) is low. Sexual activity was thought to be a likely contributor to myocardial infarction in only 0.9 percent of 858 men in one study (Muller, Munder et al. 2009). Thus, the absolute increase in risk caused by sexual activity is low (one chance in a million for a healthy man). According to data from the National Center for Health Statistics and the Framingham Heart Study, the rate of death from myocardial infarction or stroke for men in the age range in which erectile dysfunction is common is approximately 170 per million men per week. Therefore, it appears that sildenafil therapy is safe for most men. Nevertheless, given that most of the men who died had underlying cardiovascular disease; cardiovascular status should be carefully assessed before treatment. The combination of nitrates and sildenafil has resulted in severe hypotension and 16 deaths in the United States. Therefore, nitrate therapy is an absolute contraindication to sildenafil therapy (Lue T F 2000).

Sildenafil is absorbed well during fasting, and the plasma concentrations are maximal within 30 to 120 minutes (mean, 60). It is eliminated predominantly by hepatic metabolism, and the terminal half-life is about four hours. The recommended starting dose is 50 mg taken one hour before sexual activity. The maximal recommended frequency is once per day. On the basis of effectiveness and side effects, the dose may be increased to 100 mg or decreased to 25 mg (Lue T F 2000). There is no specific contraindication to use of sildenafil (Viagra) in transplant patients so long as standard precautions are taken regarding concomitant coronary artery disease.

Oral vardenafil (Phosphodiesterase-5 Enzyme Inhibitor) therapy has a high efficacy and a low incidence of adverse events for kidney transplant recipients with ED (Yang, Ju et al. 2008). Vardenafil enhances the effect of NO by inhibiting phosphodiesterase type 5 (PDE-5), which is responsible for degradation of cGMP in the corpus cavernosum; when sexual stimulation causes local release of NO, inhibition of PDE-5 by vardenafil causes increased levels of cGMP in the corpus cavernosum, resulting in smooth muscle relaxation and inflow of blood to the corpus cavernosum. so it can prolong erectile duration of ED patients (Wang and Huang 2009); at recommended doses, it has no effect in the absence of sexual stimulation.

Transurethral administration of alprostadil (synthetic form of prostaglandin E_1) or intracavernous injection resulting in an erection sufficient for intercourse has been used successfully. The most effective intracavernous therapy used is a three-drug mixture containing papaverine, phentolamine, and alprostadil (trimix). The usual dose of trimix solution ranges from 0.1 to 0.5 ml. The rate of response to this solution is as high as 90 percent (Bennett 1991). In case of drug treatment failure, penile prosthesis can be considered even in transplanted patients (Lasaponara, Pasquale et al. 2009; Phe, Roupret et al. 2009).

3. Female reproduction

3.1 Menstrual cycle

The menstrual cycle is a hormonally controlled process of events occurring through the hypothalamic-pituitary-ovarian axis and reflected by the histological changes in the endometrium.

The normal menstrual cycle is a tightly coordinated cycle of stimulatory and inhibitory effects that results in the release of a single mature oocyte from a pool of hundreds of thousands of primordial oocytes.

The menstrual cycle lasts 25 to 30 days in most women. It is divided into two successive phases: the follicular phase and the luteal phase. By convention, the day of menstruation is designated as day 1 of the menstrual cycle. The luteal phase is remarkably constant in length and lasts 13 to 15 days, but length of the follicular phase is variable. The average duration of flow is 4 to 6 days but can be as few as 2 days and as many as 7 days. A flow of longer than 7 days deserves evaluation (Higham 1990).The average blood loss during one menses is about 30 mL. A flow of 80 mL or more can lead to anemia and should be evaluated (Cohen and Galbraith 2001). However, it is not necessary to measure menstrual flow; a patient's perception of abnormal menses deserves evaluation and treatment.

By definition menorrhagia is excessive and prolonged uterine bleeding at regular intervals; metrorrhagia is irregular, intermenstrual bleeding. Menometrorrhagia is heavy, prolonged, irregular bleeding at frequent, irregular intervals. Polymenorrhea is frequent, regular episodes of uterine bleeding at intervals of less than 21 days. Oligomenorrhea is irregular bleeding occurring at prolonged intervals of more than 35 days. Amenorrhea is absence of uterine bleeding (Sciarra J 2001).

There is relatively little cycle variability among women between the ages of 20 and 40 years. In comparison, there is significantly more cycle variability for the first 5 to 7 years after menarche and for the last 10 years before cessation of menses (Treloar 1967).

3.2 Menstrual cycle irregularities in end stage renal disease

Menstrual problem is common among women with renal insufficiency. It is partly because of abnormal bleeding time due to platelet dysfunction and also because of failure to ovulate or sustain adequate corpus luteum function.

Amenorrhea is common by the time the patient reaches end-stage renal disease. The menstrual cycle typically remains irregular with scanty flow after the initiation of maintenance dialysis, although normal menses are restored in some women(Holley 1997) In others, menorrhagia develops, sometimes leading to significant blood loss and increased transfusion requirements.

Oligo/ anovulation is the major factor for these menstrual cycle abnormalities in uremic women. Uremia is associated with hypothalamic-pituitary-gonadal dysfunction.

Leptin is one of the responsible factors involving in this cycle abnormality. In general, serum leptin levels are significantly elevated in patients with renal failure, particularly when compared to age and body mass index (BMI)-matched controls (Wolf 2002). Leptin appears to be one of several factors that influence the maturation of the gonadotropin-releasing hormone (GnRH) pulse generator.

Hyperprolactinemia is common in women with chronic renal failure due to increased secretion and decreased metabolic clearance of this hormone (Sievertsen 1980). The elevated prolactin levels may impair hypothalamic-pituitary function and contribute to sexual dysfunction and galactorrhea in these patients. Although kidney transplantation greatly improves menstrual pattern, but irregular bleeding is still a major problem among women with a transplanted kidney. In a study on 114 women with a transplanted kidney we found normal menstruation in 49%, oligo/ hypomenorrhea or amenorrhea in 31.3% and hypermenorrhea in 19.8% (Lessan-Pezeshki, Ghazizadeh et al. 2004).

In order to reduce the chance of endometrial hyperplasia that results from chronic stimulation of the endometrium with estradiol, medroxyprogesterone acetate (Provera), 10 mg/day orally for 5 days is prescribed. Patients with adequate endogenous estrogens will bleed within 3 to 5 days after medication, indicating adequate endogenous estrogen stimulation of the endometrium. Patients with relatively low levels of endogenous estrogens may have a limited response to the progesterone challenge.

3.3 Sexual dysfunction in uremic women

Sexual desire or drive is defined as the frequency or intensity with which a person desires to participate in sexual activity. Both organic and psychological variables contribute to this interest. Hormones can act on sexual behavior indirectly by influencing general mood. They can influence sexual interest levels by their peripheral action, such as by increasing genital vasocongestion and sexual sensation or by enhancing the sexual attractiveness of the female by means of smell. Women receiving chronic dialysis tend to experience decreased libido and reduced ability to reach orgasm.

Uremic patient's sexual difficulties are often worsened by hemodialysis, with a lowered frequency of intercourse, reduced sexual desire, and an increased incidence of sexual failure (Thurm JA 1976). Initial treatment goals for uremic women with sexual dysfunction include increasing the adequacy of dialysis, and correcting the anemia of chronic renal failure.

Amenorrheic dialysis patients may have low estradiol levels; this may lead to vaginal atrophy and dryness, thereby resulting in discomfort during intercourse. Such patients may benefit from local estrogen therapy or vaginal lubricants. Successful transplantation is clearly the most effective means to restore normal sexual desire in women with chronic renal failure (Diemont 2000). Sexual desire increases significantly after successful transplantation in most patients, however improvement in frequency of sexual activity and overall sexual satisfaction is not as high as sexual desire.

Low dose testosterone may be effective but, due to potential toxicity, is rarely used. The administration of bromocriptine may help restore sexual function in those with hyperprolactinemia.

3.4 Pregnancy in end stage renal disease

Fertility is reduced in the presence of end-stage renal disease. Conception is rare for women on dialysis, and occurs at a rate of one in every 200 patients (Rizzoni, Ehrich et al. 1992). Pregnancy is often diagnosed late because of menstrual irregularities; thus, early spontaneous abortion may be overlooked. The diagnosis of pregnancy may be difficult in women with end-stage renal disease; particularly because serum levels of beta-human chorionic gonadotropin (beta-hCG) may be increased in the absence of pregnancy. The main risks for a fetus include death, prematurity, and growth retardation. A review by Hou of 37 pregnancies associated with chronic renal dialysis found that 75% to 80% resulted in spontaneous abortion, stillbirth, or neonatal death. (Hou S 1987) Placental abnormalities included abruption, infarction, and microscopic areas of necrosis. No developmental abnormalities were reported, and the incidence of congenital abnormalities appeared to be no greater than for normal pregnancies.

Hypertension is a major problem and may prove very difficult to control. Forty-nine percent of the patients reviewed by Hou became hypertensive during pregnancy. The infants of hepatitis carriers should receive hepatitis B immune globulin and vaccine in the first 72 hours to avoid becoming carriers.

Since 1976, chronic ambulatory peritoneal dialysis (CAPD) has been increasingly used to manage end-stage renal failure. It has several theoretical advantages over hemodialysis for the management of pregnant patients (Mahanty, Cherikh et al. 2001). A more constant intrauterine environment without rapid shifts in fluid, solutes, and electrolytes may benefit a fetus, Redrow compared eight pregnancies managed with peritoneal dialysis with seven managed with hemodialysis (Redrow 1988). Hypotensive episodes appear to be less frequent, hematocrits higher, and control of insulin and glucose levels more exact in the group on peritoneal dialysis. Further experience is needed to determine if this is the preferred mode of dialysis in pregnancy. If peritoneal dialysis is used, the exchange volumes should be decreased (eg, to 1.5 liters) and the frequency should be increased (Jungers and Chauveau 1997).

3.4.1 Management

An increased dose of dialysis appears to be beneficial, with reports of Kt/V values of 6 to 8, on hemodialysis 5-6 days per week (Henrich WL 2004), with the BUN being maintained at under 50 mg/dL or even under 45 mg/dL. Ameliorating the uremic milieu can avoid polyhydramnios, help control hypertension, and improve maternal nutrition. Increased doses of erythropoietin are required to maintain hemoglobin levels in an acceptable range (10 to 11 g/dl) and transfusions are sometimes required (Chao 2002). Protein intake should be 1 g/kg per day plus an additional 20 g/day for fetal growth. Diet should be supplemented with water soluble vitamins and zinc. Metabolic acidosis and hypocalcemia should be corrected. Careful uterine and fetal monitoring during hemodialysis, such as assessment of the fetal heart rate (particularly during the last portion of a session), combined with measures aimed at preventing dialysis-induced hypotension should be performed. In many cases, patients are hospitalized around week 20 of gestation for management of blood pressure, dialysis fluid balance, nutrition and anemia.

If peritoneal dialysis is used, the exchange volumes should be decreased (eg, to 1.5 liters) and the frequency should be increased.

3.5 Pregnancy in renal transplantation

Fertility is usually restored in women with renal transplants and pregnancy is common, occurring in 12% of women at childbearing age in one series (Sturgiss and Davison 1995). Pregnancy success rate exceeds 90% after the first trimester. The recovery of fertility is less common in women who undergo transplantation close to the end of their childbearing years (Hou S 1987). The first reported successful pregnancy occurred in a recipient of a kidney transplant from an identical twin sister performed in 1958 (Murray 1963). Since then, there have been hundreds of successful pregnancies reported in renal transplant recipients (Davison JM 1987). During the last decade there has been a steady increase in the number of pregnancies following renal transplantation (Sgro, Barozzino et al. 2002).

Pregnancy in transplant recipients provides an opportunity to investigate biological processes that may have an impact on graft outcome as well as pregnancy outcome. For example, immunologic adjustments are believed to be involved in implantation as well as a successful acceptance of the allogenic fetus by their mother (Matthew RW 2005).

3.5.1 Effect of pregnancy on graft function

Although pregnancy can cause an increase in the glomerular filtration rate, which could theoretically lead to hyperfiltration and resultant glomerulosclerosis, the hyperfiltration of pregnancy is flow related, with no concomitant increase in intraglomerular pressure (Denton and Baylis 2007).

In cyclosporine treated patients, graft dysfunction after pregnancy was seen in patients with higher mean serum creatinine levels and lower mean cyclosporine doses prior to conception (ArmentiVT, Radomski JS et al. 2000). Overall, in the majority of recipients studied, pregnancy does not appear to cause excessive or irreversible problems with graft function if the function of transplant organ is stable prior to pregnancy (Armenti, Constantinescu et al. 2008).

The long-term effect of pregnancy on renal function is less clear. Two small studies in which matched nonpregnant controls were used found conflicting results: no deleterious effect in one with 15 year follow-up; and an increase in the plasma creatinine concentration of 0.5 to

0.7 mg/dL at 3 to 12 months in the other (Salmela, Kyllonen et al. 1993; Sturgiss and Davison 1995). The latter report also suggested that a second pregnancy might carry a greater risk, as renal function deteriorated in three of seven women (Salmela, Kyllonen et al. 1993).

The incidence of acute rejection is not greater than expected for non-pregnant transplant patients. The incidence of acute rejection during pregnancy and three months after delivery varies between 9 and 14.5% in the published series. Rejection is sometimes difficult to diagnose and an ultrasound-guided biopsy may be helpful to diagnose acute pyelonephritis, recurrent glomerulonephritis, and severe pre-eclampsia. Renal biopsy should be performed before starting anti-rejection therapy, and high steroid doses are the first line of treatment. It has been suggested that acute rejection during the puerperium may be due to a return to a normal immune status or to a rebound effect from the altered gestational immune responsiveness. Therefore, immunosuppression should be re-adjusted immediately after delivery.

3.6 Immunosuppressive drugs in pregnancy

Immunosuppression in pregnancy is a concern from the perspective of both maternal and fetal safety issues. Blood volume and volume of distribution increase during pregnancy thus blood levels of immunosuppressive drugs are often lower, though there is no evidence that effective immunosuppression is inadequate if prepregnancy doses are used. We currently have limited information regarding the toxicities and teratogenic potentials of these agents, although our knowledge has recently increased as more women maintained on immunosuppressive therapy for solid organ transplants have opted to become pregnant.

3.6.1 Glucocorticoids

The most commonly used glucocorticoids are the short acting agents; prednisone, prednisolone and methyl prednisolone. Radiolabaled prednisone and prednisolone can cross the placenta, but maternal / cord blood ratios are approximately 10:1 (Beitins 1972). In utero exposure to high-dose steroid and immunosuppressive agents does not seem to be associated with an increased incidence of congenital anomalies in the offspring of pregnant women with a renal transplant. Adrenal insufficiency and thymic hypoplasia have occasionally been described in the infants of transplant recipients, but these problems are unlikely if the dose of prednisone has been decreased to 15 mg . Cases of cleft palate, mental retardation, have also been described in humans after in utero corticosteroid exposure. Glucocorticoid therapy during pregnancy can result in premature rupture of the membranes (PROM) and intrauterine growth restriction. The increased risk of PROM with prednisone therapy likely reflects the inhibitory effects of glucocorticoids on fetal membrane extracellular matrix synthesis. Alternatively, PROM may be the result of prednisone's stimulatory effects on fetal membrane, placental, and decidual corticotropin releasing hormone. Furthermore, pregnancy-induced hypertension, gestational diabetes, and osteoporosis can be exacerbated.

Doses of prednisone greater than 20 mg/d have been associated with serious maternal infection, however treatment of rejection with steroids, if necessary, should not be avoided during pregnancy (Lessan-Pezeshki M 2002).

Current data suggest that steroids and immunosuppressive agents in the doses used to prevent graft rejection in transplant recipients are well tolerated by the fetus. Long-term

studies are required to determine whether there may be other effects, particularly an increase in the incidence of malignancies or abnormalities in the subsequent generation.
FDA rates the risk of prednisone use in pregnancy as C which implies that "Risks can not be ruled out".

3.6.2 Azathioprine

Azathioprine is an antimetabolite, an imidazole derivative of 6- mercaptopurine . It is commonly used during pregnancy in transplant recipients. Radioactive labeling studies in humans have shown that 64 - 93 percent of azathioprine administered to mothers appears in fetal blood as inactive metabolites (Sarikoski 1973). Azathioprine can cause transient gaps or breaks in lymphocyte chromosomes. Germ cells and other tissues have not been studied. In the adult, azathioprine is metabolized to 6- mercaptopurine. The immature fetal liver lacks the enzyme inosinate pyrophosphorylase, needed for conversion, and the fetus is relatively protected from the effects of the drug (Lessan-Pezeshki M 2002). The desired drug dose of azathioprin is 2 mg/kg/day or less. In high doses (6 mg/kg), azathioprine is teratogenic in animals. In human studies low birth weights, prematurity, jaundice, respiratory distress syndrome and aspiration have been reported in kidney transplant recipients. Azathioprine has been associated with a dose related myelosuppression in the fetus, but leukopenia is not usually a problem in the neonate if the maternal white blood count is maintained at greater than 7500 /mm3 (Armenti, Constantinescu et al. 2008).
FDA rated azathioprine use during pregnancy as D which implies that "positive evidence of risk exists but potential benefit may outweigh the risk"

3.6.3 Cyclosporine

Cyclosporine is a small cyclic polypeptide of fungal origin that inhibits calcineurin. There is little or no transplacental passage of cyclosporine in rodents (Safwenberg, Backman-Bave et al. 1977). In comparison, there are conflicting reports on the transfer of cyclosporine across the human placenta. Studies in pregnant rats have generally shown no effect of cyclosporine on organogenesis, although some renal proximal tubular cell damage can occur (Bailie, Elder et al. 2007). Human data showed that administration of cyclosporine was associated with low birth weights and a higher incidence of maternal diabetes, hypertension and renal allograft dysfunction. Cyclosporine metabolism appears to be increased during pregnancy and higher doses may be required to maintain plasma levels in the therapeutic range (Murirhead 1992). In women several years post-transplant with stable renal function, the pre-pregnancy dose can be continued. Some of the pregnancies in cyclosporine- treated women were complicated by preeclampsia. Cyclosporine increases production of thromboxane and endothelin, which have both been implicated in the pathogenesis of preeclampsia. Because of this, some physicians have suggested that the dose be limited to 2 to 4 mg/kg per day (Lindheimer Md and 1992).
Although the safety of cyclosporine is not well established in pregnancy, but it does not appear to be a major teratogen, as suggested by the results of a meta-analysis of 15 studies (Bar Oz 2001).
FDA rates the risk of cyclosporine use in pregnancy as C.

3.6.4 Tacrolimus

Tacrolimus is another calcineurin inhibitor. Experience with tacrolimus in pregnancy is limited. Among 100 pregnancies in 84 women treated with tacrolimus, of whom 27 percent

were renal transplant recipients, 68 progressed to a live birth, with 60 percent of deliveries being premature (Kaniz and 2000). It has been associated with neonatal hyperkalemia. As with cyclosporine, patients taking tacrolimus require frequent monitoring of renal function and drug levels. During pregnancy, the hepatic cytochrome p450 enzymes may be inhibited, which can lead to increased serum level of tacrolimus. The dose may therefore have to be significantly reduced to prevent toxicity (sometimes as much as 60 %) (Lessan-Pezeshki M 2002).
FDA rates the risk of tacrolimus use in pregnancy as C.

3.6.5 Mycophenolate Mofetil (MMF)

MMF is a selective antimetabolite which impairs lymphocyte function by blocking purine biosynthesis via inhibition of the enzyme inosine monophosphate dehydrogenase. Mycophenolate was developed as a replacement for azathioprine for maintenance immunosuppression. It is not nephrotoxic, and has less bone marrow toxicity than azathioprine.
MMF has been reported to cause head and eye malformations in the offspring of rat. Reported experience in human pregnancy with MMF is limited. There have been birth defects in few cases, but current data are insufficient to determine incidence of specific malformation. Among the 14 MMF-exposed offspring that has been reported, the underlying maternal conditions were kidney transplantation (N=7), lupus nephritis (N=4), liver transplantation, heart transplantation, and recurrent erythema multiforme. All were exposed in early pregnancy. The most distinctive malformation was moderate-to-severe microtia or anotia in 12, with external auditory canal atresia in 9. Other common craniofacial malformations and minor anomalies included orofacial clefts, hypertelorism, coloboma, and micrognathia. Six had cardiovascular malformations, of which three were either conotruncal or aortic arch defects (Anderka, Lin et al. 2009).
The manufacturer of MMF recommends that women of child-bearing age should have a negative pregnancy test prior to the initiation of therapy. We currently recommend that allograft recipients who wish to conceive should change from MMF to azathioprine, if there are no contraindications to the switch. MMF should be stopped 6 weeks prior to conception.
FDA rates the risk of MMF use in pregnancy as D.

3.6.6 Sirolimus

Sirolimus is a macrolide antibiotic compound that is structurally related to tacrolimus. Following entry into the cytoplasm, sirolimus binds to the FK binding protein and presumably modulates the activity of the mammalian target of rapamycin (mTOR). The mTOR inhibits interleukin-2 mediated signal transduction, resulting in cell cycle arrest in the G1-S phase (Danovitch GM 2005). It causes delayed ossification in animal reproductive studies, and its use is contraindicated in human until more data are available. Its use should also be discontinued at least 6 weeks prior to attempted conception.
In general, we recommend that women post-transplant who wish to conceive be switched prior to conception from sirolimus to cyclosporine. Upon delivery, it is recommended to switch the mother back to her basal immunosuppression in view of the potential benefits of the newer agents to prevent late acute rejection and chronic allograft nephropathy.

FDA rates the risk of sirolimus use in pregnancy as C.

3.6.7 OKT3 and polyclonal antibodies

OKT3 is a mouse antibody licensed for antirejection therapy, being directed against the CD3 antigen that is closely associated with the T cell receptor. It crosses the placenta. The National Transplantation Pregnancy Registry (NTPR) has reported the treatment of five women with OKT3 during pregnancy, with four surviving infants (Eisenberg 1997). The effect of polyclonal antibodies on the developing fetus is not known, but the IgG component would be expected to cross the placenta.

3.6.8 Intravenous Immune Globulins (IVIG)

Pooled human gamma-globulin preparations which were initially developed for the treatment of humoral immune deficiency disorders, proving to be invaluable in certain defined situations in clinical transplantation when used alone or in combination with plasmapheresis, such as antibody mediated rejection (Danovitch GM 2005). IgG is selectively transported across the placenta and the amount transferred increases with gestational age and dose. No cases of human deficiency virus (HIV) transmission have been reported with the use of IVIG, but adverse effects include thrombosis, alopecia, liver function disturbances, transient neutropenia, chills, nausea, flushing, tightness of chest and anaphylactic reaction in those with IgA antibodies.

There is little information regarding the teratogenicity of IVIG in animals. One report showed that IVIG was well tolerated in pregnant mice with induced antiphospholipid antibody syndrome (Bakimer 1993). In humans, IVIG appears to cross the placenta after 32 weeks of gestation, even after modification that alters the Fc binding sites (Hockel 1986). There have been no reports of fetal malformations in humans. However, IVIG is not completely benign, since hemolytic disease of the newborn and transmission of hepatitis C has been reported in selected cases.

3.6.9 Leflunomide

Leflunomide is an antimetabolite with both immunosuppressive and antiviral activities. It has been used successfully in the treatment of polyoma virus nephropathy (Danovitch GM 2005). It has marked teratogenic properties.

FDA rates its use during pregnancy as X. This medication should not be used during pregnancy or breast feeding.

3.7 Management of pregnancy in kidney transplant patient's guidelines:

All women of childbearing age should be counseled concerning the possibility and risks of pregnancy after kidney transplantation. Women who are not rubella immune should receive the rubella vaccine before transplantation, because live virus vaccines are contraindicated post transplantation (Hou S and 1999). Women are usually advised to wait at least one year after living related donor transplantation and two years after cadaveric renal transplantation (Lessan-Pezeshki M 2002). However, waiting 5 or more years may result in impaired renal function post partum that fails to recover, because of gradually deteriorating renal function secondary to chronic allograft nephropathy.

Criteria that should be ideally met before conception are shown in table 1.

At least 1 year post transplantation
Stable renal function with creatinine< 1.5 mg/dl
No recent episodes of acute rejection
BP ≤ 140/90 mmHg on medications
Proteinuria <500 mg/ day
Prednisone ≤ 15 mg/day
Azathioprine ≤ 2 mg /kg/day
Cyclosporine 2- 4 mg/ kg/ day
Normal allograft ultrasound

Table 1. Criteria for transplant recipients contemplating pregnancy

3.7.1 Management of preeclampsia and chronic hypertension

Preeclampsia is the most common complication, affecting 30% of pregnancies in renal transplant recipients, especially those with pre-transplant hypertension. Women with mild to moderate hypertension should be watched closely, warned about signs of early superimposed preeclampsia.

In transplant recipients, changes in urinary protein excretion, plasma uric acid, platelet count, or liver function tests seem to be less useful as markers of preeclampsia than in the normal population. Blood pressure, renal function, proteinuria and weight should be monitored every 2-4 weeks, with more attention during the third trimester. Anti-hypertensive agents should be changed to those tolerated during pregnancy.

3.7.2 Antihypertensive drugs used in pregnancy

Safety and efficacy of Alpha Methyldopa are supported in several randomized trials and in 7.5 years follow up study of children born to treated mothers.

Beta Blockers; especially Atenolol and Metoprolol, appear to be safe and efficacious in late pregnancy; but fetal growth retardation has been noted when treatment was started in early or midgestation (Lindheimer MD.Davison JM 2001).

Hydralazine is safe and used frequently as adjunctive therapy with α methyldopa and β blockers.

Calcium Channel Blockers such as Nifedipine, Nicardipine and Verapamile have been used in severe hypertension. They do not appear to be associated with any increase in congenital anomalies when used in the first trimester.

Calcium channel blockers may potentiate the hypotensive effects and neuromuscular blockade of magnesium and the interaction should be kept in mind when the drugs are used in women with a possibility of developing preeclampsia (Dynder 1988).

Labetalol appears to be as effective as methyldopa, but there is little follow up information on children born to mothers treated with this drug.

The second and third trimester exposure to ACE inhibitors and AT1 antagonists may be associated with serious adverse fetal effects. Most of these problems have been disturbances of fetal and neonatal renal function, such as oligohydramnios, neonatal anuria, renal failure and death (Pryde 1993). The fetal outcome is generally good in women who present in early pregnancy while taking an ACE inhibitor if the drug is stopped.

Continued administration of an ACE inhibitor during pregnancy is contraindicated (Shotan 1994).

The use of thiazide diuretics has been approved in women with chronic hypertension if prescribed before gestation; however, the recommendation is against their use in preeclamptic women, who often manifest decreased intravascular volumes and poor placental perfusion.

3.7.3 Management of infection

Pregnancy is associated with suppression of the adaptive immune system. There is evidence that pregnant women in general are more susceptible to infection. Infection also is an important consideration in any patient receiving immunosuppressive drugs, including transplant patients.

3.7.3.1 Bacterial

Urinary tract infections are the most common bacterial infections and occur in up to 40% of pregnant transplant recipients, and are particularly common in patients who develop end-stage renal disease due to pyelonephritis. These women should have monthly screening urine cultures (Armenti, Constantinescu et al. 2008), if asymptomatic bacteriuria is present; the patient should be treated for 2 weeks and may be treated with suppressive doses of antibiotics for the rest of the pregnancy (Lessan-Pezeshki M 2002). If there is a need for invasive procedures such as fetal monitoring with scalp electrodes or intrauterine pressure monitoring, prophylactic antibiotics are recommended. Aseptic technique should be used for even minor surgery and steroid therapy augmented.

3.7.3.2 Viral

Cytomegalovirus (CMV) remains the most frequent cause of viral infection post transplantation, however if the patient waits the recommended time after transplantation to become pregnant, she has passed the peak time of risk for CMV infection.

Infection in the fetus can be diagnosed by culturing the amniotic fluid. Titers of anti-CMV IgG and IgM during pregnancy are recommended, Ganciclovir has caused birth defects in animals when administered at twice human dose (Hou S and 1999). Herpes Simplex Virus (HSV) infection before 20 weeks gestation is associated with an increased rate of abortion. A positive HSV cervical culture at term is an indication for cesarean section. This can minimize the risk for neonatal herpes. Acyclovir can be safely used in pregnancy (Andrew 1992).

Continuous exposure to CsA in utero seems to impair T-, B- and NK-cell development and function in neonates. This effect is prolonged throughout the first year of life. In addition, low levels of serum immunoglobulins occur at the same time. This leads to suggest a delayed administration of classical vaccinations (after the first 6 months of life) in view of the potential risks of both sub-optimal immunologic responses, and adverse events after the administration of live, attenuated vaccines in infants born from young female organ transplant recipients (Schen 2002).

An infant born to an HBSAg - positive mother should be given hepatitis B immunoglobulin within 12 hours of birth and HBV vaccine at another site within 48 hours followed by a booster injection at 1 and 6 month.

The combination of immunoglobulin and vaccine offers protection for more than 90% of infants.

Vertical transmission is believed to be low (<7%) with hepatitis C unless the patient is also infected with the human immunodeficiency virus (Lessan-Pezeshki M 2002).

3.7.4 Labor and delivery

The incidence of pre-term delivery is 50%, because of presence of preeclampsia, renal function deterioration, fetal distress, premature rupture of membrane and premature labor. Intrauterine uterine growth retardation showing small-for-age babies is present in 20% of pregnancies. In general, successful fetal outcome is related to better renal function at conception. Despite immunosuppressive therapy there is no increase of fetal abnormalities.

A transplanted kidney rarely obstructs labor, vaginal delivery is recommended in most transplant recipient women. Cesarean section should be performed only for standard obstetric reasons. Delivery should occur in a specialized centre. Care must be taken to avoid fluid overload and infection. At the time of delivery, instrumentation should be minimized. Patients with renal insufficiency may be particularly at risk for water retention secondary to oxytocin (Lessan-Pezeshki M 2002).

In the perinatal period, the steroid dose should be augmented to cover the stress of labor and to prevent postpartum rejection. Hydrocortisone, 100 mg every 6 hours, should be given during labor and delivery. In the puerperium, renal function, proteinuria, blood pressure, cyclosporine/tacrolimus blood levels and fluid balance should be closely monitored.

3.7.5 Breastfeeding

Breastfeeding is discouraged for patients taking any immunosuppressive drugs. Cyclosporine measurement in maternal blood and breast milk revealed a mean breast milk/ maternal blood level ratio of 84% (Munoz-Flores- thiagarajan and 2001).

Azathioprine is also appears in breast milk, these levels can be toxic to a newborn, and nursing is not recommended. Similar recommendations exist for tacrolimus or any other immunosuppressive agents.

In summary, Because the outcome of pregnancy in transplantation are so different than those in chronic dialysis, it is advisable to treat end-stage renal disease patients with transplantation and wait until renal function has been stable for 1 to 2 years before undertaking a planned pregnancy. Such planned pregnancies offer the mother and fetus the best chance of favorable outcome. Before any woman with a renal transplant embarks on a pregnancy, she should be counseled by an obstetrician and transplant physician. Pregnancy appears to have no significant effect on graft function or survival; however, an important concern is that a mother may not survive to bring up the child that she bears. (Davison JM 1987)

3.8 Contraception for transplant patients:

Most female transplant recipients are unaware that transplantation has reversed the relative infertility associated with end-stage renal disease. The incidence of unwanted pregnancy among female kidney transplant recipients is significantly higher than general population. An unplanned pregnancy puts this special group at higher risk; either an induced abortion or continuing the pregnancy without a preconceptional evaluation could be harmful (Lessan-Pezeshki and 2004). Outcomes for unwanted pregnancies are inferior to outcomes for planned pregnancies, so it is strongly advised that every sexually active transplant recipient attend a family-planning counseling session. Contraceptive counseling should be provided before transplantation surgery, because ovulatory cycles may begin within 1 to 2 months after transplantation in women with grafts that are functioning well. Women who do not desire pregnancy should be protected by an effective method of contraception. Surgical contraception (sterilization) should be considered for those who have completed their family. Tubal ligation can be performed at the time of transplantation surgery. Vasectomy is also an effective form of permanent contraception with little morbidity. The risk for infection may be increased with the use of an intrauterine device in immuno-compromised patients, and their efficacy decrease because of anti-inflammatory effects of immunosuppressive agents (Zerner J, Doil KL et al. 1981). New devices containing levonorgestrel are more effective than previous copper containing devices, with fewer side effects (Fong and Singh 1999).

Depot medroxyprogesterone acetate injection at three months interval is another effective method of contraception for these patients but return of fertility after discontinuation is not fast and loss of bone mineral density is a concern with its long-term use.

Although low dose estrogen progesterone oral contraceptive preparations are not contraindicated for transplant patients, but they should be used with caution because they may cause or aggravate hypertension or precipitate thromboembolism, especially in the context of cyclosporine immunosuppression. Calcineurin inhibitors levels should also be monitored soon after the contraceptive is started. Because of unfounded fear of using contraceptive pills, a significant number of kidney transplant recipients use less effective methods such as coitus interruptus. In our study on unwanted pregnancy we found that 92% of women with unwanted pregnancies were using coitus interruptus as the only method of contraception (Ghazizadeh 2005). Progestin-only pill is an option for women who have contraindication to use estrogen but their failure rate is higher than combined oral contraceptive pills. Barrier contraceptives such as male condom are the safest modality but depend on user compliance for efficacy. It provides some protection against sexually transmitted diseases. Patients should know about emergency contraception in case of a broken condom. Two tablets of 0.75 mg of Levonorgestrel pills are administered within 72 hours of unprotected intercourse. Considering the above mentioned issues, unplanned pregnancy should be avoided by proper use of effective contraception.

4. Conclusion

Chronic kidney disease affects reproductive and sexual functions in both sexes. Although adequate dialysis will improve this dysfunction to some extent, but successful kidney transplantation has a better impact on fertility and reproductive functions.

Reproductive success is a common, expected outcome for male and female recipients of kidney transplant. One of the most impressive aspects of successful renal transplantation in the young person is the ability of the male patient to father a child and the female patient to give birth to a healthy baby. There are, however, important maternal and fetal complications that need to be considered to provide optimal care to the mother and her infant.

5. References

Delano, B. (1989). "Improvements in quality of life following treatment with r-HuEPO in anemic hemodialysis patients." Am J Kidney Dis(14): 14.

Diemont, W., Vruggink, PA, Meuleman, EJ, et al. (2000). "Sexual dysfunction after renal replacement therapy." Am J Kidney Dis 35: 845.

Finkel, D., Phillips, JL, Snyder, PJ. (1985). "Stimulation of spermatogenesis by gonadotropins in men with hypogonadotropic hypogonadism." N Engl J Med(313): 651.

Grossman, E., Swan, SK, Muirhead, GJ, et al. (2004). "The pharmacokinetics and hemodynamics of sildenafil citrate in male hemodialysis patients." Kidney Int(66): 367.

Hockel, M., Kaufmann, R, (1986). "Placental transfer of class G immunoglobulins treated with B-propiolactone (P-PL) for intravenous application a case report." J Perinat Med 14: 205.

Holdsworth, S., Atkins, RC, de Kretser, DM. (1977). "The pituitary-testicular axis in men with chronic renal failure." N Engl J Med (296): 1245.

Holdsworth, S., de Kretser, DM, Atkins, RC (1978). " A comparison of hemodialysis and transplantation in reversing the uremic disturbance of male reproductive function." Clin Nephrol(10): 146.

Holley, J., Schmidt, RJ, Bender, FH, et al. (1997). "Gynecologic and reproductive issues in women on dialysis." Am J Kidney Dis 29: 685.

Ifudu, O. (1998). "Care of patients undergoing hemodialysis." N Engl J Med(339): 1054.

Levitan, D., Moser, SA, Goldstein, DA, et al. . . (1984). "Disturbances in the hypothalamic-pituitary-gonadal axis in male patients with acute renal failure." Am J Nephrol (4): 99.

Lim, V., Fang, VS. (1976). "Restoration of plasma testosterone levels in uremic men with clomiphene citrate." J Clin Endocrinol Metab(43): 1370.

Rosas, S., Joffe, M, Franklin, E, et al. (2003). "Association of decreased quality of life and erectile dysfunction in hemodialysis patients." Kidney Int(64): 232.

Sawin, C., Longcope, C, Schmitt, GW, Ryan, RJ. (1973). "Blood levels of gonadotropins and gonadal hormones in gynecomastia associated with chronic hemodialysis. ." J Clin Endocrinol Metab 36: 988.

Sievertsen, G., Lim, VS, Nakawatase, C, Frohman, LA, (1980). "Metabolic clearance and secretion rates of human prolactin in normal subjects and patients with chronic renal failure. ." J Clin Endocrinol Metab 50: 846.

Turk, S., Karalezli, G, Tonbul, HZ, et al. (2001). "Erectile dysfunction and the effects of sildenafil treatment in patients on haemodialysis and continuous ambulatory peritoneal dialysis." Nephrol Dial Transplant(16): 1818.

Wolf, G., Chen, S, Han, DC, Ziyadeh, FN, (2002). "Leptin and renal disease." Am J Kidney Dis 39: 1.

Anderka, M. T., A. E. Lin, et al. (2009). "Reviewing the evidence for mycophenolate mofetil as a new teratogen: case report and review of the literature." Am J Med Genet A 149A(6): 1241-8.

Andrew, E., Yankaskas, BC, Cordero, JF, Schoeffler, K, Hampp, S: (1992). "Acylovir in pregnancy registry: six years experience." Obstet Gynecol(79): 7-13.

Armenti, V. T., S. Constantinescu, et al. (2008). "Pregnancy after transplantation." Transplant Rev (Orlando) 22(4): 223-40.

ArmentiVT, Radomski JS, et al. (2000). "Report from the National Transplantation Pregnancy Registry(NTPR) outcome of pregnancy after transplantation." Clin Transpl 123-34.

Bailie, G. R., S. J. Elder, et al. (2007). "Sexual dysfunction in dialysis patients treated with antihypertensive or antidepressive medications: results from the DOPPS." Nephrol Dial Transplant 22(4): 1163-70.

Bakimer, R., Guilburd, B, Zurgil, N, Schoenfeld, Y, (1993). "The effect of intravenous gamma globulin on the induction of experimental antiphospholipid syndrome. ." Clin Immunol Immunopathol 69: 97.

Bar Oz, B., Hackman, R, Einarson, T, Koren, G, (2001). " Pregnancy outcome after cyclosporine therapy during pregnancy: a meta-analysis." Transplantation 71(8): 1051-5.

Beitins, I., Bayard, F, Ances, IG, et al. (1972). "The transplacental passage of prednisone and prednisolone in pregnancy near term." J Pediatr (81): 936.

Bennett, A., Carpenter, AJ, Barada, JH, (1991). "An improved vasoactive drug combination for a pharmacological erection program. ." J Urol 146 1564-5.

Berek, J. S. (2002). Novak's Gynecology, Lippincott Williams & Wilkins.

Biller BM; Molitch ME; Vance ML; Cannistraro KB; Davis KR; Simons JA; Schoenfelder JR; Klibanski A (1996). "Treatment of prolactin-secreting macroadenomas with the once-weekly dopamine agonist cabergoline." J Clin Endocrinol Metab 81(6): 2338-43.

Chao, A., et al (2002). "Pregnancy in women who undergo longterm dialysis." Am J Obstet Gynecol 187: 152-156.

Cohen, D. and C. Galbraith (2001). "General health management and long-term care of the renal transplant recipient." Am J Kidney Dis 38(6 Suppl 6): S10-24.

Cowden, E., Ratcliff, WA, Ratcliff, JG, et al (1981). "Hypothalamic-Pituitary function in uremia." Acta Endocrinol 98: 488.

Danovitch GM (2005). Handbook of Kidney Transplantation, Lippincott Williams&Wilkins.

Davison JM (1987). "Renal transplantation and pregnancy. ." Am J Kidney Dis 9: 374.

De Celis, R. and N. Pedron-Nuevo (1999). "Male fertility of kidney transplant patients with one to ten years of evolution using a conventional immunosuppressive regimen." Arch Androl 42(1): 9-20.

de Vries, C., Gooren, LJG, Oe, PL. (1984). "Hemodialysis and testicular function." Int J Androl(7): 97.

Denton, K. and C. Baylis (2007). "Physiological and molecular mechanisms governing sexual dimorphism of kidney, cardiac, and vascular function." Am J Physiol Regul Integr Comp Physiol 292(2): R697-9.

Diemont, W., Vruggink, PA, Meuleman, EJ, et al. (2000). "Sexual dysfunction after renal replacement therapy." Am J Kidney Dis (35): 845.

Dynder, S., Cardwell, MS, (1988). "Neuromuscular blockade with magnesium sulfate and nifedipine." Am J Obstet Gynecol(161): 35-36.

Eid, M. M., I. A. Abdel-Hamid, et al. (1996). "Assessment of sperm motion characteristics in infertile renal transplant recipients using computerized analysis." Int J Androl 19(6): 338-44.

Eisenberg, J., Armenti, VT ,Mc Grovy, CH, et al (1997). "National transplantation pregnancy registry(NTPR) : Use of muromonab-CD3(OKT3) during pregnancy in female transplant recipients." Am Soc Transplant phys(20): 108.

Esteban de la Rosa, R. J., J. A. Bravo Soto, et al. (2003). "Influence of age, sex, and hepatitis C virus infection on peripheral blood lymphocyte subsets in stable kidney transplantation." Transplant Proc 35(8): 2905-7.

Fong, Y. F. and K. Singh (1999). "Effect of the levonorgestrel-releasing intrauterine system on uterine myomas in a renal transplant patient." Contraception 60(1): 51-3.

Ghazizadeh, S., Lessan-Pezeshki, M, Khatami, MR, Mahdavi, M, (2005). "Unwanted Pregnancy in Kidney Transplant Recipients in Iran." Transplantation Proceedings 37(7): 3085-3086.

Hagen C, O. K., McNeilly AS (1976). "Prolactin and the pituitary gonadal axisin male uremic patients on regular dialysis. ." Acta Endocrinol (Copenh)(82): 29.

Henrich WL (2004). Principles and Practice of Dialysis, Lippincott Williams&Wilkins.

Higham, J., O'Brien, PMS, Shaw, RM, (1990). "Assessment of menstrual blood loss using pictorial chart." Br J Obstet Gynaecol 97: 734.

Hou S (1987). " Pregnancy in women requiring dialysis for renal failure." Am J Kidney Dis 9 368.

Hou S and (1999). "Pregnancy in chronic renal insufficiency and end stage renal disease. ." Am J Kidney Dis (33): 235.

Issac, R., et al (1978). " Effect of parathyroid hormone on plasma prolactin men." (47): 18.

Juenemann, K.-P., Lue, TF, Luo, JA, Benowitz, NL, Abozeid, M, Tanagho, EA. (1987). "The effect of cigarette smoking on penile erection." J Urol 138 438-41.

Jungers, P. and D. Chauveau (1997). "Pregnancy in renal disease" Kidney Int 52: 871-885.

Kaczmarek, I., Groetzner, J, Adamidis, I, Landwehr, P, (2004). "Sirolimus impairs gonadal function in heart transplant recipients. ." Am J of Transplantation 4: 1084.

Kaniz, A., Harabacz, I, Cowirick, IS, et al. and (2000). "Review of the course and outcome of 100 pregnancies in 84 women treated with tacrolimus. ." Transplantation proceeding(70): 1718.

Lasaponara, F., G. Pasquale, et al. (2009). "[Penile prosthesis implantation in kidney-transplanted patients.]." Urologia 76(2): 95-97.

LeRoith, D., Danovitz, G, Trestian, S, Spitz, IM. (1980). "Dissociation of pituitary glycoprotein response to releasing hormones in chronic renal failure." Acta Endocrinol (Copenh)(93): 277.

Lessan-Pezeshki M (2002). "Pregnancy After Renal Transplantation, Points to Consider " Nephrol Dial Transplant 17: 703-707.

Lessan-Pezeshki, M., S. Ghazizadeh, et al. (2004). "Fertility and contraceptive issues after kidney transplantation in women." Transplant Proc 36(5): 1405-6.

Lessan-Pezeshki, M., Ghazizadeh, S, Khatami, M, R, Mahdavi, M, Razeghi, E, Seifi, S,Ahmadi, F, Maziar,S, and (2004). "Fertility and contraceptive issues after kidney transplantation in women " Transplantation proceeding (36): 1405-1406.

Lim, V., Kathpalia, SC, Henriques, C. (1978). "Endocrine abnormalities associated with chronic renal failure." Med Clin North Am 62:. 1341.

Lindheimer Md, K. A. and (1992). "Pregnancy in the renal transplant patients." Am J Kidney Dis (19): 173.

Lindheimer MD.Davison JM, K. A. (2001). "The kidney and hypertension in pregnancy: twenty exciting years." Semin Nephrol 21 (2): 173-189.

Lue T F (2000). "Erectile dysfunction." The New England Journal of Medicine 342(24): 1802, 12.

Mahanty, H. D., W. S. Cherikh, et al. (2001). "Influence of pretransplant pregnancy on survival of renal allografts from living donors." Transplantation 72(2): 228-32.

Matthew RW (2005). Medical Management of Kidney transplantation, Lippincott Williams & Wilkins.

Miller, N., Gold, MS. (1988). "The human sexual response and alcohol and drugs." J Subst Abuse Treat 5: 171-7.

Mirone, V., N. Longo, et al. (2009). "Renal transplantation does not improve erectile function in hemodialysed patients." Eur Urol 56(6): 1047-53.
Muller, I., M. Munder, et al. (2009). "Polymorphonuclear neutrophils and T lymphocytes: strange bedfellows or brothers in arms?" Trends Immunol 30(11): 522-30.
Munoz-Flores- thiagarajan, K., Easterling, T, Davis, C, Bond, EF. and (2001). " Breast-feeding by a cyclosporine- treated mother." Obstet Gynecol(97): 816 -8.
Murirhead, N., Sabharwal, AR, reider, MJ, et al (1992). "The outcome of pregnancy following renal transplantation- the experience of a single center." Transplantation proceeding(54): 429.
Murray, J., Reid, DE, Harrison, JH, et al (1963). "Successful pregnancies after human renal transplantation." N Engl J Med: 269:346.
Nevins, T. E. and D. L. Dunn (1992). "Use of ganciclovir for cytomegalovirus infection." J Am Soc Nephrol 2(12 Suppl): S270-3.
Olshan, A., Mattison, DR, Zwanenburg, TS, (1994). "International Commission for Protection against Environmental Mutagens and Carcinogens. Cyclosporine A: review of genotoxicity and potential for adverse human reproductive and developmental effects. Report of a working group on the genotoxicity of cyclosporine A,." Mutat Res 317: 163-173.
Palmer, B. (1999). "Sexual dysfunction in uremia." J Am Soc Nephrol (10): 1381.
Pece, S., et al , (1979). "Prolactin in chronic renal failure, hemodialysis and transplant patients " Proc Eur Dial Transplant Assoc (16): 700.
Phe, V., M. Roupret, et al. (2009). "[Erectile dysfunction and renal chronic insufficiency: etiology and management]." Prog Urol 19(1): 1-7.
Price, D., Gingell, JC, Gepi-Attee, S,Wareham, K, (1998). "Sildenafil: Study of a novel oral treatment for erectile dysfunction in diabetic men." Diabet Med 15: 821-5.
Procci, W., Goldstein, DA, Adelstein, J, (1981). "Sexual dysfunction in the male patient with uremia; a reappraisal." Kidney Int 19: 317.
Pryde, P., Sedman, AB, Nugent, CE, Barr, M Jr. (1993). "Angiotensin converting enzyme inhibitor fetopathy." J Am Soc Nephrol (3): 1575.
Ramirez, G., O`Neil, W, Jubiz, W, et al (1976). "Thyroid dysfunction in uremia: evidence for thyroid and hypophyseal abnormalities." Am Intern Med 84: 627.
Redrow, M., Cherem, L, Elliott, J, Mangalat, J, (1988). "Dialysis in the management of pregnant patients with renal insufficiency." Medicine 67(4): 199-208.
Rizzoni, G., J. H. Ehrich, et al. (1992). "Successful pregnancies in women on renal replacement therapy: report from the EDTA Registry." Nephrol Dial Transplant 7(4): 279-87.
Safwenberg, J., U. Backman-Bave, et al. (1977). "The effect of blood transfusions on cadaver kidney transplants--an analysis of patients transplanted in Uppsala." Scand J Urol Nephrol Suppl(42): 59-61.
Salmela, K. T., L. E. Kyllonen, et al. (1993). "Impaired renal function after pregnancy in renal transplant recipients." Transplantation 56(6): 1372-5.
Sarikoski, S., Seppala, M. (1973). " Immunosupression during pregnancy: transmission of azathioprine and its metabolites from the mother to the fetus." Am J Obstet Gynecol(115): 1100.
Schaefer, F., R. Stanhope, et al. (1989). "Pulsatile gonadotropin secretion in pubertal children with chronic renal failure." Acta Endocrinol (Copenh) 120(1): 14-9.

Schen, F., Stallone, G, Schena, A, Manfredi, G, Derosa, C, Procino, A, Di Paolo, S. (2002). "Pregnancy in renal transplantation: immunologic evaluation of neonates from mothers with transplanted kidney." Transpl Immunol 9(2-4): 161-4.
Schrier RW (2001). Diseases of the kidney and urinary tract, Lippincott Williams&Wilkins.
Sciarra J (2001). Gynecology &Obststrics, Lippincot Williams & Wilkins.
Seethalakshmi, L., Diamond, DA, Malhotra, RK, Mazanitis, SG, Kumar, S, Menon, M, (1988). "Cyclosporine induced testicular dysfunction: a separation of the nephrotoxic component and an assessment of a 60-day recovery period. ." Transplant Proc 20 (Suppl 3): 1005-1010.
Seethalakshmi, L., Flores, C, Carboni, AA, Bala, R, Diamond, DA, Menon, M, (1990). "Cyclosporine: its effect on testicular function and fertility in the prepubertal rat. ." J Androl 11: 17-24.
Seethalakshmi, L., Flores, C, Diamond, DA, Menon, M, (1990). "Reversal of the toxic effects of cyclosporineA (CsA) on male reproduction and kidney function of rats by simultaneous administration of hCG and FSH." J Urol 144: 1489-149.
Seibel, I., Poli De, Figueiredo CE, Teloken, C, Moraes, JF. (2002). "Efficacy of oral sildenafil in hemodialysis patients with erectile dysfunction." J Am Soc Nephrol (13): 2770.
Sgro, M. D., T. Barozzino, et al. (2002). "Pregnancy outcome post renal transplantation." Teratology 65(1): 5-9.
Shotan, A., Widerhorn, J, Hurst, A, Elkayam, U, (1994). "Risks of angiotensin converting enzyme inhibition during pregnancy: experimental and clinical evidence, potential mechanisms and recommendations for use." Am J Med(96): 451.
Steele, T., Wuerth, D, Finkelstein, S, et al. (1996). "Sexual experience of the chronic peritoneal dialysis patient." J Am Soc Nephrol(7): 1165.
Stewart-Bentley, M., Gans, D, Horton, R. (1974). "Regulation of gonadal function in uremia." Metabolism (23): 1065.
Sturgiss, S. N. and J. M. Davison (1995). "Effect of pregnancy on the long-term function of renal allografts: an update." Am J Kidney Dis 26(1): 54-6.
Thurm JA (1976). " Effect of chronic renal disease on sexual functioning." Med Asp Human Sex 10: 81.
Toorians, A. W., E. Janssen, et al. (1997). "Chronic renal failure and sexual functioning: clinical status versus objectively assessed sexual response." Nephrol Dial Transplant 12(12): 2654-63.
Treloar, A., Boynton, RE, Behn, BG, Brown, BW, Brown BW, (1967). "Variation of the human menstrual cycle through reproductive life." Int J Fertil 12: 77.
Wang, H. Y. and Y. F. Huang (2009). "Vardenafil for refractory erectile dysfunction: the latest advances." Zhonghua Nan Ke Xue 15(11): 1035-8.
Yang, J., W. Ju, et al. (2008). "Efficacy and safety of vardenafil for kidney transplant recipients with erectile dysfunction." Zhonghua Nan Ke Xue 14(10): 911-3.
Zerner J, Doil KL, et al. (1981). "Intrauterine contraceptive device failures in renal transplant patients." J Reprod Med. 26(2): 99-102.
Zuber, J., D. Anglicheau, et al. (2008). "Sirolimus may reduce fertility in male renal transplant recipients." Am J Transplant 8(7): 1471-9.

14

Management of Bone Disease in Kidney Transplant Recipients

Rubin Zhang and Brent Alper
Department of Medicine, Tulane University Health Sciences Center,
New Orleans, Louisiana
USA

1. Introduction

There are several types of bone disease that are commonly seen in kidney transplant recipients. These include pre-existing uremic osteodystrophy, osteopenia, osteoporosis, bone fracture, osteonecrosis and bone pain syndrome (Brandenburg et al., 2004; Cohen et al., 2004; Julian et al., 1991; Zisman and Sprague, 2006). Kidney transplant recipients are now living longer than ever, and thus, proper prevention and management of bone disease has become an increasingly important part of their long-term care. Complications from post-transplant bone disease not only cause significant morbidity, but also increase the cost of care, hospitalization, and mortality (Abbott et al., 2001; Duriex et al., 2002; Jeffrey et al., 2003; Vatour et al., 2004; Zhang et al., 2008).

Bone disease after kidney transplant is a multifactorial process that includes continuing bone loss superimposed on pre-existing renal osteodystrophy (Brandenburg et al., 2004; Cohen et al., 2004; Zisman & Sprague, 2006; Zhang et al., 2008). There can be several different bone histologies and no single clinical biomarker can distinguish between the various bone disorders (Cruz et al., 2004; Cueto-Manzano et al., 2003; Monier-Faugere et al., 2000; Rolla et al., 2006). Bone biopsy, the gold standard for diagnosis and most accurate tool to guide clinical management is not commonly undertaken due to its invasive nature and difficulty with proper interpretation. The clinical disease spectrum includes four distinct phases: 1) pre-transplant osteodystrophy, 2) post-transplant bone loss exacerbated by a number of factors including immunosuppressive medications, 3) late stabilization with a functioning allograft, and 4) a return to uremic osteodystrophy when the renal allograft fails. This chapter will review the complex pathophysiology of the various types of bone diseases after kidney transplantation and explore the current evidence for their prevention and treatment.

2. Pre-existing uremic osteodystrophy

There are several different types of pre-existing renal osteodystrophy that may be encountered in kidney transplant patients including osteitis fibrosa cystica, adynamic bone disease, osteomalacia, osteopenia or osteoporosis.

2.1 Osteitis fibrosa cystica

Persistent secondary or tertiary hyperparathyroidism (HPT), reported in up to 30-50% of renal transplant patients, can lead to osteitis fibrosa cystica, a form of high turnover bone disease (Heaf et al., 2003). High bone turnover is usually associated with cortical bone loss and weakening its mechanical function (Malluche et al., 2010). Bone biopsy characteristically shows increased bone resorption, extensive osteoclastic activity and endosteal fibrosis (Malluche et al., 1994). High serum calcium (Ca), high phosphorus (Phos), low active vitamin D, high parathyroid hormone (PTH), and elevated alkaline phosphatase (AP) and osteocalcin are common. Alkaline phosphatase and osteocalcin are secreted by osteoblasts and can serve as useful clinical markers of high bone turnover. The cornerstone of treatment aims to suppress PTH secretion by a variety of methods including dietary phosphate restriction and use of phosphate binders, the use of the calcimimetic agent, cinacalcet, or surgical parathyroidectomy (Block et al., 2004; Chertow et al., 2002; Eknoyan et al., 2003; Teng et al., 2003).

2.2 Adynamic bone disease

This condition is usually caused by over-suppression of PTH and other growth factors, including gonadal hormones, growth hormone, and insulin-like growth hormone-1 (Brandenburg et al., 2004; Eknoyan et al., 2003; Zisman & Sprague, 2006). Bone biopsy findings include a low bone formation rate as assessed by tetracycline fluorescence-labeling, little or no evidence of cellular activity, a paucity of osteoblasts and osteoclasts, and thin osteoid seams (Malluche et al., 1994). Low bone turnover is frequently associated with loss of cancellous bone and abnormal mineral metabolic activity. Inability to maintain mineral homeostasis may contribute to cardiovascular and soft tissue calcifications, which may explain the high mortality rate in patients with low bone turnover (Malluche et al., 2010). Patients may have a high serum Ca, a relatively low PTH and low AP levels. Groups at highest risk include the elderly, diabetics, patients previously on peritoneal dialysis, those on calcium-containing phosphate binders, and those with over-suppressed PTH by vitamin D analogues. The prevention and treatment of adynamic bone disease is avoidance of over suppression of PTH secretion (Eknoyan et al., 2003). Historically, excessive aluminum accumulation was a major cause of adynamic bone disease in ESRD patients before the strict water purification and the avoidance of aluminum-containing phosphate binders were adopted (Zhang et al., 2008).

2.3 Osteomalacia

Osteomalacia in post-transplant patients has numerous causes including a deficit in bone mineralization due to hypophosphatemia, malnutrition, vitamin D deficiency, or aluminum toxicity (Brandenburg et al., 2004; Eknoyan et al., 2003; Zisman & Sprague, 2006). Characteristic findings on bone biopsy include wide unmineralized osteoid seams, low bone formation, absence of osteoblasts and osteoclasts and endosteal fibrosis (Malluche et al., 1994). Patients may have low serum Ca and Phos levels but PTH and AP levels are frequently within normal limits or slightly high. The gold standard for the diagnosis of osteomalacia from aluminum toxicity is aluminum staining of the bone biopsy (Eknoyan et al., 2003; Malluche et al., 1994). However, a useful, noninvasive clinical test in patients suspected to have chronic aluminum toxicity is desferoxamine stimulation of aluminum release. Treatments are targeted toward the underlying causes and include Ca and vitamin

D supplementations. The treatment of osteomalacia from aluminum toxicity is desferoxamine administration or kidney transplantation (Malluche et al., 1984; Zhang et al., 2008).

2.4 Osteopenia and osteoporosis

These conditions are usually diagnosed by bone mineral density (BMD) measurement with dual energy X- ray absorptiometry. Many patients undergoing transplant already have low bone mineral density. Thus, it is not surprising that low BMD (osteopenia and osteoporosis) is very common in kidney transplant recipients (Braun et al., 1999; Gallego et al., 2006). Common risk factors include older age, female gender, Caucasian race, chronic disease, immobility and malnutrition. In addition, hypogonadism is very common, but not routinely screened for or treated among the ESRD population. Chronic metabolic acidosis and uremic osteodystrophy can also contribute to bone loss (Brandenburg et al., 2004; Eknoyan et al., 2003; Zisman & Sprague, 2006).

2.5 Other bone disease

Dialysis-related amyloidosis is caused by β_2 -microglobulin deposition as amyloid fibrils, leading to chronic inflammatory response, destructive arthropathy and lytic bone lesions. The articular symptoms associated with this disorder rapidly improve after renal transplantation. Although new cystic lesions are unusual, resolution of existing cysts is unusual (Zhang et al., 2008).

2.6 Clinical course

Patients often have a combination of the different type of bone diseases as described above, commonly termed mixed bone diseases. Due to the dynamic nature of renal osteodystrophy, it is not uncommon for one type of bone disease to evolve into another type of bone disease, depending on the clinical setting and management (Cohen et al., 2004; Eknoyan et al., 2003; Zisman & Sprague, 2006).

The nature and evolution of pre-existing renal osteodystrophy after kidney transplant has yet to be fully established, largely due to a lack of serial histological studies by bone biopsy in this population. Several small studies do provide some insight into this issue. In a histological study of 20 patients who had bone biopsies before and 6 months after kidney transplant were compared (Cruz et al., 2004). Five of the 12 patients with adynamic bone disease recovered completely and the remaining cases had some improvement. Five of 8 patients with high-turnover bone disease developed low-turnover bone disease (4 with adynamic bone disease, 1 with osteomalacia). In a long-term study of 57 patients followed for a mean of 5.6 years after kidney transplant, 56% of patients were demonstrated to have decreased cancellous bone volume, 46% of patients had low bone turnover, and 59.7% of patients had reduced bone formation indices. High bone turnover was rarely seen, despite the fact that 63% of patients had elevated serum creatinine levels (monier-Faugere et al., 2000). In another report of 25 patients at least 5 years after transplant with good renal allograft function, bone biopsy revealed mixed bone disease in 10 patients, adynamic bone in 7 patients, high turnover bone in 4 patients, and normal bone in 3 patients (Cueto-Manzano et al., 2003). These studies suggest that pre-transplant renal osteodystrophy may not resolve completely, but often persists or evolves into a different disease process, depending on the allograft function, PTH level, immunosuppressive medications, and clinical management.

3. Post-transplant bone loss

During the first 6 to 12 months after kidney transplant, there is a rapid bone loss. After this time period, patients may either continue to lose bone at a slower rate, stabilize, or improve BMD depending on numerous factors including medication usage, overall health, and renal function (Brandenburg et al., 2004; Julian et al., 1991; Zisman & Sprague et al., 2006). A recent study reported 66% of patients with functioning renal allografts have osteopenia or osteoporosis (Gallego et al., 2006). Even after 20 years of kidney transplantation, 31% of patients had osteopenia and 41 % had osteoporosis (Braun et al., 1999). In another study of 63 kidney transplant recipients underwent yearly BMD measurements of the lumbar spine between 3 and 68 months posttransplant, BMD was significantly lower compared with healthy controls at all times. BMD measurements revealed a biphasic pattern. Between 3 and 10 months, a significant decrease in lumbar BMD occurred. However, no further significant bone loss was noted after the first year, and BMD remained relatively stable but at significantly lower levels compared with healthy controls (Brandenburg et al., 2004).
The possible causes of bone loss after kidney transplant are numerous and usually multiple factors are present in each patient. These factors include pre-existing continued uremic osteodystrophy as discussed above, immunosuppressive drugs, persistent HPT, hypophosphatemia, poor allograft function, loop diuretics, acidosis, smoking, alcohol abuse, hypogonadism, aging, chronic disease, physical inactivity/immobilization, and poor nutrition (Cohen et al., 2004; Cunningham, 2005; Gallego et al., 2006; Zisman & Sprague, 2006).

3.1 Immunosuppressive drugs

Rapid bone loss is very common in the first several months after kidney transplant, primarily caused by steroid usage, either as a large dose of steroids prescribed as a part of induction therapy or for the treatment of acute rejection episodes. The predominant effect of glucocorticoids on the skeleton is that of reduced bone formation. The decline in bone formation may be due to direct inhibition of osteoblast proliferation and increased apoptosis of osteoblasts and mature osteocytes. Glucocorticoids also increase bone resorption by increasing osteoclastogenesis. In addition, glucocorticoids decrease secretion of androgens and estrogens, primarily mediated by inhibition of gonadotropin secretion, and increase secretion of PTH (Brandenburg et al., 2004; Braun et al., 1999; Cunningham, 2005; Monier-Faugere et al., 2000; Van den Ham et al., 2003). There is some evidence that cyclosporine may increase bone turnover in animal study (Epstein, 1996). However, the effect of cyclosporine on bone metabolism in humans is less clear, being confounded by the presence of other illnesses or drugs that affect bone, particularly glucocorticoids. Tacrolimus appears to have less adverse effect on bone than cyclosporine (Marcen et al., 2006). The effects of other immunosuppressive medicines such as mycophenolate mofetil and sirolimus on bone remodeling remain unknown. The use of potent antibody induction therapy and modern maintenance agents can promote steroid-free or steroid-minimization protocol, which may exert protective effect on bone.

3.2 Hyperparathyroidism and hypercalcemia.

Elevated PTH levels usually decline, initially rapidly, then slowly after kidney transplant. About 30% of patients may still have elevated PTH levels beyond 1 year despite the presence of normal renal function and vitamin D metabolism (Heaf et al., 2003). These patients likely have tertiary HPT due to the nodular transformation from a polyclonal hyperplasia into a monoclonal adenoma. The risk factors may include higher PTH level before transplant, longer time on dialysis and older age. Persistent HPT after transplant leads to continuing bone loss (Gallego et al., 2006; Heaf et al., 2003). A recent study of 201 transplant recipients reported a biphasic pattern of serum calcium levels with hypocalcemia immediately after kidney transplant and subsequent development of hypercalcemia (Evenepoel et al., 2009). It is well known that hypercalcemia can cause acute renal graft dysfunction from vascular constriction and volume depletion. Persistent hypercalcemia was shown to correlate with interstitial microcalcifications in renal graft and poor graft survival (Gwinner et al., 2005). Hypercalcemia can also cause calciphylaxis, neurological and other systemic symptoms. Persistent HPT, resorption of calcium deposits in soft tissues and normalization of active vitamin D metabolism likely contribute to the development of hypercalcemia after kidney transplant (Cunningham, 2005; Heaf et al., 2003; Kandil et al., 2010).

3.3 Hypophosphatemia

Renal phosphate wasting and hypophosphatemia are very common (up to 90%) in the early post transplant period, though they tend to resolve over time (Eknoyan et al., 2003; Levi, 2001). Persistent hyperparathyroidism and elevated phosphotonin fibroblast growth factor 23 (FGF23) are the main causes of hyperphosphaturia. Other possible causes include steroid therapy, reduced intestinal phosphorus absorption, reduced proximal tubular Na/Pi co-transporter expression or increased tubular sensitivity to PTH (Heaf et al., 2003; Levi, 2001; Zhang et al., 2008). Serum FGF23 level was found to be the best predictor of serum phosphate nadir after kidney transplant. The resolution of hyperphosphatoninism correlated with diminished renal phosphorus wasting 1 year after successful kidney transplant (Evenepoel et al., 2007, 2008). Phosphate supplements are usually given, but frequently are not effective in correcting severe hypophosphatemia. Administration of calcimimetic agent cinacalcet was reported to significantly decrease renal phosphate wasting, which was associated with suppressed serum PTH level, but not FGF23 level (Serra et al., 2008). Interestingly, dipyridamole can improve renal tubular phosphate reabsorption and increase serum phosphate levels in these patients (Balal et al., 2005).

3.4 Vitamin D receptor (VDR) genotype.

There are several variants and genotypes of the VDR reported. Compared with Bb and BB alleles, the bb allele was associated with a significantly increased recovery of BMD from 3 to 12 months after kidney transplant with a 7% of BMD increase in lumbar spine. More rapid resolution of both HPT and histological osteitis fibrosa after kidney transplant was also documented in patients with the "favorable" VDR bb allele (Torres et al., 1996).

3.5 Hypogonadism

The majority of ESRD patients are hypogonadal and gonadal hormones remain low in both female and male patients after kidney transplant. Steroids have been suggested to play a role. Reports show that about 50 % of male patients have low testosterone levels after kidney transplant. Aging and postmenopausal status worsen bone loss and increase the risk of bone fracture after kidney transplant (Cunningham, 2005; Cohen et al., 2004; Eknoyan et al., 2003; Epstein, 1996; Zisman & Sprague, 2006).

4. Prevention and treatment of bone loss

The 2009 Kidney Disease: Improving Global Outcome (KDIGO) clinical practice guideline provides recommendations for the evaluation, prevention, and treatment of bone disorder in renal transplant patients (KDOQI, 2009). The same measures that are used to prevent osteoporosis in the general population also apply to transplant recipients. General recommendations should include the following: all patients should receive counseling regarding smoking cessation, early mobilization after transplantation and fall prevention.

4.1 Vitamin D

Vitamin D deficiency (e.g., 25-hydroxyvitamin D level less than 20 ng/ml) is very common in kidney patients, including CKD, ESRD and kidney transplant recipients. Large dose vitamin D (50,000 units of vitamin D2 or D3) given weekly is more effective than the over-the-counter low dose vitamin D in correcting deficiency. Despite of the successful kidney transplant, the active 1, 25 hydroxyvitamin D levels are lower than the expected (Fleseriu & Licata, 2007). Correcting vitamin D deficiency by supplement can increase the serum level of active 1, 25 hydroxyvvitamin D (Amin et al., 2007). After kidney transplantation, all patients should receive 1000 mg/day of calcium and 800 IU/day of vitamin D in absence of hypercalcemia (Cunningham, 2005; Cohen et al., 2004; 2003; Epstein, 1996; Torres et al., 2004; Zisman & Sprague, 2006). Studies have found that BMD increases in treated patients and decreases in untreated patients, with a difference of 6-7% being seen 1 year after kidney transplant. Active vitamin D calcitriol or its analogues should be considered when a patient has a GFR of < 30 ml/min, secondary HPT or malabsorption. Serum Ca, Phos and PTH levels need to be monitored periodically and the dose of vitamin D adjusted accordingly (Jeffery et al., 2003; Torres et al.2004). The other benefic effects of vitamin D on immune system and cardiovascular health are being elucidated. It is with the hope that vitamin D may have the potential for reducing infectious complications while decreasing the risk of rejection after kidney transplant.

4.2 Gonadal hormones

Many premenopausal women and men undergoing solid organ transplantation have hypogonadism, most often related to the effects of glucocorticoids and chronic illness. In men and women undergoing transplantation, testosterone and estrogen-progestin replacement, respectively, have been shown to slow bone loss (Eknoyan et al. 2003; Cunningham, 2005). Hormonal replacement therapy (HRT) or selective estrogen-receptor modulators should be used for postmenopausal recipients after kidney transplant if there is no contraindication. Testosterone may also be considered for men with documented hypogonadism and osteoporosis (Eknoyan et al. 2003; Cunningham, 2005; Zhang et al., 2008).

4.3 Parathyroidectomy

After kidney transplant, HPT frequently undergoes spontaneous regression as both renal function and vitamin D metabolism return to normal. However, as many as 30% of patients may have persistently high PTH levels, often due to the development of a nodular monoclonal adenoma (Heaf et al., 2003). About 5% of kidney transplant recipients, with a reported range of 1 to 20%, undergo a surgical parathyroidectomy. The indications for surgery vary among the transplant centers, but the two major indications for parathyroidectomy in renal transplant patients are severe symptomatic hypercalcemia (> 11.5 mg/dl), usually occurring in the early post transplant period, and persistent hypercalcemia more than 1 year after transplant (Kandil et al.,2010; Zhang et al., 2008). BMD usually increases after surgical correction of HPT (Eknoyan 2003; Heaf et al., 2003; Jeffery et al., 2003; Levi, 2001). Parathyroidectomy was reported to be associated with an inferior graft function and worsening graft survival (Schwarz et al., 2007; Schmid et al., 1997). We retrospectively analyzed 794 kidney transplants performed at our center with at least 3 years of follow-up, 49 of them had persistent HPT after kidney transplant. Patients with HPT and non- HPT had similar 3-year graft survival. Parathyroidectomy was associated with a decreased estimated glomerular filtration rate at 3 years. However, there was no statistical difference in 3-year graft survival. Our experience suggests that parathyroidectomy is a safe and effective therapy for persistent HPT in renal transplant recipients (Kandil et al.,2010).

4.4 Calcimimetics

Cinacalcet, a calcimimetic compound, has been increasingly studied and used to treat persistent HPT and its associated hypercalcemia after kidney transplant. All studies in transplant patients have found that serum calcium concentration decreases with cinacalcet therapy (Black et al., 2003; El-Amm et al., 2007; Kamar et al., 2008; Kruse et al., 2005; Leca et al., 2006; Serra et al., 2005; Srinivas et al., 2006; Szwarc et al., 2006). However, the effect of cinacalcet on PTH and serum phosphorus levels varies across studies with no decrease in PTH level reported in two studies, while PTH decreased in the rest. Serum phosphorus level increased in most and did not change in three studies (Kruse et al., 2005; Srinivas et al., 2006). A recent study of 9 patients reported a favorable effect of cinacalcet on BMD (Bergua et al., 2008). Although large studies from dialysis patients demonstrate its safety, there is limited data in transplant patients. Cinacalcet was found to have moderate effect on tacrolimus pharmacokinetics, but not on cyclosporine or mycophenolate in renal transplant recipients (Falck et al., 2008). Thus, cinacalcet is not officially approved for usage in transplant patients yet.

4.5 Minimizing steroids

It is recommended to rapidly taper to a maintenance dose of 5 -7.5mg of prednisone daily, if possible, to minimize the bone loss and osteotoxic effects. Further, steroid-free protocols should be considered for patients with pre-transplant osteopenia or osteoporosis (Braun et al., 1999; Cunningham, 2005; Gallego et al., 2006; Van de Ham et al., 2003). Steroid withdrawal at 6 months has been reported to improve BMD at 1 year after kidney transplant. However, this was done in highly selected adult patients. There is no good data that later steroid withdrawal (after 1 year) is beneficial for the purpose of bone building (Eknoyan et al., 2003; Epstein, 1996). Recently, a prospective study comparing steroid -free and steroid-treated children found that the BMD Z-scores significantly decreased in steroid-free groups with or without prophylaxis with vitamin D analogue alphacalcidiol. However, steroid-treated group, who also received ibandronade prophylaxis, maintained BMD Z-scores over 2 year of follow-up (Grenda et al., 2011).

4.6 Bisphosphonates

Bisphosphonate therapy, that increases osteoclast apoptosis and reduces active osteoclasts and bone resorption, has been widely used to treat postmenopausal and steroid-induced osteoporosis. There are consistent studies reporting that it can also effectively prevent and treat bone loss in kidney transplant recipients. A BMD difference of up to 9% has been reported after 1 year's treatment compared with control group without bisphosphonate treatment (Coco et al., 2003; Fan et al., 2003; Hass et al., 2003). In addition, in a follow-up study of 4 years, intravenous pamidronate (0.5mg/kg) given at the time of transplant and at 1 month later could provide long-term protection of BMD (Fan et al., 2003). However, adynamic bone disease was commonly observed after bisphosphonate treatment (Coco et al., 2003). Low turnover bone diseases are common in dialysis patients and additional suppression of bone remodeling without stimulation of new bone formation may not improve the mechanical strength and quality of bone (Coco et al., 2003; Cruz et al., 2004; Zhang et al., 2008). This may explain why the prevention of bone loss with bisphosphonates has not been shown to effectively decrease bone fracture rate in kidney transplant recipients yet.

4.7 Calcitonin

Although calcitonin is effective in preventing bone loss in postmenopausal women, its effectiveness in post-transplant bone loss is uncertain. One report noted that intranasal salmon calcitonin 200 IU every other day can prevent early bone loss as effectively as alendronate and alfacalcidol in renal transplant recipients (El-Agroudy et al., 2005). But other studies have failed to demonstrate superiority to calcium supplementation in transplant recipients (Bone et al., 2004; Palmer et al., 2005; Valimaki et al., 1999).

4.8 Teriparatide

Recombinant human parathyroid hormone (PTH, teriparatide) has been shown to improve BMD in patients with glucocorticoid-induced and postmenopausal osteoporosis (Black et al., 2003; Neer et al., 2001). It has been approved by the FDA for treating osteoporosis in general population, but not in organ transplant patients. A recent study of 26 kidney transplant recipients with daily teriparatide injections demonstrated a stabilization of BMD in the femoral neck and increased cortical width. But there was no improvement in bone turnover or bone mineralization as measured by histology (Cejka et al., 2008). Thus, its use in this setting remains experimental.

5. Post-transplant bone fracture

Bone fracture is a devastating complication for transplant patients. It impairs their quality of life, increases the cost of care and hospital stay, and may even cause death. Common fracture sites are the legs, vertebral bodies, hips and ribs (Abbott et al., 2001; Nisbeth et al., 1999; Vautour et al., 2004). The risk of fracture is greatest in the first 6 months after kidney transplant, but continues over the long term, as bone loss slows 6-24 months after transplantation (Vautour et al., 2004). The cumulative bone fracture rate has been reported as high as 17 to 20% (Abbott et al., 2001; Nisbeth et al., 1999; Vautour et al., 2004). Higher fracture rates are seen in the elderly, females, diabetics, and simultaneous kidney pancreas transplant recipients (Abbott et al., 2001; Nisbeth et al., 1999; Vautour et al., 2004). The high bone fracture rate is thought to be the consequence of continuing bone loss that is superimposed on preexisting uremia osteodystrophy. Development of osteoporosis places kidney transplant recipients at increased risk for bone fractures (Brandenburg et al., 2004; Cohen et al., 2004; Cunningham, 2005). It is important to note that no medicine has been proven to decrease fracture risk in the kidney transplant patients yet.

6. Osteonecrosis

Osteonecrosis or avascular necrosis commonly affects the femoral head, knee, shoulder or elbow, and usually appears 6 to 24 months after kidney transplant. It is characterized by the ischemic death of bone marrow cells and osteocytes and loss of trabeculae. Clinical presentation is mainly joint pain that worsens with weight bearing. It may affect up to 15% of kidney transplant recipients (Lausten et al., 1998). In a cohort study of over 42,000 kidney recipients, the cumulative incidence of hospitalization for osteonecrosis was 7.1 episodes per 1,000 patient-years (Abbott et al., 2002). Steroid usage, especially a high cumulative dose of steroid or pulse steroid therapy is implicated as the main etiology. Other risk factors are pre-existing bone disease, diabetes and lupus nephritis (Abbott et al., 2005; Teng et al., 2000). The best diagnostic test for avascular necrosis is MRI, as plain film X-rays and bone scanning are less sensitive. Treatment includes resting, core decompression, vascularized bone grafts, or joint replacement, depending on the clinical severity.

7. Post-transplant bone pain syndrome

About 10 to 20% of transplant recipients experience bone pain, usually diffuse, particularly in the lower extremities. Both of the calcineurin inhibitors, cyclosporine and tacrolimus, have been implicated as the possible cause (Goffin et al., 2003; Grotz et al., 2001). Calcium channel blockers have been demonstrated to reduce bone pain (Barbarosa et al., 1995; Goffin et al., 2003). This suggests that calcineurin inhibitor -associated intraosseous vasoconstriction and ischemia may underlie the pathophysiology of this syndrome.

8. Clinical approach

Therapy for post-transplant bone disease needs to be individualized with physicians assessing the risk factors of bone loss in each patient and creating a plan for long-term bone care. It is recommended that a baseline BMD should be documented before or at the time of kidney transplant, with the BMD being repeated at 3 to 6 months after transplantation and then every 12 months for those with an abnormal BMD (Brandenburg et al., 2004; Cohen et al., 2004; Cunningham, 2005; Eknoyan et al., 2003).

All patients should be screened for vitamin D deficiency. Vitamin D deficiency or insufficiency should be treated with large dose of regular vitamin D, which follows with a maintenance dose of vitamin D supplement. All patients should receive counseling regarding smoking cessation, early mobilization after transplantation, and fall prevention. For patients with baseline BMD consistent with osteopenia or osteoporosis, calcium and vitamin D supplements should be started after kidney transplant. Further, all patients with evidence of hypogonadism should receive HRT if it is not contraindicated. Bisphosphonate should be considered and used with caution for patients with baseline osteoporosis, a history of fracture with minimal trauma, or at high risk for fracture. If baseline BMD is normal, then calcium, vitamin D and HRT should be considered as prophylaxis of bone loss in high-risk patient groups such as the elderly, diabetics, or combined kidney and pancreas transplant recipients.

If BMD is declining after transplant from baseline despite calcium, vitamin D and HRT, then bisphosphonates or calcitonin may be considered. We suggest bisphosphonates, rather than calcitonin, as there is more efficacy data with biphosphonates. Both oral and intravenous bisphosphonates have been shown to be effective in this setting. The decision should be based upon individual patient preferences and ability to take oral medications. Calcitonin can replace bisphosphonates if patients can't tolerate bisphosphonates or if they are contraindicated clinically. Persistent HPT should be treated with cinacalcet or parathyroidectomy surgery. Other measures include: lowering the dosages of, or discontinuing steroid if possible; treating metabolic acidosis; treating hypophosphatemia and hypocalcaemia; and limiting alcohol intake. With a failing renal allograft, patients should be managed in the same manner as any other CKD patient for recurring mineral and bone disorders, including uremic osteodystrophy.

9. Conclusion

Despite successful prevention of bone loss after transplant with several different types of medications, this effect has not resulted in the reduction of bone fracture as of yet. The bone diseases after kidney transplant have a complicated pathophysiology and various types of histology. Their clinical management is challenging and requires a comprehensive approach to address the underlying and ongoing disease processes. Bone biopsy with histomorphometric analysis is the best way to define the type of disease process and to guide our clinical management. More studies with the goal of restoring the normal bone remodeling and improving bone quality and strength are needed, so that the high incidence of facture can be successfully decreased in kidney transplant recipients.

10. References

Abbott KC, Oglesby RJ, Hypolite IO, et al. (2001). Hospitalizations for fractures after renal transplantation in the United States. *Annals of Epidemiology*; 11:450-457.

Abbott KC, Oglesby RJ, Agodoa LY. (2002). Hospitalized avascular necrosis after renal transplant in the United States. *Kidney International*; 62:2250-53.

Abbott KC, Koff J, Bohen EM, et al. (2005). Maintenance immunosuppresion use and the associated risk of avascular necrosis after kidney transplantation in the United States. *Transplantation*; 79:330-34.

Adragao T, Herberth J, Monier-Faugere MC, et al. (2009). Low bone volume- a risk factor for coronary calcification in hemodialysis patients. *Clinical Journal of American Society of Nephrology*; 4:450-5.

Amin H, Wall BM and Cooke CR. (2007). Osteomalacia and secondary hyperparathyroidism after kidney transplantation: Relationship to vitamin D deficiency. *American Journal of Medical Sciences*; 333:58-62.

Balal M, Paydas S, Seyrek N, et al. (2005). Dipyridamole for renal phosphate leak in successfully renal transplanted hypophosphatemic patients. *Clinical Nephrology*; 63:87-89.

Barbosa LM, Gauthier VJ, Davis CL. (1995). Bone pain that responds to calcium channel blockers. *Transplantation*; 59:541-544.

Bergua C, Torregrosa JV, Fuster D, et al. (2008). Effect of cinacalcet on hyercalcemia and bone mineral density in renal transplanted patients with secondary hyperparathyroidism. *Transplantation*; 86:413-7.

Black DM, Greenspan SL, Ensrud KE, et al. (2003). The effects of parathyroid hormone and alendronate alone or in combination in postmenopausal osteoporosis. *New England Journal of Medicine*; 349:1207-15.

Block GA, Martin KJ, de Francisco A, et al. (2004). Cinacalcet for secondary hyperparathyroidism in patients receiving hemodialysis. *New England Journal of Medicine*; 350:1516-25.

Bone HG, Hosking D, Devogelaer JP, et al. (2004). Ten years' experience with alendronate for osteoporosis in postmenopausal women. *New England Journal of Medicine*; 350:1189-99.

Brandenburg V, Politt D, Ketteler M, et al. (2004). Early rapid loss followed by long-term consolidation characterizes the development of lumbar bone mineral density after kidney transplantation. *Transplantation*; 77(10):1566-71.

Brandenburg VM, Westenfeld R, Ketteler M. (2004). The fate of bone after renal transplantation. *Journal of Nephrology*; 17:190-204.

Braun WE, Richmond BJ, Protiva DA, et al. (1999). The incidence and management of osteoporosis, gout and avascular necrosis in recipients of renal allografts functioning more than 20 years treated with prednisone and azathioprine. *Transplant Proceedings*; 31:1366-69.

Cejka, D, Benesch, T, Krestan, C, et al. (2008). Effect of teriparatide on early bone loss after kidney transplantation. *American Journal of Transplantation*; 8:1864-70.

Chertow GM, Burk SK, Raggi P. (2002). Sevalamer attenuates the progression of coronary and aortic calcification in hemodialysis patients. *Kidney International*; 62:245-52.

Coco M, Glicklich D, Faugere MC, et al. (2003). Prevention of bone loss in renal transplant recipients: a prospective, randomized trial of intravenous pamidronate, *Journal of American Society of Nephrology*; 14:2669-2676.

Cohen A, Sambrook P, Shane E. (2004). Management of bone loss after organ transplantation. *Journal of Bone and Mineral Research*; 19:1919-1932.

Cruz EA, Lugon JR, Jorgetti V, et al. (2004). Histological evolution of bone disease 6 month after successful kidney transplantation. *American Journal of Kidney Disease*; 44:747-756.

Cueto-Manzano AM, Konel S, Crowley V, et al. (2003). Bone histopathology and densitometry comparison between cyclosporine A monotherapy and prednisone plus azathioprine dual immunosuppression in renal transplant patients. *Transplantation*; 75:2053-2058.

Cunningham J. (2005). Posttransplant bone disease. *Transplantation*; 79:629-32.

Durieux S, Mercadal L, Orcel P, et al. (2002). Bone mineral density and fracture prevalence in long-tern kidney graft recipients. *Transplantation*; 74:496-500.

Eknoyan G, Levin A, Levin NW. K/DOQI (2003). clinical practice guidelines for bone metabolism and disease in chronic kidney disease. *American Journal of Kidney Disease*; 42(3):S12-S143.

El-Agroudy AE, El-Hussein AA, EL-Sayed M, et al. (2005). A prospective randomized study for prevention of postrenal transplantation bone loss. *Kidney International*; 67:2039-45.

El-Amm JM, Doshi MD, Singh A, et al. (2007). Preliminary experience with cinacalcet use in persistent secondary hyperparathyroidism after kidney transplantation. *Transplantation*; 83(5):546-9.

Epstein S. (1996). Post-transplantation bone disease: the role of immunosuppressive agents and the skeleton. *Journal of Bone and Mineral Research*; 11:1-7.
Evenepoel P, Van Den Bergh B, Naesens M, et al. (2009). Calcium metabolism in the early post transplant period. *Clinic Journal of American Society of Nephrology*; 4:665-72.
Evenepoel P, Meijers BKI, de Jonge H, et al. (2008). Recovery of hyperphosphatoninism and renal phosphorus wasting one year after successful renal renal transplantation. *Clinic Journal of American Society of Nephrology*; 3:1829-36.
Evenepoel P, Naesens M, Claes K, et al. (2007). Tertiary hyperphosphatoninism accentuates hypophosphatemia and suppresses calcitriol levels in renal transplant recipients. *American Journal of Transplantation*; 7:1193-200.
Fan SL, Kumar S, Cunningham J. (2003). Long-term effects on bone mineral density of pamidronate given at the time of renal transplantation. *Kidney International*; 63:2275-2279.
Falck P, Vethe NT, Asberg A, et al. (2008).Cinacalcet's effect on the pharmacokinetics of tacrolimus, cyclosporine and mycophenolate in renal transplant recipients. *Nephrology Dialysis Transplantation*; 23:1048-53.
Fleseriu M and Licata AA. (2007). Failure of successful renal transplant to produce appropriate level of 1, 25 dihydroxyvitamine D. *Osteoporosis International*; 18:363-8.
Gallego R, Oliva E, Vega N, et al. (2006). Steroid and bone density in patients with functioning kidney allografts. *Transplant Proceedings*; 38:2434-7.
Goffin E, Vande Berg B, Devogelaer JP, et al. (2003). Post-renal transplant syndrome of transient lower limb joint pain : description under a tracolimus-based immunosuppression. *Clinical Nephrology*; 59 :98-02.
Grenda R, Karczmarewicz E, Rubik J, et al. (2011). Bone mineral disease in children after renal transplantation in steroid-free and steroid-treated patients - a prospective study. *Pediatric Transplantation*; 15:205-13.
Grotz WH, Breitenfeldt MK, Braune SW, et al. (2001). Calcineurin inhibitor induced pain syndrome: a severe disabling complication after organ transplantation. *Transplant International*; 14:16-23.
Gwinner W, Suppa S, Mengel M, et al. (2005). Early calcification of renal allografts detected by protocol biopsies : causes and clinical implications. *American Journal of Transplantation* ; 5 :1934-41.
Hass M, Leko-Mohr Z, Roschger P, et al. (2003). Zoledronic acid prevents bone loss in the first 6 months after renal transplantation. *Kidney International*; 63:1130-1136.
Heaf, J, Tvedegaard, E, Kanstrup, IL, Fogh-Andersen, N. (2003). Hyperparathyroidism and long-term bone loss after renal transplantation. *Clinical Transplantion*; 17:268-10.
Jeffery JR, Leslie WD, Karpinski, et al. (2003). Prevalence and treatment of decreased bone density in renal transplant recipients: a randomized prospective trial of calcitriol versus alendronate. *Transplantation*; 76:1498-1502.
Julian BA, Laskow DA, Dubovsky J, et al. (1991). Rapid loss of vertebral mineral density after renal transplantation. *New England Journal of Medicine*; 325:544-550.
Kamar, N, Gennero, I, Spataru, L, et al. (2008). Pharmacodynamic effects of cinacalcet after kidney transplantation: once- versus twice-daily dose. *Nephrology Dialysis Transplantion*; 23:3720-4.

Kandil E, Florman S, Alabbas H, et al. (2010). Exploring the effect of parathyroidectomy for tertiary hyperparathyroidism after kidney transplantation. *American Journal of Medical Sciences*; 339:420-4.

KDIGO clinical practice guideline for the diagnosis, evaluation, prevention, and treatment of chronic kidney disease - mineral and bone disorder (CKD-MBD). (2009). *Kidney International*; S1-S130.

Kruse EA, Eisenburger U, Frey FJ, Mohaupt MG (2005). The calcimimetic cinacalcet normalizes serum calcium in renal transplant patients with persistent hyperparathyroidism. *Nephrology Dialysis Transplantation*; 20:1311-3.

Lausten GS, Lemser T, Jensen PK, et al. (1998). Necrosis of the femoral head after kidney transplantation. *Clinical Transplantion*; 12:572-57.

Leca N, Laftavi M, Gundroo A, Kohli R, Min I, Karam J, Sridhar N, Blessios G, Venuto R, Pankewycz O. (2006). Early and severe hyperparathyroidism associated with hypercalcemia after renal transplant treated with cinacalcet. *American Journal of Transplantion*; 6(10):2391-5.

Levi M. (2001). Post-transplant hypophosphatemia. *Kidney International*; 59 :2377-87.

Malluche HH, Monier-Faugere MC. (1994). The role of bone biopsy in the management of patients with renal osteodystrophy. *Journal of the American Society of Nephrology*; 4:1631-1642.

Malluche HH, Smith AJ, Abreo K and Faugere MC. (1984). The use of deferoxamine in the management of aluminum accumulation in bone in patients with renal failure. *New England Journal of Medicine*; 311:140-144.

Malluche HH, Monier-Faugere MC and Herberth J. (2010). Bone disease after renal transplantation. *Nature Reviews Nephrology*; 6 :32-40.

Marcen R, Caballero C, Pascual J, et al. (2006). Lumbar bone mineral density in renal transplant patients on neoral and tacrolimus: a four-year prospective study. *Transplantation*; 81:826-29.

Monier-Faugere MC, Mawad H, Qi Q, et al. (2000). High prevalence of low bone turnover and occurrence of osteomalacia after kidney transplantation. *Journal of the American Society of Nephrology*; 11:1093-1099.

Neer RM, Arnaud CD, Zanchetta JR, et al. (2001). Effect of parathyroid hormone (1-34) on fractures and bone mineral density in postmenopausal women with osteoporosis. *New England Journal of Medicine*; 344:1431-41.

Nisbeth U, Lindh E, Ljunghall S, et al. (1999). Increased fracture rate in diabetes mellitus and females after renal transplantation. *Transplantation*; 67:1218-1222.

Palmer SC, Strippoli GF and McGregor DO. (2005). Interventions for preventing bone disease in kidney transplant recipients: a systemic review of randomized controlled trials. *American Journal of Kidney Disease*; 45:638-49.

Rolla D, Ballanti P, Marsano L, et al. (2006). Bone disease in long-term renal transplant recipients with severe osteopenia: a cross-sectional study. *Transplantation*; 81:915-21.

Schmid T, Muller P and Spelsberg F. (1997). Parathyroidectomy after renal transplantation: a retrospective analysis of long-term outcome. *Nephrology Dialysis Transplantation*; 12: 2393-6.

Schwarz A, Rustien G, Merkel S, et al. (2007). Decreased renal transplant function after parathyroidectomy. *Nephrology Dialysis Transplantation*; 22: 584-91.

Serra AL, Schwarz AA, Wick FH, et al. (2005). Successful treatment of hypercalcemia with cinacalcet in renal transplant recipients with persistent hyperparathyroidism. *Nephrology Dialysis Transplantion*; 20(7):1315-9.

Serra AL, Wuhrmann C and Wuthrich RP. (2008). Phosphatemic effect of cinacalcet in kidney transplant recipients with persistent hyperparathyroidism. *American Journal of Kidney Disease;* 52:1151-7.

Srinivas TR, Schold JD, Womer KL, et al. (2006). Improvement in hypercalcemia with cinacalcet after kidney transplantation. *Clinical Journal of the American Society of Nephrology*; 1(2):323-6.

Szwarc I, Argilis A, Garrigue V, et al. (2006). Cinacalcet chloride is efficient and safe in renal transplant recipients with posttransplant hyperparathyroidism. *Transplantation;* 82(5):675-80.

Teng S, Chan TM, Lui SL, et al. (2000). Risk factors for avascular bone necrosis after renal transplantation. *Transplant Proceedings*; 32:1873-75.

Teng, M, Wolf M, Lowrie E, et al. (2003). Survival of patients undergoing hemodialysis with paricalcitol or calcitriol therapy. *New England Journal of Medicine*; 349:446-456.

Torres A, Machado M, Concepcion MT, et al. (1996). Influence of vitamin D receptor genotype on bone mass changes after renal transplantation. *Kidney International;* 50:1726-33.

Torres A, Garcia S, Gomez A, et al. (2004). Treatment of intermittent calcitriol and calcium reduce bone loss after renal transplantation. *Kidney International*; 65:705-712.

Valimaki MJ, Kinnunen K, Tahtela R, et al. (1999). A prospective study of bone loss and turnover after cardiac transplantation: effect of calcium supplementation with or without calcitonin. *Osteoporosis International*; 10(2):128-36.

Valimaki MJ, Kinnunen K, Volin L, et al. (1999). A prospective study of bone loss and turnover after allogeneic bone marrow transplantation: effect of calcium supplementation with or without calcitonin. *Bone Marrow Transplantion*; 23(4):355-61.

van den Ham EC, Kooman JP, Christians ML, et al. (2003). The influence of early steroid withdrawal on body composition and none mineral transplantation density in renal patients. *Transplant International*; 16:82-87.

Vautour LM, Melton LJ, Clarke BL, et al. (2004). Long-term fracture risk following renal transplantation, a population based study. *Osteoporosis International*; 15:160-167.

Zisman AL, Sprague SM. (2006). Bone disease after kidney transplantation. *Advances in Chronic Kidney Disease*; 13:35-38.

Zhang R, Alper B, Simon E, et al. (2008). Management of metabolic bone diseases in kidney transplant recipients. *American Journal of Medical Sciences*; 335:120-5.

15

Hypertension in the Kidney Transplant Recipient

Heather H. Jones and Daniel J. Salzberg
Division of Nephrology, University of Maryland Department of Medicine, School of Medicine, USA

1. Introduction

Despite normalization of renal function and improvement in volume control with kidney transplantation, the prevalence of post-transplant hypertension (HTN) is substantial. The prevalence of post-transplant HTN reported in the literature varies considerably depending on the study population and the criteria used to define HTN, although most studies report a prevalence of between 60-80% [1-3]. In one cross-sectional study of 409 adults with stable kidney allograft function, the prevalence of HTN, defined as BP > 150/90 mmHg, was 77.3% [4]. Most subjects (68.9%) required multiple antihypertensive medications. However, for patients with diabetes or estimated GFR below 60 mL/min, treatment guidelines recommend blood pressure (BP) goals below 130/80 mmHg. Applying these more stringent recommendations, the true prevalence of post-transplant HTN is likely in excess of 95%.

2. Pathogenesis and impact of immunosuppression

The exact pathogenesis of post-transplant HTN is poorly understood, as multiple factors impact its development. Important risk factors include preexisting recipient factors, donor specific factors, use of immunosuppressive agents, extra-allograft related issues, and both acute and chronic allograft dysfunction [1,2]. Ultimately, post-transplant HTN is characterized by sodium retention, enhanced sympathetic nervous system activity, renal vasoconstriction and relatively lower levels of plasma renin [5].

Post-transplant HTN demonstrates a distinctive characteristic regarding ambulatory BP monitoring, with patients having a high prevalence of nocturnal HTN [3]. In one prospective study, nearly 75% of subjects with post-transplant HTN demonstrated absence or reversal of the normal nocturnal fall in BP (i.e. non-dippers) [3]. In non-kidney transplant recipients, loss of nocturnal dip is associated with left ventricular hypertrophy, lacunar stroke and microalbuminuria [6].

3. Role of immunosuppression

Systemic steroid use contributes to the development of post-transplant HTN through various mechanisms, including sodium retention with resultant volume expansion, decreased prostaglandin biosynthesis, and increased smooth muscle pressor response [9]. In one systematic review comparing post-transplant recipients on immunosuppression regimens containing steroids versus those on steroid-sparing regimens, steroid-attributable incidence of HTN was reported to be between 2 and 17% [10]. A more recent meta-analysis of steroid avoidance or steroid withdrawal protocols examined impact on both graft and cardiovascular outcomes [11]. Steroid avoidance or withdrawal was found to be significantly related to increased risk of acute rejection and elevated creatinine at end of follow-up, with no difference in patient survival, graft loss, or death-censored graft loss. At the same time, steroid avoidance was associated with significant reduction in the risk of cardiovascular risk factors, including a 10% reduction in risk of post-transplant HTN.

However, some evidence indicates that chronic steroid use may not alter BP control. Vincenti and colleagues evaluated one-year outcomes and cardiovascular risk factors in kidney transplant recipients randomized to immunosuppressive regimens with complete steroid avoidance, early steroid withdrawal, and chronic steroid therapy. There was no difference in systolic or diastolic BP between any of the groups and no difference in the percent of patients requiring antihypertensive therapy [12].

Perhaps the most important factor in the pathogenesis of post-transplant HTN is the use of calcineurin inhibitors. Calcineurin inhibitors lead to the development of HTN through a myriad of mechanisms, including sodium retention with resultant volume expansion, enhanced sympathetic nerve activity, up-regulation of intrarenal renin biosynthesis, and vasoconstriction of the preglomerular vasculature via decreased production of vasodilatory factors and increased production of vasoconstrictive factors [5,13-14]. It has been shown that cyclosporine-induced renal vasoconstriction precedes the development of HTN [13]. Additionally, cyclosporine has been implicated as contributing to the loss of the normal nocturnal drop in BP [3].

In recent years, there has been a paradigm shift in the choice of calcineurin inhibitors from cyclosporine to tacrolimus, as short-term patient and graft survival appears to be equivalent between the two [15]. Likewise, the incidence of acute rejection is similar between the two groups when they are used in conjunction with mycophenolate mofetil. The advantage of tacrolimus over cyclosporine is a lower incidence of hyperlipidemia, hirsutism, and gingival hyperplasia. However, a difference between the two agents with regard to HTN is not as clear.

A large multi-center open label randomized controlled trial comparing cyclosporine-based versus tacrolimus-based immunosuppression regimens involving 412 kidney transplant recipients reported that at 3 years post-transplantation, the number of recipients requiring antihypertensive therapy was lower in the tacrolimus group, though this did not reach statistical significance (74.7% vs. 84.9%, $p = 0.06$) [16]. Another cross-sectional study evaluating predictors of post-transplant HTN, defined as documented diagnosis of HTN or use of antihypertensive medications, determined that significantly more patients on a cyclosporine-based regimen were prescribed 2 or more antihypertensive medications compared with those on a tacrolimus-based regimen [17].

There has been interest in the use of a mammalian-target of rapamycin (m-TOR) inhibitor-based immunosuppression regimen as an alternative to calcineurin inhibitor-based regimens, partially due to concerns over long-term effects of calcineurin-induced HTN and chronic preglomerular vasoconstriction. Thus far, the data regarding the relationship between m-TOR inhibitor use and HTN have been mixed. Comparison of a small cohort of patients on tacrolimus-based vs. sirolimus-based immunosuppression demonstrated that patients receiving sirolimus had significantly lower systolic BP on 24-hour ambulatory BP monitoring, though there was no significant difference in preserved nocturnal drop in BP [18].

However, two large randomized controlled trials evaluating the conversion of kidney transplant recipients from cyclosporine to sirolimus demonstrated no difference in BP [19-20]. The CONCEPT study, evaluating efficacy of conversion from cyclosporin to sirolimus 3-months post-transplantation in 237 kidney transplant recipients demonstrated no difference in systolic or diastolic BP one year post-transplantation [20]. There was, however, a tendency toward no need of antihypertensive medications in the sirolimus group compared to the cyclosporine group (51% vs. 38%), though this was not statistically significant. The CONVERT study, which followed a cohort of 830 subjects randomized to either sirolimus conversion or continuation of calcineurin inhibitor, found a statistically significant decrease in systolic BP at one month and in diastolic BP up to three months post-conversion [19]. However, by study endpoint two years, there was no significant difference in systolic or diastolic BP between the groups.

4. Renal artery stenosis

Transplant renal artery stenosis (tRAS) is a potentially important contributor to refractory HTN and unexplained graft dysfunction. The incidence of tRAS has been reported to range from 1 to 23%, with most of this variance attributed to differences in definition and diagnostic technique employed [21]. Most episodes of tRAS in the first three post-operative months are attributed to surgical complications, such as donor vessel trauma, intra-operative kidney malpositioning, or stenosis at the surgical anastamosis [22]. Transplant RAS occurring greater than 3 months post-transplantation is rarely related to surgical complications.

Several risk factors have been implicated in the development of late tRAS, including graft rejection, CMV infection, prolonged cold ischemia time, delayed graft function, and pediatric donor source [22-26]. A recent case-control study of 29 transplant recipients with tRAS found that CMV infection was associated with a five-fold increase in the risk for tRAS, while DGF increased tRAS risk four-fold [22].

Doppler ultrasonography may be an appropriate first-line screening test for tRAS, as it is non-invasive and avoids exposure to iodinated contrast media [21]. Sensitivity and specificity have been reported as high as 94% and 100%, respectively [27]. However, this diagnostic test is very operator-dependent, and such impressive results may not be obtained in centers without strong experience in kidney transplant imaging. Ultimately, the gold standard remains angiography.

Therapeutic options for tRAS include conservative management, angioplasty with or without stenting, and surgical repair. A recent case series compared the outcomes of these three strategies and determined that the highest success rate, defined as improvement in graft function, occurred in those who underwent primary angioplasty (36% conservative therapy, 82% angioplasty, 44% surgery) [28]. Graft survival at five years post-transplantation was also highest in the primary angioplasty group (63% conservative therapy, 86% angioplasty, 65% surgery). The primary angioplasty cohort was the only group in which a sustained improvement in BP was observed, with 63% of participants in this subgroup reaching target BP with a single agent post-procedure. However, angioplasty is not without risks. Four participants (6%) who underwent initial angioplasty had to undergo a transplant nephrectomy due to post-intervention complications, specifically uncontrolled bleeding and/or thrombosis. Furthermore, the presence of large or multiple stenoses may not be appropriate for primary angioplasty, leaving surgical intervention as the only viable option.

Another case-controlled series of patients evaluated the efficacy of angioplasty with or without stenting in participants with tRAS [22]. Both serum creatinine and BP control improved significantly post-procedure. Restenosis occurred in 27% of patients at a mean time of 26 months post-procedure, and 10% experienced immediate graft loss due to procedural complications.

Transplant RAS is an important entity to consider in subjects with new-onset or refractory HTN. It can be effectively treated in most cases with angioplasty, which appears to impact positively on graft function and potentially prolonging allograft life.

5. Outcomes

The precise role of HTN on allograft outcome has been difficult to define due to the complex interactions between HTN and worsening allograft function. Hypertension is both a cause and consequence of kidney disease. The presence of post-transplant HTN is associated with an increased risk for acute rejection, and allograft recipients who experience an episode of acute rejection have a significantly higher BP than those without rejection [29-30]. In a historical cohort study of adult allograft recipients, Mange and colleagues characterized the relationship between BP and subsequent allograft function [31]. For each 10-mm Hg increment increase in systolic, diastolic and mean BP, there was a 15%, 27% and 30% reduction, respectively, in the rate of allograft survival. Another cohort study by Opelz and colleagues demonstrated that systolic BP greater than 140 mmHg was associated with increased risk of graft failure, regardless of diastolic BP or history of acute rejection [32].

Post-transplant HTN is associated with increased mortality, chronic allograft nephropathy, acute rejection, and graft loss [7,30,32]. It is also an independent risk factor for the development of cardiovascular disease, the leading cause of death in kidney transplant recipients. The fact that more severe HTN has been associated with a higher rate of graft dysfunction, worse graft survival and a higher frequency of proteinuria is suggestive of a causative relationship [8].

6. Antihypertensive therapy

In patients with chronic kidney disease (CKD), therapy for HTN slows the progression of renal insufficiency [33]. This suggests that treatment of post-transplant HTN may likewise ameliorate the loss of allograft function. Current KDOQI guidelines recommend kidney transplant recipients maintain a target BP < 130/80, largely based on extrapolation from outcomes data in CKD patients [34]. Due to various contributing factors, post-transplantation HTN can be difficult to control. Multiple retrospective cohort analyses report a significant proportion of subjects fail to reach target BP, even with use of multiple anti-hypertensive agents. A review of the Collaborative Transplant Study, a database involving nearly 30,000 chronic transplant recipients at 400 international transplant centers, demonstrated that only 44.5% achieved systolic BP < 140 mmHg and that 24.5% achieved systolic BP < 130mmHg [32]. A smaller cohort study of 150 transplant recipients demonstrated that over 60% of patients required three or more anti-hypertensive medications and that only 40% reached the target BP of < 130/80 mmHg [35]. Although the risk of HTN is well documented, there are few published reports on the management of post-transplant HTN that clearly elucidate ideal target BP or choice of individual antihypertensive agents [22].

7. Calcium channel blockers

Calcium channel blockers (CCB) are effective medications to lower BP in kidney transplant recipients. In the general population, they have proven to be robust agents to lower BP regardless of age, gender, ethnicity, and salt intake, which may explain why they are also effective in the kidney transplant population (36). In addition, they also appear to reverse some of the intra-renal vasoconstriction caused by calcineurin inhibitors (*36-38*). One trial of 65 transplant recipients receiving cyclosporine-based immunosuppression randomized to the CCB or placebo at the time of transplantation demonstrated that those taking felodipine had a significantly higher renal plasma flow at 6 weeks [39]. Additionally, those randomized to the felodipine also group had lower systolic and diastolic BP, higher renal plasma flow, and higher GFR (49ml/min vs. 40ml/min, p = 0.05) at 12 weeks post-transplantation, despite a greater proportion of patients in the placebo group receiving other anti-hypertensive agents.

In a study of 123 immediate post-transplant recipients, subjects were randomized to nifedipine (CCB) or lisinopril as first line maintenance BP medication [40]. At three months post-transplantation 20% of all participants had achieved a goal diastolic BP of < 95 mmHg, with 38% in the CCB group reaching diastolic BP goal at one year. There was no difference in BP response between groups, but patients randomized to nifedipine had higher hemoglobin and lower creatinine levels compared to the lisinopril group at the study end. In an additional study comparing nifedipine and lisinopril, impact on left ventricular mass and function was assessed [41]. This study demonstrated that myocardial mass was significantly reduced in both groups one year post-transplantation, with a mean reduction of 15% in both groups. There was no statistically significant between-groups difference. The percentage of participants with persistent left ventricular hypertrophy (LVH) one year post-transplantation was similar between groups (45% nifedipine, 41% lisinopril p = NS). Another study of 99 kidney transplant recipients one year post-transplantation randomized subjects to 1 of 3 groups: (i) amlodipine (CCB) monotherapy, (ii) enalapril monotherapy, or (iii) combination amlodipine and enalapril [42]. At six months post-randomization, there was no difference amongst the three groups in terms of systolic BP or number of antihypertensive agents used. However, participants assigned to amlodipine monotherapy demonstrated improved creatinine clearance but no change in proteinuria, as compared with either angiotensin converting enzyme (ACE)-inhibitor monotherapy or combination. Results of this study should be interpreted with some caution, as they did not reach the target number of participants for adequate power.

A recent meta-analysis of randomized controlled trials involving antihypertensive agent use in renal transplant recipients was conducted [43]. This analysis concluded that use of a CCB versus placebo did not reduce the risk of death but did reduce the risk of graft lost by 25% at 12-months post-transplantation. Additionally, subjects receiving CCB had significantly higher estimated glomerular filtration rate (eGFR). When compared to ACE-inhibition. There was no difference detected in death, graft loss, or cardiovascular event risk.

8. Renin-angiotensin system blockade

Use of renin-angiotensin system (RAS) blockers in kidney transplant recipients was initially limited due to a number of concerns, including ineffectiveness in BP control, potential exacerbation of anemia, potential for inducing hyperkalemia, and the risk of precipitating acute kidney injury, [44-46]. The concern for ineffective BP control with renin-angiotensin blockade was related to the fact that post-transplant HTN, characterized by a low renin, volume expanded state, has been compared with the Goldblatt single-kidney, one-clip model of HTN, which potentially would not be very responsive to these agents [47]. However, this concern has not been borne out clinically, as multiple studies have demonstrated that RAS blockers have efficacy in reducing BP in post-transplant HTN [48].

Renin-angiotensin system blockade has now become commonplace in many transplant centers. Before 1990, approximately 9% of post-transplant subjects received treatment with an ACE inhibitor, which increased to roughly 47% in 2003 [49]. In the same retrospective review, only 38.5% (781 subjects) had never received an ACE inhibitor or an angiotensin receptor blocker (ARB). Six-hundred thirty eight subjects (31.4%) used ACE inhibitor or ARB therapy for the entirety of their follow-up, and 612 subjects (30.1%) received this therapy during various times of follow-up [49].

Furthermore, there are multiple theoretical benefits supporting the use of RAS blockers in the treatment of post-transplant HTN, such as (i) decreasing intraglomerular capillary pressure, (ii) decreasing the production and expression of the potentially damaging growth factors, (iii) decreasing proteinuria, (iv) for primary and secondary prevention of adverse cardiovascular outcomes, (v) decreasing cyclosporine nephrotoxicity, and (vi) blocking angiotensin type 1 (AT_1) receptor antibodies that may be associated with vascular rejection [50-51]. In the general population, RAS blockers have been shown to reduce both primary and secondary cardiovascular events [52]. Despite these theoretical benefits for their RAS blocker use, there are no prospective studies demonstrating the advantage of RAS blockers for the protection against allograft loss or for prolonging patient survival.

The largest study to date that has evaluated the efficacy of a RAS blocker is the SECRET trial, a multi-center double-blind randomized placebo-controlled trial involving 500 participants from several transplant centers in Europe [53] This trial was designed to evaluate the effects of Candesartan (ARB) therapy compared with placebo, on mortality, cardiovascular events, and graft failure. The study was discontinued prematurely due to a lower than expected event rate in both groups, which precluded conclusions regarding the primary endpoints. However, analysis of secondary endpoints revealed that reductions in BP and proteinuria were greater in the ARB group, but this was associated with a decrease in creatinine clearance and hemoglobin There was no significant difference in cardiovascular or graft outcomes between the two groups, though the overall event rate was quite low (5.1% with candesartan vs. 5.3% with placebo).

A much smaller study involving fifty recipients of living unrelated kidney transplants at least six months prior to enrollment were randomized to losartan (ARB) 50 mg daily or placebo for one year [54]. Of note, the subjects were not proteinuric at randomization. There was no difference in number of antihypertensives prescribed between the two groups and no difference in creatinine clearance at study end. However, systolic BP was significantly lower in the ARB group at 12 months (113mmHg vs. 126mmHg).

Although insufficient data exist to determine the impact of RAS blockade on overall cardiovascular outcomes, a small study has evaluated the impact of ACE inhibitor therapy on echocardiographic findings [55]. Evaluation of 74 transplant recipients randomized to lisinopril (ACE) or placebo and followed for 18 months demonstrated a significant decrease in left ventricular mass index in the ACE group while no difference was observed in the placebo group. There was no difference between the groups in terms of systolic BP, serum creatinine, urinary protein excretion, or number of antihypertensive agents used. The decrease in left ventricular mass index was observed exclusively in those concomitantly treated with ACE and cyclosporine, as opposed to tacrolimus. This small study is one more piece of evidence corroborating data from the general population, suggesting that drugs that block the RAS are capable of regressing left ventricular hypertrophy, both as part of their hemodynamic effect, but also through BP independent mechanisms. It is likely that regression of LVH may be a beneficial prognostic event that patients achieve with an appropriate BP control and an optimal class of antihypertensive therapy, with a potential for reducing adverse cardiovascular events. This study parallels efforts in older trials in the general population, illustrating the advantages of a RAS blocking drugs in the reduction of proteinuria and the risk for cardiovascular events and renal disease progression. Sadly, compelling data are still lacking in the kidney transplant population.

Although the number of randomized controlled trials regarding RAS blockade in transplant recipients has increased in recent years, much of the available data are from retrospective studies and systematic reviews. In one retrospective review of more than 2,000 recipients of kidney transplants at the University of Vienna, investigators noted that the ten-year patient survival rates were 74% in patients receiving either an ACE inhibitor or an ARB as part of their antihypertensive regimen and only 53% in patients not receiving these agents (49). Their results were even more remarkable when one considers that the group receiving the RAS blockers were older, required a higher number of antihypertensive medications, and were more likely to have type 2 diabetes and evident cardiovascular disease, when compared to the group not receiving these agents. Although selection bias limits the power of this study, the data are intriguing and suggest that there may be an important advantage to employ RAS blocking drugs as part of an antihypertensive regimen in an effort to reduce cardiovascular events.

Heinze and colleagues (49), studied 436 kidney transplant recipients who had delayed graft function. Approximately half of those patients (n=181) were given either an ACE inhibitor or ARB at the time of transplantation. Those patients who received RAS blocker had improved ten-year graft survival, when compared to those who were not treated with RAS blockers (44% vs. 32%, respectively). Hiremath and colleagues (56) performed a systematic review of 21 randomized trials of 1,549 patients to determine the effect of ACE inhibitor or ARBs on graft function and patient survival after kidney transplantation. In this analysis, drugs that block the RAS were associated with a significant decrease in GFR (-5.8 mL/min), proteinuria (-470 mg/day), and hematocrit (-3.5%)(51,57). However, there was insufficient data to determine their impact on patient or graft survival. Authors suggested that there may be a trade off between the beneficial effects of proteinuria reduction and potential cardiac protection with the development of possible anemia and lowered GFR.

9. Beta-blockade

Since kidney transplant patients are at much greater risk for cardiovascular events compared to the general population (58), due to both traditional and non-traditional Framingham Heart Study risk factors, beta-blocker use is often advisable. This may be important both during the peri-operative period to protect against myocardial ischemia, but also in the long-term management of HTN and cardiovascular disease. However, these agents have not been extensively studied. A recent meta-analysis of randomized controlled trials involving antihypertensive therapy in renal transplant recipients identified four studies involving beta-blockers [43]. Currently, there is insufficient data to determine relative benefits and harms of these agents. However, data from these studies indicate that beta-blockers are effective in BP reduction without appreciable impact on renal function, proteinuria, or left ventricular mass [59-61].

10. Alpha-blockers

In addition to their antihypertensive effects, alpha-blockers are often used to facilitate prostatic relaxation. This is particularly important in many older patients who may have occult prostatic hypertrophy, or some degree of bladder detrusor neuropathy due to diabetes. However, these agents, in general, tend to cause significant orthostatic symptoms, and have not been proven to reduce mortality (62). Both doxazosin and prazosin have been shown to decrease HTN in transplant recipients, although the literature remains sparse (63-64).

11. Conclusion

Taken together, the clinical trials of antihypertensive therapeutics in kidney transplant subjects illustrates that BP can be controlled. However, it usually requires multiple drugs. Although the data is not definitive, it appears that CCB and or RAS blockers should be included in an effective antihypertensive regimen. Subjects at risk for, or who have known coronary disease, may also derive benefit from beta-blockers. More studies are needed to define optimal levels of BP control and ideal combination of agents to facilitate better long-term patient and graft survival in kidney transplant recipients.

12. References

[1] Raine AE. Does antihypertensive therapy modify chronic allograft failure? Kidney Int Suppl. 1995;52:S107-11.
[2] Sanders CE Jr, Curtis JJ. Role of hypertension in chronic renal allograft dysfunction. Kidney Int Suppl. 1995;52:S43-7.
[3] Oliveras A, Vazquez S, Hurtado S, et al. Ambulatory blood pressure monitoring in renal transplant patients: modifiable parameters after active antihypertensive treatment. Transplant Proc. 2004;36: 1352-4.
[4] Budde K, Waiser J, Fritsche L, et al. Hypertension in patients after renal transplantation. Transplant Proc. 1997; 29: 209-11.
[5] McNally PG, Feehally J. Pathophysiology of cyclosporin A nephrotoxicity: experimental and clinical observations. Nephrol Dial Transplant. 1992;7:791-804.
[6] Lipkin GW, Tucker B, Giles M, Raine AE. Ambulatory blood pressure and left ventricular mass in cyclosporin- and non-cyclosporin-treated renal transplant recipients. J Hypertens. 1993; 11: 439-42.
[7] Sorof JM, Sullivan EK, Tejani A, Portman RJ. Antihypertensive medication and renal allograft failure: a North American Pediatric Renal Transplant Cooperative Study report. J Am Soc Nephrol. 1999; 10: 1324-30.

[8] Kasiske BL, Anjum S, Shah R, et al. Hypertension after kidney transplantation. Am J Kidney Dis. 2004; 43: 1071-81.
[9] Whitworth J. Mechanisms of glucocorticoid-induced hypertension. Kidney Int. 1987; 31: 1213-1224.
[10] Veenstra D, Best J, Hornberger J, Sullivan S, Hricik D. Incidence and long-term cost of steroid-related side effects after renal transplantation. Am J Kidney Dis. 1999; 33: 829-839.
[11] Knight S, Morris P. Steroid avoidance or withdrawal after renal transplantation increases the risk of acute rejection but decreases cardiovascular risk. A meta-analysis. Transplantation. 2010; 89: 1-14.
[12] Vincenti F, Schena F, Paraskevas S, et al. A randomized multicenter study of steroid avoidance, early steroid withdrawal, or standard steroid therapy in kidney transplant recipients. Am J Transplant. 2008; 8: 307-316.
[13] Conte G, Dal Canton A, Sabbatini M, et al. Acute cyclosporine renal dysfunction reversed by dopamine infusion in healthy subjects. Kidney Int. 1989; 36: 1086-92.
[14] Textor S, Taler S, Canzanello V, et al. Posttransplantation hypertension related to calcineurin inhibitors. Liver Transplantation. 2003; 6: 530.
[15] Tanabe K. Calcineurin inhibitors in renal transplantation: What is the best option? Drugs. 2003; 63: 1535-1548.
[16] Jensik S. and FK 506 Kidney Transplant Study Group. Tacrolimus (FK 506) in kidney transplantation: Three-year survival results of the US multicenter, randomized comparative trial. Transplant Proc. 1998; 30: 1216-1218.
[17] Bohlke M. Barcellos F, Rocha M. et al. Predictors of hypertension following successful renal transplantation: A population-based study. Transplantation Proc. 2009; 41: 3743-3746.
[18] Steigerwalt SP, Brar N, Dhungel A, et al. Improved 24-hour blood pressure control with sirolimus versus calcineurin inhibitor based immunosuppression in renal transplant recipients. Transplant Proc, 2009; 41: 4184-4187.
[19] Schena F, Pascoe M, Alberu J, et al. Conversion from calcineurin inhibitors to sirolimus maintenance therapy in renal allograft recipients: 24-month efficacy and safety results from CONVERT trial. Transplantation 2009; 87: 233-242.
[20] Lebranchu Y, Thierry A, Toupance O, et al. Efficacy on renal function of early conversion from cyclosporine to sirolimus 3 months after renal transplantation: Concept study. Am J of Transplant. 2009; 9: 1115-1123.
[21] Bruno S, Remuzzi G, Ruggenenti P. Transplant renal artery stenosis.J Am Soc Nephrol. 2004 Jan;15(1):134-41.
[22] Audard V. Matignon M. Hemery F, et al. Risk factors and long-term outcome of transplant renal artery stenosis in adult recipients after treatment by percutaneous transluminal angioplasty. Am J Transplant. 2006; 6: 95-99.
[23] Wong W, Fynn SP, Higgings RM, et al. Transplant renal artery stenosis in 77 patients: Does it have an immunological cause? Transplantation. 1996; 61: 215-219.
[24] Pouria S, State O, Wong W, Hendry B. CMV infection is associated with transplant renal artery stenosis. QJM. 1998; 91: 185-189.
[25] Sankari B, Geisinger M, Zelch M, et al. Post-transplant renal artery stenosis: Impact of therapy on long-term kidney function and blood pressure control. J Urology. 1996; 155: 1860-1864.

[26] Patel N, Jindal R, Wilkin T et al. Renal artery stenosis in renal allografts: Retrospective study of predisposing factors and outcome after percutaneous transluminal angioplasty. Radiology. 2001; 219: 663-667.
[27] Loubeyre P, Cahen R, Grozel F, et al. Transplant renal artery stenosis. Evaluation of diagnosis with magnetic resonance angiography compared with color duplex sonography and arteriography. Transplantation. 1996; 62: 446-450.
[28] Ghazanfar A, Tavakoli A, Augustine T, et al. Management of transplant renal artery stenosis and its impact on long term allograft survival: A single centre experience. Nephrol Dial Transplant. 2011; 26: 336-343.
[29] Cosio FG, Pelletier RP, Pesavento TE, et al. Elevated blood pressure predicts the risk of acute rejection in renal allograft recipients. Kidney Int. 2001 Mar;59(3):1158-64.
[30] Cosio FG, Pelletier RP, Sedmak DD, et al. Renal allograft survival following acute rejection correlates with blood pressure levels and histopathology. Kidney Int. 1999 Nov;56(5):1912-9.
[31] Mange KC, Cizman B, Joffe M, Feldman HI. Arterial hypertension and renal allograft survival. JAMA. 2000 Feb 2;283(5):633-8.
[32] Opelz G, Wujciak T, Ritz E. Association of chronic kidney graft failure with recipient blood pressure. Collaborative Transplant Study. Kidney Int. 1998 Jan;53(1):217-22.
[33] Mimran A, Ribstein J. Angiotensin-converting enzyme inhibitors versus calcium antagonists in the progression of renal diseases. Am J Hypertens. 1994 Sep;7(9 Pt 2):73S-81S.
[34] K/DOQI clinical practice guidelines on hypertension and antihypertensive agents in chronic kidney disease. AJKD. 2004; 43: S1-S290.
[35] Malyszko J, Malyszko J, Bachorzewska-Gajewska H, et al. Inadequate blood pressure control in most kidney transplant recipients and patients with coronary artery disease with and without complications. Transplant Proc. 2009; 41: 3069-3072.
[36] Sennesael JJ, Lamote JG, Violet I, Tasse S, Verbeelen DL. Divergent effects of calcium channel and angiotensin converting enzyme blockade on glomerulotubular function in cyclosporine-treated renal allograft recipients. Am J Kidney Dis 1996 May;27:701-8.
[37] Curtis JJ, Laskow DA, Jones PA, et al. Captopril-induced fall in glomerular filtration rate in cyclosporine-treated hypertensive patients. J Am Soc Nephrol 1993:1570-4.
[38] van der Schaaf MR, Hene RJ, Floor M, Blankestijn PJ, Koomans HA. Hypertension after renal transplantation. Calcium channel or converting enzyme blockade? Hypertension 1995; 25:77-81.
[39] Madsen J, Sorensen S, Hansen H, Pedersen E. The effect of felodipine on renal function and blood pressure in cyclosporine-treated renal transplant recipients during the first three months after transplantation. Nephrol Dial Transplant. 1998; 13: 2327-2334.
[40] Midtvedt K, Hartmann A, Holdaas H, Fauchald P. Efficacy of nifedipine or lisinopril in the treatment of hypertension after renal transplantation: A double-blind randomized comparative trial. Clin Transplant. 2001; 15:426-431.
[41] Midtvedt K, Hartmann A, Foss A, et al. Sustained improvement of renal graft function for two years in hypertensive renal transplant recipients treated with nifedipine as compared to lisinopril. Transplantation. 2001 Dec 15;72:1787-92.

[42] Halimi JM, Giraudeau B, Buchler M, et al. Enalapril/amlodipine combination in cyclosporine-treated renal transplant recipients: A prospective randomized trial. Clin Transplant. 2007; 21:277-284, 2007.

[43] Cross N, Webster A, Masson P, O'Connell P, Craig J. Antihypertensives for kidney transplant recipients: Systematic review and meta-analysis of randomized controlled trials. Transplantation. 2009; 88: 7-18, 2009.

[44] Vlahakos DV, Canzanello VJ, Madaio MP, Madias NE. Enalapril-associated anemia in renal transplant recipients treated for hypertension. Am J Kidney Dis. 1991;17:199-205.

[45] Curtis JJ, Luke RG, Whelchel JD, et al. Inhibition of angiotensin-converting enzyme in renal-transplant recipients with hypertension. N Engl J Med. 1983 17;308:377-81.

[46] Andres A, Morales E, Morales JM, et al. Efficacy and safety of valsartan, an angiotensin II receptor antagonist, in hypertension after renal transplantation: a randomized multi-center study. Transplant Proc. 2006; 38:2419-23.

[47] Kornerup HJ, Pedersen EB, Fjeldborg O. Kidney transplant artery stenosis. Interrelationship between blood pressure, kidney function, renin-aldosterone system and body sodium content. Proc Eur Dial Transplant Assoc. 1977;14:377-85.

[48] del Castillo D, Campistol JM, Guirado L, et al. Efficacy and safety of losartan in the treatment of hypertension in renal transplant recipients. Kidney Int Suppl. 1998;68:S135-9.

[49] Heinze G, Mitterbauer C, Regele H, et al. Angiotensin-converting enzyme inhibitor or angiotensin II type 1 receptor antagonist therapy is associated with prolonged patient and graft survival after renal transplantation. J Am Soc Nephrol. 2006;17:889-99.

[50] Traindl O, Falger S, Reading S, et al. The effects of lisinopril on renal function in proteinuric renal transplant recipients. Transplantation. 1993;55:1309-13.

[51] el-Agroudy AE, Hassan NA, Foda MA, et al. Effect of angiotensin II receptor blocker on plasma levels of TGF-beta 1 and interstitial fibrosis in hypertensive kidney transplant patients. Am J Nephrol. 2003;23:300-6.

[52] Weir MR. Providing end-organ protection with renin-angiotensin system inhibition: the evidence so far. J Clin Hypertens (Greenwich) 2006; 8: 99-105.

[53] Philipp T, Martinez F, Geiger H, et al. Candesartan improves blood pressure control and reduces proteinuria in renal transplant recipients: Results from SECRET. Nephrol Dial Transplant. 2010; 25: 967-976.

[54] Nouri-Majalan N, Ghafari A, Moghaddasi S. Effect of angiotensin II type-1 receptor blockers on stable allograft kidneys: Prospective randomized study. Transplant Proc. 2009; 41: 2832-2834.

[55] Paoletti E, Cassottana P, Amidone M et al.: ACE inhibitors and persistent left ventricular hypertrophy after renal transplantation: a randomized clinical trial. Am J Kidney Dis 50:133-142, 2007.

[56] Hiremath S, Fergusson D, Doucette S, Mulay AV, Knoll GA. Renin angiotensin system blockade in kidney transplantation: a systematic review of the evidence. Am J Transplant 2007; 7: 2350-60.

[57] Cieciura T, Senatorski G, Rell K, Baczkowska T, Paczek L, Gradowska L, et al. Influence of angiotensin-converting enzyme inhibitor treatment of the carotid

artery intima-media complex in renal allograft recipients. Transplant Proc 2000Sep; 32:1335-6.
[58] Premasathian NC, Muehrer R, Brazy PC, Pirsch JD, Becker BN. Blood pressure control in kidney transplantation: therapeutic implications. J Hum Hypertens. 2004; 18: 871-7.
[59] Tylicki L, Biedunkiewicz B, Chamienia A, et al. Randomized placebo-controlled study on the effects of losartan and carvedilol on albuminuria in renal transplant recipients. 2006; Transplantation. 81: 52-56.
[60] Suwelack B, Gerhardt U, Hausberg M, Rahn K, Hohage H. Comparison of quinipril versus atenolol: Effects on blood pressure and cardiac mass after renal transplantation. American Journal Cardiology 2000; 86: 583-585.
[61] Hausberg M, Barenbrock M, Hohage H, et al. ACE inhibitor versus beta-blocker for the treatment of hypertension in renal allograft recipients. Hypertension. 1999; 33: 862-8.
[62] Ruggenenti P, Perico N, Mosconi L, et al. Calcium channel blockers protect transplant patients from cyclosporine-induced daily renal hypoperfusion. Kidney Int. 1993; 43: 706-11.
[63] Curtis J, Bateman F. Use of prazosin in management of hypertension in patients with chronic renal failure and in renal transplant recipients. British Med J. 1975; 4: 432-434.
[64] Martinez-Castelao A, Hueso M, Sanz V, et al. Treatment of hypertension after renal transplantation: Long-term efficacy of verapamil, enalapril, and doxazosin. Kidney Int. 1998; 68: S-130-S-134.

16

Diagnosis and Treatment of Status Epilepticus in a Pediatric Renal Recipient

Gao Hong-jun, Luo xiangdong, Liang Taisheng, Liang Fangfang et al.
Department of Transfusion Research, The Rui Kang Affiliated Hospital of Guangxi Traditional Chinese Medical University, Nanning, China

1. Introduction

Organ transplant traces its origins to a landmark operation by Murray in Boston in 1954 in which an identical twin received a donated sibling kidney. Since that seminal procedure, advances in tissue matching, improvements in surgical technique, and new and more-powerful immunosuppressive agents have increased the number and types of transplants that can be done. Advances in immunology and transplant technique have allowed longer survival for transplant recipients, but this has resulted in the emergence of several neurologic problems.

The kidney is the most frequently transplanted organ with more than 10 000 transplants occurring per year worldwide. Since that historic operation, kidney transplants have developed into the best-accepted therapy for most causes of end-stage renal failure. The 1-year survival rate is close to 100%, with an 85% to 95% graft survival rate. However, despite these advances, neurologic complications after renal transplants occur approximately 30% of the time . Several characteristics of renal transplant patients make overall complication rates in these persons different from those of other organ transplant recipients. Many renal transplant patients have some degree of vascular compromise either as a result of their underlying disease (eg, hypertension, diabetes) or because of emboli associated with underlying atherosclerosis or heart disease. After transplant, neurologic complications may develop secondary to the transplant itself, the immunosuppressive agent, or a previously known organ parenchymal failure.Under the effect of immunosuppression and other factors, renal transplant recipients are likely to be afflicted with epilepsy, the attack rate of which can reach almost 20% among pediatric patients. However, at present there are insufficient statistics to explain the cause of this danger.[1] Status epilepticus, also called grand mal seizures, can have a serious effect on the prognosis of renal transplant recipients. In particular, the first few attacks after kidney transplantation may have a serious effect on renal transplant recipients.

2. Briefing of case history

2.1 Object

A 17-year-old female patient was hospitalized because of dizziness and fatigue of more than 2 months' duration and with no obvious precipitating factor. Without timely treatment, she soon experienced syncope. She was hospitalized and examined, judged to have high blood pressure and a serum creatinine (SCr) level of 1374.9 μmmol/L, diagnosed with chronic glomerulonephritis and uremia, and treated with hemodialysis.

2.2 Preoperative diagnosis and treatment

After being hospitalized, the patient was treated with regular hemodialysis and underwent a series of preoperative therapeutic measures including blood pressure control, anemia improvement, and weight control. On the 40th preoperative day, the patient developed acute loss of consciousness, expressionless eyes, foaming at the mouth, and convulsion of the limbs, all of which lasted for about 5 min. Cerebral MRI was performed, but no abnormalities were detected. The patient was then diagnosed with symptomatic epilepsy. Carbamazepine was initially administered at a dosage of 0.1 g twice a day; the concentration was checked at regular intervals to adjust the dosage. After 2 weeks, the patient was treated with maintenance therapy at a dosage of 0.1 g once a day. This therapy was successful and the patient was never again afflicted with epilepsy. The patient confirmed that there had been no record of epilepsy in her previous case history.

2.3 Surgery

Renal transplantation was performed. The transplanted kidney secreted urine normally during establishment of its blood supply, but the postoperative urine amount gradually decreased until it reached a low of only 368 mL at the 14th postoperative hour. Ten hours postoperatively, reversed blood flow was observed in the transplant renal vein by color Doppler ultrasound, which suggested the presence of renal vein thrombosis (RVT). Thus, removal of the RVT was immediately implemented. After the operation, the patient was treated with urokinase thrombolysis and heparin anticoagulant therapy. As a result, transplant renal function rapidly returned to normal with urine volume maintaining a level of 4000 to 5000 mL/d and no worsening of the creatinine level. The patient was not disturbed and experienced no discomfort.

2.4 The patient's postoperative condition

2.4.1 Conditions on postoperative days 3 and 4

During these 2 days, the general condition of the patient was well and she was able to perform the Q & A. With the exception of pain associated with the surgical incision, the patient reported no discomfort. Urine volume was normal, being maintained at approximately 5000 mL/d. The heparin anticoagulant therapy was performed with a continuous infusion of liquaemin for 24 h. On the fourth postoperative day, anticoagulation therapy was stopped based on PT and APTT levels, and conventional postoperative antirejection therapy was implemented.

The application of immunosuppressants: Clinical use immunosuppressive often need to use a combination of, in order to improve the treatment effect, at the same time could reduce harmful side effects. Currently renal transplantation is relatively commonly used combination for: cyclopsorin or tacrolimus + azathioprine or? For Macaulay phenolic ester + laser

Meat.this one IST tacrolimus (FK506) + mycophenolate mofetil (MMF) + prednisone was implemented postoperatively. Tacrolimus (FK506) is from streptomycestsknbaenisis actinomycete glycolysis extracted a productKind of 23 ring big ring lactone antibiotics, which has strong immunosuppression function, its strength is about the meal A ring spore 50 to 100 times. mouthTake quickly absorb, main absorption parts in small intestine, absorption process similar ring spore meal A. Blood drug peak concentration appeared in oral within 0.5 ~ 3Hours, half-life 3.5 to 40.5 hours, average 8.7 hours, mainly by liver P4503A cell metabolism, by bravery pigment systemJuice and urinary excretion. Mainly by inhibiting intracellular calcium and calcium calmodulin and dependence on serine/threonine phosphatase neural calcium protein(the activation, blocking calcineurin) IL - 2 gene transcription, inhibiting cell activation. Oral starting dose for0.1 ~ 0.3 mg/kg d.), then according to the blood drug concentration to make adjustments. Valley value concentration 1 months for 8 ~ 12ng/ml, Within 6 ~ 8ng/ml, later maintain in 4 ~ 6ng/ml above. FK506 common side effects have diabetes, neurological side effects (including tremor, insomnia, limb abnormalities, etc), and kidney Toxicity, gastrointestinal reaction. MMF oral after being absorbed, quickly, being exactly convert bioactive Mycophenolate (MPA), plasma can't detect MMF, average oral bioavailability nearly 94%, MPA in liver be metabolized to MPAG rkatsiteli grapes (MPA), renal excretion through, MPA half-life nearly 18 hours. MPA is single phosphate hypoxanthine dehydrogenase (IMPDH) reversible, a non-competitive inhibitors, restrain guanine nucleotide classic synthesis methods, lymphocyte proliferation is blocked in the cell cycle S period, thus giving full play of lymphocyte immunosuppression effect. MMF Aza alternative medicine as often and ring spore meal A or tacrolimus, corticosteroids, dose doxycline for 0.5 g ~ 1.0 g/times every oral 2 times. MMF major adverse reaction was gastrointestinal reaction and hematopoietic system of toxic (leukopenia, thrombocytopenia).

2.4.2 Conditions on postoperative days 5 to 11

At 4:30 a.m. on the fifth day, the patient experienced acute paroxysmal convulsions of her lower right extremity with no obvious precipitating factor; the convulsions subsequently spread to both upper and lower extremities. Her entire body was afflicted with persistent tonic convulsions and she experienced loss of consciousness, expressionless eyes, frothing at the mouth, and gatism, all of which lasted approximately 2 min. The patient was given a pressure pad to protect her tongue and was treated with intravenous and luminal intramuscular injections of diazepam and oral carbamazepine, which had no obvious effect. The patient experienced the aforementioned typical signs of epilepsy at intervals ranging from 30 min to 2 h. These typical epileptic seizures occurred 10 times in 24 h. Given the frequency of status epilepticus and the unusually severe drug effect, the patient underwent a neurological consultation and was treated with a continuous intravenous drip of 500 mL 5% glucose + 100 mg diazepam at 10 mL/h. The patient fell into somnolence and her symptoms improved. During treatment with diazepam, although no typical epileptic attacks occurred, atypical epileptic seizures occurred 10 times in the form of twitching of the corners of the mouth and right upper extremity. On the sixth postoperative day, there were still no typical epileptic attacks with continuous use of diazepam. With a decreasing dose of diazepam, the patient was in a superficial coma, afflicted with hypomyotonia, and had an inability to move the right side of her body. A head CT scan revealed a nodule with an unclear outline in the left frontal lobe, around which patches of edema were observed. Patches of edema were also observed in the right semioval center, and the left tricorn was narrowed by the pressure. The midline shifted toward the left, resulting in edema of the brain tissue.(Fig1.2.3)

The patient's tranquilization was continued, and she was treated for dehydration and diuresis and given supportive therapy for the right side of her body. From the seventh postoperative day, the patient was in a lighter comatose state but was afflicted with type 1 respiratory failure and pulmonary infection. Thus, she was given a breathing machine and anti-infective treatment.

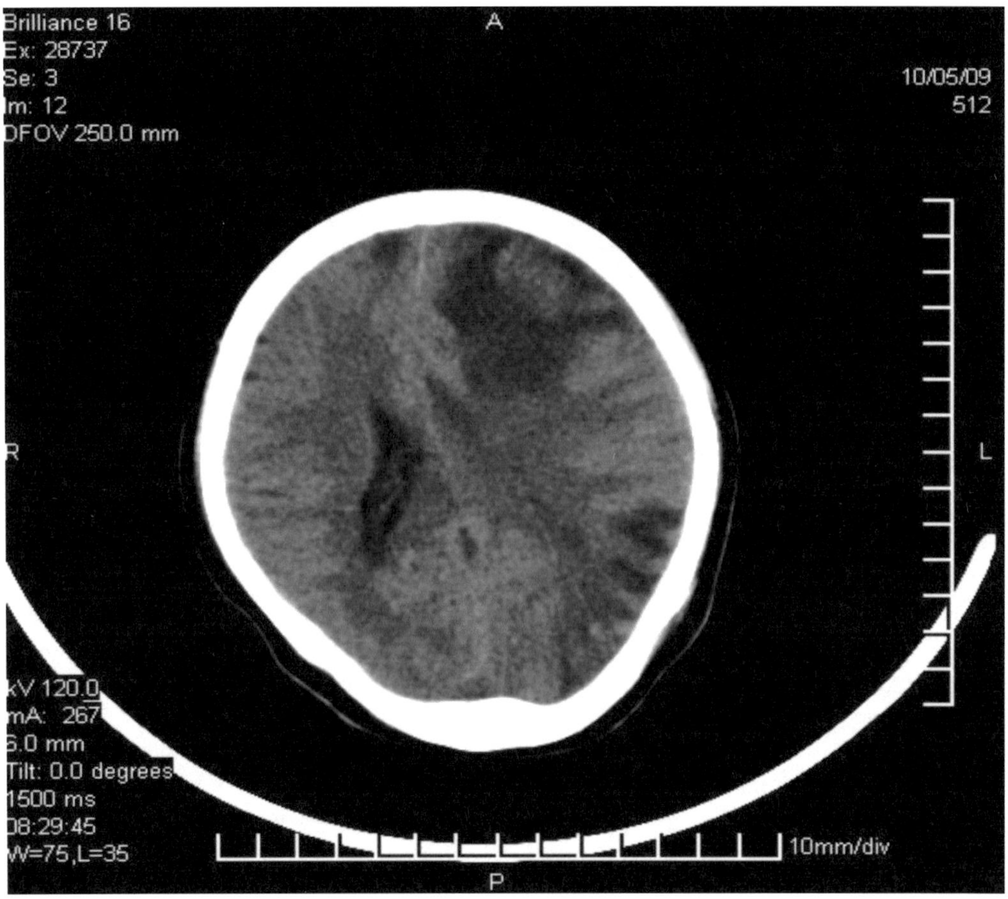

Fig 1.

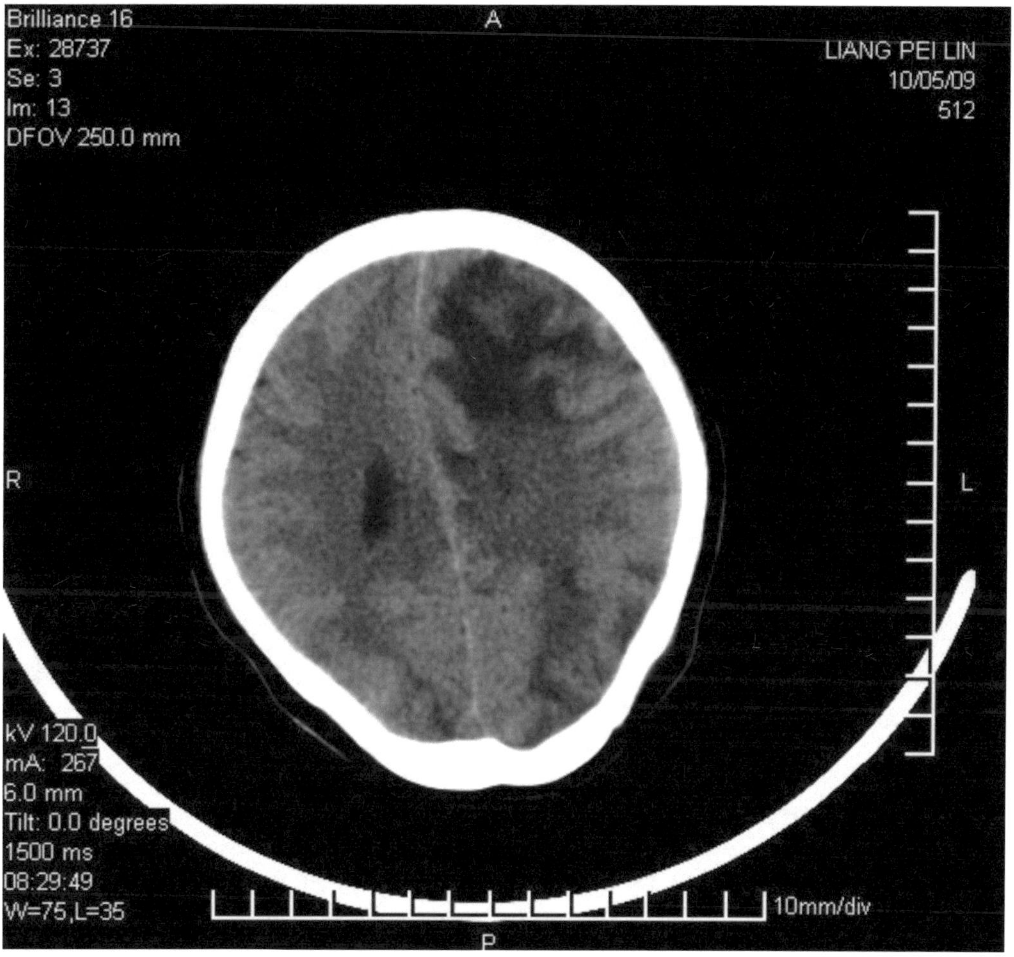
Brilliance 16
Ex: 28737
Se: 3
Im: 13
DFOV 250.0 mm
A
LIANG PEI LIN
10/05/09
512
R
L
kV 120.0
mA: 267
6.0 mm
Tilt: 0.0 degrees
1500 ms
08:29:49
W=75,L=35
10mm/div
P

Fig. 2.

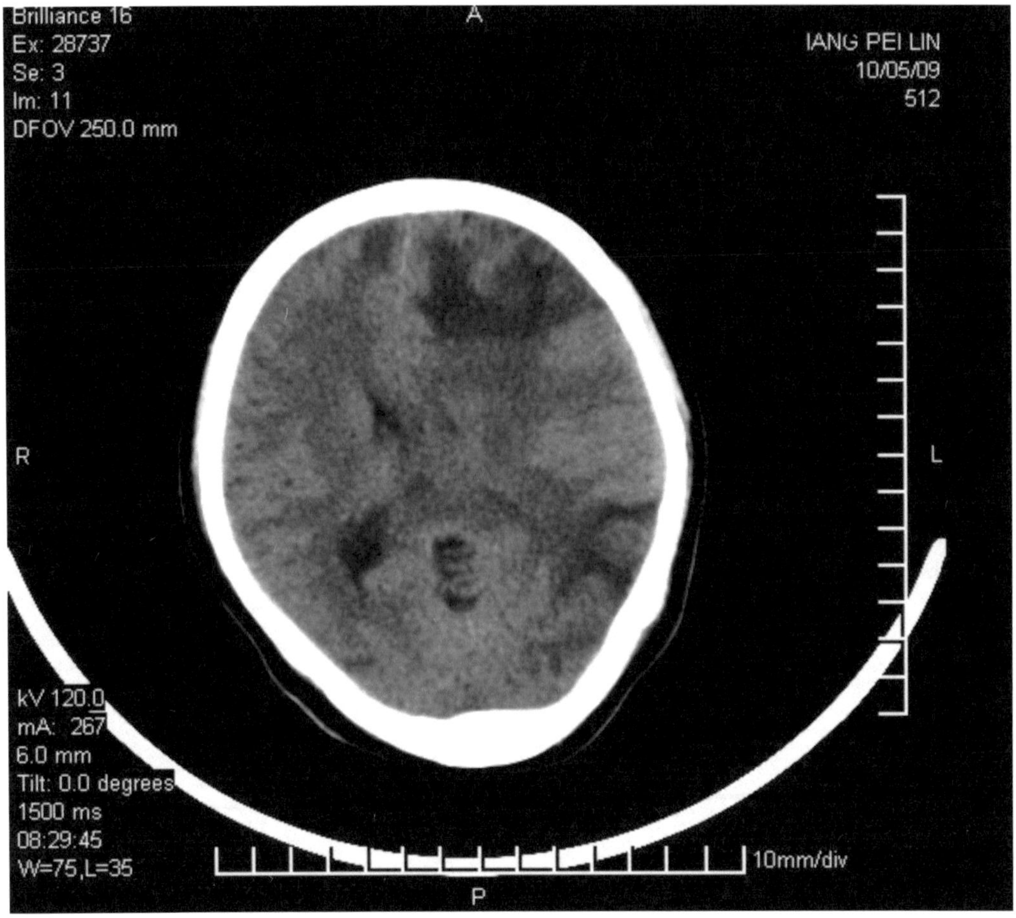

Fig. 3.

2.4.3 Conditions on postoperative days 12 to 30.

On the 12th postoperative day, the patient's condition improved with a gradual recovery of consciousness and myodynamia of the extremities. The muscular tension level of the left extremities was low, while that of the right was zero. On the 15th postoperative day, the breathing machine was removed; the muscular tension level of the left extremities returned to normal, and that of the right was five. Head CT revealed large patches of low-density areas in the semioval center of the left frontal lobe, and the left ventricle was under a small amount of pressure(Fig4.5).The patient was able to perform early ambulation, but discordance of the right extremities was still observed. Head CT on the 27th postoperative day revealed the persistence of irregular low-density areas in the left frontal lobe, and the left frontal angle had moved back slightly. With normal movement of the extremities, an almost-normal muscular tension level of the left extremities, and elimination of the pulmonary infection, the patient was cured and discharged from the hospital.

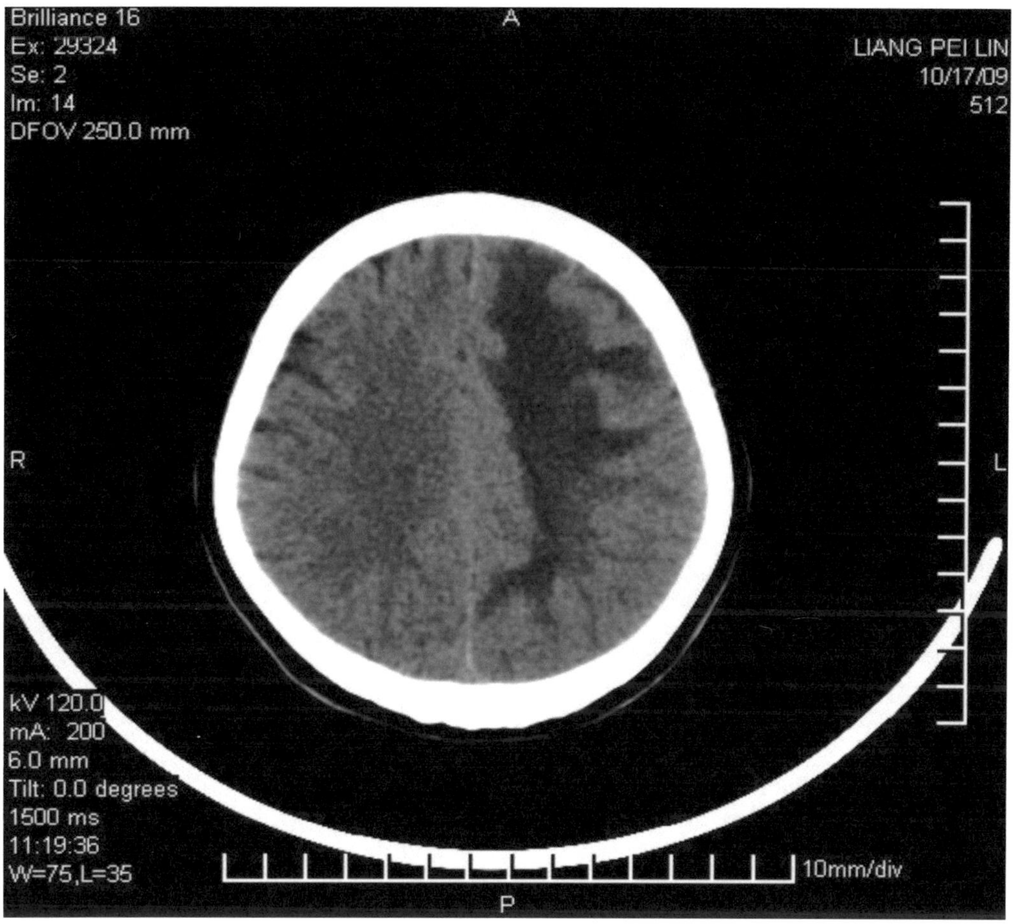
Brilliance 16
Ex: 29324
Se: 2
Im: 14
DFOV 250.0 mm
A
LIANG PEI LIN
10/17/09
512
R
L
kV 120.0
mA: 200
6.0 mm
Tilt: 0.0 degrees
1500 ms
11:19:36
W=75,L=35
10mm/div
P

Fig. 4.

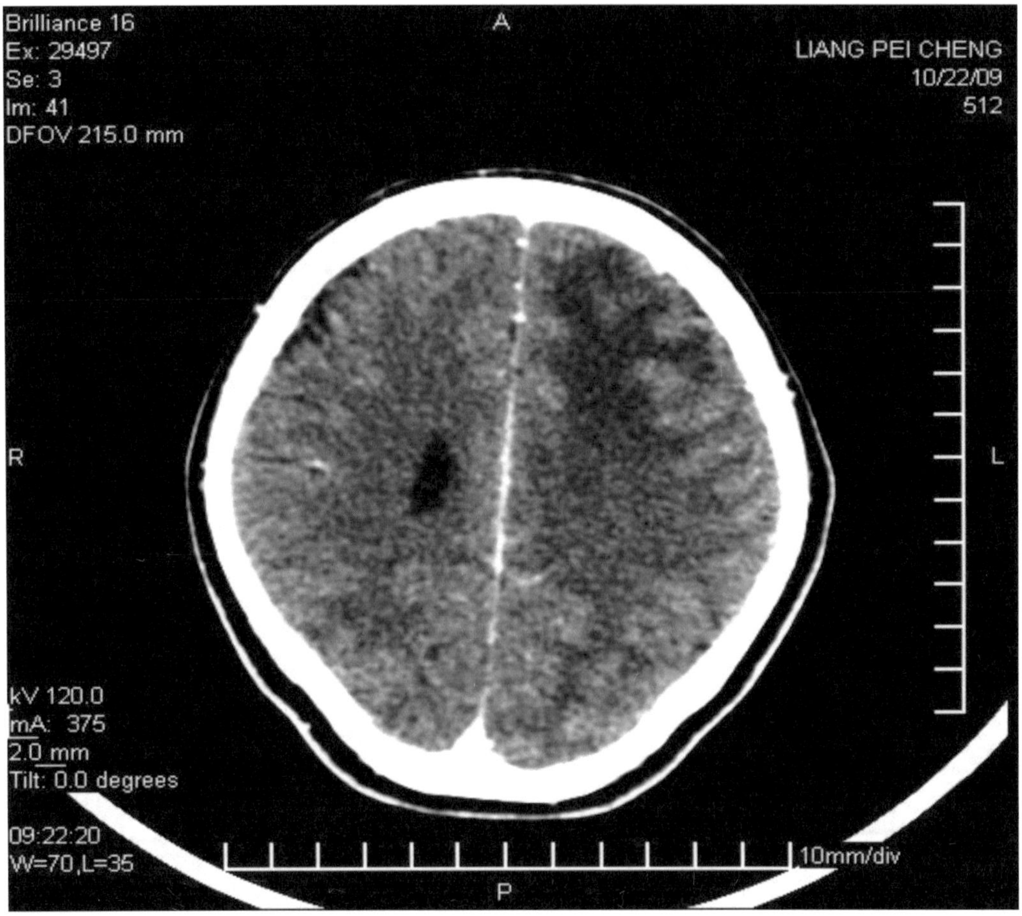

Fig. 5.

2.4.4 Follow-ups from hospital discharge to present.

At present, the general health condition, spirit, and appetite are good; the transplant kidney functions well; no neurological sequelae remain; and no abnormalities exist on head CT.

2.5 The application of immunosuppressive agents.

One aliquot of rabbit antihuman thymocyte globulin was used on the day of the operation, and another was used the following day. During the operation, 350 mg methylprednisolone was administered *via* intravenous injection, and in the following 3 days, the use of methylprednisolone was continued at a dosage of 350 mg in the first 2 days and 200 mg on the third day. IST tacrolimus (FK506) + mycophenolate mofetil (MMF) + prednisone was implemented postoperatively. Oral administration of FK506 at a dosage of 5 to 7 mg/kg/d and MMF at a dosage of 0.5 mg twice daily was begun one day preoperatively. Because of carbamazepine's effect on FK506, the amount of FK506 was increased to achieve the target concentration.

2.6 Others Case report form view

Germany T. Manz report:

A 56-year-old man with end-stage renal disease due to autosomal dominant polycystic kidney disease had continuous ambulatory peritoneal dialysis for 2 years and intermittent haemodialysis for an additional 5 years. In March 1998 his 49-year-old wife donated a kidney to him for renal transplantation. Immunosuppressive treatment consisted of prednisone, antithymocyte globulin, cyclosporin, and mycophenolate mofetil. There was delayed recovery of transplant function because of cyclosporin toxicity 1 month after transplantation. Cyclosporin dosage was reduced and mycophenolate dosage was tapered to 2 g/day for 1 month. Four months after transplantation cyclosporin was replaced by tacrolimus because of gingival hyperplasia and a raised serum creatinine. The blood levels of cyclosporin and tacrolimus were within therapeutic ranges. The patient's course was unremarkable until 6 months post-transplantation, when his condition deteriorated progressively, and was complicated by drowsiness, headache, impaired co-ordination and speech impediment. Axial T2 and post-contrast T1 MRI scans (Figure 1•) showed multiple 'target'-appearing ring enhancing masses in the right basal ganglia with slightly perifocal vasogenic oedema, and left frontal subcortical with central hypodensity consistent with necrosis.

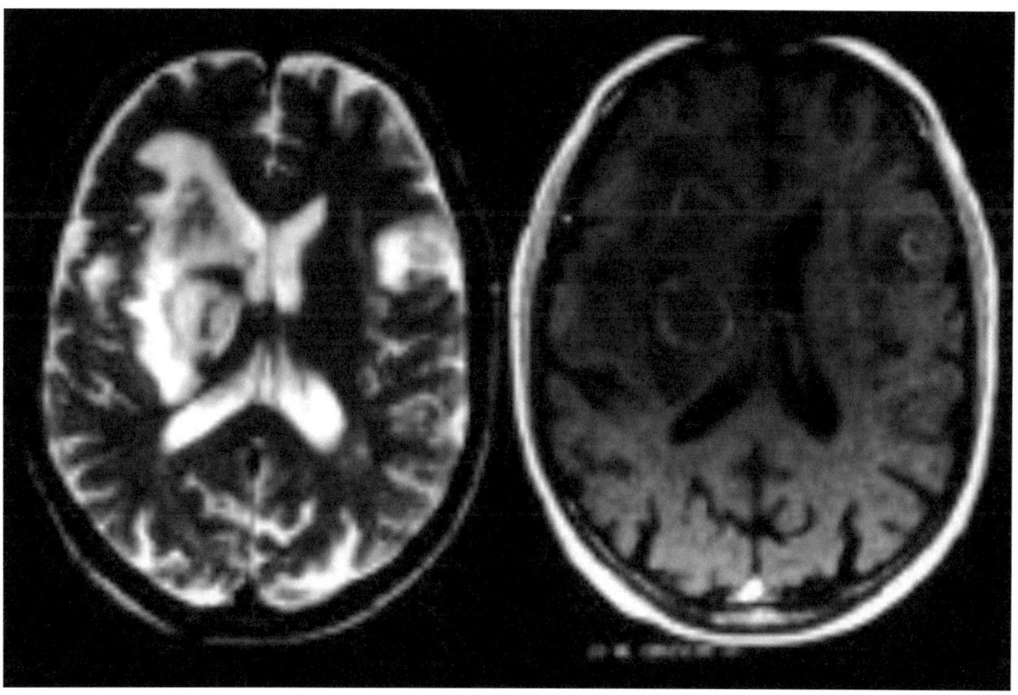

Fig. 6. Axial T2 and post-contrast T1 MR scans on admission show multiple 'target'-appearing ring enhancing masses in right basal ganglia with perifocal vasogenic oedema, and left frontal subcortical with central hypodensity consistent with necrosis.

London 's Marjan Chegounchi also report:

A 42 years old man of mixed race with an African father had originally presented with severe hypertension and renal failure. Renal biopsy showed severe vascular pathology but no primary glomerular disease. He underwent a cadaver renal transplant (111 mis-match) in July 2002 and received tacrolimus and prednisolone. The kidney functioned immediately. On day 8 (d8) with a plasma creatinine that had not fallen below 180 µmol/l and tacrolimus concentration consistently 15 ng/ml (target concentration 10–15 ng/ml), he had a renal biopsy that showed acute rejection (Banff IIa). He received intravenous methylprednisolone and Cellcept 500 mg bd was added. The creatinine fell to125 µmol/l.
Eight weeks after transplantation (d59) he was admitted to another hospital following a road traffic accident. Whilst driving he had experienced sudden onset of drowsiness with headache and numbness in his fingers and toes. He temporarily lost consciousness and collided with another vehicle. Computed tomography (CT) scan of his head showed no abnormality and he was discharged home the following day. The following week he was readmitted (d66). He had a month history of persistent frontal headache, relieved by simple analgesic. He was intermittently confused and unable to recognize members of his family. This was associated with unsteady gait and slurred speech. During these episodes he appeared withdrawn and somewhat blank. Episodes lasted 1–8 hours. He had had one grand mal convulsion witnessed at home. There was no previous history or family history of neurological disease. On admission, he was afebrile with blood pressure of 120/75. He had no focal neurological deficit and no meningism. Cerebrospinal fluid (CSF) examination was normal: microscopy, Gram and Zeihl-Nielson stain, cytology, virology, glucose, protein, cultures and India-ink for cryptococcus were unremarkable. Blood cultures, blood count, Chest and skull X-ray were normal. Electroencephalogram (EEG) revealed sharpening and spikes independently in both temporal lobes consistent with temporal lobe partial epilepsy. The magnetic resonance imaging (MRI) of brain showed multiple areas of low signal intensity (T1-weighted FLASH) in the pons, medulla oblongata, basal ganglia and also in the cerebral hemispheres (figure 1). These lesions were reported as 'consistent with small vessel ischemia secondary to hypertension'. The diagnosis of partial epilepsy was made and he was started on lamotrigine. His renal function remained stable. Magnesium was consistently at the lower limit of normal range 0.6 mmol/l (normal range 0.6 - 1.1 mmol/l), cholesterol 4.5 mmol/l (2.3 - 5.2 mmol/l). The tacrolimus level was kept within range 8–15 ng/dl.
He was readmitted three weeks later (d113) having had further fits. He was agitated, psychotic with visual hallucinations. No focal neurology was found and he rapidly became obtunded with a Glasgow coma score of 6–8/15. Repeat CT and MRI were unchanged. Lumbar puncture revealed high open pressure and raised protein 1.3 g/l but CSF analysis was otherwise normal. Repeat EEG was consisted with complex partial status epileptics with "frequent frontal notched theta activity". He was treated with antibiotic and antifungal agents and phenytoin infusion. There was no improvement in his condition and a diagnosis of tacrolimus-induced neurotoxicity was made (tacrolimus 10 ng/ml). Tacrolimus was switched to cyclosporine. Over the next few days he showed rapid and progressive improvement. He recovered fully and was discharge home. He has had no further seizure activity nor neurological symptoms since tacrolimus had been stopped. He continues to do well. A MRI scan performed in 2004 no longer showed the earlier lesions.

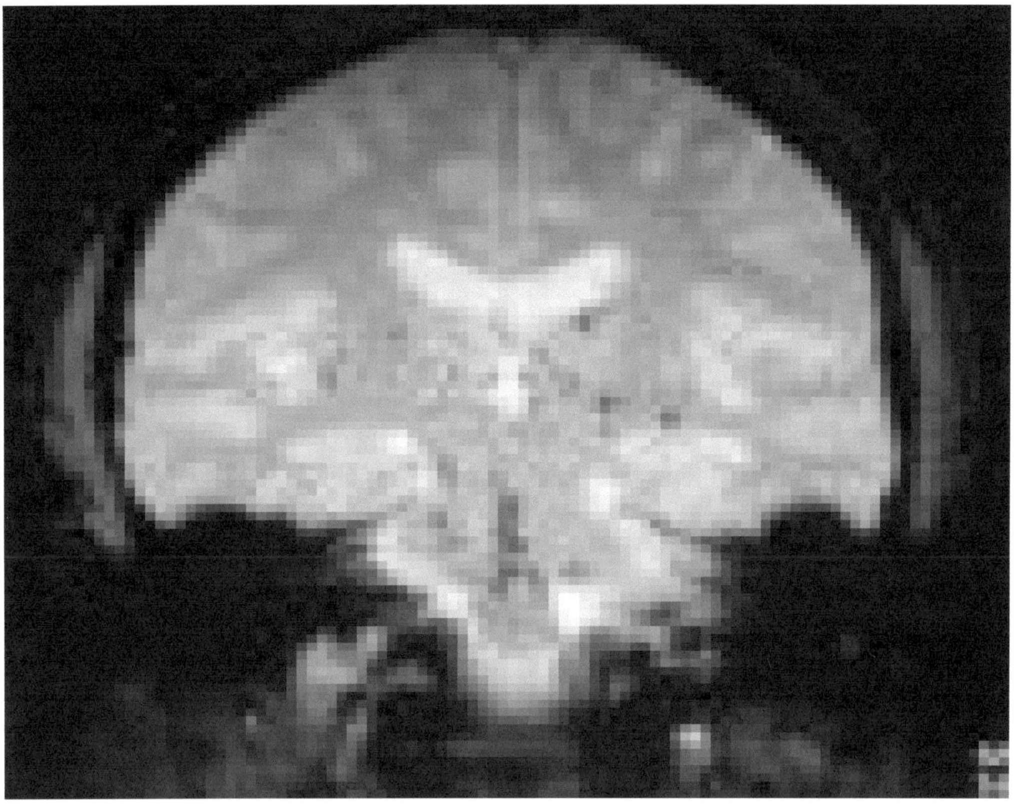

Fig. 7. MRI Brain. There are multiple areas of low signal intensity in the pons, medulla oblongata, basal ganglia and also in the cerebral hemispheres (MRI Brain T1).

3. Discussion

Status epilepticus is a pathological condition characterized by continuous and frequent seizures and is classified as a neurological emergency. According to conventional standards, status epilepticus consists of attacks lasting more than 30 min or repeated attacks during which consciousness is lost. New diagnostic criteria have recently been proposed by Lowenstein and other experts:[1] among adults and children older than 5 years of age, generalized convulsive status epilepticus refers to a continuous seizure of more than 5 minutes in duration or more than 2 seizures at a time; during the seizure, the patient's consciousness is lost. A common clinical, and the most dangerous, form is the persistent state of the generalized tonic-clonic seizure. Symptoms are a sudden loss of consciousness, muscle twitching, foaming (sometimes with blood) at the mouth, frequent apnea, cyanosis, dilated pupils, a diminishing papillary light response, and gatism. The seizure is long in duration or occurs repeatedly. If not quickly controlled, it may be life-threatening or cause perpetual brain damage. Status epilepticus is mainly caused by improper drug decrease and withdrawal, sudden changes in medication, or nonstandard times of antiepileptic treatment administration; it may also be induced by infection, mental factors, fatigue, pregnancy, drinking, and other causes. Infection, birth injury, and congenital malformation are the main causes in infancy and childhood. Common causes in young adults include traumatic brain injury, intracranial masses, and parasitic diseases, while stroke, brain tumors, trauma, and degenerative diseases are the main causes in the elderly.

Nilgul Yardimci 's report: they evaluated 132 patients who had undergone a renal transplant. Ninety-seven of the recipients (73.5%) were men and 35 (26.5%) were women (M:F=2.77:1). The mean age of the recipients was 34.32 /0.90 years (range, 18-66 years). One hundred forty-two transplants were done; 10 patients had a retransplant. Among these 142 transplants, 36 grafts (25%) were taken from a deceased donor, and 106 (75%) were obtained from a living donor (deceased:living donor=1:3).

The most common renal diseases leading to renal transplant were hypertension (19 patients, 14.4%), vesicoureteral reflux (15 patients, 11.4%), and glomerulonephritis (membranoproliferative, 7 patients [5.3%]; mesangioproliferative, 6 patients [4.5%], and focal segmental glomerulosclerosis, 10 patients [7.6%]). In 28 patients (21.2%), the cause of end-stage renal disease was unknown. The mean duration of renal disease before renal transplant was 63.11 ?5.74 months (range, 1-444 months); of these, 115 had received dialysis for a mean of 35.57 ?3.24 months (range, 1-156 months). Thirty-five patients (26.5%) had received continuous ambulatory peritoneal dialysis for a mean of 24.68 ?3.6 months (range, 1-84 months; total, 863.96 months); 89 patients (67.4%) had undergone hemodialysis for a mean of 36.26 ?3.70 months (range, 1-144 months; total, 3227.72 months). Seventeen patients had not received any type of dialysis. At the time of transplant, 103 patients (78%) had hypertension, and 21 (15.9%) had hyperlipidemia. The mean follow-up was 17.26 ?0.89 months (range, 2 weeks to 40 months; total, 2279.50 months).

Neurologic complications were observed in 18 patients (13.6%; mean age, 33.83 ?2.37 years; range, 20-59 years). Those 18 individuals experienced a total of 20 episodes of neurologic complications (2 separate episodes in 2 of the patients). The observed 20 neurologic complications were classified as follows: headache (10 episodes; 55.6%), seizure (3 episodes; 16.7%), cerebral infarcts (2 episodes; 11.1%), tremor (2 episodes; 11.1%), encephalopathy (1 episode; 5.6%), sinus thrombosis (1 episode; 5.6%), and posterior leukoencephalopathy syndrome (1 episode, 5.6%). Immunosuppressive agents were the primary cause of 16 of the 20 episodes of neurologic complications. Encephalopathy due to hyponatremia (1 patient), sinus thrombosis (1 patient), and stroke (2 patients) were the other causes of neurologic complications.

Of the 10 episodes with headache, 7 patients had been receiving cyclosporine for a mean of 6.04 ?2.99 months (range, 2 days to 23 months), 2 patients had been receiving sirolimus for a mean of 10.5 ?6.5 months (range, 4-17 months), and 1 patient had been receiving tacrolimus for 7 months. When cyclosporine blood levels of these patients with headache were analyzed, cyclosporine concentrations were within normal limits in 4 patients, and they were higher than normal in 3 patients. Tacrolimus and sirolimus blood concentrations all were within normal limits in the other patients with headache.

observed seizures in 3 patients, each of whom had been receiving cyclosporine, tacrolimus, or sirolimus. None of the patients had seizures before the transplant. The first patient had a seizure during the first month after transplant, and the blood concentration of cyclosporine was 305 ng/mL. The second patient had been taking tacrolimus for 1 month; the blood level at the time seizure occurred was 19 ng/mL. The third patient had been taking sirolimus for 3 months; the concentration at the time of the symptom was 17 ng/mL. At the time of the seizure, there were no electrolyte disturbances or clinical events that could precipitate seizures. Functioning of the kidneys was within normal limits. Plasma sodium and magnesium concentrations were within normal ranges. None of these patients had a fever,

and none was on any other medication that could cause a convulsion. The results of brain magnetic resonance imaging scans all were normal, with no evidence of a mass lesion.
Tremor developed in 2 patients who had been taking cyclosporine for a mean of 0.62 /0.37 months (range, 1 week to 1 month). The cyclosporine blood concentration was within normal limits in 1 patient and higher than normal in the other. However, tremor was so severe in these patients, that cyclosporine had to be switched to another calcineurin inhibitor. One patient developed posterior leukoencephalopathy syndrome after taking tacrolimus for 11 months (blood concentration, 5.5 ng/mL). The patient clinically presented with altered mental functioning and seizures associated with symmetrical, posterior, hemispheric edema, which was apparend on cranial magnetic resonance imaging.
We observed encephalopathy due to hyponatremia (118 mmol/L) in 1 patient. Cerebrovascular infarcts were present in 2 patients, and a sinus thrombosis was observed in 1 patient.
Neural complications in renal transplant recipients are likely to occur at any stage of the postoperative period and have an incidence of 30% to 60%. Both the neural complication incidence and the mortality have a great effect on renal transplant recipients.[2-4] The characteristics of neural complications caused by renal transplants are distinct from those caused by other organ transplants, and include limb tremors, insomnia, dysphoria, coma, and convulsions. Epilepsy also occurs among renal transplant recipients,[5] and the incidences among adults and children are 11.4% and 17.6%, respectively.[6] In cats with end-stage renal failure that have undergone renal transplants, the incidence of epilepsy may reach 28.9%.[7]
Many factors can lead to epilepsy after transplantation, among which electrolyte disturbance is the most common.[8] Characteristics include early epileptic attacks, usually in the 72nd postoperative hour; a high urine volume at 10 000 mL/d; rapid recovery of renal function; and the return of SCr to a normal level at the first epileptic attack. Epilepsy can be easily controlled by correction of electrolyte disturbances with supplementation of blood calcium, magnesium, and sodium and intramuscular injections of diazepam. However, the causes of status epilepticus might be linked to withdrawal of antiepileptic drugs (AEDs) and intoxication[9] of the calcineurin inhibitors cyclosporine and tacrolimus. Epilepsy can be caused by intoxication of cyclosporine and tacrolimus,[10] the incidences of which are 2% to 6%[11-14] and 5.6% to 11.6%.[15] Antirejection therapy can be impacted by the use of larger doses of hormones, by which the patient's mental state can be changed and epilepsy can be easily triggered. This type of epilepsy has more severe symptoms, easily causes acute respiratory distress syndrome, and maintains a high mortality; it is also very difficult to cure, often requiring tracheal cannulation and positive end-expiratory pressure with a breathing machine. The aforementioned patient was afflicted by epilepsy once during the month before the transplant. Because of AED withdrawal, the impact of MMP, and the use of tacrolimus, children and young adults with a history of epilepsy are afflicted with epilepsy more frequently, and its persistent state is caused by neurological diseases under the combined action of hormones and physiological changes. It was found by Gleeson through 3-year follow-ups of patients with epileptic seizures during the perioperative period during AED withdrawal, the patients were never afflicted with epilepsy.[16]
Many renal transplant patients have some degree of vascular compromise, either as a result of their underlying disease (hypertension, diabetes) or because of emboli associated with underlying atherosclerosis or heart disease (5). The most common posttransplant neurologic complications in this patient population are cerebrovascular events; these occur in

approximately 9% of all renal transplant patients. infarcts in 2 patients (1.5%). Stroke may occur in about 8% of renal transplant patients.

An increased risk of venous thromboembolism also has been demonstrated after renal transplant. Commonly reported sites have been deep vein thrombosis, pulmonary thromboembolism, and vascular thrombosis involving the graft. Cerebral venous thrombosis has not been reported thus far. assessed transverse sinus thrombosis in 1 patient (0.8%).Tremor is another common complication, which is frequently seen after transplant; sometimes present in up to 40% of patients . Tremor is mostly the consequence of immunosuppressive treatment. The most pronounced neurotoxic effect is induced by the calcineurin inhibitors, tacrolimus and cyclosporine. The spectrum of neurologic disturbances caused by calcineurin inhibitors ranges from mild symptoms such as paraesthesia, tremor, headache, or flushing, to severe changes that can cause a lethal outcome. In our study, we evaluated 2 patients (1.5%) with tremor while taking cyclosporine. To control tremor, the drug must be switched to another calcineurin inhibitor. In fact, tremor in most of the recipients is the result of immunosuppressive agents. However, if severity of the tremor is not significant and does not worsen the patient's quality of life, there is a tendency to ignore the symptom (because survival of the graft is the ultimate goal in immunosuppressive therapy). In the current study, we observed only 2 tremors; however, these were severe enough to warrant a change in the immunosuppressive protocol. The slight tremor in the other recipients probably had been underestimated in the patients' records.Posterior leukoencephalopathy syndrome is most commonly seen in patients with hypertensive encephalopathy, eclampsia, renal failure, or use of immunosuppressive agents (20). In the transplant population, posterior leukoencephalopathy synrome is a well-known complication of immunouppressive therapy with cyclosporine and tacrolimus . In the current study, we observed 1 patient (0.8%) with posterior leukoencephalopathy syndrome. *Posterior leukoencephalopathy syndrome* is a term first used by Hinchey and associates (20) to describe a group of disorders that present clinically with headache, seizures, visual disturbances, and altered mental function associated with symmetrical posterior hemispheric edema. The cause of posterior leukoencephalopathy syndrome is not fully undertood but is believed to be due to a breakdown in cerebral autoregulation that results in leakage of fluid into the interstitium, which is detected as vasogenic edema. (21) Encephalopathy is a severe adverse effect of cyclosporine and tacrolimus, occurring in approximately 5% of patients taking the drugs. These patients may present with a decreased level of consciousness, headache, dysarthria, depression, mania, cortical blindness, visual hallucinations, and seizures . (22)The syndrome is usually found in patients with elevated blood calcineurin inhibitor levels; however, other factors, such as hypoholesterolemia, hypomagnesemia, hypoatremia, high-dose steroids, hypertension, and uremia may be involved as well. We observed encephalopathy due to hyponatremia in 1 patient (0.8%); the encephalopathy resolved after the hyponatremia ameliorated. In the current study, we did not evaluate any malignancies or central nervous system infections that are other frequent causes of neurologic complications in transplant recipients.

The grand mal seizures after renal transplantation were usually serious. However, the patient was cured without neurological sequelae, and the transplant kidney recovered very well. Experience with this diagnosis and treatment regimen has been gained in the following 4 respects. First, while the patient's life must be saved, transplant renal function must be maintained and delayed graft function (DGF) must be prevented, which is the core of successful treatment. Changes in the patient's blood pressure and heart rate can be caused by epileptic seizures. In particular, status epilepticus has a more serious effect on the circulatory system, easily triggering DGF because of the adverse effect on transplant renal function. Once DGF has been triggered, the whole treatment will be more difficult. Second, accurate judgment of the causes of epilepsy is critical to effective diagnosis and treatment. Different causes, such as brain tumors, cerebrovascular accident, and drug-induced factors, require different treatments. However, the treatment should be simplified in case the patient's condition is complicated. Third, when epilepsy occurs during the perioperative period, immunosuppressive agents[17, 18] should be appropriately adjusted. Because of the interaction between AEDs and antirejection drugs, blood concentrations of cyclosporine and tacrolimus can be dramatically lowered by the carbamazepine. Thus, blood concentrations of carbamazepine and tacrolimus should be monitored so that the adjustment of immunosuppressive agents can be performed in time. Finally, comprehensive measures should be taken to prevent other complications and reduce adverse effects in the therapeutic process. Aspiration can easily be caused by seizures, and status epilepticus requires patients to stay in bed; both increase the possibility of pulmonary infection. In addition, central respiratory problems can be caused by severe cerebral problems. The importance of prevention and cure of pulmonary infection is determined by the complexity, refractory characteristics, and high mortality of pulmonary infection after transplant.

The improvement of surgical techniques of organ transplantation and specific nursing practices that can reduce mortality and morbidity make it possible to perform many organ transplantations. The postoperative period of organ transplantation mostly focuses on infection prevention and antirejection treatment. Most neural complications are atypical and have not been given enough attention. However, a certain amount of morbidity and mortality is still attributed to serious neural complications. On one hand, neural complications in some renal transplant recipients are caused by postoperative diseases. On the other hand, neurotoxicity caused by immunotherapy medication can also lead to a series of complications. The adverse effects of the immune overreaction to cyclosporine and tacrolimus should be noted.[19] Many factors, acting alone or in combination, can cause epileptic seizures after renal transplantation. Thus, for prevention and cure, great importance should be attached to comprehensive treatment. Drugs that can trigger epileptic seizures should be avoided. If epileptic seizures take place, the pathogenesis should be determined and symptomatic therapy begun.

4. References

[1] Lowenstein DH, Bleck TP, Macdonald RL. It's time to revise the defi-nition of status epilepticus. Epilepsia, 1999, 40 (1) : 120 - 122

[2] Bruno A, Adams HP Jr. Neurologic problems in renal transplant recipients. Neurol Clin. 1988;6:305-325.

[3] Mart ez AJ. The neuropathology of organ transplantation:comparison and contrast in 500 patients. Pathol Res Pract. 1998; 194:473-486.

[4] Schwechheimer K, Hashemian A. Neuropathologic findings after organ transplantation. An autopsy study. Gen Diagn Pathol. 1995;141:35-39.

[5] Hamiwka LD, Midgley JP, Hamiwka LA.Seizures in children after kidney transplantation: has the risk changed and can we predict who is at greatest risk? Pediatr Transplant. 2008 Aug;12(5):527-30.

[6] Awan A Q , Lewis MA , Postleth waite R J ,et al. Seizures fol-lowing renal transplantation in childhood. Pediatr-Nephrol ,1999 ,13 :275 - 279.
[7] Mathews K G, Gregory C R. Renal transplants in cats :66 cas-es. J Am Vet Med Assoc, 1997 ,211 :1432 - 1436.
[8] Wan Jun R., Zi Dong L, Xiao Ping W. 2 Cases of Epilepsy Tonic - Clonic Seizures after Renal Transplantation. Chinese Journal of Organ Transplantation.2002;23:235 - 235
[9] Patchell RA. Neurological complications of organ transplantation. Ann Neurol. 1994;36:688-703
[10] Appignani BA, Bhadelia RA, Blacklow SC, Wang AK, Roland SF, Freeman RBJ: Neuroimaging findings in patients on immunosuppressive therapy: experience with tacrolimus toxicity. *AJR Am J Roentgenol* 1996, 166:683-688.
[11] Racusen LC, Famiglio LM, Fivush BA, Olton DS, Solez K. Neurologic abnormalities and mortality in rats treated with cyclosporine A. Transplant Proc. 1988;20(suppl 3):934-936.
[12] Graham RM. Cyclosporine: mechanisms of action and toxicity. Cleve Clin J Med. 1994; 61:308-313.
[13] Gijtenbeek JM, van den Bent MJ, Vecht CJ. Cyclosporine neurotoxicity: a review. J Neurol. 1999;246:339-346.
[14] Walker RW, Brochstein JA. Neurologic complications of immunosuppressive agents. Neurol Clin. 1988;6:261-278
[15] Sevmis S, Karakayali H, Emiroglu R, Akkoc H, Haberal M. Tacrolimus-related seizure in the early postoperative period after liver transplantation. Transplant Proc. 2007;39:1211-12
[16] Gleeson JG, duPlessis AJ, Barnes PD, Riviello JJJ.Cyclosporin A acute encephalopathy and seizure syndrome in childhood: clinical features and risk of seizure recurrence. J Child Neurol 1998, 13:336-344
[17] Yardimci N, Colak T, Sevmis S, Benli S .Neurologic complications after renal transplant Exp Clin Transplant. 2008 Sep;6(3):224-8..
[18] Senzolo M, Ferronato C, Burra P.Neurologic complications after solid organ transplantation. Transpl Int. 2009 Mar;22(3):269-78.
[19] Yardimci N, Colak T, Sevmis S, Benli S.Neurologic complications after renal transplant. Exp Clin Transplant. 2008 Sep;6(3):224-8.
[20] Hinchey J, Chaves C, Appignani B, et al. A reversible posterior leukoencephalopathy syndrome. N Engl J Med. 1996;334:494-500.
[21] Mukherjee P, McKinstry RC. Reversible posterior leukoencephalopathy syndrome: evaluation with diffusion-tensor MR imaging. Radiology. 2001;219:756-765.
[22] Adams DH, Ponsford S, Gunson B, et al. Neurological complications following liver transplantation. Lancet. 1987;1:949-951.

Part 4

Graft Function

17

Chronic Allograft Nephropathy

Harzallah Kais
Faculty of Medicine of Tunis/Military Hospital of Tunis
Tunisia

1. Introduction

Since the first successful kidney transplantation in 1954 between Identical twins, a new modality to treat patients with terminal kidney insufficiency was born. Although the results in the first decades were modest, continuous development has characterized this captivating field. A major advance was the introduction of the new immunosuppressant cyclosporine A in the early 1980s. The fundament of its success was the aptitude to improve kidney graft survival significantly over the first year, and calcineurin inhibitors are the cornerstone of immunosuppression even in the present decade.
Chronic allograft nephropathy is a histopathological diagnosis used to denote features of chronic interstitial fibrosis and tubular atrophy within the renal allograft. It remains the most common cause of graft dysfunction and loss after renal transplantation.
The term Chronic allograft nephropathy was proposed in 1991, and it replaced the previously used term "chronic rejection". The intention was to unify chronic histological changes seen under light microscopy, such us interstitial fibrosis, tubular atrophy, transplant glomerulopathy and vasculopathy. The pathophysiology behind each of these features may nevertheless be different. The processes involved are approached by dividing them roughly into immunological and non-immunological factors, although they may be interrelated.
In this chapter we will discuss the histological features, the pathogenesis, the different etiologies and the therapeutic possibilities in cases of chronic allograft nephropathy.

2. Epidemiology of chronic allograft nephropathy

Prevalence of chronic allograft nephropathy at 2 years was reported in a prospective multicenter trial that compared cyclosporine against Tacrolimus (Solez et al., 1998), in which 72.3 % and 62.0 % of biopsies exhibited CAN, respectively. There was no difference in chronic histology between the therapeutic arms, but CAN at 2 years was associated with older donor age, early acute rejection, and episodes of acute CNI nephrotoxicity. Functional studies unfortunately underestimate significantly the incidence of histological graft injury. One study found that 94 % of grafts has histological evidence of interstitial fibrosis and tubular atrophy at 1 year (Nankivell et al., 2003). This same study found that much of the progressive chronic damage was related to Calcineurin inhibitors, even though the levels of these drugs had been maintained well within the defined target range.

3. Histopathology of chronic allograft nephropathy

Previously, chronic allograft rejection was considered the main aetiological factor for chronic graft loss, as features of cellular inflammatory immune infiltrates, identified on kidney biopsies, were suggestive of injury from immunological changes within the graft. This classification changed with the implementation of the Banff 97 working classification of renal allograft pathology criteria, which integrated features of the Chronic Allograft Damage Index (Racusen et al., 1999) and Cooperative Clinical Trials in Transplantation systems (Isonemi et al., 1994). This led to the standardization and semiquantification of these lesions. Then, the term chronic allograft nephropathy replaced chronic allograft rejection.

The histological features that define chronic allograft nephropathy in the kidney transplant allograft include interstitial fibrosis and tubular atrophy, as mentioned above, as well as features of glomerulosclerosis with an aspect of double contours in the glomerular basement membrane, arteriolar hyalinosis and arteriolosclerosis (Fig 1) (Nankivell et Chapman, 2006).

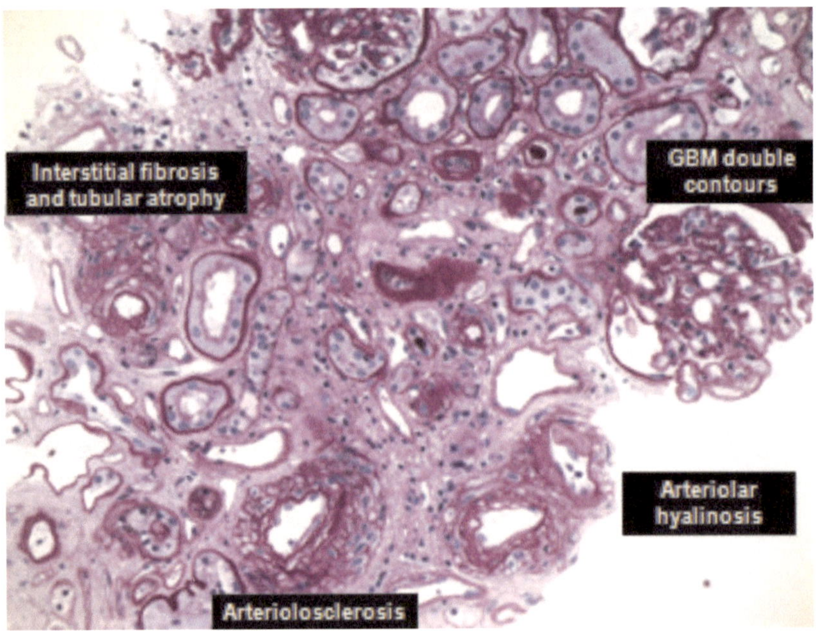

Fig. 1. Histological manifestations of chronic allograft nephropathy

Chronic allograft nephropathy is graded as mild, moderate or severe based on the severity of chronic interstitial fibrosis and tubular atrophy and the area of cortex affected in the biopsy specimen. Interstitial fibrosis, denoted as ci, is scored by the area fibrosed and ranges from mild (ci1 6–25%) to severe (ci3 >50%). Tubular atrophy refers to the loss of tubular height and increased luminal size of the tubules and is denoted as ct (ct0–ct3). Tubular atrophy and interstitial fibrosis are often nonspecific by themselves (Table 1).

Chronic transplant glomerulopathy refers to the thickening of the glomeruli and is quantified by the percentage of glomeruli developing "double contours" of peripheral capillary loops and is denoted as cg (cg0–cg3). Arteriolar hyalinosis, as suggested by the term, denotes thickening of arterioles within the kidney based on the amount of periodic-acid-Schiff-positive hyalinosis and is denoted as ah (ah0–ah3), often implying calcineurin inhibitor nephropathy. More in-depth quantification of all of these criteria is readily available (Racusen et al., 1999).

Grade	Histology	Interstitial Fibrosis	Tubular Atrophy
I	Mild	ci1* 6-25 % of cortical area	ct1 Up to 25 % of cortical tubules
II	Moderate	ci2 26-50 %	ct2 26-50 %
III	Severe	ci3 > 50 %	ct3 > 50 %

Table 1. Histologic revisted criteria of chronic allograft nephropathy

The addition of C4d staining to the Banff criteria in 2003 has allowed for the helpful diagnosis of chronic antibodymediated rejection. C4d is a positive marker of complement activation, implying the presence of antidonor antibodies and hence antibody-mediated rejection. C4d is released on binding to antibody. These antibodies bind to endothelial cells in glomerular and peritubular capillaries, suggesting antibody deposition (Fuecht et al., 1991, Nickeleitt et al., 2002) and prompting the clinician to request donor-specific antibody testing. C4d staining is regarded as positive or negative, and its position within the biopsy is recorded and graded by type, as acute tubular necrosis-like, capillary or arterial (Racusen et al., 2003). C4d has a role in acute rejection, early unexplained primary graft non function and chronic dysfunction where transplant glomerulopathy is present (Nickeleitt et al., 2002). The evidence for chronic allograft nephropathy as the leading cause for progressive renal failure and graft loss is supported by both transplant registry and protocol biopsy data. Graft loss secondary to the progressive development of chronic allograft nephropathy has consistently been recorded within Australian–New Zealand (ANZDATA) transplantation registries (Chang et al., 2007). Although histological confirmation of chronic allograft nephropathy by biopsy is variable, reports from all databases show progressive transplant loss attributable to CAN continuing to the present day despite improved changes to immunosuppression regimens. Cohort studies using protocol biopsies performed from day of transplant to 10 years posttransplantation consistently demonstrate the evolution and progression of CAN (Fernando et al., 2004, Nankivell et al., 2003, 2004c, Schwarz et al, 2005). Larger studies have helped identify aetiological factors involved in chronic graft injury.
In particular, the 10-year protocol biopsy study on adult patients with kidney–pancreas transplants defined the occurrence of severe rejection, of subclinical rejection and in some cases true chronic rejection, as evidenced by tubulointerstitial damage, with increasing evidence of progressive nephropathy from calcineurin inhibitors. Histological lesions of grade 1 chronic allograft nephropathy present in up to 94.2% of adult patients at 1 year posttransplant (Nankivell et al., 2003, 2004c), and grades progressively worsen up to 10 years.

4. Pathogenesis of chronic allograft nephropathy

The pathogenesis of chronic allograft nephropathy is still not fully elucidated, although several theories have been suggested (Häyry et al., 1993, Halloran et al., 1999, Paul et al.,

1999, Joosten et al., 2004). Chronic allograft nephropathy is thought to initiate from a series of challenges to the allograft. Injury to the graft begins even before the effect of the alloresponse: donor brain death, warm ischemia, cold ischemia, and ischemia/reperfusion injury all result in increased immunogenicity in the graft, causing increased inflammatory alloresponse after the revascularization of the allograft. Series of injuries continues during the first weeks after transplantation; acute tubular necrosis, acute rejection episodes, calcineurin inhibitors nephrotoxicity, and infections in the graft, among others, contribute to the injury of the transplanted kidney. All this occurs against the background of foreign MHC antigens and often in a kidney from an older donor with some extent of age associated changes and limited capacity of restoration from injury.
Renal injury is thought to result in an inflammatory response; recipient lymphocytes and monocytes enter the graft and produce cytokines, which stimulate inflammatory and mesenchymal cells to produce excess growth factors, resulting in proliferation of myofibroblasts and smooth muscle cells in the vascular wall and increased of collagen synthesis in fibroblasts. This process is thought to lead to scar formation; excess interstitial fibrosis, tubular atrophy and vascular intimal thickening represent the stereotypic histopathological picture seen in endstage renal diseases.

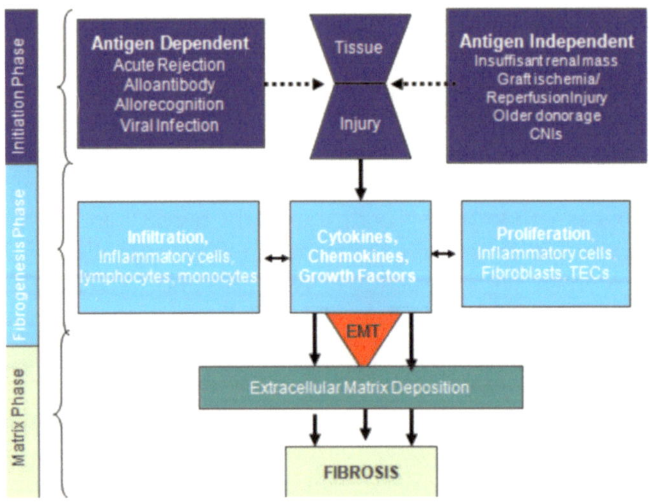

Fig. 2. Major risk factors of chronic allograft nephropathy

Whether the initial injury in the graft occurs in the vascular wall, resulting in the proliferation of the vascular wall and narrowing of the lumen, followed by tubulointerstitial lesions due to growth factor response and partly ischemia (Häyry et al., 1993), or whether the initial event is tubular cell injury, resulting in growth factor response, tubular atrophy, interstitial fibrosis, and finally vascular narrowing, is still under discussion (Paul et al., 1999). Nankivell et al. (2003) support the hypothesis that interstitial fibrosis and tubular atrophy were the first manifestations of chronic allograft nephropathy and preceded vasculopathic changes. Most of the histopathological changes of chronic allograft nephropathy are also seen in the aging kidney. This fact and knowledge of the limited cell cycle capacity has led to the theory that cellular or tissue senescence might play a role in the pathogenesis of chronic allograft nephropathy (Halloran et al., 1999).

Continuous injury to an aging graft may result in exhaustion of the replicative cells and inability to repair injury and remodel the tissue in an adequate way. This is thought to lead to the histopathological lesions seen in chronic allograft nephropathy.

5. Diagnosis of chronic allograft nephropathy

Clinically, chronic allograft nephropathy is characterized by a slow but variable loss of function, starting 3 months after implantation, often in combination with proteinuria generally in the non nephritic range and hypertension (Paul et al., 1999).
The progressive decline in renal function measured by increasing serum creatinine, or the development of overt proteinuria, is often the first indication alerting the clinician to the presence of chronic allograft nephropathy. Evaluation of large registry data, however, has shown that serum creatinine has limited predictive value for subsequent graft loss (Kaplan et al., 2003). A single reference range for serum creatinine can be misleading and often underestimates the deterioration of renal function, especially at glomerular filtration rate between 30 and 70 mL/min (Levey et al., 1999). If clinicians wait until their individual patients start showing rising creatinine levels, then a considerable amount of damage will already have been done and it may be too late for successful intervention (Chapman et al., 2005).

6. Risk factors of chronic allograft nephropathy

6.1 Immune-dependent factors

6.1.1 HLA mismatches

HLA antigens present in the donor but absent in the recipient are counted as HLA-mismatches. HLA-A, -B and -DR mismatches have been associated with poor graft survival. Although organ allocation relies on several non-immunological and logistic factors, a close HLA match is desirable. It was clearly demonstrated that the greater the number of mismatches, the poorer the graft survival at 5 years of follow-up (Opelz et al. 1999) The importance of HLA-mismatch in the era of modern immunosuppression (i.e. tacrolimus, mycophenolate mophetil, induction therapies) was evaluated in the largest European study, where the results of two eras: 1985–1994 and 1995–2004, were compared. A total of 135,970 cadaver kidney transplants were followed up for 5 years. Although the survival rates improved over the years, HLA mismatches still had a clear impact. A multiregression analysis of factors contributing to graft survival revealed that the impact of HLA-mismatches on graft survival was equally strong in the two decades compared (Opelz & Döhler 2007).

6.1.2 Sensitization

The main routes of sensitization are blood transfusion, pregnancy and transplantation.
Alloantibodies were first implicated in chronic rejection of human allografts (Russel 1970) with the occurrence of chronic allograft arteriopathy only in patients who developed de novo antidonor antibodies (human leukocyte antigen (HLA)). Terasaki et al. (2007) detected an association of circulating HLA antibodies with an increased risk of long-term graft loss. Halloran et et al. (1990) showed that acute renal allograft rejection in patients with donor-specific anticlass 1 HLA antibodies had distinct pathological features. An advance finding was the demonstration of the complement fragment C4d in peritubular capillaries (PCT) in

patients with acute rejection (Feucht et al., 1991). This was tied to circulating donor-specific antibodies and graft pathology by Collins et al., (1999), and confirmed by many others, leading to the introduction of the diagnosis "acute antibody-mediated rejection" in the BANFF classification. Mauyyedi et al. (2002) then connected the dots and discovered that glomerulopathy or arteriopathy was liked to C4d deposition in peritubular capillaries and donor-specific alloantibody. For this condition, a new term was proposed with "chronic humoral rejection". Several groups had confirmed these findings and it's clear that about 50 % of patients with transplant glomerulopathy or arteriopathy have C4d deposition in peritubular capillaries (Sis et al., 2007, Calvin et al., 2007).

6.1.3 Chronic humoral rejection

In 2005, the Banff consensus conference added a new category "chronic active antibody-mediated rejection" to its classification with the criteria given in table 2 (Solez et al., 2007).

Morphological features
Duplication of glomerular basement membrane (cg1-3)
Multilaminated PTC basement membrane
Arterial intimal fibrosis without elastosis
Interstitial fibrosis with tubular atrophy with or without PTC loss
Diffuse C4d positivity along PTC
Presence of donor-specific antibody

Abbreviation: PTC, perittubular capillary

Table 2. Banff criteria for chronic antibody-mediated rejection

Recent studies have indicated that chronic humoral rejection is common in unselected indication biopsies, found in one 10-year series in 9.3 % of 771 cases (Farris, 2009). The onset of chronic humoral rejection is typically late, after the first year, and the prevalence rises progressively to about 20 % in the fifth year. Proteinuria is common but not invariable (~50 % have > 1 g per day proteinuria). Renal function is often abnormal, but can remain stable for considerable time periods (years) (Kieran et al., 2009).The strongest risk factor identified to date is the existence of pretransplant donor-specific antibodies, but most cases occur in patients without a history of presensitization or even an episode of acute humoral rejection. Serologically, the most interesting aspect of chronic humoral rejection is the strong association with class II DSA (Gloor et al., 2007) which is not a characteristic of acute humoral rejection.

The major features of chronic humoral rejection are duplication of the glomerular basement membrane ("transplant glomerulopathy"), multilamination of peritubular capillaries basement, mononuclear cells in glomeruli and peritubular capillaries, and loss of normal glomerular capillary endothelial fenestrations (Colvin et al., 2006). In addition to multilamination of basement membranes, loss of peritubular capillaries has been demonstrated in patients with chronic graft injury and this correlates inversely with serum creatinine (Ishii et al., 2005). It is possible that the loss of capillaries is related to endothelial-mesenchymal transition (Zeisberg et al., 2007).

6.1.4 Acute rejection

Historically, acute rejection episodes that are severe, recurrent, or that occur late have been associated with inferior outcomes. The strong correlation between late acute rejection and chronic allograft rejection, as well as late graft loss, has been reported consistently (Nankivell et al., 2001, Sijpkens et al., 2003). The risk of graft loss is different for acute rejections that are functional reversible on treatment compared with those with functional deterioration (Meier-Kreische et al., 2004). In the mean time however, higher risk donors and recipients have also been transplanted in more recent times. An impaired ability to tissue restoration in these kidneys, as has been described for acute cellular or Banff grade I rejection in kidneys from older donors, may at least partly explain the observed lack of functional reversibility (de Fijter et al., 2001).

6.1.5 Subclinical rejection

The term subclinical rejection refers to allografts with stable renal function that display an interstitial infiltrate and tubulitis.

There is increasing evidence that subclinical rejection may represent an important factor in predicting early graft loss (Nankivell et al., 2004b, Veronese et al., 2004). The prevalence of subclinical rejection is maximal during the initial 3 months, progressively declines in the first year, but may persist in a small number of patients after the first year (Nankivell et al., 2004b). According to the Banff criteria, approximately 1 out 3 subclinical rejection episodes are classified as being of interstitial acute rejection grade 1, and 2 out of 3 are classified as borderline changes (Nankivell et al., 2004d).

The largest observational study to date of 961 renal transplant biopsies performed on 119 consecutive simultaneous pancreas kidney transplant recipients reported an subclinical rejection prevalence of 60.8, 45.7, and 25.8 % at 1 month, 3 months, and 1 year, respectively (Nankivell et al., 2003). In renal recipients, the prevalence of subclinical rejection in 3-month protocol biopsies has been observed at between 23 and 43 %, but its difficulty to directly compare these results because of differences in histological interpretation, histocompatibility, patient selection, and immunosuppressive regimens (Nankivell et al., 2001, Rush, DN et al., 1994, 1995, Shapiro et al., 2001, Shishido et al., 2003). A prevalence of 18 % at 3 months was reported in deceased donor kidney transplant recipients on Tacrolimus, azathioprine, and prednisone (Jurewicz, WA 1999), whereas in patients on tacrolimus, mycophenolate mofetil, and prednisone, the prevalence was only 2.6 % (Gloor et al., 2002). A recent randomized, multicenter study in renal transplant patients, considered to have a low risk profile of acute rejection, receiving tacrolimus, mycophenolate mofetil, and prednisone reported a low overall prevalence of subclinical rejection (4,6 %) (Rush, D 2007). Treatment of subclinical rejection in the biopsy arm of this study with high-dose steroids, however, did not result in beneficial outcomes, at least in the short term.

6.2 Non Immune-dependent factors

6.2.1 Donor age and cellular senescence

It is generally accepted (Halloran et al., 1999, Basar et al., 1999, Oppenheimer et al., 2004) that increased donor age is associated with reduced actuarial graft survival, increased rate of delayed graft function, and earlier onset of chronic allograft nephropathy.

In vitro studies have shown that cellular senescence can be categorized in either replicative, stress- or aberrant signaling-induced senescence (Itahana et al., 2004).

Replicative senescence (so called "mitotic clock") is associated with shortened telomeres in human (Harley et al., 1990). After a variable number of mitotic divisions, cells cannot pass from G1 to S phase of their cycle as a consequence of DNA loss corresponding to telomere shortening.

A recent study (Westhoff et al., 2010) demonstrated in a telomere-deficient mouse model that telomere shortening was associated with reduced replicative capacities and a compromised ability of tubular cells to respond adequately to acute kidney injury. Although intriguing, the precise role of replicative senescence on the onset of chronic allograft nephropathy remain unclear.

Stress- and aberrant signaling induced senescence is secondary to extrinsic stress and characterized by an increased expression of the cyclin-dependant kinase inhibitor p16, a cell cycle regulator, and the activation of the p53 pathway (Zindy et al., 1997). It has been shown that markers of the senescent cellular phenotype, such as p161NK4a, cyclogenase 1, or HSP A5, are overexpressed in allografts with chronic allograft nephropathy, suggesting the implication of some features of aging on graft impairment (Chkhotua et al., 2003. Melk et al., 2004).

6.2.2 Brain death

Brain death, in addition to other unspecific injuries of organs at the time of transplantation, is considered as the main reason for the superior clinical survival of living donor transplants, even when disadvantaged for human lymphocyte antigen compatibility (Gasser et al., 2000).

It's supposed that there's, in kidneys from brain dead donor, an augmented inflammatory and dentritic cell response compared with kidneys from living donor (Timsit et al., 2010).

6.2.3 Ischemia

Consequences of ischemia/reperfusion injury correlate with chronic allograft nephropathy in clinical and experimental studies. A retrospective study based on the United Network for Organ Sharing database showed that prolonged cold ischemia was a significant risk factor for late allograft loss (Salahudeen et al., 2004). Increased graft immunogenicity, accelerated host immune responses, and fibrotic changes due to increased matrix synthesis are currently evocated as mechanisms correlating ischemia/reperfusion injury and chronic allograft nephropathy.

Iischemia/reperfusion injury leads to an increased expression of both class I and class II major histocompatibility complex molecules in the allograft (Shoskeet al., 1996), as well as to accelerated dendritic cell differentiation and increased rates of acute rejection through either direct or indirect allorecognition (Ke et al., 2005). In addition, ischemia/reperfusion injury upregulates the expression of adhesion molecules and leukocyte recruitment in the graft leading to a sustained host immune response (Farhood et al., 1995, Osborn et al., 1990).

6.2.4 Calcineurin Inhibitors nephrotoxicity

Calcineurin inhibitors are pleomorphic nephrotoxins affecting every histological compartment of the transplanted kidney. The classical calcineurin inhibitors lesions (Benigni et al., 1999, Mihatsch et al. 1988, Davies et al., 2000) include de novo or increasing arteriolar hyalinosis and striped fibrosis, supported by microcalcification unrelated to other causes such as tubular necrosis and hyperparathyroidism (Gwinner et al., 2005). Ciclosporine A and Tacrolimus nephrotoxicity and increasingly common late after transplantation (Nankivell et al., 2003, Solez et al., 1998). Arteriolar hyalinosis is the most reliable diagnostic marker of calcineurin inhibitors nephrotoxicity (Solez et al., 1993). Confirmation of the diagnosis can be made by exclusion of donor hyalinosis detectable on implantation biopsy, diabetes and hypertensive nephrosclerosis (distinguished by subendothelial hyalinosis, elastic lamina reduplication and medial hyperplasia in larger arteries (Mihatsch et al., 1988, Mihatsch et al., 1995). Severe arteriolar hyalinosis causes vascular narrowing and downstream ischemic glomerulosclerosis (Nankivell et al., 2004c)

6.2.5 Recurrent glomerulonephritis

Recurrent glomerulonephritis is diagnosed by exclusion of donor-transmitted disease and de novo glomerulonephritis, and currently accounts for 8.4% of allograft loss by 10 years in recipients with renal failure from glomerulonephritis (Briganti et al., *2002*). The clinical course and severity of recurrent glomerular disease often recapitulates the patient's native disease (Chadban et al., 2001) except for vasculitis or lupus nephritis, which are usually controlled by transplant immunosuppression. Focal segmental glomerulosclerosis (20–50% recurrence rates) and dense deposit disease (50–90% recurrence) have the worst prognosis; compared with membranous glomerulonephritis (29–50% recurrence), membranoproliferative glomerulonephritis type 1 (20–33% recurrence) or IgA nephropathy, which recurs in up to 58% but with less clinical impact (Chadban et al., 2001). Diabetic glomerulopathy can also recur in allografts, usually after many years.

6.2.6 Infections

Infectious diseases affect graft and patient survival and contribute to the development of chronic allograft nephropathy. This group of diseases includes nephropathy due to polyoma (BK) virus infection, direct and indirect effects of cytomegalovirus (CMV) infection, and bacterial infections. Rarer infections causes of chronic allograft nephropathy include cryoglobulinemia associated with hepatitis C, Epstein-Barr virus (EBV)-associated posttransplant lymphoproliferative disease (PTLD), and direct cytotoxicity from adenoviral infection or parvovirus B19.

6.2.6.1 BK virus

BK virus is an endemic polyoma virus of high prevalence, low morbidity, long latency and asymptomatic reactivation in immunocompentent individuals (Hirsch et al., 2003, Mannon et al., 2004). Prospective screening studies suggest that 50 % or more of patients develop BK viruria after transplantation, with a peak incidence in the first 3-12 months (Nickeleit et al., 2000b, White et al., 2008, Koukoulaki et al., 2009). However only 1-5 % of viruric patients go on to develop nephropathy (Smith et al., 2007, Kim et al. 2005). When BK virus-associated nephropathy (BKVAN) occurs, reported rates of graft loss have ranged from 10 to 80 % (Nickeleit et al., 2000a. Weiss et al., 2008). Although early reports suggested a link with Tacrolimus and mycophenolate-based regimens, it seems likely that the risk of BKVAN relates to the total burden of immunosuppression rather than to any specific drug (Rahamimov et al., 2003, Nickeleit et al., 2000a).

Some authors reported that the injury of the renal allograft may have an important role in the pathogenesis of BKVAN (Drachenberg et al., 2005). The association found between human lymphocyte antigen mismatching and BKVAN supports the hypothesis (Awadalla et al., 2004).

6.2.6.2 Cytomegalovirus

The extent of the contribution of cytomegalovirus infection to chronic allograft nephropathy remains controversial. Cytomegalovirus infection has been shown to upregulate class I and class II major histocompatibility complex molecules on T lymphocytes and renal parenchymal cells. This effect is likely to be a cytokine-mediated phenomenon because of upregulation of proinflammatory cytokines such as interferon-γ. The immediate early gene product of cytomegalovirus shares a sequence homology with human lymphocyte antigen DR (Beck et al., 1988). Cytomegalovirus infection also blocks p53 (an important cell cycle regulatory protein), which may inhibit apoptosis and promote graft vasculopathy (Garcia et al., 1997). Other potential indirect effects of cytomegalovirus include upregulation of antiendothelial antibodies contributing to graft vascular injury (Toyoda et al., 1997) and upregulation of adhesion molecules (Helantera et al., 2005), leading to enhanced adhesion of host, leukocytes to graft endothelium, and thereby promoting allograft injury and/or rejection. These indirect effects of cytomegalovirus are thought to affect graft survival principally through an increased risk of acute rejection.

Although the combination of cytomegalovirus infection and acute rejection has an adverse effect on graft survival, whether cytomegalovirus infection contributes to graft failure, in the absence of acute rejection remains unclear. There is some evidence, mainly from animal models, suggesting a direct role for cytomegalovirus in mediating chronic allograft nephropathy.

Cytomegalovirus infection has been shown to have both proinflammatory and profibrotic effects. In rodents, cytomegalovirus upregulates transforming growth factor-β, platelet-derived growth factor (which stimulates smooth muscle proliferation and fibroblast activity), and connective growth factor (Inkinen et al., 2001, Inkinen et al., 2003, Helantera et al., 2006). Clinical studies have demonstrated similar effects in man (Helantera et al., 2005). Cytomegalovirus infection is also known to induce macrophage scavenger receptors and phenotypic changes in vascular smooth muscle cells, which have been shown to contribute to vasculopathy in cardiac allografts (Carlquist et al., 2004).

6.2.6.3 Urinary tract infection (UTI)

Urinary tract infection is a common complication following renal transplantation (Prat et al., 1985, Abbott et al., 2001). Graft pyelonephritis is well recognized to cause graft dysfunction but the longer-term impact is less clear (Pelle et al., 2007). A review of US registry data suggested that late urinary tract infections are not benign but they may be associated with an increased risk of death and graft loss (Abbott et al., 2004).

7. Management of chronic allograft nephropathy

The multiple pathophysiological causes of injury suggest that no single action will suffice, but instead, it is more likely that several therapies and approaches will be needed to abrogate specific etiological insults. These may include multiple, specific antagonists which are targeted to drivers of fibrogenesis, and well as indirect therapy targeting control of hypertension, hyperlipemia, infections etc.

7.1 Optimal immunosuppression

Prevention of chronic allograft nephropathy is presently one of the main goals in renal transplantation for the improvement of kidney graft survival. Refinements in immunosuppressive protocols, both controlling alloimmune responses and avoiding calcineurin inhibitor nephrotoxicity, are mandatory.

Ideally, optimal immunosuppression to prevent chronic allograft nephropathy should provide low rates of acute rejection, low rates of subclinical rejection and should be based on non-nephrotoxic agents able to preserve renal function.
Because calcineurin inhibitors nephrotoxicity, which seems common in the long term, has been considered as one of the main contributors to chronic allograft nephropathy, the prevention of chronic allograft nephropathy has been mainly attempted by reducing/avoiding the use of calcineurin inhibitors.
Unfortunately, sparing calcineurin inhibitors strategies have been associated in several trials with an increased rate of acute rejection without significant improvement in renal function and no impact on graft survival.

7.1.1 Mycophenolate mofetil (MMF)-based strategies

The impact of avoiding of calcineurin inhibitors based on the immunosuppressive potency of mycophenolate mofetil was associated with controversial results. The first study conducted 10 years ago combined daclizumab, mycophenolate mofetil and steroids (Vincenti et al., 2001). The lack of calcineurin inhibitors resulted in an incidence of acute rejection of 48 % during the first 6 months after Tx, and at the end of the first year, more than 60 % of patients were on calcineurin inhibitors. The CAESAR study compared 2 arms. The first arm associated a triple therapy with conventional doses of cyclosporine A, mycophenolate mofetil and steroids and the second arm involving daclizumab, low-dose Cyclosporin A (trough level 50-100 ng/ml) and steroids with the discontinuation of cyclosporine A 6 months after the transplantation in this arm (Ekberg et al., 2007). Renal function was not significantly different between the 2 groups and there was a trend toward higher creatinine clearance in the low-dose cyclosporine A group. In contrast, the cyclosporine A withdrawal group did not have better renal function, and there was a rebound of acute rejection after cyclosporine A withdrawal that could have counterbalanced the renal benefits of cyclosporine elimination. Other studies with planned conversion from Calcineurin inhibitors to antimetabolites in de novo renal transplant recipients also resulted in an increase in acute rejection and biopsy-proven chronic rejection (Smak Gregoor et al., 2000, 2002). In established stable patients treated with mycophenolate mofetil, discontinuation of cyclosporine A was followed by significant improvement in renal function at 1 year after this therapeutic change (Abramowicz et al, 2005), but with more patients losing their graft because of immune-mediated rejection at 5 years. In the Symphony study (Ekberg et al., 2007), the control arm with standard cyclosporine A and the low-dose cyclosporine A group had the same drug doses as in the CAESAR study. In addition, two more groups with reduced doses of Tacrolimus (target levels 3-7 ng/ml) or low sirolimus (target levels 4-8 ng/ml) were also enrolled in this large study of more than 1600 patients. The mean calculated GFR was higher in patients receiving low-dose Tacrolimus (65,4 ml/min) than in the other three groups. The rate of biopsy-proven acute rejection (BPAR) was lower in patients receiving low-dose Tacrolimus (12,3 %) than in those receiving standard-dose cyclosporine A (25,8 %), low-dose cyclosporine A (24,0 %), or low-dose sirolimus (37,2 %). Allograft survival differed significantly between the four groups ($p=0.02$) and was highest in the low-dose Tacrolimus group (94,2 %), followed by the low-dose cyclosporine A group (93.1 %), the standard-dose cyclosporine A group (89.3 %), and the low-dose sirolimus group (89.3 %). The 3-year data of this study was published recently (Ekberg et al., 2009) and showed that the differences between treatment groups were often no longer significant and renal function remained stable during the follow-up, suggesting that low-dose Tacrolimus with mycophenolate mofetil may avoid the negative effects on renal function commonly reported for standard calcineurin inhibitors regimes despite the potential patient's selection and uncontrolled treatment modifications.

7.1.2 Mammalian target of rapamycin (mTOR) inhibitor-based strategies

The conversion from calcineurin inhibitors to mTOR inhibitors has been followed by variable success (Flechner et al., 2008). Conversion in cases with a significantly deteriorated renal function and proteinuria does no help to stabilize graft function. Indeed, all these concepts have been consolidated after a large prospective study with more than 800 maintenance patients of conversion from calcineurin inhibitors to sirolimus (Schena et al., 2009). In this trial, the efficacy and safety of converting maintenance renal transplant recipients from calcineurin inhibitors to sirolimus were evaluated. The primary end points were calculated GFR (stratified at baseline: 20-40 vs > 40 ml/min) and the cumulative rates of BPAR, graft loss, or death at 12 months. Enrollment in the 20-40 ml/min stratum was halted prematurely because of higher incidence of safety and points in the sirolimus conversion arm. The intent-to-treat analyses at 12 and 24 months showed no significant treatment difference in GFR in patients with baseline GFR higher than 40 ml/min stratum. On-therapy analysis of this cohort showed significantly higher GFR at 12 and 24 months after sirolimus conversion. Rates of BPAR, graft survival, and patient survival were similar between groups. Median urinary protein-to-creatinine ratios (UPr/Cr) were similar at baseline but significantly increased after sirolimus conversion. *Post hoc* analyses identified a subgroup of patients with baseline GFR > 40 ml/min and UPr/Cr ≤ 0.11, whose risk-benefit profile was more favorable after conversion than for the overall sirolimus conversion cohort. Thus, selection of suitable candidates is fundamental to get the profit of calcineurin inhibitors withdrawal with mTOR inhibitors. Consequent from the results of these trials on conversion from calcineurin inhibitors to mTOR inhibitors, it is generally accepted that elective and planned conversion may be the best approach to stabilize renal function.

Switching immunosuppressive therapy from cyclosporine A-mycophenolate sodium (MPS) and therapy with everolimus-steroids at 6 months after renal transplantation is effective in preventing rejection with ameliorating renal function has been shown in a recent published interim analysis (Bemelman et al., 2009).

It's important to note that the immense majority of studies attempting de *novo* introduction or conversion to mTOR inhibitors have displayed significant discontinuation rates because of drug-related adverse effects.

All the recent data suggest the importance of defining the right target levels for mTOR inhibitors and an adequate management of the overlapped toxicities of their use with antimetabolites.

7.1.3 Belatacept-based strategies

Belatacept is a second generation CTL4-Ig costimulator blocker with a high avidity for CD86 and CD80 molecules and prevents T-cell activation (Larsen et al. 2005). This drug may be very interesting in the development of safe calcineurin inhibitors-free regimens to preserve renal function. Thus, in a phase II multicenter trial (Vincenti et al., 2005), therapy with cyclosporine A, MMF, and steroids plus basiliximab was compared with belatacept in two therapeutic regimens (more intensive (MI) and less intensive (LI)) depending on the dose and frequency of belatacept administrations, in association with mycophenolate mofetil , steroids and basiliximab. Belatacept was used as in induction treatment since the first day of the transplantation and next given as a maintenance immunosuppressant. The belatacept-treated arms, had a similar low incidence of acute rejection (18 and 19 %) at 6 months, compared with the cyclosporine A arm. This trial demonstrated, particularly at 12 months, lower incidence of chronic allograft nephropathy in protocol biopsies, better renal function in terms of measured GFR, and a more favorable cardiovascular risk profile in the costimulation blockade arm in comparison with the standard cyclosporine A and mycophenolate mofetil combination.

This trial was followed by two phase III pivotal trials (Durrbach et al., 2010, Vincenti et al., 2010) in patients receiving kidneys from conventional donors (BENEFIT) or extended criteria donors (BENEFIT-EXT). The Belatacept dose regimens, M1 and L1, were similar to those in phase II trials. The data of these 2 studies indicate that the renal benefits on function and structure are even more evident in optimal renal allografts, and that an induction and maintenance immunosuoppression based on belatacept may prevent long term graft deterioration. The incidence of acute rejection was similar across the groups and < 20 %, except for the MI in the BENEFIT study, suggesting the L1 regimen provides the best risk/benefit balance. Safety data from these studies have shown a higher incidence of post-transplant lymphoproliferative disease in patients treated with belatacept, which was associated with the use of polyclonals, concomitant cytomegalovirus infection, and recipient's seronegativity for Epstein-Barr virus.

7.2 Non-immune interventions

The discrepancy between significant improvements in the prevention of acute rejection and failure to ameliorate long-term outcomes suggests that non-immunological injuries may have an important role in the occurrence of chronic allograft nephropathy (Remuzzi et al., 1998). Functional and structural changes of chronic renal allograft failure share similarities with those observed in other forms of chronic progressive kidney disease, in which decline of functioning nephron mass has been considered the key event. The existence of a single transplanted kidney supplies only half the number of nephron commonly available to a healthy subject. This implies workload per nephron to maintain body homeostasis (Brenner 1985). Graft injury is the result of glomerular hypertension and hyperfiltration in surviving units, which in turn leads to graft injury (Azuma et al., 1997). Other aggressions act against transplanted kidney like surgical and ischemic injury, acute rejection, and chronic toxicity of calcineurin inhibitors (Naesens et al., 2009) and mTOR inhibitors (Tomlanovich et al., 2007). Strategies developed to preserve renal function in patients with chronic kidney disease are mandatory to improve renal graft outcome in the long term.

7.2.1 Control of blood pressure

Hypertension is frequent among renal transplant recipients and can be observed even starting from the first week after transplantation, mainly when doses of calcineurin inhibtors and steroids are elevated (Tedla et al. 2007). The prevalence of hypertension has changed from between 40 to 60 % in the pre-cyclosporine era to up to 80-90 % after the introduction of cyclosporine (Schwenger et al., 2001, Curtis et al., 1992).

There are no randomized, controlled trials comparing different antihypertensive drugs or optimal BP goals in transplant recipients. On the basis of large clinical trials in nontransplant patients with or without kidney disease, the Kidney Disease Outcomes Quality Initiative (KDIGO) guidelines recommend BP goals of 125/75 mmHg for transplant recipients with proteinuria and 130/85 mmHg in the absence of proteinuria (Bakris et al., 2000).

The first step of treatment should be based on non-pharmacologic interventions such weight reduction, exercise, smoking cessation, and dietary sodium restriction. Reach target levels of BP and proteinuria required frequently a simultaneous initiation of non-pharmacologic and pharmacologic treatment (Svetkey et al., 2005).

The choice of antihypertensive class depends on the individual patient. Calcium channel blockers can be used as first line therapy, especially in the early period of the transplantation because they are effective in counteracting the vasoconstrictive effect of high-dose calcineurin inhibitors (Harper et al., 1992).

In opposition, in proteinuric chronic kidney disease patients, dihydropiridinic-calcium channel blocker has been associated with increased risk of renal disease and death (Wright Jr et al., 2002, Agodoa et al., 2001).

The use of angiotensin-converting enzyme inhibitors and angiotensin II receptor blockers in renal transplant recipients is now more frequent (Ram et al., 2008). This fact is due to the cardioprotective and renoprotective effects of renin-angiotensin system (RAS) blockade in the general population (Braunwald et al., 2004) and in patients with chronic kidney disease (Ruggenenti et al., 1997).

A particular caution should be taken when using these agents in kidney transplant patients, as in the presence of artery stenosis of the graft the use of RAS inhibitors may dramatically increase the risk of kidney function impairment and hyperkalemia (Salzberg et al., 2007).

However, the multifactorial nature of hypertension in transplanted patients often requires multiple drugs, including α- or β-blockers, centrally acting drugs, and diuretics (Ojo et al., 2006).

7.2.2 Proteinuria

The prevalence of proteinuria in kidney transplant patients ranges between 10 and 25% (Kasiske, et al., 2000). The three most common causes of persistent proteinuria after kidney transplantation are chronic graft injury, recurrent glomerulonephritis, and drug related nephrotoxicity (Bear et al., 1988). Calcineurin inhibitors have been considered as the immunosuppressive drugs with the highest risk of nephrotoxicity. Recently, increasing evidence has suggested a potential nephrotoxicity also with mTOR inhibitors. Indeed, they have been associated with an increased risk of proteinuria, possibly resulting from a direct toxicity on glomerular and tubular epithelial cells (Tomlanovich et al., 2007).

Proteinuria represents also a strong independent risk factor for graft loss (Bear et al., 1988). It's a marker of progressive renal injury and contributes to progression of kidney dysfunction and fibrosis through aberrant proximal tubule protein uptake and direct tubular cell toxicity (Remuzzi et al., 2006).

RAS inhibitors have been shown to be efficient in reducing proteinuria and progression of renal disease in experimental models of renal mass reduction and in patients with chronic nephropathies (Remuzzi et al., 2006). Interestingly, RAS inhibitor therapy may exert renoprotection independently from its effect on proteinuria. Indeed, AT1 receptors mediate inflammation and are involved in the profibrotic action exhibited by potent cytokines (Ruiz-Ortega et al., 2006). Angiotensin II is also synthesized by the proximal renal tubule cells and

exhibits powerful hemodynamic and non-hemodynamic effects, all implicated in the progression of chronic kidney disease (Brewster et al., 2004).
A recent analysis of 2031 patients, who received their first renal allograft at the Medical University of Vienna between 1990 and 2003, showed that RAS inhibitor therapy was associated with a significantly higher patient (74 versus 53%, P=0.001) and graft (59 versus 43%, P¼0.002) survival at 10 years after transplant as compared with non-RAS inhibitor therapy (Heinze et al., 2006). This is at variance with a previous systematic review of 21 studies consisting of 1549 patients on the effect of RAS inhibitor therapy after kidney transplantation that failed to show any beneficial effect on patient and graft survival over a median follow-up of 27 months (Hiremath et al., 2007).

7.2.3 Hyperlipemia

Hyperlipidemia is a frequent finding in kidney transplant recipients, affecting 60% of patients (Kasiske et al., 2000). Its pathogenesis is multifactorial and includes posttransplantation weight gain and the use of immunosuppressive drugs, such as mTOR inhibitors and steroids (Tsimihodimos et al., 2008). Particularly, higher triglyceride levels have been associated with poorer graft outcomes (Del Castillo et al., 2004).
Therapeutic agents to control low-density lipoprotein cholesterol and triglycerides include statins as well as fenofibrates. Intriguingly, statins have been implicated as nephroprotective agents beyond their lipid-lowering ability because of their potential to regulate fibrogenic mechanisms, as well as their impact on endothelial dysfunction (Perico et al., 2008). The Assessment of Lescol in Renal Transplantation (ALERT) trial randomized 2102 renal transplant recipients with total cholesterol 156–351 mg/dl to fluvastatin or placebo over a 5-year follow-up period. Treatment was safe and effective in lowering total and low-density lipoprotein cholesterol (Holdaas et al., 2003). Moreover, although the trial had insufficient power to detect a significant reduction in the primary end point of cardiac death, non-fatal myocardial infarction, or coronary intervention procedure, there was a significant 35% reduction in the secondary end point of cardiac death and non-fatal myocardial infarction with fluvastatin. The treatment, however, had no effect on graft survival or function. Yet, a recent randomized controlled study in 89 kidney transplant recipients showed a beneficial effect of fluvastatin (80 mg/day) over placebo on the incidence of transplant vasculopathy (7 versus 33%; p=0.02) over 6 month followup (Seron et al., 2008).
Attractively, experimental and clinical evidence suggest that statins may have an additive beneficial effect with RAS inhibitors on kidney graft outcomes (Perico et al., 2008).

8. Immune monitoring and biomarkers to predict chronic allograft nephropathy

Chronic allograft nephropathy continues to plague kidney allografts, in spite of potent immunosuppressive therapies. Both immune-dependent and -independent factors continue to contribute to failure. A number of promising observations made in human kidney recipients suggest unique protein and genetic signatures that may identify biomarkers of injury, as well as potential targets of therapy. Technical advances such as gene cDNA microarrays, proteomics and metabonomics will multiply the number of potential etiologies and mechanisms of chronic allograft nephropathy. Discrimination between clinically important versus statistically significant factors yielding small effects will be essential.

Transcriptional changes may be detectable prior to histologically apparent fibrosis, and discrimination of inflammatory infiltrates according to the constellation of expressed genes, promises to both improve diagnoses and optimize treatment strategies (Mannon et al., 2010).

9. Conclusion

Chronic kidney allograft abnormalities represent the effects of cumulative damage from a series of time-dependent stressors, which are combined with an allograft healing response and modified by immunosuppression. Early tubulointerstitial damage results from ischemia-reperfusion injury, acute tubular necrosis, acute and subclinical rejection and calcineurin inhibitor nephrotoxicity, superimposed upon donor abnormalities. Later, microvascular and glomerular Injury increases frequently as a result of calcineurin inhibitors nephrotoxicity, but also from hypertension, immune-mediated vascular hyperplasia, transplant glomerulopathy and occasionally from recurrent or de novo glomerulonephritis. Additional mechanisms of chronic allograft nephropathy include internal structural disruption of the kidney, cortical ischemia, inability to resolve chronic inflammation, senescence, cytokine excess, epithelial-to-mesenchymal induced fibrosis, hypertension and other stressors. Early detection (Fig 4) appears to be critical issue for this disorder. The role of protocol biopsy and management of subclinical rejection are under study. Treatment options are nonspecific and limited. Various immunosuppressive strategies avoiding or limiting calcineurin inhibitors, biologics and anti-proliferatives are under study. Despite marked improvements in short graft survival and reduction in acute rejection rates, long term graft function remains a critical issue. Current immunosuppressive regimens do not adequately address the causes of long-term allograft dysfunction and loss calcineurin inhibitors-sparing regimens are urgently required

10. References

Abbott, KC, Oliver III, JD, Hypolite, I (2001). Hospitalizations for bacterial septicemia after renal transplantation in the United States. *American Journal of Nephrology* 21, 120–127.

Abbott, KC, Swanson, SJ, Richter, ER (2004). Late urinary tract infection after renal transplantation in the United States. *American Journal of Kidney Diseases* 44, 353–362.

Abramowicz, D, Manas, D, Lao, M, Vanrenterghem, Y, Del Castillo, D, Wijngaard, P, Fung (2002). Cyclosporine Withdrawal Study Group. Cyclosporine withdrawal from a mycophenolate mofetil containing immunosuppressive regimen in stable kidney transplant recipients: a randomized, controlled study. *Transplantation* 74: 1725–1734.

Abramowicz, D, Del Carmen Rial, M, Vitko S, del Castillo, D, Manas, D, Lao, M, Gafner, N, Wijngaard, P et al (2005). Cyclosporine Withdrawal Study Group. Cyclosporine withdrawal from a mycophenolate mofetil containing immunosuppressive regimen: results of a five-year, prospective, randomized study. *Journal of American Society of Nephrology* 16: 2234–2240.

Agodoa, LY, Appel, L, Bakris, GL, Beck G, Bourgoignie J, Briggs JP, Charleston J, Cheek, D, Cleveland, W, Douglas, JG, Douglas, M, Dowie, D, Faulkner, M, Gabriel, A, Gassman, J, Greene, T, Hall, Y, Hebert, L, Hiremath, L, Jamerson, K, Johnson CJ,

Kopple J, Kusek J, Lash J, Lea J, Lewis JB, Lipkowitz M, Massry S, Middleton, J, Miller, ER 3rd, Norris, K, O'Connor, D, Ojo, A, Phillips, RA, Pogue, V, Rahman, M, Randall, OS, Rostand, S, Schulman, G, Smith, W, Thornley-Brown, D, Tisher, CC, Toto, RD, Wright JT, Jr, Xu, S; African American Study of Kidney Disease and Hypertension (AASK) Study Group (2001). Effect of ramipril vs amlodipine on renal outcomes in hypertensive nephrosclerosis: a randomized controlled trial. *The journal of the American Medical Association* 285: 2719–2728.

Awadalla, Y, Randhawa, P, Ruppert, K, Zeevi, A, Duquesnoy, RJ (2004). HLA mismatching increases the risk of BK virus nephropathy in renal transplant recipients. *American Journal of Transplantation* 4: 1691–1696.

Azuma, H, Nadeau, K, Mackenzie, HS, Brenner, BM, Tilney, NL (1997). Nephron mass modulates the hemodynamic, cellular, and molecular response of the rat renal allograft. *Transplantation* 63: 519–528.

Bakris, GL, Williams, M, Dworkin, L, Elliott, WJ, Epstein, M, Toto, R, Tuttle, K, Douglas, J, Hsueh,W, Sowers, J (2000). Preserving renal function in adults with hypertension and diabetes: a consensus approach. National Kidney Foundation Hypertension and Diabetes Executive Committees Working Group. *American Journal of Kidney Diseases* 36: 646–661.

Basar, H, Soran, A, Shapiro, R, Vivas, C, Scantlebury, VP, Jordan, ML, Gritsch, HA, McCauley, J, Randhawa, P, Irish, W, Hakala, TR, Fung JJ (1999). Renal transplantation in recipients over the age of 60: the impact of donor age. *Transplantation* 67: 1191–1193.

Bear, RA, Aprile, M, Sweet, J, Cole, EH (1988). Proteinuria in renal transplant recipients: incidence, cause, prognostic importance. *Transplantation Proceedings* 20: 1235–1236.

Beck, S & Barrell BG (1988). Human cytomegalovirus encodes a glycoprotein homologous to MHC class-I antigens. *Nature* 331: 269–272.

Bemelman, FJ, de Maar, EF, Press, RR, van Kan, HJ, ten Berge, IJ, Homan van der Heide, JJ, de Fijter, HW (2009). Minimization of maintenance immunosuppression early after renal transplantation: an interim analysis. *Transplantation* 88: 421–428.

Benigni, A, Bruzzi, I, Mister, M, Azzollini, N, Gaspari, F, Perico, N, Gotti, E, Bertani, T, Remuzzi, G (1999). Nature and mediators of renal lesions in kidney transplant patients given cyclosporine for more than one year. *Kidney International* 55 (2): 674.

Braunwald, E, Domanski, MJ, Fowler, SE, Geller, NL, Gersh, BJ, Hsia, J, Pfeffer, MA, Rice, MM, Rosenberg, YD, Rouleau, JL; PEACE Trial Investigators (2004). Angiotensin-convertingenzyme inhibition in stable coronary artery disease. *New England Journal of Medicine* 351: 2058–2068.

Brenner BM (1985). Nephron adaptation to renal injury or ablation. *American Journal of Physiology* 249: F324–F337.

Brewster UC, Perazella MA (2004). The renin-angiotensin-aldosterone system and the kidney: effects on kidney disease. *American Journal of Medicine* 116: 263–272.

Briganti, EM, Russ, GR, McNeil, JJ, Atkins, RC, Chadban, SJ (2002). Risk of renal allograft loss from recurrent glomerulonephritis. *New England Journal of Medicine* 347 (2): 103.

Carlquist, JF, Muhlestein, JB, Horne, BD, Hart, NI, Lim, T, Habashi, J, Anderson, JG, Anderson, JL (2004). Cytomegalovirus stimulated mRNA accumulation and cell surface expression of the oxidized LDL scavenger receptor, CD36. *Atherosclerosis* 177: 53–59.

Chadban S (2001). Glomerulonephritis recurrence in the renal graft. *Journal of the American Society of Nephrology* 12 (2): 394.
Chang, SH, Russ, GR, Chadban, SJ, Campbell, SB, McDonald, SP (2007). Trends in kidney transplantation in Australia and New Zealand 1993-2004. *Transplansplantation* 15;84(5):611-8.
Chapman, JR O'Connell PJ, Nankivell BJ (2005). Chronic renal allograft dysfunction. *Journal of the American Society of Nephrology* 16(10):3015-26.
Chkhotua, AB, Gabusi, E, Altimari, A, D'Errico, A, Yakubovich, M, Vienken, J, Stefoni, S, Chieco, P, Yussim, A, Grigioni, WF (2003). Increased expression of p16(INK4a) and p27(Kip1) cyclin-dependent kinase inhibitor genes in aging human kidney and chronic allograft nephropathy. *American Journal of Kidney Diseases* 41: 1303–1313.
Collins, AB, Schneeberger, EE, Pascual, MA, Saidman, SL, Williams, WW, Tolkoff-Rubin, N, Cosimi, AB, Colvin, RB (1999). Complement activation in acute humoral renal allograft rejection: diagnostic significance of C4d deposits in peritubular capillaries. *Journal of the American Society of Nephrology* 10(10):2208-14.
Colvin, RB (2006). Renal transplant pathology. In: Jennette JC, Olson JL, Schwartz MM, Silva FG (eds). *Heptinstall's Pathology of the Kidney*, 6th edn, vol. 2. Lippincott-Raven: Philadelphia, pp 1347–1490.
Colvin RB (2007). Antibody-mediated renal allograft rejection: diagnosis and pathogenesis. *Journal of American Society of Nephrology* 18(4):1046-56.
Curtis JJ (1992). Cyclosporine and posttransplant hypertension. *Journal of American Society of Nephrology* 2: S243–S245.
Davies, DR, Bittmann I, Pardo J (2000). Histopathology of calcineurin inhibitor-induced nephrotoxicity. *Transplantation* 69(12 Suppl): SS11.
de Fijter, JW, Mallat, MJ, Doxiadis, II, Ringers, J, Rosendaal, FR, Claas, FH, Paul, LC (2001). Increased immunogenicity and cause of graft loss of old donor kidneys. *Journal of American Society of Nephrology* 12(7):1538-46.
Del Castillo, D, Cruzado, JM, Manel Díaz, J, Beneyto Castelló, I, Lauzurica Valdemoros, R, Gómez Huertas, E, Checa Andrés, MD (2004) et al. The effects of hyperlipidaemia on graft and patient outcome in renal transplantation. *Nephrology Dialysis Transplantation*; 19(Suppl 3): iii67–iii71.
Drachenberg, CB, Papadimitriou, JC, Mann, D, Hirsch, HH, Wali, R, Ramos, E (2005). Negative impact of human leukocyte antigen matching in the outcome of polyomavirus nephropathy. *Transplantation* 80: 276–278.
Durrbach, JM Pestana JM, Pearson T, Vincenti F, Garcia VD, Campistol J, Rial Mdel C, Florman S, Block A, Di Russo G, Xing J, Garg P, Grinyó J (2010). A Phase III Study of Belatacept Versus Cyclosporine in Kidney Transplants from Extended Criteria Donors (BENEFIT-EXT Study). *American Journal of Transplantation* 10(3):547-57.
Ekberg, H, Grinyó, J, Nashan, B, Vanrenterghem, Y, Vincenti, F, Voulgari, A, Truman, M, Nasmyth-Miller, C, Rashford, M (2007a). Cyclosporine sparing with mycophenolate mofetil, daclizumab and corticosteroids in renal allograft recipients: the CAESAR Study. *American Journal of Transplantation* 7: 560–570.
Ekberg, H, Tedesco-Silva, H, Demirbas, A, Vítko, S, Nashan, B, Gürkan, A, Margreiter, R, Hugo, C, Grinyó, JM, Frei, U, Vanrenterghem, Y, Daloze, P, Halloran, PF; ELITE-Symphony Study (2007b). ELITE-Symphony Study. Reduced exposure to

calcineurin inhibitors in renal transplantation. *New England Journal of Medicine* 357: 2562–2575.

Ekberg, H, Bernasconi, C, Tedesco-Silva, H, Vítko, S, Hugo, C, Demirbas, A, Acevedo, RR, Grinyó, J, Frei, U, Vanrenterghem, Y, Daloze, P, Halloran, P (2009). Calcineurin inhibitor minimization in the Symphony study: observational results 3 years after transplantation. *American Journal of Transplantation* 9: 1876–1885.

Farhood, A, McGuire, GM, Manning, AM, Miyasaka, M, Smith, CW, Jaeschke, H (1995). Intercellular adhesion molecule 1 (ICAM-1) expression and its role in neutrophil-induced ischemia-reperfusion injury in rat liver. *Journal of Leukocyte Biology* 57: 368–374.

Farris, AB, Gaut, J, Wong, W, Della Pelle, P, Brousaides, N, Collins, AB, Saidman, S, Schneeberger, EE, Smith, RN, Colvin, RB (2009). Pathology, serology and clinical characteristics of 68 patients with chronic humoral renal allograft rejection. *Laboratory Investigations* 22(Suppl 1): 302A–303A.

Fernando, GC (2004). Development of chronic allograft nephropathy (CAN) in low risk kidney transplant recipients. *American Journal of Transplantation* 4:278.

Feucht, HE , Felber, E, Gokel, MJ, Hillebrand, G, Nattermann, U, Brockmeyer, C, Held, E, Riethmüller, G, Land, W, Albert, E (1991). Vascular deposition of complement-split products in kidney allografts with cell-mediated rejection. *Clinical and Experimental Immunology* 86(3):464-70.

Flechner, SM, Kobashigawa, J, Klintmalm, G (2008). Calcineurin inhibitor-sparing regimens in solid organ transplantation: Focus on improving renal function and nephrotoxicity. *Clinical Transplantation* 22: 1–15.

Garcia, JF, Piris, MA, Lloret, E, Orradre, JL, Murillo, PG, Martínez, JC (1997). p53 expression in CMV-infected cells: association with the alternative expression of the p53 transactivated genes p21/WAF1 and MDM2. *Histopathology* 30: 120–125.

Gasser, M, Waaga, AM, Laskowski, IA, Tilney, NL (2000). The influence of donor brain death on short and long-term outcome of solid organ allografts. *Annals of Transplantation* 5: 61–67.

Gloor, JM, Cohen, AJ, Lager, DJ, Grande, JP, Fidler, ME, Velosa, JA, Larson, TS, Schwab, TR, Griffin, MD, Prieto, M, Nyberg, SL, Sterioff, S, Kremers, WK, Stegall, MD (2002). Subclinical rejection in tacrolimus-treated renal transplant recipients. *Transplantation* 27;73(12):1965-8.

Gloor, JM, Sethi, S, Stegall, MD, Park, WD, Moore, SB, DeGoey, S, Griffin, MD, Larson, TS, Cosio, FG (2007).Transplant glomerulopathy: subclinical incidence and association with alloantibody. *American Journal of Transplantation* 7(9):2124-32.

Gwinner, W, Suppa S, Mengel M, Hoy L, Kreipe HH, Haller H, Schwarz A (2005). Early calcification of renal allografts detected by protocol biopsies: causes and clinical implications. *American Journal of Transplantation* 5 (8): 1934.

Halloran, PF, Wadgymar, A, Ritchie, S, Falk J, Solez, K, Srinivasa, NS (1990). The significance of the anti-class I antibody response. I. Clinical and pathologic features of anti-class I-mediated rejection. *Transplantation* 49(1):85-91.

Halloran, PF, Melk A, Barth, C (1999). Rethinking chronic allograft nephropathy: the concept of accelerated senescence. *Journal of American Society of Nephrology* 10: 167–181.

Harley, CB, Futcher, AB, Greider CW (1990). Telomeres shortening during ageing of human fibroblasts. *Nature*; 345: 458–460.

Harper, SJ Moorhouse J, Veitch PS, Horsburgh T, Walls J, Bell PR, Donnelly PK, Feehally J (1992). Nifedipine improves immediate, and 6- and 12-month graft function in cyclosporin A (CyA) treated renal allograft recipients. *Transplant International* 5(Suppl 1): S69–S72.

Häyry, P, Isoniemi, H, Yilmaz, S, Mennander, A, Lemström, K, Räisänen-Sokolowski, A,Koskinen, P, Ustinov, J, Lautenschlager, I, Taskinen, E et al. (1993). Chronic allograft rejection. *Immunology Reviews* 134:33-81.

Heinze, G, Mitterbauer , C, Regele, H, Kramar, R, Winkelmayer, WC, Curhan, GC, Oberbauer, R (2006). Angiotensin-converting enzyme inhibitor or angiotensin II type 1 receptor antagonist therapy is associated with prolonged patient and graft survival after renal transplantation. *Journal of the American Society of Nephrology;* 17: 889–899.

Helantera, I, Loginov, R, Koskinen, P, Törnroth, T, Grönhagen-Riska, C, Lautenschlager, I (2005). Persistent cytomegalovirus infection is associated with increased expression of TGF-beta1, PDGF-AA and ICAM-1 and arterial intimal thickening in kidney allografts. *Nephrology Dialysis Transplantation* 20: 790–796.

Helantera, I, Teppo, AM, Koskinen, P, Törnroth, T, Grönhagen-Riska, C, Lautenschlager, I (2006). Increased urinary excretion of transforming growth factor-beta(1) in renal transplant recipients during cytomegalovirus infection. *Transpant Immunology* 15: 217–221.

Hiremath, S, Fergusson D, Doucette S. (2007). Renin angiotensin system blockade in kidney transplantation: a systematic review of the evidence. *American Journal of Transplantation;* 7: 2350–2360.

Hirsch HH & Steiger J (2003). Polyomavirus BK. *Lancet Infectious Diseases* 3(10):611-23.

Holdaas, H, Fellstrom, B, Jardine, AG (2003). Effect of fluvastatin on cardiac outcomes in renal transplant recipients: a multicentre, randomised, placebo-controlled trial. *Lancet* 361: 2024–2031.

Inkinen, K, Soots, A, Krogerus, L (2001). Cytomegalovirus infection enhances connective tissue growth factor mRNA expression in a rat model of chronic renal allograft rejection. *Transplantation Proceedings* 33: 379.

Inkinen, K, Holma, K, Soots, A (2003). Expression of TGF-beta and PDGF-AA antigens and corresponding mRNAs in cytomegalovirus-infected rat kidney allografts. *Transplantation Proceedings* 35: 804–805.

Ishii, Y, Sawada, T, Kubota, K, Fuchinoue, S, Teraoka, S, Shimizu, A (2005). Loss of peritubular capillaries in the development of chronic allograft nephropathy. *Transplantation Proceedings* 37(2):981-3.

Isonemi, H, Takinen, E, Hayry, P (1994). Histological chronic allograft damage index accurately predicts chronic renal allograft rejection. *Transplantation* 58: 1195, 1994.

Itahana, K, Campisi, J, Dimri, GP et al. (2004). Mechanisms of cellular senescence in human and mouse cells. *Biogerontology* 5: 1–10.

Joosten, SA, van Kooten, C, Sijpkens, YW, de Fijter, JW, Paul, LC (2004). The pathobiology of chronic allograft nephropathy : immune-mediated damage and accelerated aging. *Kidney International* 65(5):1556-9.

Jurewicz, WA (1999). Immunological and nonimmunological risk factors with tacrolimus and Neoral in renal transplant recipients: an interim repot. *Transplantation Proceedings* 31(7A):64S-66S.

Kaplan, B, Schold, J, Meier-Kriesche, HU (2003). Poor predictive value of serum creatinine for renal allograft loss. *American Journal of Transplantation* 3(12):1560-5.

Kasiske, BL, Vazquez, MA, Harmon, WE (2000). Recommendations for the outpatient surveillance of renal transplant recipients. *Journal of American Society of Nephrology* 15: S1–S86.

Ke, B, Shen, XD, Gao, F (2005). The CD154-CD40 T-cell co-stimulation pathway in liver ischemia and reperfusion inflammatory responses. *Transplantation* 79: 1078–1083.

Kieran, N, Wang, X, Perkins, J, Davis, C, Kendrick, E, Bakthavatsalam, R, Dunbar, N, Warner, P, Nelson, K, Smith, KD, Nicosia, RF, Alpers, CE, Leca, N, Kowalewska, J (2009). Combination of peritubular c4d and transplant glomerulopathy predicts late renal allograft failure. *Journal of the American Society of Nephrololgy* 20(10):2260-8.

Kim, HC, Hwang, EA, Han, SY (2005). Polyomavirus nephropathy after renal transplantation: a single centre experience. *Nephrology (Carlton)* 10: 198–203.

Koukoulaki, M, Grispou, E, Pistolas, D (2009). Prospective monitoring of BK virus replication in renal transplant recipients. *Transplant Infectious Diseases* 11: 1–10.

Larsen, CP, Pearson, TC, Adams, AB (2005). Rational development of LEA29Y (belatacept), a high-affinity variant of CTLA4-Ig with potent immunosuppressive properties. *American Journal of Transplantation* 5: 443–453.

Levey, AS, Bosch, JP, Lewis, JB, Greene, T, Rogers, N, Roth, D (1999). A more accurate method to estimate glomerular filtration rate from serum creatinine: a new p^rdiction equation. Modification of Diet in Renal Disease Study group. *Annals of Internal Medicine* 16;130(6):461-70.

Mannon RB (2004). Polyomavirus nephropathy: what have we learned? *Transplantation* 15;77(9):1313-8.

Mannon RB (2010). Immune monitoring and biomarkers to predict chronic allograft dysfunction. Kidney International 78 Suppl 119:S59-65.

Mauiyyedi, S, Crespo, M, Collins, AB, Schneeberger, EE, Pascual, MA, Saidman, SL, Tolkoff-Rubin, NE, Williams, WW, Delmonico, FL, Cosimi, AB, Colvin, RB (2002). Acute humoral rejection in kidney transplantation: II. Morphology, immunopathology, and pathologic classification. *Journal of the American Society of Nephrology* 13(3):779-87.

Meier-Kriesche, HU, Schold, JD, Srinivas, TR, Kaplan, B (2004). Lack of improvement in renal allograft survival despite a marked decrease in acute rejection rates over the most recent era. *American Journal of Transplantation* 4(3):378-83.

Melk, A, Schmidt, BM, Takeuchi, O (2004). Expression of p16INK4a and other cell cycle regulator and senescence associated genes in aging human kidney. *Kidney International* 65: 510–520.

Mihatsch, MJ, Thiel, G, Ryffel, B (1988). Histopathology of cyclosporine nephrotoxicity. *Transplantation Proceedings* 20(3 Suppl 3): 759.

Mihatsch, MJ, Ryffel B, Gudat F (1995). The differential diagnosis between rejection and cyclosporine toxicity. *Kidney International Suppl* 95; 52: S63.

Naesens, M, Kuypers, DR, Sarwal, M (2009). Calcineurin inhibitor nephrotoxicity. *Clinical Journal of the American Society of Nephrology* 4: 481–508.

Nankivell, BJ, Fenton-Lee, CA, Kuypers, DR, Cheung, E, Allen, RD, O'Connell, PJ, Chapman, JR (2001). Effect of histological damage on long-term kidney transplant outcome. *Transplantation* 27;71(4):515-23.

Nankivell, BJ, Borrows RJ, Fung CL, O'Connell PJ, Allen RD, Chapman JR et al (2003). The natural history of chronic allograft nephropathy. *New England Journal of Medicine* 349:2326–2333.

Nankivell, BJ, Borrows, RJ, Fung, CL, O'Connell, PJ, Allen, RD, Chapman, JR (2004a). Evolution and pathophysiology of renal-transplant glomerulosclerosis. *Transplantation* 78 (3): 461-468.

Nankivell, BJ, Borrows, RJ, Fung, CL, O'Connell, PJ, Allen, RD, Chapman, JR (2004b). Natural history, risk factors, and impact of subclinical rejection in kidney transplantation. *Transplantation* 78:242–249.

Nankivell, BJ, Borrows, RJ, Fung, CL, O'Connell, PJ, Chapman, JR, Allen, RD (2004c). Calcineurin inhibitor nephrotoxicity: longitudinal assessment by protocol histology. *Transplantation* 78:557–565.

Nankivell, BJ, Borrows, RJ, Fung, CL, O'Connell, PJ, Chapman, JR, Allen, RD (2004d). Delta analysis of posttransplantation tubulointerstitial damage. *Transplantation* 78:434–441.

Nankivell, BJ & Chapman, JR (2006). Chronic allograft nephropathy: current concepts and future directions. *Transplantation* 15;81(5):643-54.

Nickeleit, V, Hirsch, HH, Zeiler, M (2000a). BK-virus nephropathy in renal transplants-tubular necrosis, MHC-class II expression and rejection in a puzzling game. *Nephrology Dialysis Transplantation* 15: 324–332.

Nickeleit, V, Klimkait, T, Binet, IF (2000b). Testing for polyomavirus type BK DNA in plasma to identify renal-allograft recipients with viralnephropathy. *New England Journal of Medicine* 342: 1309–1315.

Nickeleitt, V, Zeiler, M, Gudat, F, Thiel, G, Mihatsch, MJ (2002). Detection of the complement degradation product C4d in renal allografts: Diagnostic and therapeutic implications. *Journal of American Society of Nephrology* 13:242–251.

Ojo, AO (2006). Cardiovascular complications after renal transplantation and their prevention. *Transplantation* 82: 603–611.

Opelz, G, Wujciak T, Döhler B, Scherer S, Mytilineos J (1999). HLA compatibility and organ transplant survival : Collaborative Transplant Study. *Reviews in Immunogenetics* 1(3):334-42.

Opelz, G & Döhler B (2007). Effect of human leukocyte antigen compatibility on kidney graft survival: comparative analysis of two decades. *Transplantation* 27;84(2):137-43.

Oppenheimer, F, Aljama, P, Asensio Peinado, C (2004). The impact of donor age on the results of renal transplantation. *Nephrology Dialysis Transplantation* 19(Suppl 3): 11–15.

Osborn, L (1990). Leukocyte adhesion to endothelium in inflammation. *Cell* 62: 3–6. Paul, LC (1999). Chronic allograft nephropathy: An update. *Kidney International* 56(3):783-93.

Pelle, G, Vimont, S, Levy, PP (2007). Acute pyelonephritis represents a risk factor impairing long-term kidney graft function. *American Journal of Transplantation* 7: 899–907.

Perico, N, Benigni, A, Remuzzi, G (2008). Present and future drug treatments for chronic kidney diseases: evolving targets in renoprotection. *Nature Reviews Drugs Discovery* 7: 936–953.

Prat, V, Horcickova, M, Matousovic, K (1985). Urinary tract infection in renal transplant patients. *Infection* 13: 207–210.

Racusen, LC, Solez K, Colvin, RB, Bonsib, SM, Castro, MC, Cavallo, T, Croker, BP, Demetris, AJ, Drachenberg, CB, Fogo, AB, Furness, P, Gaber, LW, Gibson, IW, Glotz, D, Goldberg, JC, Grande, J, Halloran, PF, Hansen, HE, Hartley, B, Hayry, PJ, Hill, CM, Hoffman, EO, Hunsicker, LG, Lindblad, AS, Yamaguchi,Y. The Banff 97 working classification of renal allograft pathology. *Kidney International* 55: 713–723.

Racusen, LC, Colvin, RB, Solez, K, Mihatsch, MJ, Halloran, PF, Campbell, PM, Cecka, JM, Cosyns, JP, Demetris, AJ, Fishbein, MC, Fogo, AB, Furness, P, Gibson, IW, Glotz, D, Hayry, P, Hunsickern, LG, Kashgarian, M, Kerman, R, Magil, AJ, Montgomery, R, Morozumi, K, Nickeleit, V, Randhawa, P, Regele, H, Seron, D, Seshan, S, Sund, S, Trpkov, K (2003). Antibody mediated rejection criteria: An addition to the Banff 97 classification of renal allograft rejection. *American Journal of Transplantation* 3:708–714.

Rahamimov, R, Lustig, S, Tovar, A (2003). BK polyoma virus nephropathy in kidney transplant recipient: the role of new immunosuppressive agents. *Transplantation Proceedings* 35: 604–605.

Ram, CV (2008). Angiotensin receptor blockers: current status and future prospects. *American Journal of Medicine* 121: 656–663.

Remuzzi, G & Perico, N (1998). Protecting single-kidney allografts from long-term functional deterioration. *Journal of American Society of Nephrology* 9: 1321–1332.

Remuzzi, G, Benigni, A, Remuzzi ,A (2006). Mechanisms of progression and regression of renal lesions of chronic nephropathies and diabetes. *Journal of Clinical Investigation* 116: 288–296.

Ruggenenti, P, Perna, A, Mosconi, L (1997). Randomised placebo-controlled trial of effect of ramipril on decline in glomerular filtration rate and risk of terminal renal failure in proteinuric, non-diabetic nephropathy. The GISEN Group (Gruppo Italiano di Studi Epidemiologici in Nefrologia). *Lancet* 349: 1857–1863.

Ruiz-Ortega, M, Ruperez, M, Esteban, V (2006). Angiotensin II: a key factor in the inflammatory and fibrotic response in kidney diseases. *Nephrology Dialysis Transplantation* 21: 16–20.

Rush, D, Arlen, D, Boucher, A, Busque, S, Cockfield, SM, Girardin, C, Knoll, G, Lachance, JG, Landsberg, D, Shapiro, J, Shoker, A, Yilmaz, S (2007). Lack of benefit of early protocol biopsies in renal transplant patients receiving TAC and MMF: a randomized study. *American Journal of Transplantation* 7(11):2538-45.

Rush, DN, Henry, SF, Jeffery, JR, Schroeder, TJ, Gough, J (1994). Histological findings in early routine biopsies of stable renal allograft recipients. *Transplantation* 57(2):208-11.

Rush, DN, Jeffery, JR, Gough, J (1995). Sequentiel protocol biopsies in renal transplant patients. Clinico-pathological correlations using the Banff schema. *Transplantation* 27; 59(4):511-4.

Russell, PS & Winn HJ (1970). Transplantation. I. *New England Journal of Medicine* 2; 282(14):786-93.

Salahudeen, AK, Haider, N, May, W (2004). Cold ischemia and the reduced long-term survival of cadaveric renal allografts. *Kidney International* 65: 713–718.

Salzberg, DJ (2007). Is RAS blockade routinely indicated in hypertensive kidney transplant patients? *Current Hypertension Reports* 9: 422–429.

Schena, FP, Pascoe, MD, Alberu, J (2009). Sirolimus CONVERT Trial Study Group Conversion from calcineurin inhibitors to sirolimus maintenance therapy in renal allograft recipients: 24-month efficacy and safety results from the CONVERT trial. *Transplantation* 87: 233–242.

Schwarz, A, Mengel, M, Gwinner, W, Radermarcher, J, Hiss-Kreipe, H, Haller, H (2005) Risk factors for chronic allograft nephropathy after renal transplantation: A protocol biopsy study. *Kidney International* 67:341–348.

Schwenger, V, Zeier, M, Ritz, E (2001). Hypertension after renal transplantation. *Current Hypertension Reports* 3: 434–439.

Seron, D, Oppenheimer, F, Pallardo, LM (2008). Fluvastatin in the prevention of renal transplant vasculopathy: results of a prospective, randomized, double-blind, placebo-controlled trial. *Transplantation* 86: 82–87.

Shapiro, R, Randhawa, P, Jordan, ML, Scantlebury, VP, Vivas, C, Jain, A, Corry, RJ, McCauley, J, Johnston, J, Donaldson, J, Gray, EA, Dvorchik, I, Hakala, TR, Fung, JJ, Starzl, TE (2001). An analysis of early renal transplant protocol biopsies--the high incidence of subclinical tubulitis. *American Journal of Transplantation* 1(1):47-50.

Shishido, S, Asanuma, H, Nakai, H, Mori, Y, Satoh, H, Kamimaki, I, Hataya, H, Ikeda, M, Honda, M, Hasegawa, A (2003). The impact of repeated subclinical acute rejection on the progression of chronic allograft nephropathy. *Journal of American Society of Nephrology* 14 (4):1046-52.

Shoskes, DA & Halloran, PF. Delayed graft function in renal transplantation: etiology, management and long-term significance. *Journal of Urology* 155: 1831–1840.

Sijpkens, YW, Doxiadis, II, van Kemenade, FJ, Zwinderman, AH, de Fijter, JW, Claas, FH, Bruijn, JA, Paul, LC (2003). Chronic rejection with or without transplant vasculopathy. *Clinical Transplantation* 17(3):163-70.

Sis, B, Campbell, PM, Mueller, T, Hunter, C, Cockfield, SM, Cruz, J, Meng, C, Wishart, D, Solez, K, Halloran, PF (2007). Transplant glomerulopathy, late antibody-mediated rejection and the ABCD tetrad in kidney allograft biopsies for cause. *American Journal of Transplantation* 7(7):1743-52.

Smak Gregoor, PJ, van de Se´vaux RG, Ligtenberg G (2000). Randomized study on the conversion of treatment with cyclosporine to azathioprine or mycophenolate mofetil followed by dose reduction. *Transplantation* 70: 143–148.

Smak Gregoor, PJ van Gelder, T, van Besouw, NM et al. (2002). Withdrawal of cyclosporine or prednisone six months after kidney transplantation in patients on triple drug therapy: a randomized, prospective, multicenter study. *Journal of American Society of Nephrology* 13: 1365–1373.

Smith, JM, Dharnidharka, VR, Talley, L (2007). BK virus nephropathy in pediatric renal transplant recipients: an analysis of the North American Pediatric Renal Trials and Collaborative Studies (NAPRTCS) registry. *Clinical Journal of American Society of Nephrology* 2: 1037–1042.

Solez, K, Axelsen, RA, Benediktsson, H (1993). International standardization of criteria for the histologic diagnosis of renal allograft rejection: the Banff working classification of kidney transplant pathology. *Kidney International* 44 (2): 411.

Solez, K, Vincenti, F, Filo, RS (1998). Histopathologic findings from 2-year protocol biopsies from a U.S multicenter kidney transplant trial comparaing tacrolimus versus cyclosporine : a report of the FK506 Kidney transplant Study Group.. *Transplantation* 27; 66(12):1736-40.

Solez, K, Colvin, RB, Racusen, LC, Sis, B, Halloran, PF, Birk, PE, Campbell, PM, Cascalho, M, Collins, AB, Demetris, AJ, Drachenberg, CB, Gibson, IW, Grimm, PC, Haas, M, Lerut, E, Liapis, H, Mannon, RB, Marcus, PB, Mengel, M, Mihatsch, MJ, Nankivell, BJ, Nickeleit, V, Papadimitriou, JC, Platt, JL, Randhawa, P, Roberts, I, Salinas-Madriga, L, Salomon, DR, Seron, D, Sheaff, M, Weening, JJ et al. (2007). Banff '05 Meeting Report: differential diagnosis of chronic allograft injury and elimination of chronic allograft nephropathy ('CAN'). *American Journal of Transplantation* 7(3):518-26.

Svetkey, LP, Erlinger, TP, Vollmer, WM (2005). Effect of lifestyle modifications on blood pressure by race, sex, hypertension status, and age. *Journal of Human Hypertension* 19: 21–31.

Tedla, F, Hayashi, R, McFarlane (2007). Hypertension after renal transplant. *Journal of Clinical Hypertension (Greenwich)* 9: 538–545.

Terasaki, PI, Ozawa, M, Castro, R (2007). Four-year follow-up of a prospective trial of HLA and MICA antibodies on kidney graft survival. *American Journal of Transplantation* 7(2):408-15.

Timsit, MO, Yuan, X, Floerchinger, B, Ge, X, Tullius, SG (2010). Consequences of transplant quality on chronic allograft nephropathy. *Kidney International* 78 Suppl 119:S54-8.

Tomlanovich, SJ & Vincenti, F (2007). Sirolimus: defining nephrotoxicity in the renal transplant recipient. *Clinical Journal of American Society of Nephrology* 2: 198–199.

Toyoda, M, Galfayan, K, Galera, OA (1997). Cytomegalovirus infection induces anti-endothelial cell antibodies in cardiac and renal allograft recipients. *Transplant Immunology* 5: 104–111.

Tsimihodimos, V, Dounousi, E, Siamopoulos, KC (2008). Dyslipidemia in chronic kidney disease: an approach to pathogenesis and treatment. *American Journal of Nephrology* 28: 958–973.

Veronese, FV, Noronha, IL, Manfro, RC, Edelweiss, MI, Goldberg, J, Gonçalves, LF (2004). Prevalence and immunohistochemical findings of subclinical kidney allograft rejection and its association with graft outcome. *Clinical Transplantation* 18(4):357-64.

Vincenti, F, Ramos, E, Brattstrom, C (2001). Multicenter trial exploring calcineurin inhibitors avoidance in renal transplantation. *Transplantation*; 71: 1282–1287.

Vincenti, F, Larsen, C, Durrbach, A (2005). Belatacept Study Group. Costimulation blockade with belatacept in renal transplantation. *New England Journal of Medicine* 353: 770–781.

Vincenti, F, Charpentier, B, Vanrenterghem, Y (2010). A Phase III Study of Belatacept-based Immunosuppression Regimens versus Cyclosporine in Renal Transplant Recipients (BENEFIT Study). *American Journal of Transplantation* 10(3): 535-546.

Weiss, AS, Gralla, J, Chan, L (2008). Aggressive immunosuppression minimization reduces graft loss following diagnosis of BK virus associated nephropathy: a comparison of two reduction strategies. *Clinical Journal of American Society of Nephrology* 3: 1812–1819.

Westhoff, JH, Schildhom, C, Jacobi, C (2010). Telomere shortening reduces regenerative capacity after acute kidney injury. *Journal of American Society of Nephrology* 21: 327–336.

White, LH, Casian, A, Hilton, R. (2008). BK virus nephropathy in renal transplant patients in London. *Transplantation* 85: 1008–1015.

Wright Jr, JT, Bakris, G, Greene, T (2002). Effect of blood pressure lowering and antihypertensive drug class on progression of hypertensive kidney disease: results from the AASK trial. *The journal of the American Medical Association* 288: 2421–2431.

Zeisberg, EM, Tarnavski, O, Zeisberg, M, Dorfman, AL, McMullen, JR, Gustafsson, E, Chandraker, A, Yuan, X, Pu, WT, Roberts, AB, Neilson, EG, Sayegh, MH, Izumo, S, Kalluri, R (2007). Endothelial-to-mesenchymal transition contributes to cardiac fibrosis. *Nature Medicine* 13(8):952-61.

Zindy, F, Quelle, DE, Roussel, MF (1997). Expression of the p16INK4a tumor suppressor versus other INK4 family members during mouse development and aging. *Oncogene* 15: 203–211.

18

Antibody-Mediated Kidney Allograft Rejection

Xu Haiyan and He Xiaozhou
Third Affiliated Hospital of Soochow University, Changzhou, China

1. Introduction

Successful kidney transplantation improves the quality of life and increases survival when compared with long-term dialysis. Renal transplantation is now a well established and the preferred treatment for most patients with end-stage renal disease (ESRD). In recent years, the short-term effects of kidney transplantation have been greatly achieved due to the improvement in immunosuppression medicines, better genotyping technology and monitoring methods. However, the long-term outcome of kidney transplantation has not been improved for long period. Among the various influencing factors, antibody-mediated kidney allograft rejection is now widely recognized as a major problem which decreases the long-term outcome. How many kinds of antibodies involved in the antibody-mediated rejection (AMR)? How do these antibodies produce? How do these antibodies injure the transplantated kidney function? How to eliminate these antibodies? How about the clinical effects when the new agents were applied? All these questions are being gradually and deeply studied.

2. Anti-HLA and MHC-class I related chain A antibody

At present, anti-HLA antibody (Lefaucheur et al., 2010) and anti-MHC-class I related chain Antibody (Zou et al., 2009) are the main cytotoxic antibodies, resulting in kidney allograft rejection and long-term kidney allograft survival.

2.1 Anti-HLA antibody

HLA (the human leukocyte antigen system) is the name of the major histocompatibilty complex (MHC) in humans. MHC molecules are divided into 2 main classes: HLA class I antigens (HLA-A, -B, and –C), presented on the surface of all nucleated cells and platelets; and HLA class II antigens (HLA-DR, -DQ, -DP, -DM and –DO), expressed on professional antigen-presenting cells, but also on the surface of vascular endothelial cells and renal tubular epithelial cells. There lie high polymorphism degree of the HLA system (more than 1600 alleles), so the individuals do not present identical sets of HLA antigens. After solid organ transplantation, HLA polymorphism confers immunological identity to the recipients, thus, the immune system can distinguish between self and non-self, and non-self may represent targets for the immune system. T cellular-mediated rejection (TCMR) and/or AMR will be initiated. As for AMR, donor specific anti-HLA antigens -I and -II alloantibodies would be produced.

The presence of alloantibodies against donor HLA-I and HLA-II antigens has been associated with hyperacute and accelarated graft rejection. Since HLA typing is strictly requested before renal transplantation (RTx), whatever cadaveric RTx, or living related or non-related RTx, the incidence of hyperacute and accelarated graft rejection have been greatly decreased.
However, some evidences suggest that donor specific antibody (DSA) is common in RTx recipients after 1 year of operation, which may be explained by the HLA polymorphism.

2.2 Anti-MHC-class I related chain A antibody (MICA)

MHC-class I related chain (MIC) has been reported to be an important polymorphic alloantigen system, consisting of MICA and MICB, and distributing on the peripheral blood lymphocytes, tissue endotheliocytes, and umbilical endotheliocytes, which also play a role in renal allograft rejection. Specific anti-MICA antibody can be found in sera of transplanted patients with allograft rejection (Zou et al, 2007). And the statistical analysis indicated that, anti-MICA antibodies were associated with the failure of a renal graft, regardless of good HLA typying (0 or 1 HLA mis matched) and PRA =0.
One report showed that, despite negative pretransplantation T- and B- lymphocyte flow cytometric crossmatches and blood group identity, two cases of hyperacute humoral rejection of living related kidney grafts happened (Grandtnerova et al, 2008). Retrospectively, antiendothelial IgG antibodies were detected on a panel of umbilical cord cells in the first case, and IgM antibodies against donor endothelial precursor cells were detected using a new endotheilal cell crossmatch kit in the second case. Standard crossmatch methods using donor lymphocytes failed to detect these pathogenic antibodies and did not predict the danger of hyperacute rejection.
Now, MIC typying is still not carried out in clinic. Were the antiendothelial IgG and IgM antibody all belonging to anti-MICA antibody? This question may be worth investigating.

2.3 Subtypes of alloantibodies

IgM-alloantibody and IgG-alloantibody are all common in the peripheral blood and intragraft of recipients, and they are all involved in kidney allograft rejection.
IgM antibodies against donor HLA antigens can be found before transplantation and also produced both early and late in the post-transplant course. IgM antibodies against donor HLA appear to be associated with decreased survival of kidney and heart allografts.
IgG1/IgG3 and IgM can specially bind to alloantigens, activate complement system, and play their immunological action. While IgG2 only weakly activate complement system, and IgG4 does not activate complement system. IgG1/IgG3 and IgM probably participate in AMR by this pathway.
This viewpoint is concordant to the observed evidence. For example, three cases of successful living donor kidney transplantation, showed strongly positive B lymphocyte flow cytometry owing to highly reactive DSA directed to HLA II antigens. IgG solid-phase subtypes analysis suggested that, more than 50% of these antibodies were represented by non-complement binding IgG2/IgG4 subtypes (Lobashevsky et al., 2010).
Now, new technologies are quickly developed. Some new methods based on solid phase multiplex platforms, such as ELISA, flow cytometry and luminex, have been applied in clinic. These methods can detect binding of serum antibodies to specific antigens independently of complement activation. And, using additional anti-IgM/IgG antibodies,

these new technologies can distinguish between IgM and IgG anti-HLA antibodies. Additionally, it can discriminate between HLA class I and class II antibodies, and more, single antigen methods allow identification of a unique HLA specificity.
With the help of development in detection technology, clinician can obtain more precise information and make rational decision.

2.4 Potential mechanism

After these antibodies are produced, they will attack their targets represented by the graft endothelial cells, complement system would be activated, coagulation cascade happened and other inflammation factors would be produced. This procedure may be the most classical procedure of AMR.
The microcirculation characteristic of microcirculation changes of AMR include of:
(1) Microcirculation inflammation (glomerulitis (g), peritubular capillaritis (ptc))(Einecke et al., 2009); (2) Microcirculation deterioration (transplant glomerulopathy (cg), medangial matrix increase (mm)); (3) Peritubular capillary basement membrane multilayering (ptcm-score) ; (4) Diffuse C4d positivity.
A key element in the pathology of AMR is capillaritis, which is associated with glomerulitis and anti-HLA antibodies. Over time it seems likely that capillaritis will induce peritubular capillary basement membrane multilayering as a time dependent feature of late AMR.

3. Antibody-producing cells

3.1 Characterization of intra-graft B cells

During renal allograft rejection, cluster-forming $CD20^+$ B cells in the rejected graft are likely derived from the recipient and composed of mature B cells. These cells are activated ($CD79a^+$), some of them contain memory B cells ($CD27^+$) and do not correlate with intra-graft C4d deposition or with donor-specific antibody detection.
Furthermore, several non-cluster forming $CD20^-$ B-lineage $CD38^+$ plasmablasts and plasma cells infiltrate in the rejected grafts and these cells strongly correlated with circulating donor-specific antibody, and to a lesser extent with intra-graft C4d.
Both $CD20^+$ B cells and $CD38^+$ cells correlated with poor response of the rejection to steroids. Reduced graft survival is associated with the presence of CD20 cells in the graft.
And, a specific subset of early lineage B cells appears to be antigen-presenting cells and which may support a steroid-resistant T-cell-mediated cellular rejection when these cells present in the rejected graft. Late lineage interstitial plasmablasts and plasma cells may also support AMR. These studies suggest that detailed analysis of interstitial cellular infiltrates may allow better use of B-cell lineage specific treatments to improve graft outcomes.

3.2 Plasma cells and memory B cells

Now the exact cellular mechanisms responsible for AMR are still not known. It seems likely that both pre-existing plasma cells and the conversion of memory B cells to new plasma cells play a role in the increased DSA production (Stegall et al., 2010).
There indeed normally exists very little amount of long-lived plasma cells, but they may not be able to produce enough pathological alloantibodies to injury the kidney allograft. Plasma cells, DSA and C4d are associated with each other in renal transplants developing chronic rejection by sequential graft biopsies detection. Bone-marrow-derived long-lived plasma

cells appear to be a major source of donor-specific alloantibody in sensitized renal transplant recipients. Memory B cells appear to be important in early acute AMR, but few basic have been performed.

3.3 Potential survival factor: BAFF

Some factors may survive the plasma cells or enhance the production of pathological alloantibodies. B cell activating factor belonging to TNF superfamily (BAFF) may be one of the most potential survival factors. BAFF is also termed Blys, TALL-1, zTNF4, THANK and TNFSF13b, is a nomotrimer, member of the TNF superfamilies, expressed on the cell surface or cleaved and secreted. BAFF specifically binds to BAFF receptor (BAFF-R, also known as BR3 (Thompson, et al., 2001)), and BAFF can also bind to other two receptors, transmembrane activator and calcium-modulator and cyclophilin ligand interactor (TACI) and B-cell maturation antigen (BCMA), shared with another TNF ligand, a proliferation-inducing ligand (APRIL) (Day, et al., 2005).

BAFF is expressed by monocyte-derived cells, such as monocytes, macrophages, dendritic cells, and activated T lymphocytes, which plays an important role in immune response (Mackay, F. and Schneider, P. 2009). The discovery of BAFF has shed new light on the importance of finely tuned B cell survival for B cell tolerance during B cell maturation and activation. Excessive production of BAFF is associated with the development of autoimmune diseases, because transgenic (Tg) mice that overproduce BAFF develop severe autoimmune disorders resemble systemic lupus erythematosus (SLE) and Sjogren's syndrome (SS) in humans, possibly as a result of improper B cell survival, predominantly affecting the maturing splenic transitional type 2 (T2) and the marginal zone (MZ) B cell populations. BAFF-induced autoimmunity in BAFF Tg mice appears to be highly dependent on B cells and possibly the production of autoantibodies. High levels of BAFF have been found in the blood of patients with autoimmune diseases, particularly SLE and SS. And BAFF is also found on T lymphocytes infiltrating labial salivary glands from patients with SS.

3.3.1 BAFF and rituximab

Rituximab can specially delete $CD20^{+}$ B lymphocytes, gradually applied to induce immunosuppression state at present. The impact of rituximab therapy on tertiary lymphoid organs associate with chronic active antibody-mediated rejection, a prototypic humoral chronic inflammatory condition. In certain patients, inflammatory microenvironment provides BAFF-dependent paracrine survival signal to B-cells in tertiary lymphoid organs, allowing them to escape rituximab-induced apoptosis, thereby thwarting therapeutic efficiency (Thaunat et al. 2008).

3.3.2 BAFF and alemtuzumab

BAFF is increased in renal transplant patients following treatment with alemtuzumab (Bloom et al. 2009). Alemtuzumab is an anti-CD52 monoclonal antibody that can deplete T and B cells and is used as induction therapy for renal transplant recipients. However without long-term calcineurin inhibitor (CNI) therapy, alemtuzumab-treated patients have a prospensity to develop alloantibody and may undergo AMR.

These data suggest associations between BAFF signal and AMR in alemtuzumab-treated patients.

3.3.3 BAFF and renal transplantation

In view of special bioactivity of BAFF, experiments have been carried through to explore the expression characteristic of BAFF and its potential bioactivity in renal allograft rejection, and some significant results were obtained.

3.3.3.1 BAFF expression and serum PRA

The FACS (Fluorescence Activated Cell Sorter) results indicated that, cell surface BAFF was abnormally highly expressed on peripheral T lymphocytes of some kidney transplant recipients, especially in those recipients for more than 5 years (Fig.1).

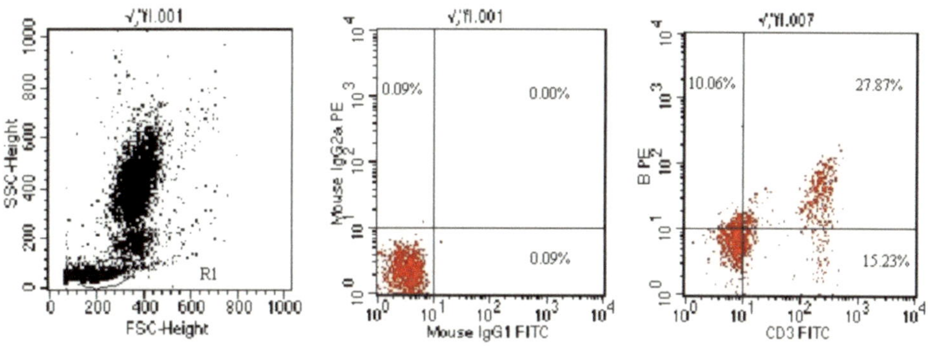

Fig. 1. BAFF expression on CD3+ T lymphocytes in RTx recipients after 5 yrs' operation

The real-time PCR (Polymerase Chain Reaction) results showed that BAFF mRNA levels gradually increased along with the prolonged transplantation time, and BAFF mRNA levels were consistent with BAFF protein levels in different groups (Fig.2).

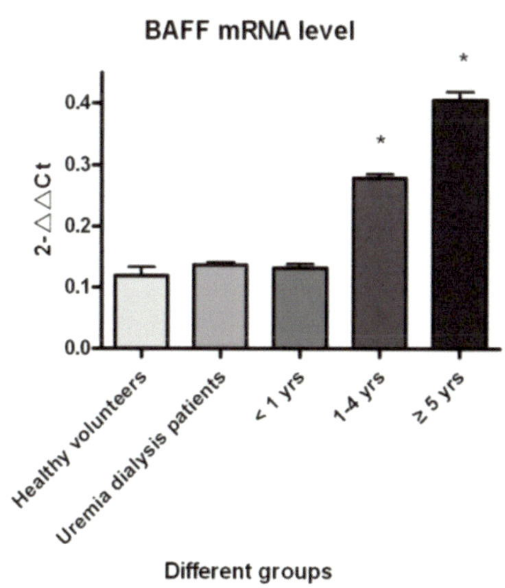

Fig. 2. BAFF mRNA levels in peripheral blood monocytes of RTx recipients after operation with different periods (<1 yr, 1-4 yr and ≥5 yr)

Healthy volunteers and uremia dialysis patients as controls
To investigate the correlation of transplanted renal function and BAFF expression, transplanted renal function was stratified and these data were statistically analyzed. In abnormal renal function group, BAFF was abnormally highly expressed on peripheral T lymphocytes, and the expression level was about as high as that in ≥ 5 years group. And there was statistically significant association between anti-HLA I & II antibodies level and BAFF expression level (Tab.1).

		anti-HLA I & II antibodies
CD257	Person Correlation	.587**
	Sig (2-tailed)	.008

Table 1. The correlation analysis of BAFF expression and serum PRA (panel reactive antibody)

The results indicated that BAFF expression was correlated with gradually decreasing transplant renal function, and BAFF may be involved in immune regulating network of kidney transplantation, which was the first report about BAFF and kidney transplantation.

3.3.3.2 BAFF and its receptors in the allograft rejection tissues

To further investigate the role of BAFF in AMR in renal transplantation, the correlation of BAFF and C4d deposition in excised transplanted kidney and protocol biopsies were investigated. The results showed that, BAFF could not only be found in renal allograft tissues, including AR and IF/TA (Interstitial Fibrosis/Tubular Atrophy) tissues, but also was highly expressed in these allograft sections, compared to protocol biopsy sections. BAFF can regulate the development of transitional B lymphocytes and survival of plasmacytoid lymphocytes, which implies that the BAFF signal may participate in AMR. To test this presumption, C4d and IgG were also detected in these allograft sections by immunohistochemistry. The results showed that BAFF expression significantly correlated with C4d deposition. The intensity and percentage score of BAFF were similar to those of C4d. BAFF mainly distributed in the perinephric tubular epithelial cell cytoplasm and cytomembrane, similar to the distribution of C4d. There was IgG deposition in BAFF high-expression sections, but its intensity and percentage score were much weaker than BAFF. IgG deposition was also mainly distributed in the perinephric tubular epithelial cell cytoplasm and cytomembrane.
The patients' clinical materials were shown in Tab.2. And the representative examples of immunohistochemical (IHC) staining of BAFF and C4d in renal allograft rejection tissues were listed in Fig. 3.

groups		**gender** Male/ female	**Age (year) (means±SD)**	**PRA(%)**	**HLA-DR non-matched level**	**POD(day, means±SD)**
Graft failure	AR(n=10)	6/4	39±10 (19~58)	17±4.1	0.8±0.6 (0~2)	9±8
	UAC(n=9)	4/5	42±8 (32~56)	5±4.2	0.7±0.7 (0~2)	1875±784
Graft normal	Protocol renal biopies (n=10)	7/3	37±5 (26~48)	7.4±3.5	0.7±0.7 (0~2)	17±4

Table 2. All the accepted patients' clinical materials

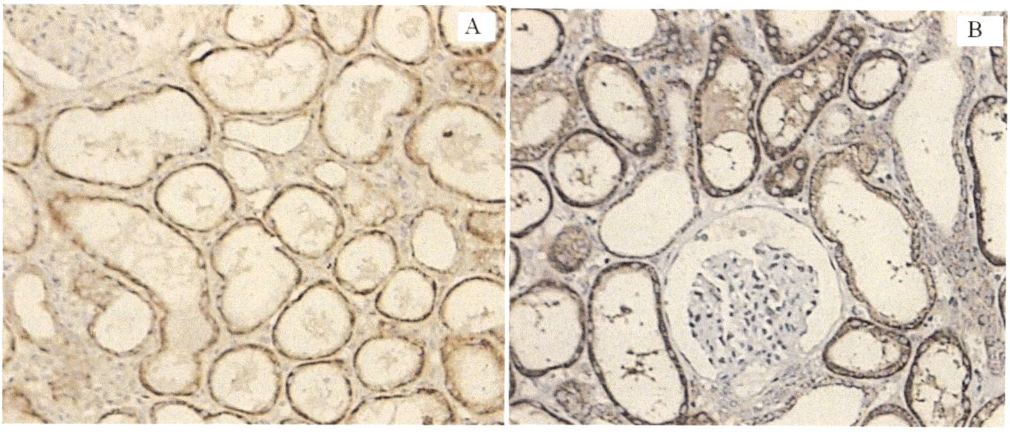

Fig. 3. Representative examples of immunohistochemical staining of BAFF and C4d in renal allograft rejection (original mannification 200X).Positive staining was observed as a dark brown color. Renal allograft rejection tissues showed strong expression of C4d (A) and BAFF (B).

We performed further study by IHC to investigate the receptors of BAFF involved in the renal allograft rejection. The TACI, BCMA and BAFF-R (BAFF receptor, BR3) were all detected. And the APRIL, much high homogenicity with BAFF, was also done. Meanwhile, the plasma cell marker CD138 was also investigated.

The obtained data showed that, high immunogenicity of BAFF, APRIL and their receptors, TACI, BCMA and BAFF-R, and CD138 can be found in renal allograft rejection tissues (including of acute and chronic rejection) (Fig.4), while these molecules all have low immunogenicity in other etiological tissue (excluding of acute and chronic rejection).

All data were analyzed according to C4d expression. In C4d negative group, BAFF, BAFF-R, BCMA and CD138 were all low immunogenicity, while APRIL and TACI have high immunogenicity. In C4d positive group, BAFF, BAFF-R, BCMA, APRIL, TACI and CD138 were all high immunogenicity. The statistical analysis suggested that, the expression of BAFF, BAFF-R, BCMA and CD138 significantly correlated with C4d deposition (Fig.5). These results suggest that BAFF signal may participate in AMR, and APRIL signal may simultaneously participate in cell-mediated and antibody-mediated rejection.

4. Diagnosis of AMR

4.1 Diagnosis of acute AMR

AMR may occur early or late, may be acute or chronic and is associated with poor renal allograft function and survival. According to the speed of rejection, three AMR conditions are now recognized: hyperacute, subacute and chronic AMR.

The following items are required in diagnosis of acute AMR:

1. Histopathological evidence of either acute tubular injury (with no other identifiable cause for it), glomerulitis, endothelitis or capillaritis with neutrophil or mononuclear cell infiltratem capillary thrombosis;
2. Serologica evidence of circulating antibodies;
3. Diffuse C4d positivity in peritubular capillaries (PTC).

These diagnosis criteria are based on Banff 2005 guidelines, in which, C4d deposition in the peritubular capilary (PTC) is considered as the mark of AMR.

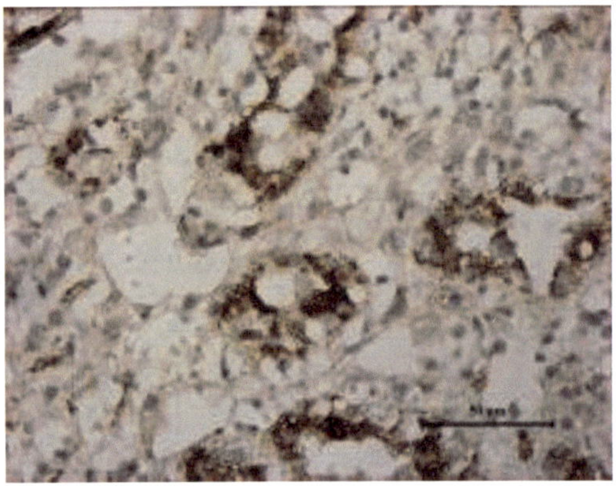

(A) CD256 (×400)

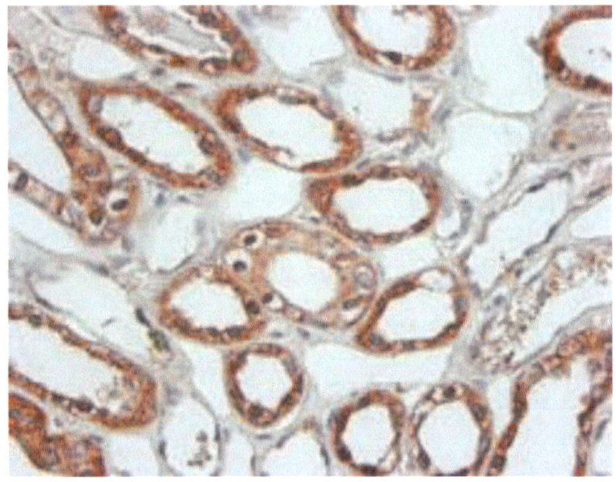

(B) TACI (×400)

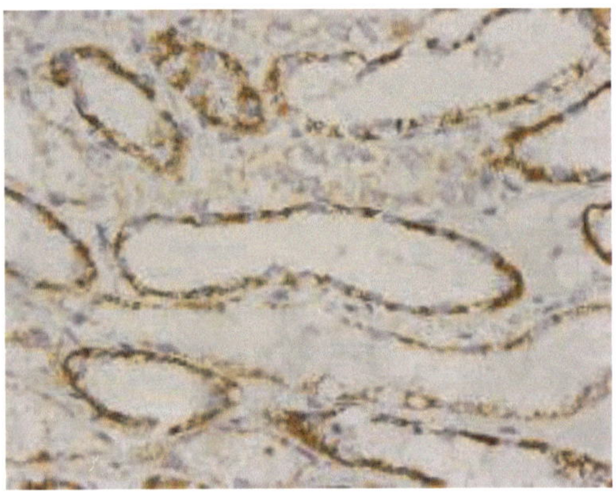

(C) BAFF-R (×400)

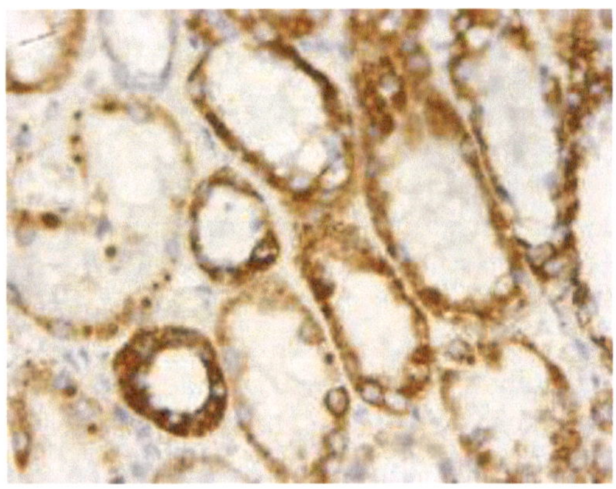

(D) BCMA (×400)

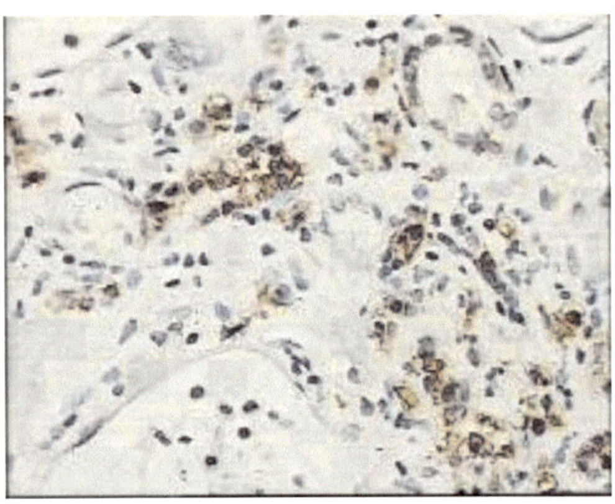

(E) CD138 (×400)

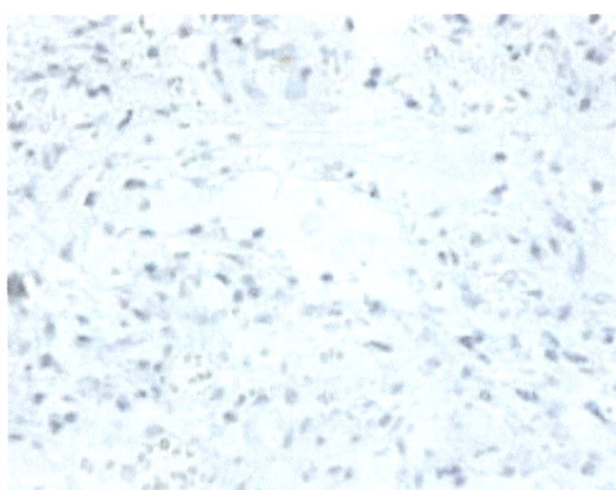

(F) IgG isotype (×400)

Fig. 4. The representative IHC staining results of APRIL, TACI, BAFF-R, BCMA and CD138 were listed (×400). The APRIL, BAFF-R,BCMA and CD138 signal were developed with 3,3'-diaminobenzidine tetrahydrochloride (DAB), the dark brown particles were the positive signal. And TACI signal was developed with 3-amino-9-ethycarbozole (AEC), the red particle was the positive signal. (F): the IgG isotype of the used antibodies.

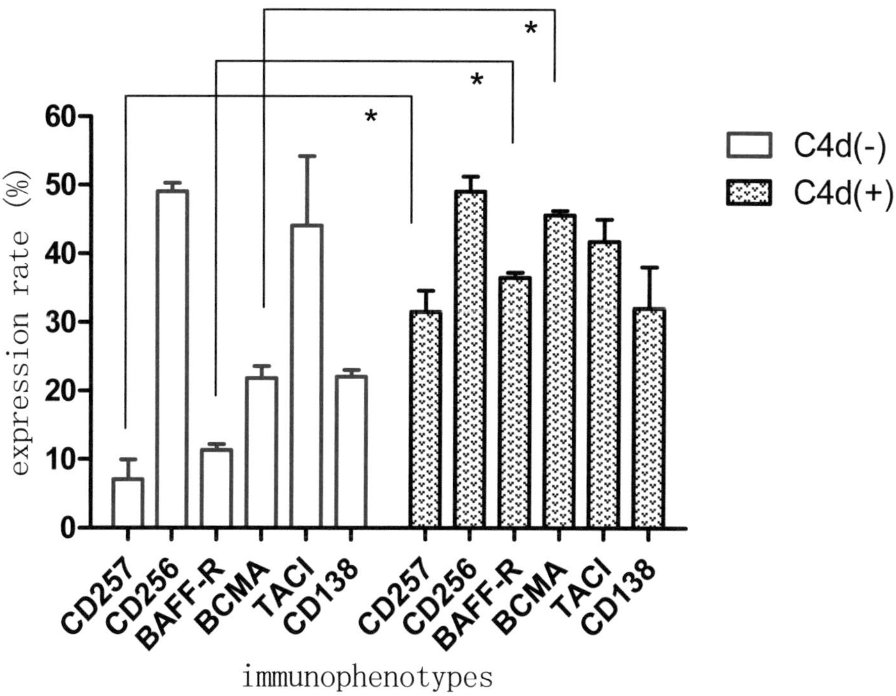

Fig. 5. All data was analyzed according to C4d immunoreactivity, C4d(-) represented C4d negative group and C4d(+) represented C4d positive group. There were significant difference of the expression rate of BAFF, BAFF-R and BCMA between C4d(-) group and C4d(+) group. $P<0.05$ was considered as statistical significance. * $P<0.05$.

4.2 Suspicious for AMR

However, C4d staining is found to be not completely useful in diagnosis of AMR with the advancement of knowledge about AMR. For example, C4d staining in post-reperfusion renal biopsy is not useful for the early detection of AMR when CDC crossmatching is negative (David-Neto et al., 2010). In ABO-incompatible transplant cases, AMR is difficult to be diagnosed by C4d analysis.

Banff 09 meeting discussed several aspects of solid organ transplants with a special focus on antibody mediated graft injury, and revised the diagnosis indexes.

Because C4d may not be sensitive in the diagnosis of AMR: many cases of transplant glomerulopathy with anti-HLA are C4d negative (Sis et al., 2009). Therefore, the recent update of the Banff classification introduced the diagnostic category "**suspicious for AMR**" if C4d (in the presence of antibody) or alloantibody (in the presence of C4d) cannot be demonstrated but morphologic evidence of antibody-mediated tissue injury is present. Moreover, in microarray studies, expression of endothelial transcripts was increased in biopsies with DSA and associated with graft loss even in C4d negative biopsies.

4.3 Remained questions

The risk for graft loss is not captured well by the current Banff diagnoses because many cases with AMR features (anti-HLA and microcirculation changes) were C4d negative and thus

given other diagnosis. However, when AMR is redefined as the presence of HLA antibody and microcirculation changes, regardless of C4d status, it is the most frequent phenotype associated with subsequent graft loss. In contrast, nonspecific scarring (IFTA), calcineurin inhibitor toxicity and TCMR are rare diagnosis in grafts that subsequently failured. Thus, antibody-mediated microcirculation injury accounts for the majority of kidneys presenting with indications for biopsy and subsequently failing, but many cases are C4d negative.
Subclinical AMR seems to be complicated by a substantial proportion of positive-crossmatch transplantations even in the absence of allograft dysfunction, and may result in chronic histological abnormalities and shorten allograft function (Loupy et al., 2009).
So, although much advancement have been obtained in diagnosis, there is still absent of specific marker to aid the diagnosis and therapeutic of AMR.

5. Therapeutic strategies of AMR

Once AMR happen, it requires intensive therapy, but no standard treatment has been established now. To eliminate the alloantibodies and antibody-producing cells are the main strategy of AMR treatment.

5.1 Therapeutic strategies of acute AMR

Now, several strategies are being routinely applied, such as plasmapheresis, high-dose intravenous immunoglobulin (IVIG) and plasmapheresis (PP) with low-dose IVIG. Some new interventions have been applied in clinic, such as the use of rituximab (anti-CD20 chimeric antibody)(Rodriguez et al. 2010; Takagi et al., 2010), bortezomib (a proteasome inhibitor-mediated plasma cell depletion)(Raghavan et al. 2010; Walsh et al., 2010), and eculizumab (recombinant human C5-inhibitor)(Lonze et al., 2010; Tillou et al.,2010), for preventing acute AMR. These methods are promising therapeutic avenues currently under investigation.
IVIG has many ideal advantages as a therapy for AMR.

1. It can down regulate B-cell activation and antibody production.
2. It can induce anti-inflammatory cytokines and contain blocking antiidiotyic antibodies to anti-HLA antibodies;
3. IVIG has the unique ability to block complement-mediated injury through inhibition of C3 activation.

Rituximab (anti-CD20 chimeric antibody) can deplete B cells and interfere with antigen-presenting cell (APC) activity of B cells subsequently decreasing T-cell activation,
Bortezomib is one kind of proteasome inhibitors. The preliminary results indicate that bortezomib therapy provides effective reduction in DSA levels with long-term suppression in transplant recipients.
Bortezomib therapy's advantages:

1. It provides effective treatment of AMR and TCR with minimal toxicity.
2. It provides sustained reduction in iDSA and non-iDSA levels.

While, other center reported that, Bortezomib treatment did not significantly decrease DSA within the 150-day posttreatment period in any patient; lack of efficacy on long-lived plasma cells. So, one cycle of bortezomib alone does not decrease DSA levels in sensitized kidney transplant recipients in the time period studied. These results underscore the need to evaluate this new desensitization agent properly in prospective, randomized and well-controlled studies (Sberro-Soussan et al., 2010).

5.2 Therapeutic strategies of subacute and chronic AMR

Now, there seems to have not any good methods to treatment the subacute and chronic AMR. Although subacute and chronic AMR are not immediately result in the graft loss, they cause chronic histological injury and shorten allograft function. Many evidences have suggested that AMR is the important factor influencing the long-term of kidney allograft. Thus, great efforts are still needed to resolve this problem.

6. Conclusion

In summary, recent advances in the diagnosis and treatment of AMR has allowed for significant improvements in the outcome of a condition usually associated with rapid graft failure. However, much work needs to be done to better understand the immunologic processes leading to AMR and how current therapies can be best used to effectively prevent and treat it.

7. References

Bloom, D.; Chang, Z.; Pauly, K.; et al. (2009) BAFF is increased in renal transplant patients following treatment with alemtuzumab. *Am J Transplant*. Vol. 9(8):1835-45.

David-Neto, E.; David, DS.; Ginani, GF.; et al. (2010) C4d staining in post-reperfusion renal biopsy is not useful for the early detection of antibody-mediated rejection when CDC crossmatching is negative. *Nephrol Dial Transplant*. 2010, Vol 26(4):1388-92.

Day, ES.; Cachero, TG.; Qian, F.; et al. (2005) Selectivity of BAFF/Blys and APRIL for binding to the TNF family receptors BAFFR/BR3 and BCMA. *Biochemistry*. Vol.44(6):1919-31.

Einecke, G.; Sis, B.; Reeve, J.; et al. (2009) Antibody-mediated microcirculation injury is the major cause of late kidney transplant failure. *Am J Transplant*. Vol.9(11):2520-31.

Lefaucheur, C.; Loupy, A.; Hill, GS.; et al. (2010) Preexisting donor-specific HLA antibodies predict outcome in kidney transplantation. *J Am Soc Nephrol*. Vol.21(8):1398-406.

Lonze, BE.; Dagher, NN.; Simpkins, CE.; et al. (2010) Eculizumab, bortezomib and kidney paired donation facilitate transplantation of a highly sensitized patient without vascular access. *Am J Transplant*. Vol.10(9): 2154-60.

Lobashevsky, A.; Rosner, K.; Goggins, W.; et al. (2010) Subtypes of immunoglobulins (Ig)-G antibodies against donor class II HLA and cross-match results in three kidney transplant candidates. *Transpl Immunol*. Vol.23(1-2):81-5.

Loupy, A.; Suberbielle-Boissel, C.; Hill, GS.; et al. (2009) Outcome of subclinical antibody-mediated rejection in kidney transplant recipients with preformed donor-specific antibodies. *Am J Transplant*. Vol.9(11): 2561-70.

Mackay, F. and Schneider, P. (2009) Cracking the BAFF code. *Nature Reviews / Immunology*. Vol 9:491-502.

Rodriguez, F.; Rincon, A.; Bucalo, L.; et al. (2010) Treatment of acute antibody-mediated rejection: a single-center experience. *Transplant Proc*. Vol.42: 2848-50.

Raghavan, R.; Jeroudi, A.; Achkar, K.; et al. (2010) Bortizomib in kidney transplantation. *J Transplant*. 2010.pii:698594.

Sherro-Soussan, R.; Zuber, J.; Suberbielle-Boissel, C.; et al. (2010) Bortezomib as the sole post-renal transplantation desensitization agent does not decrease donor-specific anti-HLA antibodies. *Am J Transplant*. Vol.10(3):681-6.

Sis, B.; Jhangri, GS.; Bunnag, S.; et al. (2009) Endothelial gene expression in kidney transplants with alloantibody indicates antibody-mediated damage despite lack of C4d staining. *Am J Transplant*. Vol.9(10):2312-23.

Stegall, MD.; Gloor, JM. ((2010) Decipering antibody-mediated rejection: new insights into mechanisms and treatment. *Curr Opin Organ Transplant*. Vol.15(1):8-10.

Takagi, T.; Ishida, H.; Shirakawa, H.; et al. (2010) Evaluation of low-dose rituximab induction therapy in living related kidney transplantation. *Transplantation*. Vol.89(12):1466-70.

Thaunat, O.; Patey, N.; Gautreau, C. et al. (2008) B cell survival in intragraft tertiary lymphoid organs after rituximab therapy. *Transplantation*. Vol. 85(11): 1648-53.

Thompson, JS.; Biller, SA.; Qian, F.; et al. (2001) BAFF-R, a newly identified TNF receptor that specially interacts with BAFF. *Science*. Vol.293(5537):2108-11.

Tillou, X.; Poirier, N.; Le Bas-Bernardet, S.; et al. (2010) Recombinant human C1-inhibitor prevents acute antibody-mediated rejection in alloimmunized baboons. *Kidney Int*. Vol.78(2):152-9.

Walsh, RC.; Everly, JJ.; Brailey, P.; et al. (2010) Proteasome inhibitor-based primary therapy for antibody-mediated renal allograft rejection. *Transplantation*. Vol.89(3):277-84.

Zou, Y.; Stastny, P.; Susal, C.; et al. (2007) Antibodies against MICA antigens and kidney-transplant rejection. *N Engl J Med*. Vol. 357(13):1293-300.

Zou Y and Stastny P. (2009) The role of major histocompatibility complex class I chain-related gene A antibodies in organ transplantation. *Curr Opin Organ Transplant*. Vol.14(4):414-8.

19

Pathogenesis and Preventive Strategies of Chronic Dysfunction of Renal Allograft

Wenqian Huo, Keqin Zhang, Chengguo Ge, Gang Wu,
Fengshuo Jin, Gang Yuan and Qiansheng Li
*Department of Urology, Institute of Surgery Research, Daping Hospital,
Third Military Medical University, Chongqing,
China*

1. Introduction

Novel immunosuppressants have decreased the incidence rate of acute rejection significantly, but fail to prevent chronic allograft dysfunction (CAD). Around 40% patients develop CAD gradually in several months or several years after renal transplantation. They present with progressive deterioration of long-term allograft function and allograft failure, and end up with resuming dialysis. It has also been demonstrated that CAD may increase the cardiovascular mortality after renal transplantation. Therefore, it is crucial for promoting long-term allograft survival to investigate the pathogenesis and preventive and therapeutic strategies of CAD. CAD, formerly termed chronic rejection (CR), is also known as late graft loss (LGI) or chronic allograft nephropathy (CAN), since it involves both immune factors (transplantation antigen dependent) and non-immune factors (transplantation antigen independent).

CAD refers to progressive functional impairment of allograft, with pathologic changes including tubular atrophy, interstitial fibrosis, progressive glomerulosclerosis, and arterial fibrous intimal thickening and arteriole hyalinosis. These pathologic changes include immune and non-immune injury to allograft. Chronic rejection is usually associated with acute rejection or subclinical rejection, HLA mismatch, panel reactive antibodies (PRA), and donor specific antibodies (DSA). In contrast, non-immune allograft injury is usually associated with calcineurin inhibitors (CNI), preexisting delayed graft function (DGF), hypertension, hyperlipidemia, proteinuria, viral infection, chronic obstruction and chronic pyelonephritis. In addition, CAD includes recurrent kidney disease, de novo nephritis, posttransplantation lymphoproliferative diseases (PTLD). Many of the above-mentioned factors that lead to CAD usually exist simultaneously; thus, the pathologic manifestations of CAD are complex and not specific, making the treatment of CAD difficult. In short, there are many factors influencing the incidence and development of CAD, and the pathogenesis of CAD remains largely unclear. Microcirculation injury mediated by donor specific antibodies is thought to be the major cause for long-term allograft dysfunction.

2. Risk factors for CAD

2.1 Transplantation antigen dependent risk factors

Epidemiologic study indicated that patients with acute rejection are more likely to develop chronic rejection than those without. The frequency, histologic type and time of onset of acute rejection are closely associated with allograft dysfunction. In particular, frequent and delayed (more than one year) acute rejection is likely to result in allograft dysfunction. Gulanikar et al. reported that the risk for CAD was 9% in patients developing acute rejection once after renal transplantation, was 38% in those developing acute rejection twice, and was 50% in those developing acute rejection thrice, and that early-stage acute vascular rejection was more harmful than acute interstitial rejection. Van et al. reported that the the 5-year kidney survival rates were 34%, 71%, and 74% in patients developing acute vascular rejection, acute interstitial rejection, and without acute rejection in the 3 months after transplantation. It was reported that acute rejection may increase the expression of platelet-derived growth factor (PDGF) and its receptor on arterial smooth muscle cells. PDGF is one of the main stimulators for interstitial cell proliferation in CAD. Hence, PDGF may play a role in acute rejection and CAD.

1. HLA match

Major Histocompability Complex (MHC) mismatch is a crucial risk factor for CAD. The long-term allograft survival rate is the highest for cadaveric renal transplantation with perfect MHC match, and CAD does not occur following homogenic transplantation. Among HLA-A, B, and DR, group A is not so important as groups B and D. Mismatch of both loci of group B is likely to lead to acute rejection and subsequent chronic rejection. In the presence of mismatch of one locus of group B and one locus of group DR, 82% of type I helper T cells proliferate; in the absence of mismatch, only 6% proliferate. Meanwhile, in the presence of mismatch, the release of allogenic antigen peptide increases by 10 folds. The long-term allograft survival rates differ significantly with different number of mismatching MHC sites, suggesting the importance of transplantation antigen dependent factors in the development of CAD.

2. Antibodies

The main mechanism for CAD is believed to relate to allograft stimulated production of anti-donor specific circulating antibodies. As currently available immunosuppressants mainly suppress T cells, antibodies might be a main factor for chronic rejection. In chronic allograft rejection, there are many antibody-secreting plasma cells in the kidney, and these antibodies are against mesenterial cells, focal adhesion plaques, molecules synthesized and secreted by activated mesenterial cells or basement membrane antigen. Interfering recombination activation gene 2(RAG-2) will lead to T and B cell defect, and immunoglobin transmembrane domain-encoding gene defect will preclude the production of mature B cells and antibodies. In both cases, allograft atherosclerosis will not occur. In addition, macrophage dysfunction and defect of MHC class II antigen mitigate atherosclerosis, and defects of MHC class I antigen, CD8 positive cells and NK cells exacerbate atherosclerosis.

Hypersensitivity to panel reactive antibodies (PRA) correlates highly to acute rejection. PRA or the reaction rate of donor lymphocytes to recipient serum is frequently used to predict the risk for acute rejection. Preoperative PRA being more than 10% correlates significantly to the three-year allograft survival rate. Anti-lymphocyte antibody was detected in 28.2% patients with chronic rejection, and of them, 57% were found to have anti-HLA antibody. In vitro study confirmed that monoclonal antibody against type I HLA molecule induced the expression of fibroblast growth factors receptor on endothelial cells and smooth muscle cells. Allogenic antibodies exhibit the same effect, and they promote glomerulosclerosis and fibrosis. Antibodies against occult epitopes may cause chronic damage, and elevated levels of antibodies against molecules contributing to tissue injury will lead to excessive fibrosis during tissue repair.

3. TGF-β1 pathway

It was demonstrated that molecules recognized by antibodies following transplantation, biglycans and modified molecules also bind to TGF-β1. TGF-β1 is the main cytokine regulating CAD fibrosis. Sharma et al. reported that TGF-β1 mRNA expression correlates significantly to kidney allograft interstitial fibrosis and CAD. Angiotensin II receptor antagonists were shown to reduce plasma TGF-β1 level by 50%, suggesting the potential of angiotensin II receptor antagonists to prevent CAD. Meanwhile, urine TGF-β1 secretion is obviously higher in CAD patients than in patients with stable renal function.

2.2 Transplantation antigen independent risk factors

Non-immune factors and multiple risk factors jointly lead to chronic rejection-like changes of allograft. Rats survived for long term following homogenic renal transplantation. In case of renal function damage, macrophage infiltration and cytokine upregulation were observed in the allograft, just like chronic rejection changes following allogenic renal transplantation. After an allograft with functional impairment was transplanted back into the donor, early-stage renal damage may restore normal, but late-stage damage will continue to deteriorate, demonstrating that early-stage chronic rejection depends on allogenic antigens and is reversible, while late-stage injury does not depend on allogenic antigens and is irreversible.

1. Early-stage ischemia /reperfusion injury

Renal allografts will undergo a series of ischemic events during organ harvesting, preservation, and transplantation. The longer the ischemia time, the more serious the reperfusion related injury. During 2- 5 d of ischemia/reperfusion injury, the expression of leukocyte and endothelial cell adhesion molecules, endothelin, MHC class II molecules, interferin γ and TNF-α is upregulated in kidney tissue, which is complicated by increased oxyradical production and T cells and macrophages in the allograft. Connolly et al. reported that prolonged cold ischemia affected the short-term and long-term survival of cadaveric renal allograft adversely, and that the benefit of HLA match for allograft survival was offset by prolonged cold ischemia. Ischemia /reperfusion injury damages the kidney through the following mechanisms: ① microcirculation disturbance, early-stage renal function loss or delayed renal function, tubular necrosis, TGF-p increase, interstitial fibrosis; ② oxyradical caused acute vascular endothelial cell injury and arterial sclerosis; ③ activation of T lymphocytes, causing subclinical immune reaction, arteritis, nephron reduction, monocyte/macrophage infiltration and interstitial fibrosis.

2. Cytomegalovirus

CMV infection of allograft endothelial cells will lead to chronic rejection quickly. CMV may enhance MHC expression, which leads to the production of anti-endothelial cell antibody and endothelial cell damage. In clinical practice, if acute rejection is refractory to immunosuppressants, and if there are a number of memory CD8+T cells in peripheral blood and evidence of asymptomatic CMV infection, anti-CMV treatment is usually effective to improve renal function. The mechanism is as follows: the immediate early gene of CMV encodes homologous protein, which cross-reacts to HLA-DR-β chain, thus enhancing the recipient's immune reaction to donor antigens. CMV encodes a glycoprotein, which is homologous to the heavy chain of MHC class I antigen and can react to the light chain of MHC class I antigen. Active CMV infection, along with VCAM-1 expression enhancement and leukocyte adhesion and infiltration on capillary endothelial cells will influence allograft function for long term. In addition, in CMV infection, inflammatory cytokines aggavate endothelial cell damage and vascular pathologic changes.

3. Drug toxicity

Cyclosporin (CsA) and Tacrolimus (FK-506) are both CNI-type immunosuppressants. When they relieve early-stage acute rejection significantly, CNI induced long-term kidney toxicity may be an important cause for accelerating CAD progress. As a result, the long-term survival of allograft may decrease. Chronic nephrotoxicity of CNI is characterized by interstitial fibrosis, hyalinization of small artery and tubular vacuolar degeneration in the kidney. The causes of nephrotoxicity include kidney vasospasm, release of endothelin-β, and excessive expression of transforming growth factor-β (TGF-β) and vascular endothelial growth factor (VEGF). It has been demonstrated recently that allograft function may be protected and allograft survival be prolonged by early reduction or withdrawal of CNIs and administration of Sirolimus (SRL) following renal transplantation, without the risk of increasing acute rejection (AR). In addition, the combination of nephrotoxicity-free immunosuppressants, e.g., SRL and Mycophenolate mofetil helps to delay the incidence of CAD.

4. Nephron reduction

Nephron reduction due to various causes leads to glomerular hyperfiltration, early-stage compensated glomerular hypertrophy and increased exudation, kidney dysmetabolism, and allograft failure. Nephron reduction may be associated with the following factors: ① donor/recipient mismatch of body size, or inappropriate ratio of kidney weight /body weight. For instance, an allograft from a donor weighing 50kg is transplanted into a recipients weighing more than 90kg, which means nephron reduction and may result in renal functional impairment; ② the donor is too young (less than three years) or too old (more than 60 years). If the donor is too young, the nephron is immature and cannot tolerate the perfusion pressure for adult kidneys. If the donor is too old, there may be vascular sclerosis and nephron reduction in the kidney; ③ sex difference. The three-year survival rate of allografts from female donors is 5% lower than from male donors.

5. Hyperlipidemia

Food rich in cholesterol and hyperlipidemia synergize in kidney injury, and they change macrophage function, and lead to secretion of vasoactive substances and cell proliferation, thus aggravating kidney damage. Controlled intake of protein can temporarily stabilize allograft function in patients with chronic rejection. Cholesterol-rich apoprotein B and triglyceride are independent risk factors for chronic rejection, and they induce arterial sclerosis and enhance oxidization. Oxidized low-density lipoprotein may lead to proliferation and migration of smooth muscle cells and aggravate vasculopathy.

6. Other risk factors

The following factors are shown to associate with chronic rejection: ① blood pressure elevation is associated with allograft failure. However, which occurs first is still unclear; ② smoking may promote allograft vasculopathy and CAD. Little investigational work has been done in this regard; ③ epidemiologic survey has revealed that continuous proteinuria occurs in approximately 20% of patients following transplantation, and two thirds of these patients suffer from CAD. Chronic allograft damage resulting from proteinuria is an important risk factor for CAD, possibly because of persistent protein loss, failure of epithelial cell repair, and epithelial atrophy and secondary tissue fibrosis.

3. Pathologic classification of CAD

Allograft fibrosis and sclerosis are main pathologic changes in CAD, which can be observed in any anatomical structures of allograft. There may also be progressive proliferation and focal sclerosis of glomerular matrix, and intimal thickening of small artery and capillary in the kidney due to fibrosis and hyaline substance aggregation. Peritubular capillaries may develop multilayered basal lamina, and there may be thickening of glomerular capillary walls with reduplication of basement membrane and mesangial interposition. Gradual accumulation of interstitial matrix leads to interstitial fibrosis (IF), collagen scars, interstitial capillary loss and tubular atrophy (TA).

Allograft fibrosis is the final common pathway of multi-factorial injury. Therefore, chronic rejection alone cannot explain the pathogenesis of fibrosis. Chronic allograft nephropathy (CAN) was used to describe chronic allograft fibrosis. Nevertheless, CAN is not an etiologic diagnosis. Thus, in 2005, the Banff consensus conference recommended adopting need-based diagnosis and abandoning the concept of 'CAN'. According to the Banff 2005 meeting report, possible causes of IF/TA include drug toxicity (especially calcineurin inhibitor toxicity), bacterial or viral infection, hypertension, obstruction, recurrent and de novo glomerular and tubulointerstitial diseases, as well as chronic rejection. Pathologic changes vary depending on different etiologic factors, and they should be discriminated.

Macroscopic examination reveals no obvious allograft changes at the early-stage of CAD, but obvious shrinkage, thickening and adhesion of renal capsule, with scars of various sizes on the uneven, pale surface of kidney at the late-stage of CAD. Small scarring kidney is hard and has a thin cortex. Histopathologic changes include glomerular, interstitial, tubular and vascular changes.

1. Transplant glomerulopathy

Transplant glomerulopathy is mainly characterized by glomerular basement membrane thickening, glomerular mesenterial lysis, and accumulation of mesenterial matrix, mesenterial sclerosis, and glomerulosclerosis. However, it usually does not present with obvious proliferative reaction or dense substance deposition. In this way, it can be differentiated from membranoproliferative glomerulonephritis (Figure 1). Immune injury is generally thought to be the main cause for transplant glomerulopathy, because it correlates obviously to endothelial cell C4d deposition.

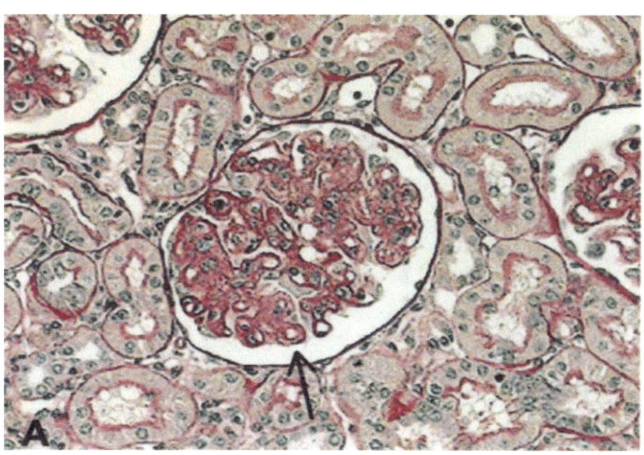

Fig. 1.

2. Interstitial fibrosis

Interstitial fibrosis is not specific to CAD, but is the final outcome of various kidney diseases. Various immune, hemodynamic and metabolic factors may lead to interstitial fibrosis. Tubular cell atrophy, diffuse interstitial infiltration of monocytes and lymphocytes, laminin and fibronectin expression increase, and gradual interstitial fibrosis may be observed (Figure 2). A number of proinflammatory and fibrogenic cytokines expressed in renal allografts may accelerate renal fibrosis, including tumor necrosis factor-α, transforming growth factor-β, platelet-derived growth factor, interferon-γ, and basic fibroblast growth factor. These factors are usually deemed early-stage markers for fibrosis.

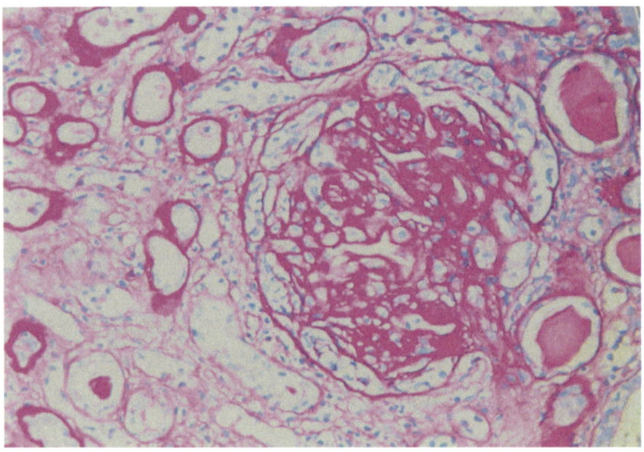

Fig. 2.

3. Tubular atrophy

Tubular atrophy (TA) is also a non-specific manifestation of various chronic kidney injuries. Ischemia/reperfusion injury, drug nephrotoxicity and immune injury may lead to TA. Generally, tubulitis is characteristics of acute cell-mediated rejection; however, whether tubulitis is the sole cause for tubular atrophy is uncertain. Tubular basement membrane loss due to acute rejection may cause late-stage tubular atrophy. At 2-3 weeks following transplantation, persistent peritubular granulomatous reaction, infiltration of tubular basement membrane by multinucleated giant cells, and partial or complete tubular atrophy can be observed (Figure 3). Therefore, immune injury may be an important factor for TA.

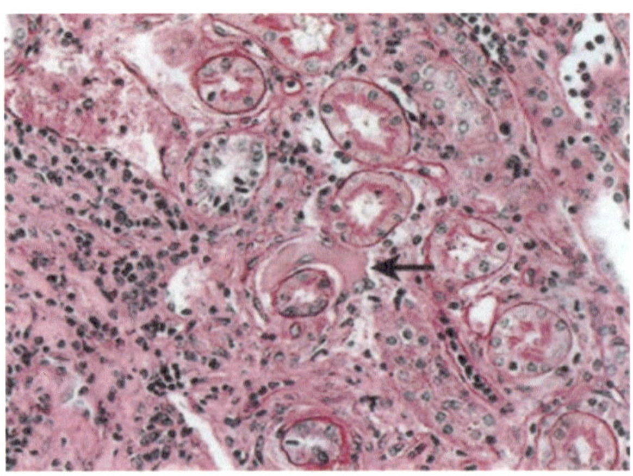

Fig. 3.

4. Transplant vasculopathy

Transplant Atherosclerosis

Transplant atherosclerosis may result from donor factors, non-immune injury (e.g., CNI nephrotoxicity) and chronic rejection. However, there are T cells or macrophages that infiltrate the affected vascular intima, which usually means vascular endothelitis (Figure 4). The incidence rate of systemic atherosclerosis increases in patients with chronic rejection, while renal failure per se does not influence the incidence of atherosclerosis greatly. Moreover, graft atherosclerosis occurs mostly in young, hypersensitive recipients or those with late-stage acute rejection. This suggests that transplant atherosclerosis is closely associated with immune injury. The specification of diagnostic criteria for chronic rejection and other entities by the Banff 2005 conference was an important achievement, and the positive staining for C4d in peritubular capillaries is thought to correlate to AMR (antibody mediated rejection).

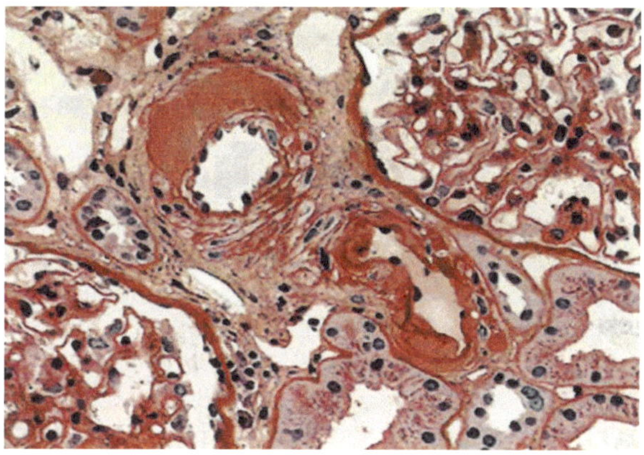

Fig. 4.

Arteriolar hyalinosis

Arteriolar hyalinosis is a characteristic feature of hypertensive nephrosclerosis, diabetic nephropathy, and chronic calcineurin renal toxicity. Hyaline change in the media of the arteriole, which may represent a consequence of myocyte necrosis, is a characteristic feature of cyclosporine-associated arteriolopathy (Figure 5). In many circumstances, such pathologic changes are not direct evidence of diagnosis, and diagnosis should be made with reference to previous pathologic findings obtained by biopsy.

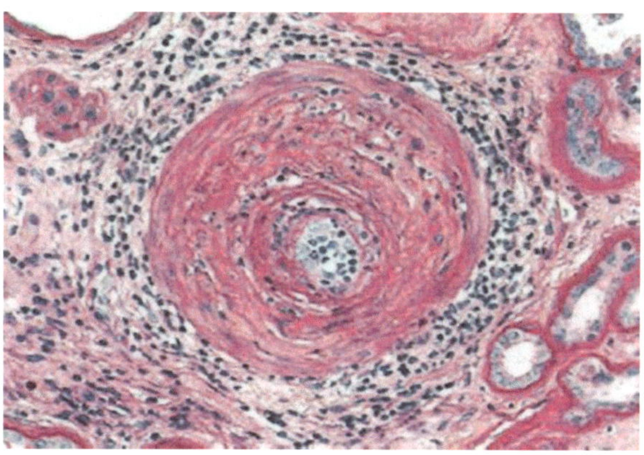

Fig. 5.

In summary, allograft fibrosis and sclerosis are caused by multiple factors, and they are the final manifestations of various acute and chronic kidney injuries. Interstitial fibrosis and tubular atrophy are non-specific. Therefore, a range of diagnostic criteria of CAD should be further investigated, and these diagnostic criteria can and should define specific lesions, thus enabling identification of pathogenic processes that affect the allograft, such as drug toxicity, bacterial or viral infection, hypertension, obstruction, recurrent or de novo renal diseases, and acute and chronic cell and/or antibody-mediated rejection.

4. Injury mechanism for CAD

4.1 Humoral immunity-mediated injury

Antibodies can contribute to transplant rejection through the classical pathways, such as activation of complements and ADCC. After antibody binding to transplantation antigens, complements are activated, followed by activation of the complement-coagulation system, which directly leads to destruction of target cells, vasodilatation, and thrombosis, resulting in allograft rejection. Athough such injury is typical for hyperacute rejection, vascular intimal thickening and presence of complements, immunoglobin and anti-endothelial cell antibody in the necrotic vascular wall have been observed in allografts with chronic rejection. There is another pathway through which T lymphocytes recognize transplantation antigens, i.e., the indirect pathway. In this indirect pathway, TCR on CD4+ T cells can recognize donor's MHC molecule allogenic antigen peptide treated and presented by APCs, also called type II helper T cell (CD4+Th2) reaction. CD4+ T cell activation by the indirect pathway reveals the priming of the rejection effector mechanism, which includes delayed hypersensitivity, cell-mediated toxicty and production of allogenic antibodies. This mechanism exacerbates acute rejection, and plays a major role in CAD. IL-4 and IL-10 produced by Th2 cells are involved in humoral immunity. Activation of helper T cell surface antigen specific TCR triggers intracellular reaction to synthesize specific new antibodies, and this plays an important role in chronic rejection. Early-stage ischemia /reperfusion injury can also activate immunity and upregulate proinflammatory mediators to produce antibodies in the recipients. For instance, in ischemic tissues, vascular endothelial cell phenotype is activated, triggering new antigen expression and leading to immune complex deposition.

4.2 Cellular immunity-mediated injury

In transplant rejection, antigen presenting cells, e.g., dendritic cells, monocytes, and macrophages are crucial for triggering immune response through: ① acquiring, processing and presentating antigens to TH/TDTH and B cells, thus activating first messengers; ② secreting second messengers, e.g., IL-1, thus leading to TH cell activation and release of IL-2, IL-4, IL-5, IL-6 and IFN-γ. Under the action of these cytokines, TDTH, Tc, and B cells that have recognized transplantation antigens begin to proliferate and differentiate into effector Tc, TDTH and antibody secreting cells, leading to transplant rejection. Tc cells directly kill target cells, and TDTH cells contribute to rejection through inducing delayed hypersensitive inflammation. At early-stage acute rejection following renal transplantation, CD4+T cells directly recognize MHC class II antigens in the allograft, and CD8+T cells directly recognize MHC class I antigens in the allograft, producing strong cell- and cytokine-mediated reactions and clinical manifestations of acute rejection. In chronic rejection, weak reactions occur through CD4+Th2 (indirect presentation as mentioned above). Donor MHC may peel from the parenchymal cells of allograft, enter blood circulation, and be phagocytized and processed by recipient's APCs, and be presented by recipient's MHC, or be taken up and processed in situ by macrophages. The recipient's APCs interalize exogenous proteins derived from the allograft, and process and present polypeptides to T cells, thus providing essential signals for lymphocyte activation. This is the classical pathway for antigen processing and presentation by the immune system. In animals immunized with donor's MHC class II antigens, allograft rejection is accelerated significantly, including serious vascular and cellular rejection, which demonstrates the role of the allogenic recognition based indirect pathway in transplant rejection. Nevertheless, immunosuppressants prevent acute rejection and induce CD4+Th2 reaction, leading to development of chronic rejection.

The intimal plaques of allograft artery in chronic rejection comprise mainly macrophages. Macrophages upregulate the expression of fibrosis factors, interleukin-1(IL-1), IL-6, TNF-a and membrane cofactor protein -1(MCP-1) and growth factors, particularly, fibroblast growth factors (bFGF) and transforming growth factors around glomeruli and vessels, thus promoting vascular wall hypertrophy, glomerulosclerosis and kidney fibrosis. Platelet derived growth factors (PDGF), intracellular adhesion molecule (ICAM) and vascular adhesion molecule -1(VCAM-1) are also present on glomerular capillary endothelial cells and other structures. Upregulation of lymphocytes function associated antigen -1(LFA-1) and very late appearing antigen -4(VLA-4), as well as infiltrating cells and cytokines in the allograft promote the waterfall effect of adhesion molecules.

In triggering immune reactions, multiple cytokines such as TNF and IFN-γ promote lymphocytes to mature and helper T cells Th1 to synthesize IL-2, IFN-γ and IL-12. Anti-inflammatory cytokines, e.g., TGF-β, lead Th2 cytokines IL-4 and IL-10 to mature, and suppress immune reactions against allogenic antigens. During rejection, all these cytokines are present in the allograft. However, in case of immune tolerance, Th1 cytokines reduce, and Th2 cytokines increase. CD4+Th2 cytokines, particularly, IL-4, IL-10 and TGF-β, suppress the synthesis of matrix metalloproteinases (MMPs) on smooth muscle and macrophages. MMPs regulate cellular matrix deposition and degradation. Hence, MMPs suppression causes vascular endothelial cell matrix to accumulate, gradually resulting in arterial sclerosis.

Although CD4+Th2 reactions dominate in chronic rejection, other cells, including endothelial cells, CD8+ T cells, NK cells and macrophages, are required to maintain chronic rejection. For instance, CD8+T cells can activate allogenic class I antigens crosslinking on endothelial cells to produce IL-4, IL-10 and TGF-β. Crosslinking of allogenic antibodies to class I antigen molecules on endothelial cell surface will lead to activation and synthesis of TGF-β, PDGF and FGF.

4.3 Allograft structural component reactivity

Various structural components of allograft exhibit different reactivity at early-stage and late-stage following transplantation. In chronic rejection, vascular obstruction results from repeated activation, injury, proliferation and repair of endothelial cells and deposition of extracellular matrix proteins. Vascular wall injury is caused by homogeneous immune reactions because early-stage antigens or proinflammatory factors (e.g., leukotriene, oxyradicals) upregulate complements and adhesion molecules. Allograft arteriosclerosis is associated with autoimmune reactions induced by heat shock protein produced by activated endothelial cells. Changes in the phenotype of activated endothelial cells cause cell denudation and exposure of subendothelial collagen to platelets and plasma proteins, which promotes focal coagulation and thrombosis. Ischemic tissues produce various coagulants, and injured or activated endothelial cells release cytokines, chemical inducers, mediators, thromboxanes, leukotriene and growth factors, including PDGF, platelet-activating factor, NOSi and elastin. Chemical inducers and adhesion molecules promote circulating leukocytes to migrate to the site of injury, and then to vascular wall and perivascular space. Inflammatory reactions caused by cytokines and growth factors result in vascular smooth muscle proliferation and migration, tissue deformation, and vascular involvement. In chronic rejection, there are focal or diffuse glomerular changes, and macrophage infiltration may accelerate early-stage glomerular injury to develop into glomerulosclerosis. Glomerulosclerosis and vascular luminal narrowing lead to gradual renal functional impairment and systemic hypertension. As a result, remnant nephrons are subject to glomerular hyperfiltration and fibrosis, and finally lose function. Non-specific interstitial fibrosis and tubular atrophy stem from organ injury. Therefore, in the presence of early-stage injury following organ transplantation, despite persistent administration of immunosuppressants, renal function may be impaired gradually over several months to several years, and these changes correlate to the reactivity of various structural components of allograft.

4.4 Recurrent and de novo allograft disease

Recurrent glomerulonephritis posttransplantation refers to glomerulonephritis of allograft following renal transplantation, which is pathologically identical to glomerulonephritis of autologous kidney. De novo glomerulonephritis posttransplantation refers to glomerulonephritis of allograft following renal transplantation, which is pathologically different from glomerulonephritis of autologous kidney or the pathology of allograft prior to transplantation. The key to diagnose recurrent and de novo glomerulonephritis lies in the availability of biopsy findings of the autologous kidney and allograft prior to transplantation. In effect, glomerulonephritis is virtually recurrent in all cases. The incidence of recurrent nephropathy of allograft correlates obviously to the histologic type of kidney before transplantation and the time following transplantation. Some glomerular diseases are likely to recur, e.g., mesenterial capillary nephritis, and IgA nephropathy, with the incidence rate of 50-90%. However, these recurrent diseases are unnecessarily influence allograft function seriously. Generally, renal function impairment progresses slowly, with long stable periods. Tables 1-2 list common recurrent and de novo allograft diseases. Currently, most investigations focus on the incidence rate, risk factors and clinical manifestations of recurrent allograft nephritis. Clinically, large doses of immunosuppressants are administered to prevent allograft rejection, but allografts may develop recurrent nephritis, demonstrating that currently available immunosuppressants cannot suppress the incidence of preexisting glomerular diseases. Novel immunosuppressants e.g., MMF and Rapamycin, can suppress cell proliferation in vitro, but their efficacy for recurrent glomerular disease has not been established. Therefore, further investigating the treatment of recurrent and de novo nephritis will deepen the understanding of the pathophysiology of autologous glomerulonephritis and immune pathogenesis of allograft rejection.

Pathologic classification	Recurrent rate (%)	Allograft loss rate (%)
FSGS	20~40	25
IgA nephropathy	50	5~10
Membranous nephropathy	20	5~10
MPGN-I	25	5~10
MPGN-II	90	20
HUS	10~50	10~50
HSPN	30~80	10
Wegener's granuloma	5~20	5~20
Anti-GBM disease	<10	<1
Lupus nephritis	5~10	<5

FSGS: focal segmental glomerulosclerosis, MPGN: membranoproliferative nephritis, HUS: hemolytic uremic syndrome, HSPN: anaphylactoid purpura nephritis

Table 1. Recurrent rate and allograft loss rate of allograft nephritis

Pathologic classification Incidence rate (%)
Etiologies
Allograft nephropathy 5 Rejection? T cell mediated endothelial cell injury? viral infection?
De novo membranous nephropathy 2 Rejection related? de novo antigens produced after allograft injury form immune complexes in situ
De novo HUS 1~3 Calcium channel blockers, allograft ischemia, transplant rejection
De novo MPGN ? 2 HCV, cryoglobulin? deposition of HCV antigens in glomeruli
Alport syndrome
Anti-GBM disease Rare IgG product related to type IV collagen α chain

Table 2. Common de novo allograft diseases

4.5 Posttransplantation lymphoproliferative disease

PTLD is one of the serious complications after organ and marrow transplantation, which presents with lymphocyte proliferation disorder and formation of lymphoma. The probability of PTLD in renal transplantation patients is 20 times that in normal populations. Nevertheless, the incidence rate of PTLD is relatively low (1 %-10%) in renal transplantation patients. PTLD usually affects lymph nodes, the allograft, small intestine and central nervous system, and it occurs mostly in the 2 years following transplantation. PTLD localized to the allograft usually occurs earlier than that outside the allograft. PTLD occurs earlier in patients positive for EB virus than in those negative for EB virus. PTLD mostly stems from B lymphocytes (approximately 87%), and sometimes from T lymphocytes (12%). PTLD stemming from B lymphocytes is mostly complicated by EB virus positivity, while only 38% of PTLD stemming from T lymphocytes is complicated by EB virus positivity. Although PTLD may originate from the donor's cells or the recipient's cells, it mainly originates from the donor's cells. PTLD originating from the donor's cells has a better prognosis than that originating from the recipient's cells. PTLD has varied clinical manifestations, which relate mainly to the affected site and severity of pathologic changes. Common clinical manifestations include ardent fever, neutrocytopenia, anemia, anorexia, diarrhea, and stomachache. Imaging examinations are not specific for the diagnosis of

PTLD. A definite diagnosis depends on pathologic examination. When PTLD is localized to the allograft, with diffuse infiltration, but without obvious masses, it resembles allograft rejection with gradual function loss.

5. Diagnosis of CAD

5.1 Clinical manifestations

Chronic allograft rejection mostly occurs at 2 months to several years following transplantation, with clinical manifestations such as progressive impairment of allograft function, proteinuria and /or anuria, slow increase in blood creatinine (clinically termed "climbing creatinine"), hypertension, progressive anemia and allograft shrinkage.

5.2 Imaging examinations

1. Color Doppler ultrasonography

Since the allograft is shallow, ultrasonic imaging of the allograft will not be influenced substantially by organs and muscle tissue. In addition, due to great acoustic impedance difference between the kidney and surrounding tissues, allograft structures, kidney vessels, ureters and adjacent tissues are shown distinctly. Ultrasonography is able to reveal the allograft size, kidney structures, and various complications of renal transplantation. With the use of color Doppler flow imaging (CDFI) and color Doppler energy (CDE) techniques, blood flow and blood supply to the allograft, and vascular complications following transplantation can be shown clearly. In addition, under ultrasonic guide, biopsy, puncturation and drainage, and visualization are accurate, simple, safe, and non-radioactive, and unlikely to cause complications. Hence, ultrasonography is the preferred imaging modality for allograft. Under ultrasonography, CAD exhibits the following manifestations: the allograft size increases first and then decreases gradually, with a long diameter usually less than 9cm; the kidney parenchyma has enhanced and thickened echoes; the cortex becomes thinner, with indistinct borderline between the kidney parenchyma and renal sinus; at late-stage, the kidney structure is deranged. CDFI frequency spectrum indicates reduced vessels. At late-stage in serious cases, in absence of blood flow in interlobar and arcuate arteries, acute rejection cannot be excluded by ultrasonography. The renal vascular systolic peak flow rate decreases, and the end-diastolic flow rate also decreases. The renal vascular resistance differs significantly between various orders of vessels, particularly between the renal artery and arculate artery. However, the renal vascular resistance is lower than that in hyperacute rejection, accelerated rejection, and acute rejection, but higher than normal. Interstitial vascular resistance is thought to be small; hence, it may be insensitive to Doppler ultrasonography. In contrast, vascular resistance is obvious; hence, it may be sensitive to Doppler ultrasonography. If the RI is normal or less than0.7, CAD cannot be ruled out by ultrasonography. CDE indicates decreased renal vascular perfusion, particularly, in the cortex.

2. Radionuclide imaging

In CAD, the allograft is diminished, and its perfusion and excretion, particularly, uptake, are impaired. Isotope nephrogram indicates perfusion reduction.

3. Digital subtraction angiography (DSA)

In CAD, kidney arteries reduce, and they are thin and bead-like. The kidney parenchyma presents with nonuniform density and patchy changes.

4. CT and MRI

CT and MRI are atraumatic, and have high resolution for soft tissues; hence, they are complementary to other imaging methods for allograft.

5.3 Pathologic study

Currently, biopsy is the most direct, reliable tool for rejection diagnosis. In clinical practice, biopsy findings should be considered in combination with various clinical manifestations and other immunologic, biochemical and imaging findings. Percutaneous thick needle aspiration biopsy or fine needle aspiration biopsy (FNAB) are frequently adopted. If they fail to establish a diagnosis, open biopsy may be considered.

1. Fine needle aspiration biopsy (FNAB)

This method is safe, fast, highly sensitive and specific, and allows continuous observation. Under the guide by ultrasonography or palpation, a 0.7-0.8mm needle with core is inserted into the cortex of the shallower kidney pole, and 10-15tB kidney parenchyma is aspirated and mixed with 5ml heparinized RPMl 1640. The cells are harvested by centrifugation and smeared onto slides. May-Grunlvcald-Giemsa or Wright staining is performed, and cells are counted under an immersion objective. Meanwhile, blood is sampled from the fingers and cells are counted as described above. In typical specimens, there are at least 7 kidney parenchymal cells (endothelial cells, basophilic small tubular epithelial cells, large transparent tubular epithelial cells, large granular tubular epithelial cells or glomerular mesenterial cells) out of 100 inflammatory cells, or there is at least 0.25 parenchymal cell per high power field. The number of a kind of inflammatory cells in the peripheral blood is subtracted from the number of the same kind of inflammatory cells in the allograft to obtain the increament (I). The negative values are discarded. Then, the I values that represent various types of inflammatory cells multiply with a correction coefficient that reflects the contribution of the inflammatory cell type to obtain the corrected I (CI). The CI for each type of inflammatory cells is cumulated to get the total CI (TCI), which represents the extent of inflammatory reactions. Meanwhile, kidney parenchymal cells are graded according to their morphology: 0, morphologically normal; 1, swelling; 2, swelling and vacuolar degeneration; 3, swelling, vacuolization and presence of inclusion materials; 4, necrosis. FNAB specimens can also be investigated by immunocytochemical staining, e.g., peroxide-anti-peroxydase (PAP) staining, indirect immunofluorescence staining, double immunofluorescence staining, immunogold or immunosilver staining, and biotin-avidin immunostaining. FNAB is accurate for diagnosing acute cell-mediated rejection, but is useless for diagnosing CAD and vascular rejection.

2. Percutaneous thick needle aspiration biopsy

This method is the most determinant and reliable tool for differentiating allograft rejection, cyclosporin A toxicity or acute tubular necrosis. In China, the most frequently used needles are Menghini, Franklin-Vim-Silverman, Tru-Cut and Jamshidi types, which are all fit for allograft puncturation. Specimens can be aspirated from the outer edge of the midpoint of the upper and lower kidney poles or the upper kidney pole. For shallow allografts, the needle can be inserted under the guide of palpation. However, in obese patients, ultrasonography or fluoroscopy (with or without intravenous pyelography) may be adopted to guide needle insertion. In case that all these methods failed, CT guide may be considered. The complications are mainly hematuria, perirenal hematoma, arteriovenous fistula, lymphatic fistula and infection.

3. Pathologic diagnosis
   a. The allograft is slightly enlarged or normal at early-stage, and is diminished obviously at late stage. At late stage, the allograft is light and pale, with uneven surface and scars; hence, it is called "small scarring kidney". The renal capsule is obviously thickened and adhered, and cortex atrophy can be observed on the cross-section. Renal function deteriorates progressively, which is proportional to the degree of interstitial fibrosis and glomerulotubular atrophy.
   b. Histologic changes include intimal proliferation dominated proliferating vasculitis, capillary basement membrane thickening and mesenterial matrix increase. There are several pathologic types.

1. Occlusive vasculitis Small artery and arteriole are affected seriously, and interlobar and arcuate arteries may also be affected. In small interlobar artery, afferent glomerular artery and larger artery, smooth muscle and fibroblast proliferation and fibrosis of intima, intima thickening, and luminal narrowing and even obstruction can be observed. Proliferating cells are mostly intimal fibroblasts, and smooth muscle cells originate from the intima. Both cell types produce collagen fibers ultimately. In some cases, subendothelial smooth muscle cells proliferate obviously around the lumen axis, and take on a cyclic, onion-like shape, forming so-called "second tunica media". Serious arterial lesions may influence blood supply to the kidney, lead to multiple infarction, ischemic renal parenchymal atrophy, and renal interstitial sclerosis.

2. Renal interstitial sclerosis Diffuse or focal renal interstitial fibrous proliferation is the major change, which involves the cortex to the medulla. Renal interstitial matrix proliferates, with rare cells and infiltration by lymphocytes and monocytes. Tubular changes are varied, including basement membrane thickening and tubular epithelial cell regeneration. Regenerated tubular epithelial cells are large and may have multiple nuclei. Occasionally, there are single or groups of necrotic epithelial cells. Some tubules are dilated in compensation, resembling mesenchyme. Rejection glomerulonephritis or recurrent glomerulonephritis may be observed. Some patients present with obvious proliferative glomerulonephritis, with obvious increase of glomerular matrix or crescent formation.

   c. Immunofluorescence assay: IgG, IgM and C3 deposit on the glomerular capillary wall and interstitial vascular wall. In particular, in occlusive vasculitis, infiltrating inflammatory cells contain strong fluorescence-emitting IgM.
   d. Electron microscopy: The space between endothelial cells and basement membrane is widened obviously in capillary loop and electron dense substance deposits in a linear or granular manner, with obvious basement membrane thickening. There is a lot of linear and granular electron dense substance deposition along the tubular basement membrane. Mesenterial matrix and surrounding basement membrane are thickened obviously, and are curved. Collagen increases in small artery wall, and smooth muscle cells and fibroblasts proliferate. Lipid droplets increase and myofilaments decrease in the cytoplasm of smooth muscle cells, which may become fibroblasts or foam cells.
   e. Oligonucleotide microarray hybridization assay: B cell chemokine (CXCL13) and mast cells may be determined as predictors for CAD.

4. Differential diagnosis

CAD presents with glomerulosclerosis, recurrent or rejection related glomerulonephritis. Recurrent glomerulonephritis refers recurrence of preexisting nephritis in the allograft, which can be recognized through examining the recipient's original kidney specimens.

Rejection related glomerulonephritis and focal glomerulonephritis can be differentiated by vasculopathy. In serious rejection-related glomerulonephritis, glomerular capillary basement membrane is thickened obviously, which should be differentiated from membranous glomerulonephritis through PAS or PASM staining. In rejection-related glomerulonephritis, there are no spike-like deposits on the epithelial surface of basement membrane, but bilayer basement membrane. In CAD, vascular sclerosis of the allograft should be differentiated from atherosclerosis. Vascular sclerosis is characterized by typical concentric proliferation of smooth muscle and breach of internal elastic layer, but no cholesterol crystals. In contrast, atherosclerosis is characterized by deranged intimal fibers and obvious cholesterol crystals. In CAD, interstitial sclerosis is obvious sometimes, which should be differentiated from chronic interstitial nephritis. In CAD, there are renal interstitial sclerosis, rare nuclei, spare fibers, and few inflammatory cells; hence, the tissue resembles mesenchyme. In chronic interstitial nephritis, fibers are usually dense in scar tissues, with abundant nuclei and a certain number of inflammatory cells.

6. Prevention and treatment of CAD

CAD treatment

No effective treatments for CAD are available yet. The main therapeutic options include controlling blood pressure, administering immunosuppressants, stosstherapy with Methyllprednisolone (MP), intermittent intravenous infusion of Cyclophosphamide (CTX), and use of antithymocyte globulin (ATG), antilymphocyte globulin (ALG), OKT3 and OKT4 monoclonal antibodies, tripterygium glycosides, Bailing capsule, and Niaoduqing granules. The overall therapeutic effect is not good. Over recent years, many treatments have been reported. However, the overall strategy involves the rational use of immunosuppressants, preventing and treating risk factors, and prolonging the functioning life of remnant nephrons. Below are some treatments that are effective for CAD:

1. Dietary therapy Dietary therapy is one of the fundamental measures to delay renal failure in CAD. It has been established both clinically and experimentally that low protein diet and essential amino acid therapy can delay chronic renal failure in most patients. Dietary therapy is mainly aimed to minimize metabolic waste, while providing nutrients to meet basic physiologic needs. By correcting dysmetabolism of nutrients, dietary therapy can relieve the burden on remnant nephrons, correct hemodynamic disturbances, and delay the progress of kidney disease. The measures include ① low protein diet: It is generally thought that low protein diet should be prescribed for patients with chronic renal failure once the endogenous creatinine clearance rate (Ccr) falls to 55ml/min. Meanwhile, sufficient energy should be supplied. This is because high protein diet will increase kidney blood flow and the glomerular filtration rate drastically. Long-term high protein diet will result in persistent high glomerular filtration and glomerulosclerosis through cumulative effect. ② essential amino acids (EAAs): It has been demonstrated that EAAs can improve the nutritional status of patients with chronic renal failure, and can reduce the adverse effect of proteins and common amino acids on the hemodynamics of kidney, thus effectively delaying renal functional impairment. Generally EAAs should be given at week 2 of low protein diet. ⑨ low phosphorus diet and calcium supplementation: Strict control of dietary phosphorus will prevent hyperphosphatemia and secondary

hyperparathyroidism, and relieve tubular interstitial damage. Calcium supplementation should be considered for patients with hypocalcemia and controlled hyperphosphatemia. ④ Supplementation of vitamins and trace elements: Proper supplementatin of water soluble vitamins and trace elements may benefit CAD patients.

2. Cyclosporin A (CsA) The efficacy for CsA is still controversial. According to a retrospective study following up 435 cases for 14 years in the United States, the median allograft survival rate is 3 years. Compared to Azathioprine, CsA showed non-inferiority in relieving renal functional impairment. The median allograft survival rate was 11.6 years in CsA treated patients, and was 9.7 years in Aza treated patients. In animal models, CsA cannot prevent the emergence of pathologic characteristics of CAD after heart, kidney or aorta transplantation. It was also demonstrated that the use of CsA can increase the early-stage success rate obviously and the long-term survival rate as well. Long-term use of CsA is especially superior to Aza. Nevertheless, CsA may increase angiotensin and TGF-β, which is not desirable for CAD treatment. A few scholars hold that low doses of cyclosporin A (CsA) in combination with other immunosuppressants e.g., Mycophenolate mofetil (MMF), is somewhat effective for CAD.
3. FK506 Ji et al. reported that FK506 may delay the progress of CAD safely and effectively. Wang et al. reported that FK506, in place of CsA, was effective for early-stage CAD, particularly, in cases with Scr less than 400umo/L. After FK506 treatment, the Scr level decreased substantially, and hypertension and renal dysfunction improved obviously. One-year follow-up indicated that the patients' condition was stable. Nevertheless, FK506 treatment is less effective in cases with Scr more than 400umol/L. Hence, it is concluded that FK506, in place of CsA is effective for early-stage CAD. Theruvath et al. reported that the FK506+MMF immunosuppressant regimen can reduce anti-donor HLA antibody in recipients, which is of significance to prevent and treat CAD. A US-based, multi-center study primarily on renal transplantation showed that in comparison with CsA, FK506 can effectively prevent acute or glucocorticosteroids or antibody resistant allograft rejection, with increasing side effects. Among 77 patients with acute rejection, 74% of them healed after the combined use of CsA and FK506. 20 patients had obvious vasculopathy, which was refractory to antibody treatment. However, whether FK506 stabilizes allograft function for long is still unclear.
4. Mycophenolate mofetil (MMF) MMF is superior to azathioprine in the treatment of CAD. It was reported that three large clinical trials were undergoing to investigate the efficacy of MMF plus CsA plus prednisone. The dose of MMF to prevent acute rejection is 2g/d or 3g/d. Compared to the control group or the Aza treatment group, the incidence rate of acute rejection decreased obviously at 6 months postoperatively, as confirmed by biopsy. The dose of 3g/d was more effective than 2g/d. MMF may lead to abdominal discomfort, leukopenia and infection. It is now thought that MMF can reduce the incidence of acute rejection and irreversible CAD. MMF in combination with low doses of cyclosporin A (CsA) and prednisone decreased blood creatinine, cured proteinuria and improved renal function in patients with CAD. MMF was found to ameliorate CAD caused chronic renal dysfunction, particularly, mild to moderate renal dysfunction that develops in the first three years after renal transplantation. Nevertheless, long-term follow-ups should be carried out. With the use of MMF, the dose of CsA and glucocorticosteroids can be decreased to reduce the toxic or side effects

of CsA and glucocorticosteroids. The toxic or side effects of MMF are acceptable. With accumulating experience with the clinical use of MMF, the incidence rate of MMF's adverse reactions may be further decreased. CAD patients may benefit from the replacement of Azathioprine with MMF.

5. Sirolimus Sirolimus is a macrolide antibiotic produced by Streptomyces (an actinomycete). As an immunosuppressant, it resembles FK506 structurally. It is not nephrotoxic, and can reduce chronic CsA toxicity. Sirolimus suppresses vascular proliferation, and fibroblast proliferation in vitro; hence, it may prevent CAD. Sirolimus prevents allogenic CAD also through downregulation of adhesion molecule and growth factor encoding gene expression. Replacing calcineurin inhibitors with Sirolimus may delay the incidence of CAD and relieve its clinical symptoms.
6. Lelfunomide In rodent models of heart transplantation with chronic vascular rejection, Lelfunomide exhibited very significant efficacy, and it can reduce and reverse chronic vasculopathy in the allograft. Unlike other immunosuppressants, Lelfunomide will not induce diabetes. Lelfunomide has not been approved for clinical use, but it may become a new treatment for CAD.
7. Polyunsaturated fatty acids Experimental and clinical studies have demonstrated that fish oil treatment can regulate immune reaction. In rat models of heart transplantation, ω-3 polyunsaturated fatty acid can prolong the survival time of allograft obviously. However, allograft survival prolongation correlated to and the reduction of the ω-3 fatty acid content. It is possible that the ratio of dietary ω-3/ω-6 fatty acids is more important than the level of certain fatty acids. ω-3 polyunsaturated fatty acids may regulate immunity via multiple mechanisms: to suppress the effects of IL-1/TNF, to change DR antigen expression, and to reduce vascular smooth muscle cell proliferation and vascular permeability. Another study demonstrated that ω-3 polyunsaturated fatty acids (e.g., fish oil) in combination with 3-hydroxy-3-methyl-glutaryl-CoA (HMG-CoA) reductase inhibitors can reduce the incidence rate of allograft rejection, and they have no obvious toxic and adverse effects.
8. Hypolipidemic treatment HMG-CoA reductase inhibitors (e.g., Statins) are commonly used hypolipidemic agents. Regardless of the blood lipid level in patients, these drugs exhibit good protective effect. In addition to decreasing cholesterol, these drugs can stimulate vascular endothelial cells to release monoxide nitrogen, restore endothelial cell function, and improve kidney hemodynamics. They can also suppress platelet aggregation and thrombosis. It was reported that Simvastatin can reduce the incidence rate of coronary heart disease in rat models for heart transplantation, possibly through reducing the production of 7FXAz. Statins reduce the incidence rate of CAD indirectly, through protecting allograft vessels. CsA, glucocorticosteroids and rapamycin can lead to blood lipid increase. However, it is still unclear to what extent blood lipid should be increased for long. Large multicenter randomized controlled trials or systematic appraisals should be carried out to address this issue.
9. Control of hypertension It has been demonstrated that 90% of CAD patients present with various degrees of hypertension, and require antihypertensive treatment. Hypertension leads to CAD, possibly through increasing renal vascular shear stress, leading to vascular sclerosis, increasing renal vascular resistance, and finally leading to renal ischemia. CAD treatments include control of hypertension and hyperlipidemia. Angiotensin converting enzyme inhibitors or angiotensin receptor blockers can change

intraglomerular pressure and slow down renal functional impairment. Angiotensin suppression can relieve vascular fibrosis and injury in CAD.

10. Anticoagulant therapy As most patients with chronic renal failure have disturbances of blood coagulation, anticoagulant therapy can delay the progress of kidney disease. It has been demonstrated recently [39] that low molecule weight heparin can effectively improve the functional and morphologic status of CAD; however, the precise mechanism is to be elucidated. In addition, traditional Chinese medicines that can promote blood flow and remove blood stasis, e.g., Danshen and Szechwan Lovage Rhizome, exhibit certain therapeutic effects on CAD. However, these therapies need further experimental investigation and clinical observation.
11. Hyperbaric oxygen treatment Pang et al. demonstrated in animals that hyperbaric oxygen is important to prevent or relieve CAD. It was found that proteinuria was milder and the creatinine clearance rate was higher in the hyperbaric oxygen treatment group than the control group. Renal interstitial fibrosis, glomerulosclerosis, artery intimal thickening and T cell, monocyte/macrophage infiltration were milder in the hyperbaric oxygen treatment group than the control group. Therefore, it is concluded that hyperbaric oxygen is useful for CAD treatment. However, further clinical trials should be carried out in larger sample sizes.
12. Traditional Chinese medicines Glucosidorum Tripterygll Totorum and Bailing capsules are effective for CAD, and they help protect remnant nephrons and improve renal function in CAD. However, their mechanisms of action remain unclear. Further studies should be carried out to determine the pharmacokinetics, optimal medication regimen and dosage of traditional Chinese medicines.
13. Excision of renal allograft When CAD develops to renal failure and uremia, the patient needs dialysis to sustain life. The renal allograft is excised prior to discontinuation of immunosuppressants, so as to avoid the production of antibody in allograft and allow a second renal transplantation.
14. Gene therapy It may be one of the important directions in the management of CAD.

In summary, CAD should be treated comprehensively and individually.

CAD prevention

1. To optimize allograft quality Damage should be avoided during harvesting, preserving and trimming allografts. It has been demonstrated that the older the donor is, the earlier and more serious allograft glomerulosclerosis and renal interstitial fibrosis occur. Therefore, allografts should better be harvested from young donors.
2. Preoperative HLA match CAD is mainly caused by immunologic injury. Preoperative HLA match is critical to reduce CAD. It is currently thought that the UNOS six-antigen matching program is a useful tool to achieve optimal HLA match. Allografts with perfect match on the HI, A-A, B and DR loci should better be chosen.
3. To reduce ischemia /reperfusion injury The cold ischemia time should better be less than 20h. High quality vascular anastomosis and avoidance of vascular restenosis are important to reduce ischemia /reperfusion injury. In cadaveric renal transplantation, the use of 200mg recombinant human-superoxide dismutase (RH-SOD) can suppress radical-induced injury, allograft immunity, and MHCII antigen and adhesion molecule upregulation, thus relieving acute and chronic rejection.
4. To reduce acute rejection The severity, frequency and time of onset of acute rejection correlate closely to CAD, and acute rejection is the major immune factor for CAD.

Immunosuppressants have certain toxicity to allografts. Therefore, acute rejection should be prevented with most effective immunosuppressants at the smallest possible dose.

5. To improve the patient's compliance Poor compliance is found to be an important factor for allograft failure. Hence, the patient's compliance should be improved by minimizing the drug dose, educating the patient about the unwanted outcomes of irregular medication, helping the patient to schedule the medication, and establishing a close relationship with the patient.
6. To closely monitor renal function To monitor renal function closely can help physicians to supervise patients taking immunosuppressants, and to find acute rejection promptly. Both patients and physicians must bear in mind that CAD following transplantation seldom has symptoms and physical signs. Therefore, regular monitoring of blood creatinine is feasible for monitoring long-term CAD.
7. To perform biopsy regularly It has been demonstrated that low-grade tubulitis or critical acute rejection can increase the risk for CAD. If biopsy was performed regularly in the first several months following transplantation and rejection was detected and managed promptly, the creatinine level remained low in the first two years. In contrast, in the control group without receiving regular biopsy, the creatinine level was found high upon biopsy and treatment. Therefore, it is concluded that it is crucial to caution against acute and chronic rejection and prescribe kidney biopsy for more patients.
8. To manage hyperlipidemia Hyperlipidemia can promote arteriosclerosis and damage renal function. Pravastatin decreases lowly oxidized low density lipoprotein-cholesterol and triglyceride, and suppress growth factor expression and vascular smooth muscle proliferation. Therefore, to manage hyperlipidemia proactively may exert certain effect on renal arteriosclerosis.
9. To treat hypertension Cardiovascular complications are the second leading cause for death one year after renal transplantation. Both CsA and FK506 can cause hypertension. If the systolic pressure exceeds 150mmg, autoregulation of afferent glomerular artery fails, and the glomerular artery dilates, which results in the production of angiotensin-2 peptide and TGF-β. TGF-β promotes renin secretion. Various factors may reduce nephrons of the allograft, and remnant nephrons are subject to high perfusion pressure, high filtration and high secretion, thus causing glomerulosclerosis. At the early-stage of CAD, if the systolic pressure is controlled below 140mmHg, and the urine protein at 0.25-1g/d, the renal function may not deteriorate for three years. If the urine protein is kept at 1-3g/d, blood pressure may be controlled with higher doses of drugs or more drugs. If the urine protein exceeds 3g/d, blood pressure must be controlled strictly to prevent renal functional deterioration for long. In addition to antihypertensive action, Carvedil suppresses smooth muscle proliferation.
10. To prevent cytomegalovirus infection The CMV infection rate is 70% -100% in the population. Following cadaveric renal transplantation, 8% patients develops symptomatic CMV disease, and the mortality rate is 20%. When CMV disease leads to interstitial pneumonia which requires machine ventilation, the mortality rate is 90%. In the CMV infection group, the three-year allograft survival rate reduced by 30%. Active CMV replication can be detected by CMV antigen assay, LSAB assay, and monoclonal antibody determination of CMV encoded PP65 antige as early as 1-6 days prior to onset of CMV disease. CMV disease can be prevented and treated with Ganciclovir in the first three postoperative months in patients positive for CMV infection.

7. References

[1] Najafian B, Kasiske BL. Chronic allograft nephropathy. Curr Opin Nephrol Hypertens. 2008;17(2):149-55.

[2] Jevnikar AM, Mannon RB. Late kidney allograft loss: what we know about it, and what we can do about it. Clin J Am Soc Nephrol. 2008;3 Suppl 2:S56-67.

[3] Solez K, Colvin RB, Racusen LC, Sis B, Halloran PF, Birk PE, Campbell PM, Cascalho M, Collins AB, Demetris AJ, Drachenberg CB, Gibson IW, Grimm PC, Haas M, Lerut E, Liapis H, Mannon RB, Marcus PB, Mengel M, Mihatsch MJ, Nankivell BJ, Nickeleit V, Papadimitriou JC, Platt JL, Randhawa P, Roberts I, Salinas-Madriga L, Salomon DR, Seron D, Sheaff M, Weening JJ. Banff'05 Meeting Report: differential diagnosis of chronic allograft injury and elimination of chronic allograft nephropathy ('CAN') Am J Transplant. 2007;7(3):518-26.

[4] Gulanikar AC, MacDonald AS, Sungurtekin U, Belitsky P. The incidence and impact of early rejection episodes on graft outcome in recipients of first cadaver kidney transplants. Transplantation 1992;53:323–8.

[5] Issa N, Cosio FG, Gloor JM et al. Transplant glomerulopathy: risk and prognosis related to anti-human leukocyte class II antibody levels.Transplantation 2008; 86: 681–685.

[6] Jindra PT, Hsueh A, Hong L et al. Anti-MHC class I antibody activation of proliferation and survival signaling in murine cardiac allografts. J Immunol.2008; 180: 2214–2224.

[7] Haas M, Rahman MH, Racusen LC et al. C4d and C3d staining in biopsies of ABO and HLA-incompatible renal allografts: correlation with histological findings. Am J Transplant 2006; 6: 1829–1840.

[8] Lemst rom K, Koskinen P, Hayry P, et al. Molecular mechanisms of chronic renal allograft rejection. Kidney Int, 1995, (Suppl 52):2 - 10.

[9] Factors Influencing Outcome After Deceased Heart Beating Renal allograft Transplantation in the United Kingdom: An Evidence Base for a New National Kidney Allocation Policy.Transplantation: 2010, 89(4):379-386.

[10] Kaija Inkinen, Anu Soots, Leena Krogerus , Cathrien Bruggeman, Juhani Ahonen and Irmeli Lautenschlager.Cytomegalovirus increases collagen synthesis in chronic rejection in the rat.Nephrology Dialysis Transplantation, 2001, 17(5):772-779.

[11] Abramowicz D, Manas D, Lao M, et al. Cyclosporine withdrawal from a mycophenolate mofetil-containing immunosuppressive regimen in stable kidney transplant recipients: a randomized, controlled study. Transplantation. 2002;74:1725-1734.

[12] Ahmed F Hamdy, Mohamed A Bakr and Mohamed A Ghoneim. Long-term Efficacy and Safety of a Calcineurin Inhibitor-free Regimen in Live-Donor Renal Transplant Recipients. J Am Soc Nephrol.2008, 19: 1225-1232.

[13] Malek, Sayeed K.Chronic Allograft Dysfunction: A Multifactorial Problem with an Elusive Solution. Nephrology Times, 2010, 3 (6):18-19.

[14] Li C, Yang CW. The pathogenesis and treatment of chronic allograft nephropathy. Nat Rev Nephrol 2009; 5: 513–519.

[15] Lorraine C. Racusen and Heinz Regele.The pathology of CAD. Kidney International.2010, 78 (Suppl 119), 27-32.

[16] Tan JC, Workeneh B, Busque S et al. Glomerular function, structure, and number in renal allografts from older deceased donors. J Am Soc Nephrol 2009; 20: 181–188.

[17] Kambham N, Nagarajan S, Shah S et al. A novel, semiquantitative, clinically correlated calcineurin inhibitor toxicity score for renal allograft biopsies. Clin J Am Soc Nephrol 2007; 2: 135–142.
[18] Mengel M, Gwinner W, Schwarz A et al. Infiltrates in protocol biopsies from renal allografts. Am J Transplant 2007; 7: 356–365.
[19] Sis B, Jhangri GS, Bunnag S et al. Endothelial gene expression in kidney transplants with allo antibody indicates antibody-mediated damage despite lack of C4d staining. Am J Transplant.2009; 9: 2312–2323.
[20] Solez K, Colvin RB, Rcusen LC et al. Banff meeting report: differential diagnosis of chronic allograft injury and elimination of chronic allograft nephropathy (CAN) Am J Transplant, 2007; 7: 518–526.
[21] Hallgrimur Benediktsson. Histopathology of Chronic Renal Allograft Dysfunction. Transplantation Reviews. 2004, 18, (2): 80-85.
[22] Nagase H, Woessner JF Jr. Matrix metalloproteinases.J Biol Chem. 1999;274(31):21491-21494.
[23] Bigg HF, Morrison CJ, Butler CS, et al.Tissue inhibitor of metalloproteinases-4 inhibits but does not support the activation of gelatinase A via efficient inhibition of membrane type 1-matrix metalloproteinase.Cancer Res.2001;61(9):3610.
[24] Galina Pizov, Michael M Friedlaender.Immunohistochemical Staining for Proliferation Antigen as a Predictor of Chronic Graft Dysfunction and Renal Graft Loss. Nephron 2002;92:738-742.
[25] Helen Robertson, Simi Ali, Benjamin J McDonnell, Alastair D Burt and John A Kirby.Chronic Renal Allograft Dysfunction: The Role of T Cell–Mediated Tubular Epithelial to Mesenchymal Cell Transition. J Am Soc Nephrol. 2004, 15:390-397.
[26] Anthony M Jevnikar and Roslyn B Mannon, Late Kidney Allograft Loss: What We Know about It, and What We Can Do about It? CJASN, 2008, 3: 56-67.
[27] Michael Zeisberg and Eric G Neilson.Mechanisms of Tubulointerstitial Fibrosis. J Am Soc Nephrol, 2010, 21: 1819-1834.
[28] B Y Choy, T M Chan and K N Lai. Recurrent Glomerulonephritis After Kidney Transplantation. American Journal of Transplantation 2006; 6: 2535–2542.
[29] Denton MD, Singh AK. Recurrent and de novo glomerulonephritis in the renal allograft.Semin Nephrol. 2000;20(2):164-75.
[30] Claudio Ponticelli, and Richard J Glassock.Posttransplant Recurrence of Primary Glomerulonephritis. CJASN, 2010, 5 (12): 2363-2372.
[31] Worawon Chailimpamontree, Svetlana Dmitrienko, Guiyun Li, Robert Balshaw, Alexander Magil, R Jean Shapiro, David Landsberg, John Gill, Paul A Keown and the Genome Canada Biomarkers in Transplantation Group. Probability, Predictors, and Prognosis of Posttransplantation Glomerulonephritis. JASN, 2009;20 (4): 843-851.
[32] Birkeland S A, Hamilton-Dutoit S. Is posttransplant lymphoproliferative disorder (PTLD) caused by any specific immunosuppressive drug or by the transplantation per se?Transplantation. 2003, 76(6):984-988.
[33] Fellstrom B. Impact and management of hyperlipidem ia post-transplantation. Transplantation, 2000; 70 (11 supp l):SS51.

[34] Ferreira A.C., Viana H., Carvalho F., Pinto J.R., Galvão M.J., Nolasco F., andSantos J.R.Chronic Allograft Dysfunction-Is There a Treatment? Transplantation Proceedings, 2009, 41(3):874-876.

[35] Afzali B, Taylor AL, Goldsmith JA: What can we do about chronic allograft nephropathy: role of immunosuppressive modulations. Kidney Int. 2005, 1:145,

[36] Chapman JR, O'Connel PJ, Nankivell BJ: Chronic renal allograft dysfunction. J Am Soc Nephrol. 2005, 16:3015.

[37] Johnson RW, Kreis H, Oberbauer R, et al: Sirolimus allows early cyclosporine withdrawl in renal transplantation resulting in improved renal function and lower blood pressure. Transplantation. 2001, 72:777.

[38] Kruger B, Fischereder M, Jauch KW, et al:Five-year follow up after late conversion from calcineurin inhibitors to sirolimus in patients with chronic renal allograft dysfunction. Transplant Proc.2007, 39:518.

[39] Kaplan B. Overcoming barriers to long-term graft survival. Am J Kidney Dis.2006;47:S52-64.

[40] Dikow R, Becker LE, Schaier M, Waldherr R, Gross ML, Zeier M. In renal transplants with delayed graft function chemokines and chemokine receptor expression predict long-term allograft function.Transplantation. 2010, 15;90(7):771-776.

[41] Sandovici M, Deelman LE, Benigni A, Henning RH. Towards graft-specific immunosuppressantion: Gene therapy of the transplanted kidney.Adv Drug Deliv Rev. 2010, 30;62(14):1358-1368.

[42] John PV, Mohamed HS. Diagnosis and Management of Renal Allograft Dysfunction.Therapy in Nephrology & Hypertension (Third Edition), 2007, Pages 994-1008.

[43] Krüger B, Fischereder M, Jauch KW, Graeb C, Hoffmann U, Böger CA, Banas B, Obed A, Schlitt HJ, Krämer BK. Five-Year Follow-up After Late Conversion From Calcineurin Inhibitors to Sirolimus in Patients With Chronic Renal Allograft Dysfunction. Transplantation Proceedings, 2007, 39(2):518-521.

[44] Fischereder M, Graeb C, Krüger B, Kammerl MC, Zülke C, Jauch KW, Krämer BK.Conversion From Calcineurin Inhibitors to Sirolimus in Patients With Chronic Renal Allograft Dysfunction.Transplantation Proceedings, 2006, 38(5):1295-1297.

[45] Garcia R, Pinheiro-Machado PG, Felipe CR, Park SI, Silva LA, Franco MF, Tedesco-Silva H Jr, Medina-Pestana JO.Conversion From Azathioprine to Mycophenolate Mofetil Followed by Calcineurin Inhibitor Minimization or Elimination in Patients With Chronic Allograft Dysfunction.Transplantation Proceedings, 2006, 38(9):2872-2878.

20

Delayed Graft Function

Qiansheng Li, Wenqian Huo, Keqin Zhang, Gang Wu,
Fengshuo Jin, Xi Lin, Xiaojiang Jiang and Dong Gao
*Department of Urology, Institute of Surgery Research, Daping Hospital,
Third Military Medical University, Chongqing,
China*

1. Introduction

Delayed graft function (DGF) is a common complication of renal transplantation. According to a clinical data analysis of 34,647 cases of cadaveric renal transplantation documented by the Renal Transplantation Registry of the United Network Sharing (UNOS), graft function did not recover instantly after transplantation and for ever in some cases; the 1-year rate of graft loss was up to 20% in cases with poor renal function recovery; the long-term loss rate of graft was higher in cases with poor renal function recovery than those with instant graft function. The half-life time of graft is 7 years in cases with delayed graft function, and is 12 years in cases with instant graft function. Based on our 30 years of experience in renal transplantation and the literature, we reviewed the diagnosis and management of DGF.

2. Diagnostic criteria

Currently, graft function recovery is defined as follows.

1. Instant graft function (IGF): postoperative urine output >7000ml, serum creatinine recovery to normal in 3-7 days.
2. Slow graft function (SGF): postoperative urine output is normal, but serum creatinine decreases slowly, and not to normal in one week. Nevertheless, dialysis is not needed.
3. Delayed graft function (DGF): DGF can be diagnosed according to the three aspects below.
   i. **Need for postoperative dialysis:** Need for dialysis in the first week after transplant once hyperacute rejection, vascular and urinary tract complications and hyperkalemia are ruled out.
   ii. **Urine output and serum creatinine:** ① Rise in serum Cr at 6–8 h post-operatively or <300 ml of urine despite adequate volume and diuretics. ② Urine output <1 L in 24 h and <25% fall in serum creatinine from baseline in first 24 h post-transplant. ③ Urine output <75 mL/h in first 48 h or failure of serum Cr to decrease by 10% in the first 48 h. ④ Serum creatinine increases or remains unchanged or decreases <10%/day during 3 consecutive days postoperatively. ⑤ Serum creatinine >2.5 mg/dL on Day 7 or need for post-transplant hemodialysis. ⑥ Time required for the kidney to reach CrCl>10 mL/min greater than 1 week. ⑦ Failure of creatinine to decline in the first 48 h in the absence of rejection.

iii. **Urine enzymes and biopsy**: ① Urine IL-18 in first 24 h>500 pg/mg. ②Urine NGAL on Day 0 >1000 ng/mg and IL-18 on Day 0 > 500 pg/mg. ③Pre-transplant soluble IL-6R of 35 000 pg/mL. ④ Pathologic findings that support acute renal tubular necrosis.

4. No more graft function (NGF): Postoperative failure of graft function that requires dialysis.
5. Hyper delayed graft function (HDGF): In rare cases, the anuria stage persists longer than one month, even several months after renal transplantation, followed by gradual renal function recovery, a phenomenon we called HDGF. In 2000, we performed a second renal transplantation in a female patient. In this patient, the anuria stage lasted 109 days postoperatively, and urine output increased gradually, with serum creatinine decrease to normal on day 155 postoperatively. Ten years of follow-up indicated the graft function to be normal.

3. Risk factors for DGF

DGF is a complex pathologic process usually involved donor- and recipient-related factors. Donor-related factors include age, cause of death, and transplantation and cold ischemia time of graft. Recipient-related factors include rejection, anti-HLA antibody level, and times of renal transplantation, cytomegalovirus infection, obesity, body size difference with the donor, pre-transplant dialysis type, and ethnicity.

1. Donor-related factors Due to an organ shortage, organs from donors of advanced age or organs with other confounding diseases are also used as sources for organ transplantation. The quality of renal graft is crucial. Renal graft function is closely associated with the donor's age, cause of death and primary disease. Renal graft of poor quality may not survive for long because of immune or non-immune damage to the graft.

   i. Brain death Animal study has demonstrated that changes in physiology, hemodynamics, endocrinology, and histomorphology as well as early inflammation damage peripheral organs following brain death. Cytokine storm after brain death may upregulate HLA expression in the graft and make the graft susceptible to attack by preexisting anti-HLA antibody. Rejection occurred earlier in renal grafts from rats after brain death than in the control group. The survival rate of renal grafts from non-kinship living donors is much higher than that of cadaveric renal grafts. Brain death influences the quality of donor organ, increasing the incidence of DGF.

   ii. Senile donors It has been clinically shown that senility of donors is a major risk factor for DGF, and it influences the long-term survival of grafts. The UN data demonstrate that senility of donor increases the incidence of DGF significantly. For instance, the incidence of DGF is 15% if the donors' age is 20 years, and is up to 40% if the donor's age is over 65 years. The cause for such difference may lie in the fact that the number of functioning nephrons decreases in healthy individuals with aging. In addition, renal grafts may be injured by ultrafiltration following transplantation.

   iii. Cause of death The cause of death is another major risk factor influencing the long-term survival of graft. According to the UNOS data, the incidence of DGF was 18%

if the donors died of traffic accident, was 30% if the donors died of cerebrovascular accident, and was 45% in 400 non-heart-beating donors (NHBDs) (possibly related to long periods of warm ischemia).

iv. Ischemia-reperfusion injury Cessation of blood flow leads to anaerobic metabolism and adenosine triphosphate depletion in the organ. The incidence of DGF is 12% if the period of cold ischemia of renal graft is less than 12h, and is up to 45% if the period of cold ischemia exceeds 48h. In addition, the incidence of DGF is less than 10% if the donor is young and the cold ischemia time is less than 12h, and is more than 20% if the donor is senile and the cold ischemia time is short. Given the cold ischemia time of 36-48h, the incidence of DGF is up to 50% if the donor is senile and, and is only 30% if the donor is young. Animal study has shown that the donor's age and cold ischemia time exert additive effect on chronic graft rejection.

2. Recipient-related factors
   The incidence of DGF is relatively high given suboptimal HLA matching, high sensitization status and a second transplantation. The severity of immune injury depends mainly on the severity of early post-transplantation rejection. High sensitization status increases the risk of immune injury. DGF may mask rejection, but rejection may aggravate preexisting injury. It has been demonstrated that the incidence of DGF increases significantly in the presence of early graft rejection and DGF is a predictor for aggravation of rejection. Cytomegalovirus infection, obesity, type of pre-transplant dialysis, and ethnicity are all factors influencing the incidence of DGF. For instance, black recipients are more likely to develop DGF than other people. However, the mechanisms involved remain largely unknown.
3. Other factors
   i. Organ preservation: Continuous pulsatile perfusion or pulsatile perfusion plus simple cold preservation of grafts from NHBDs helps decrease the incidence of DGF and improve the long-term survival rate of graft. In NHBDs, comparison of bilateral kidneys subjected to pulsatile perfusion and simple cold preservation, respectively, showed that the incidence of DGF was 10% for grafts subjected to pulsatile perfusion, and was 30% for grafts subjected to simple cold preservation. Valero, et al analyzed in situ perfusion (ISP), total body cooling (TBC), and normothermic recirculation (NR) for grafts from NHBDs, and found that the incidence of DGF was significantly lower in grafts subjected to NR than in those subjected to ISP and TBC. The viability of grafts from NHBDs can be assessed by perfusion parameters, and be improved through infusing drugs. In 2009, Cyril Moers reported that Lifeport Transporter can significantly decrease the incidence and duration of DGF following renal transplantation, while significantly increasing the 1-years survival rate of graft. In addition, Lifeport Transporter provides useful information for professionals to make wise clinical decisions, and helps them choose renal grafts. Hence, Lifeport Transporter is an effective, economical device for renal graft preservation.

Shortening the ischemia time: Topical ischemia/reperfusion injury is the pathogenetic basis for DGF, and the severity of DGF depends on the duration of ischemia. The incidence of DGF is lower in China than in other countries. This is because the warm ischemia time (WIT) of cadaveric renal graft is usually maintained between 10 and 15min in the transplantation centers in China. The warm ischemia time should also be shortened during nephrectomy in living donors. It helps reduce the incidence of DGF to shorten the time for graft trimming and possible second warm ischemia of graft. The cold ischemia time (CIT) directly influences the incidence of DGF and graft survival. It was demonstrated that the risk of DGF increased by 23% every 6h.

Kidney preservatives: They are used to minimize topical ischemic injury. They comprise special components to relieve cellular swelling, maintain calcium homeostasis, reduce the production of oxyradicals and provide energy-rich substances. The UW preservative is superior to Euro-Collins solution in reducing the incidence of DGF. The research on preservatives is now focusing on additives to the standard formulas, e.g., Trimetazidine.

ii. Recipient management: Many patients have inadequate blood volume preoperatively, and the use of crystalline or colloid solutions under central venous pressure monitoring can reduce the incidence of DGF. The kidney is one of the organs that need plentiful blood supply, and the volume of blood supplied to the kidneys accounts for approximately 1/4 of cardiac output. The kidney is sensitive to ischemia, and the ischemia time is correlated to the severity of reperfusion-related injury. Appropriate blood pressure is a prerequisite for adequate graft perfusion. In particular, the blood pressure in the recipient prior to reperfusion determines the recovery of metabolism of graft after a series of ischemic events. A proper blood pressure ensures oxygenated blood perfusion and benefits graft functional recovery. The incidence of DGF is lower in patients receiving peritoneal dialysis prior to transplantation than those receiving hemodialysis. This may relate to decreased blood volume in patients receiving hemodialysis upon the procedure of transplantation. Therefore, sufficient fluid extension is beneficial for patients. Effective blood pressure must be maintained intra- and post-operatively, and blood pressure should better be kept 10-20mmHg (1mmHg=0.133kPa) above the basic blood pressure upon reperfusion and in the first three days postoperatively, thus ensuring effective graft perfusion. Stable blood pressure but poor graft vessel tension and anuria during operation may relate to arteriospasm that results from traction of the renal artery. Polyuria may be induce by postoperative administration of dopamine to dilate the renal artery and elevate systolic pressure.

iii. Vasodilators: During reperfusion, direct infusion of calcium channel blockers into the renal artery improves early renal function due to direct vasodilation and relief of lipid peroxide. A randomized trial has demonstrated that dilthiazem treatment of the donor or treatment of the recipient with other calcium channel blockers benefits early graft function. Atrial natriuretic peptide (ANP), a peptide hormone increasing glomerular filtration rate and urine output, improves renal function and histopathologic changes in animals with acute ischemic renal failure. After infusion of ANP increases serum creatinine clearance quickly and reduces the need for dialysis. In addition, ANP antagonizes vasoconstrictors following topical ischemic injury and promotes renal function recovery. Furosemide suppresses prostaglandin lyases and increases prostaglandin E, thus dilating renal vessels, decreasing renal vascular resistance, and increasing blood flow to the kidney, particularly to the tissues under renal cortex. Therefore, furosemide can relieve ischemic renal injury, promote renal function recovery, and decrease the incidence of DGF.

iv. HLA mismatching: Based on our data, HLA is no a risk factor for DGF, possibly because we controlled the number of HLA mismatches strictly. In addition, HLA matching directly influences the incidence of AR, and AR is one risk factor for

DGF. We also found that early urinary fistula and ureteral obstruction are not risk factors for DGF.

v. Type of dialysis: The type of pre-transplant dialysis may influence the incidence of DGF. A review of a number of cases showed that peritoneal dialysis is in favor of immediate recovery of renal function after renal transplantation, which was attributed to fluid load in the recipient. After analysis of multiple variables, e.g., DGF, ARF in patients who underwent preoperative hemodialysis (HD) or peritoneal dialysis (PD) and received the first cadaveric renal transplantation, it was found that there were 33 cases of DGF (27 cases of HD and 6 cases of PD, p=0.03, and there were 14 cases of ARF (14 cases of HD and 0 case of PD, p=0.01). The time for serum creatinine to decrease to 50% of the pre-transplant level correlates positively to the cold ischemia time and body weight increase in the recipient, and correlates negatively to the urine output in the first 24h, fluid load, and central venous pressure. PD is thought to decrease the incidence and severity of DGF after renal transplantation. Joseph, et al investigated acute rejection, DGF, graft survival, and patient survival in 325 patients who underwent preoperative HD and PD and the first cadaveric renal transplantation, and found 56 DGF cases in 183 PD patients and 58 DGF cases in 117 HD patients. The incidence of DGF was significantly higher in HD patients than in PD patients.

4. Mental disorders and interventions in DGF patients
   With technical advance in renal transplantation, mental problems in patients with renal failure or undergoing renal transplantation have drawn more and more attention. These problems include personality change, emotional disorders, mental disorders, psychological rejection, and psychosocial dysfunction. Mental problems may directly influence graft function recovery, and even lead to graft nonfunction or serious adverse events, such as non-compliance to treatment or automutilation (suicide). Therefore, it is crucial to pay close attention to the patient's mental status before and after renal transplantation and manage mental disorders promptly.

Because of biological factors, e.g., renal failure and rejection, immunosuppressant-associated adverse reactions and psychosocial factors, patients may develop various mental disorders before and after renal transplantation, including anxiety, depression, psychotic symptoms, and psychological rejection. Anxiety/depression disorder is characterized by mental stress, excessive anxiety, worry, depression, self-abasement, self-blame, and decreased interest. Some patients may present with panic attack and social anxiety disorder, and serious patients may have suicidal idea and commit suicide. Psychotic symptoms include delusion, hallucination, lack of self-awareness due to mental and somatic disorders, and detachment of the real world. Patients with psychotic symptoms may suffer from secondary behavioral disorders. These symptoms persist for varying length of time. Psychological rejection occurs mainly after renal transplantation. The patients are unable to accept the grafts mentally, and they cannot cope with the mental stress associated with transplantation. They may refuse to take anti-rejection drugs or ask for removal of the grafts. These mental disorders may cause autonomic nerve dysfunction, immune dysfunction and behavioral disorders, e.g., somatic pain, insomnia, anorexia (or apastia), and non-compliance to treatment or automutilation (suicide).

Most patients expect much from renal transplantation, and they are likely to develop mental disorders in case of DGF. There are interacting biological and psychosocial factors that underlie mental disorders.

1. Biological factors:
    i. Acute renal failure
    Following renal transplantation, ATN leads to accumulation of toxic substances which damage nerve cells directly or indirectly and influence nerve cell functions. For instance, alteration in intracerebral monamine neurotransmitters may lead to anxiety, depression and psychotic symptoms.
    ii. Immunosuppressants
    Large doses of immunosuppressants may impair the immune system, and interfere with neuroendocrine function and neurotransmitters in the brain. Neuroendocrine and neurotransmitter dysfunction serve the principal biological mechanism for mental disorders in DGF patients.
    iii. Transplantation procedure
    Renal transplantation procedure per se is a traumatic stress, which can also cause mental disorders, particularly in patients with poor physical status. In addition, perioperative administration of medications, e.g., anesthetics, is one of the causes for mental disorders in DGF patients.
2. Psychosocial factors:
    i. Personality
    Positive and optimistic attitude, good cognition assessment system and coping capacity are crucial for mental health of patients undergoing renal transplantation. Personality traits such as anxiety, paranoid idea, and disadvantage-guided thought are the personality basis for mental disorders in DGF patients.
    ii. Stressful events
    In case of accumulation of adverse life events or major adverse life events, DGF patients may suffer from serious mental trauma and mental disorders.
    iii. Psychosocial supportive system
    The psychosocial supportive system for DGF patients involves social security system, family support and other interpersonal support. Social security system includes medical insurance and psychological support (e.g., unemployment). Family support mainly involves husband-wife and parent-child relationships and socioeconomic status of family. Other interpersonal support mainly includes career, friendship and special group relationships.

Proper assessment and effective management of DGF patients with mental disorders directly influence the efficacy of medical interventions and the life quality of patients.

3. Assessment of mental disorders:
    i. The patient is interviewed face-to-face by psychiatrist and psychologist to assess his/her mental status, personality traits and life events. Meanwhile, the need for medical management and the specific interventions, e.g., psychological intervention or medical treatment, are evaluated.
    ii. Mental status scale based measurements: including measurements of mental status, personality traits, life events and life quality.
4. Prevention of mental disorders:
    i. To establish an integrated social security supportive system, including medical insurance system and government funded special social security system.

ii. To set up a team of psychiatrists or psychologists, who monitor the patients' mental status during the perioperative stage of renal transplantation, and diagnose and treat mental problems promptly.
iii. To educate DGF patients, including introducing renal transplantation related issues and possible mental problems.
5. Treatment of mental disorders:
i. Psychotherapy
Individualized psychotherapy, primarily supportive psychotherapy, is considered. Cognitive and behavioral therapy may also be utilized. In addition, volunteers who ever suffered from DGF and now have their renal function recovered normal are invited to communicate with the patients, which is the most effective modality.
ii. Drug treatment
In DGF patients with serious mental disorders, antipsychotic drugs, e.g., Olanzapine, may be prescribed. The dose must be increased gradually. In case of serious emotional disorder, e.g., anxiety-depression, particularly, high risk of suicide, antidepressant drugs should be administered immediately. SSRI and SSNI drugs may be prescribed. For patients with serious anxiety, benzodiazepines may be used. Electroshock should be considered with caution.

4. Prevention and management of DGF

DGF leads to adverse outcomes, including prolonged hospital stay, need for postoperative hemodialysis, significant increase in medical care costs, decrease in the 1-year survival rate of graft, increase in the rejection incidence, and decrease in the long-term graft survival and the short-term and long-term survival rate of patients. Various medical modalities may decrease the incidence of DGF:

1. To choose young donors and ensure good match of the graft with the recipient.
2. To reduce warm and cold ischemia time.
3. To assess the graft quality and utilize optimal renal grafts.
4. To preserve renal grafts by pulsatile mechanical perfusion.
5. To administer small doses of calcineurin inhibitors (CNIs), biological immunosuppressants and calcium channel blockers. Calcium channel blockers may regulate the immune system and reduce acute rejection. In addition, they prevent the toxic and adverse effects of CNIs and decrease blood pressure.
6. To maintain a proper level of mean arterial pressure in the recipient prior to graft reperfusion.

5. Summary

DGF is an early complication after transplantation caused jointly by immunologic and non-immunologic factors. Various novel immunosuppressants can effectively control or relieve immunologic graft injury, thus improving the short-term and long-term survival rate of grafts. However, the mechanism of pre-transplant injury to the renal graft remains largely unclear. The risk factors for DGF include the warm ischemia time, cold ischemia time, intraoperative and early postoperative hypotension, ATN, nephrotoxicity of CNIs and AR.

Further study should be carried out with large sample sizes to investigate the correlation of times of transplantation, number of HLA mismatch, early postoperative urinary fistula, ureteral obstruction, and preoperative blood transfusion with DGF. Renal graft protection has seldom been investigated. Further efforts should be made to prevent non-immunologic injury to the renal graft, so as to increase the quality of renal graft and the short-term and long-term survival rate of renal grafts.

6. References

[1] L Polyak MM, Arrington BO. Stubenbord WT, et al. The influence of pulsatile preservation on renal transplantation in the 1990s. Transplantation. 2000, 69: 249.
[2] Lane NJ, Thorniley MS, Manek S, et al. Effect of mannitol and polyethylene glycol on the action of frusemide during renal storage and transplantation. Transplantation, 1996, 62: 575. 2008. 07No.
[3] Gonwa TA, Hricik DE, Brinker K, et al. Improved renal function in sirolimus—treated renal transplant patients after-early cyclosporine elimination. Transplantation, 2002, 74: 1560.
[4] McTaggart RA, Gotflieb D, Brooks J, et al. Sirolimus prolongs recovery from delayed graft function after cadaveric renal transplantation. Am J Transplant, 2003, 3: 416.
[5] Stallone G, Di Paolo S, Schena A, et al. Addition of sirolimus to cyclosporine delays the recovery from delayed graft function but does not affect 1-year graft function. J Am Soe Nephrol, 2004, 15: 228.
[6] Boom H, Mallat MJ, de Fijter JW, et aI. Delayed graft function influences renal function, but not survival. Kidney lnt, 2000, 58: 859.
[7] Bunnapradist S, Lochlainn EN, Takemoto SK. Antibody induction therapy and their associated outcomes in cadaveric kidney transplants. Am J Transplant, 2004, 4(Suppl. 8): 264.
[8] McCormick BB. Pierrctos A, Fenteon S, et al. Review of clinical outcomes in nocturnal haemodialysis patients after renal transplantation[J]. Nephrol Transplant, 2004, 19(3): 714-719.
[9] Jacobs SC, Cho E, Foster C, et al. Laparoscopic donor nephrectomy: the University of Maryland 6-year experience EJ]. J Urol, 2004, 171(1): 47-51.
[10] Shosakes DA, Shahed AR, Kim S. Delayed graft function: Influence on outcome and strategies for prevention. Urol Clin Noah Am 2001, 28: 721—732.
[11] Fischer J, Kirste G Keller H, et al. Does ATN influence renal transplant function negatively. Transplant Proc 1 988, 20: 908.
[12] Hemandez A, Light JA, Barhyte D, et al. Ablating the ischemia reperfusion injury in non-heart-beating donor kidneys. Transplantation 1999, 67: 200-206.
[13] Ojo AO, Wolfe RA, Held, et al. Delayed graft function: risk factors an d implications for renal allograft surviva1. Transplantation 1997, 63: 968-974.
[14] Gaber LW, Gaber AO, Hathwaway DK, et al. Routine early biopsy of allograft with delayed graft function of histolopathology and transplant outcome. Clin Transplant 1 996, 1 0: 629-634.

[15] Lemay S, Rabb H, Postler G, et al. Prominent and sustained upregulation of gpl30-signaling cytokines and chemokine MIP in murine renal ischemic reperfusion. Transplantalion 2000, 69(5): 957-963.
[16] Canaud B. Leblane M. Leray Moragues H, et al. Slow continuous and daily ultrafiltration for refractory congestive heart failure. Nephrol Dial Transplant 1998, 13(14): 51 – 55.
[17] Avihingsanon Y, Ma N, PavlakisMet, et al. On the intraoperative molecular status of renal allografts after vascular reperfusion and clinical outcomes. J Am Soc Nephrol 2005; 16: 1542–1548
[18] Boom H, Mallat MJ, de Fijter JW, et al. Calcium levels as a risk factor for delayed graft function. Transplantation 2004; 77: 868–873
[19] Rodrigo E, Ruiz JC, Pinera C, et al. Creatinine reduction ratio on posttransplant day two as criterion in defining delayed graft function. Am J Transplant 2004; 4: 1163–1169
[20] Turkowski-Duhem A, Kamar N, Cointault O, et al. Predictive factors of postrenal transplant anemia. Transplant Proc 2005; 37: 1009–1011
[21] Giral-Classe M, Hourmant M, Cantarovich D, et al. Delayed graft function of more than six days strongly decreases long-term survival of transplanted kidneys. Kidney Int 1998; 54: 972–978
[22] Nickerson P, Jeffery J, Gough J, et al. Identification of clinical and histopathologic risk factors for diminished renal function 2 years posttransplant.J Am Soc Nephrol 1998; 9: 482–487
[23] Gonwa TA, MaiML, Smith LB, et al. Immunosuppression for delayedor slow graft function in primary cadaveric renal transplantation: use of low dose tacrolimus therapy with post-operative administration of anti-CD25 monoclonal antibody. Clin Transplant 2002; 16: 144–149
[24] Schmidt R, Kupin W, Dumler F, et al. Influence of the pretransplant hematocrit level on early graft function in primary cadaveric renal transplantation. Transplantation 1993; 55: 1034–1040
[25] Shoskes DA, Hodge EE, Goormastic M, et al. HLA matching determines susceptibility to harmful effects of delayed graft function in renal transplant recipients. Transplant Proc 1995; 27: 1068– 1069
[26] Mehta Tk. Quantitative detection of promoter hypermethylation as a biomarker of acute kidney injury during transplantation. Transplant Proc 2006; 38(10): 3420–6
[27] Parikh CR, Jani A, Melnikov VY, et al. Urinary interleukin-18 is a marker of human acute tubular necrosis. Am J Kidney Dis 2004; 43: 405–414
[28] Parikh CR, Jani A, Mishra J et al. Urine NGAL and IL-18 are predictive biomarkers for delayed graft function following kidney transplantation. Am J Transplant 2006; 6: 1639–1645
[29] Sadeghi M, Daniel V, Naujokat C, et al. Association of high pretransplant sIL-6R plasma levels with acute tubular necrosis in kidney graft recipients. Transplantation 2006; 81: 1716–1724
[30] Cyril M, Jacqueline M. Smits, et al. Machine Perfusion or Cold Storage in Deceased-Donor Kidney Transplantation.N Engl J Med 2009; 360:7-19

[31] T. Tsunoda, R. Yamashita, Y. Kojima, S. Takahara. Risk Factors for Depression After Kidney Transplantation. Transplantation Proceedings, 2010, 42(5):1679-1681
[32] A. Virzì, M.S. Signorelli, M. Veroux, G. Giammarresi, S. Maugeri, A. Nicoletti, P. Veroux. Depression and Quality of Life in Living Related Renal Transplantation. Transplantation Proceedings, 2007, 39(6): 1791-1793

21

Factors Related to Graft Outcome in Pediatric Renal Transplantation: a Single Center Study

Jean Herman and Rita Van Damme-Lombaerts
Department of Pediatric Transplantation
University Hospitals Leuven
Belgium

1. Introduction

Over the last decades, renal transplantation has evolved from an experimental procedure into the treatment of choice for children with end-stage renal disease. Differences in size and weight of the recipient, cause of renal failure, immune responsiveness, susceptibility to infection, pharmacokinetics of immunosuppressive drugs, and psychological aspects distinguish renal transplantation in children from adults. The longevity of an allograft is particularly important for the pediatric transplant recipient, because renal replacement therapy is necessarily a lifelong undertaking. The aim of the present study is to determine by means of a multivariable analysis the factors that significantly affect graft outcome in the paediatric transplant population. Knowledge of predictors of graft survival can be beneficial in planning the renal replacement therapy in children and improving transplantation results.

Registry studies, essentially from the North American Pediatric Renal Trials and Collaborative Studies (NAPRTCS) (Benfield et al., 1999; NAPRTCS, 2010) and from the United Network for Organ Sharing (UNOS) (Hwang et al., 2005), have been performed to analyse factors related to graft outcome in children. Registry studies have the advantage of being able to include large number of patients. However these studies usually involve heterogeneous populations with different pre-transplant selections, transplant procedures and post-transplant management. Therefore single center studies using a more homogeneous patient group and more uniform management protocols may be valuable in the analysis of transplant outcome. Nevertheless such single center studies using multivariable techniques to analyse transplant outcome are very scarce in paediatric renal transplantation (Vats et al., 2002).

We analysed all renal transplantations performed in children at our institution between 1980 and 2010 and included in our analysis various factors concerning recipient characteristics, donor characteristics, perioperative characteristics and post-transplant events.

2. Patients, materials and methods

2.1 Patients

The study population consisted of 151 kidney transplants performed between June 1980 and October 2010 in 135 children (81 boys and 54 girls) with mean age 10.7 years (± 4.9) at

transplantation. There were 132 first grafts, 15 second grafts, 3 third grafts and 1 fourth graft.
The original disease was congenital or hereditary in 74% and acquired in 26%. Thirteen children were transplanted preemptively. Kidney came from living related donors (LRD) in 33 cases (22%) and from deceased donors (DD) in 118 cases (78%). Four children underwent combined liver-kidney transplantation.
Immunosuppression consisted of an induction with antilymphocyte antibodies and a maintenance regimen with cyclosporine A (CsA) (since December 1984), azathioprine and prednisolone. Newer immunosuppressive agents were introduced more recently: tacrolimus in 1998, mycophenolate mofetyl in 1998, basiliximab and daclizumab in 1999.

2.2 Data source

Data were retrieved from the patients' medical files and from the archives and database of Eurotransplant. The follow-up period ended in February 2011.

2.3 Analytic variables and statistical analysis

The following variables were studied as potential factors affecting graft outcome:

- *Recipient characteristics*: age (years), gender, height (cm), weight (kg), body surface area (BSA, m^2), body mass index (BMI, kg/m^2), prior transplant, primary kidney disease, peak and current panel-reactive antibody percentage (PRA), ABO blood group, CMV serological status, number of prior blood transfusions (0-5 vs. >5), native nephrectomy, dialysis modality before transplantation, dialysis duration (years), time on the waiting list (years), hypertension (defined as the use of antihypertensive medications), year of transplantation.
- *Donor characteristics*: age, gender, height, weight, BSA, BMI, ABO group, CMV status, donor type (LRD vs. DD), cause of death for the deceased donors, serum creatinine level (mg/dl) at organ retrieval, diuresis (ml) during the last 24 hours and the last hour before organ retrieval.
- *Donor recipient relationships*: donor/recipient age ratio, height ratio, weight ratio, BSA ratio, BMI ratio, gender mismatch, human leukocyte antigen (HLA) mismatch, ABO mismatch (all grafts were ABO compatible but one), CMV mismatch (D+/R-, D-/R+, D+/R+, D-/R-).
- *Organ preservation and perioperative characteristics*: donor kidney preservation solution (Eurocollins (EC) vs. University of Wisconsin (UW) vs. histidine-tryptophan-ketoglutarate (HTK)), cold ischemia time (hours), warm ischemia time (minutes).
- *Immunosuppression*: induction therapy (polyclonal vs. monoclonal vs. none) and maintenance immunosuppression at time of discharge from the initial hospitalization including use of calcineurin inhibitors and type (CsA vs. tacrolimus), use of antimetabolites and type (azathioprine vs. mycophenolate mofetyl).
- *Post-transplant characteristics*: duration of initial transplant hospitalization (days), occurrence of delayed graft function (DGF) defined as the need for dialysis in the first week post-transplant, occurrence of acute rejection episodes, creatinine clearance (ml/min/1.73 m^2) at 1 year post-transplant (calculated using the Schwartz formula: creatinine clearance = 0.55*height (cm)/plasma creatinine (mg/dl)), hypertension (defined as the use of antihypertensive medications) and its severity as reflected by the

number of antihypertensive medications at 1 year post-transplant, proteinuria (>1 g/24 h) at 1 year post-transplant, hemoglobin (g/dl) at 1 year post-transplant.

Acute Rejection was defined as any rejection treatment. Acute rejection was suspected when the serum creatinine level increased to 20% above the baseline level and was biopsy proven in most cases.

Univariable analysis was performed on each of these variables using the Cox proportional hazards regression model. Variables with a p-value <0.10 in the univariable analysis were then entered into the multivariable analysis. Cox regression was applied with forward stepwise selection using likelihood-ratio tests. Variables were retained in the model at p<0.05. Acute rejection was considered as a time dependent covariate.

The hazard ratios (HR) for graft failure and corresponding 95% confidence intervals were estimated. Graft failure was defined as return to dialysis, re-transplantation or death with a functioning graft. Graft survival time was defined as the time between the date of transplantation and graft failure or the end of the study period.

Two models were constructed: one starting at the time of transplantation thus including all transplants (n=151) and one starting after the end of the first year post-transplant including transplants that functioned beyond the first year (n=140). Hypertension at 1 year, creatinine clearance at 1 year, proteinuria at 1 year (>1 g/24 h), hemoglobin at 1 year were included in the second model as additional potential predictors for graft survival after 1 year.

Patient and graft survivals were calculated with the Kaplan–Meier method.

Statistical analyses were performed using Statistica 8.1 (StatSoft Inc., Tulsa, OK., USA) and SPSS 18.0 (SPSS Inc., Chicago, IL., USA). Statistical significance was defined as p<0.05.

3. Results

3.1 Patient and graft survival

The actuarial patient survival was 97% at 1 year, 96% at 3 years, 94% at 5 years and 92% at 10 years (Figure 1). Nine patients died, three of them with a functioning graft. The cause of death was bacterial infection in four children, Pneumocystis carinii infection in one, malignant lymphoproliferative disorder in one, and a cardiovascular complication in three (two of whom died following cerebral haemorrhage and one following a myocardial infarction).

The overall actuarial graft survival was 94% at 1 year, 86% at 3 years, 80% at 5 years and 64% at 10 years (Figure 1). Mean follow-up time was 9.3 ± 6.5 years.

The actuarial graft survival at 1, 3, 5, 10 years was 94%, 90%, 83% and 68% respectively for recipients of living-related donor and 94%, 83%, 79% and 63% respectively for recipients of deceased donor (Log-Rank Test p=0.95). In children younger than 5 years the graft survival was 92% at 1 and 3 years, and 83% at 5 and 10 years; in this group the prevalence of LRD was rather high (11/24; 46%).

In total 68 grafts were lost during the study period, 9 of them during the first year post-transplant. The causes of graft loss are given in Table 1; chronic rejection being the leading cause. Non compliance was documented in 19% of the failure due to chronic rejection (9 cases). Recurrence of the initial disease was the second most frequent cause of graft failure.

The main characteristics of the study population are detailed in Table 2.

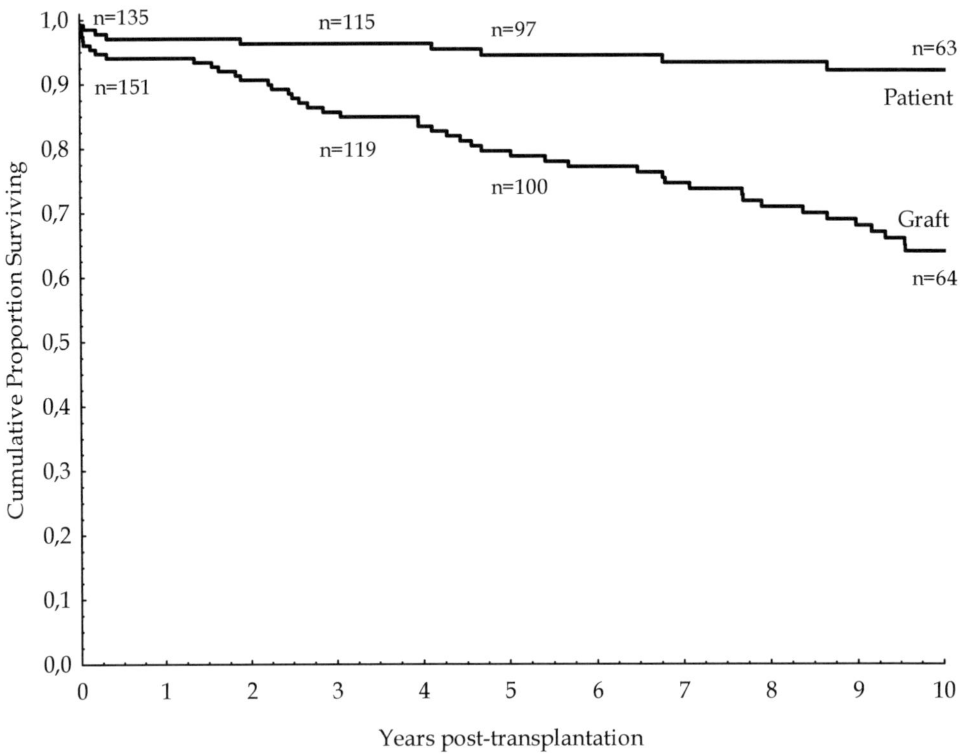

Fig. 1. Kaplan Meier plot of patient and graft survivals (n indicates the number of subjects at risk at 0, 3, 5 and 10 years).

	n	%
Chronic rejection	47	69.1
Recurrence of primary disease	8	11.8
Death with functioning graft	3	4.4
Malignancy	2	2.9
Infection	2	2.9
Technical failure	2	2.9
Primary non-function	2	2.9
Polyoma nephropathy	1	1.5
Thrombosis renal artery	1	1.5

Table 1. Causes of graft failure

	N*	Mean ± SD or n	Range or %
Recipient characteristics			
Age (year)		10.7 ± 4.7	1.3-21.9
0-4		24	15.9%
5-9		38	25.2%
≥10		56	59.0%
Gender M/F		91/60	59.6/40.4%
Weight (kg)		20.5 ± 14.5	8.4-76.4
Primary Tx/ReTx		132/19	87.4/12.6%
Primary kiney disease			
Congenital uro-nephropathy		72	47.7%
Hereditary nephropathy		40	26.5%
Acquired nephropathy		39	25.8%
Renal replacement therapy at Tx			
Hemodialysis		125	76.1%
Peritoneal dialysis		22	14.6%
Transplantation		1	0.7%
None		13	8.6%
Years of pre-transplant dialysis		1.93 ± 1.73	0-8.18
Years on waiting list	106	1.26 ± 1.12	0.04-6.25
>5 pre-transplant transfusions		62	41.1%
Current PRA>50%/Peak PRA>50%		16/33	10.6/21.9%
CMV serology: neg/pos/unknown		114/36/1	75.5/23.8/0.7%
On Antihypertensiva at time of Tx	149	81	54.4%
Donor characteristics			
Age (year)		23.8 ± 14.8	0.5-54.5
0-4		18	11.9%
5-19		48	31.8%
20-39		54	35.8%
40-55		31	20.5%
Gender M/F	150	86/64	57.3/43.7%
Weight (kg)	127	55.5 ± 23.5	7-101
Donor type			
DD/LRD		118/33	78.1/21.9%
Cause of donor death	117		
Trauma/CVA/others		71/24/22	60.7/20.5/18.8%
Donor /Recipient relationships			
Donor/Recipient Weight ratio	127	2.35 ± 1.78	0.29-8.47
Donor/Recipient BSA ratio	125	1.70 ± 0.88	0.21-4.51
Donor/Recipient BMI ratio	125	1.28 ± 0.28	0.53-2.15
CMV serology	134		
D-/R-		68	
D-/R+		23	
D+/R-		33	
D+/R+		10	

Table 2. Characteristics of the study population

	N*	Mean ± SD or n	Range or %
HLA Mismatch	150		
HLA-A		0.83 ± 0.60	
0/1/2		42/91/17	28.0/60.7/11.3%
HLA-B		1.03 ± 0.51	
0/1/2		17/111/22	11.3/74.0/14.7%
HLA-DR		0.77 ± 0.55	
0/1/2		44/97/9	29.3/64.7/6.0%
HLA-ABDR		2.62 ± 1.06	
0		7	4.7%
1		9	6.0%
2		46	30.7%
3		67	44.7%
4		15	10.0%
5		5	3.3%
6		1	0.7%
Perioperative characteristics			
Organ preservation solution	149		
Eurocollins/UW/HTK		48/64/37	32.2/43.0/24.8%
Cold ischemia time (hours) for DD	117	20.34 ± 7.70	8.40-50.47
>30 hr		10	9.3%
Warm ischemia time (min)	148	38.1 ±.11.8	15.0-95.0
>40 min		53	35.8%
Immunosuppression (IS)			
Induction	150		
Polyclonal (ALS/ATG)		92 (43/49)	61.3%
Monoclonal (anti-IL2r/OKT3)		52 (51/1)	34.7%
None		6	4%
Maintenance IS at discharge			
Cyclosporine A/Tacrolimus/No		104/31/16	68.9/20.5/10.6%
Azathioprine/MMF/No		104/45/2	68.9/29.8/1.3%
Post-transplant characteristics			
Tx hospitalization (days)		19.3 ± 12.9	7-113
Delayed graft function(DGF)		25	16.6%
Acute rejection			
Yes vs. No		69/82	45.7/54.3 %
Within the first year post Tx		58	38.4 %
Beyond the first year post Tx		23	15.7 %
Time first rejection episode (days)		46 (10-174)§	1-5474
Hemoglobin level at 1 yr (g/dl)	139	11.5 ± 1.4	6.4-14.0
Proteinuria (>1 g/24 h) at 1 yr	140	10	7.1%
Creatinine Clearance at 1 yr (ml/min/1.73 m^2)	140	72.1 ± 22.0	14.7-156.5

*N=number of transplants for whom data are available; if not specified n=151. §data given as median (interquartile range). CVA: cardiovascular accident; DD: deceased donor; DGF: delayed graft function ; LRD: Living related donor.

Table 2. Cont.

3.2 Univariable analysis of factors influencing graft outcome

Table 3 summarizes the predictors of graft outcome in univariable analysis ($p<0.10$).

Duration of pre-transplant dialysis, multiple blood transfusions pre-transplant (>5), warm ischemia time (superior to 40 min), cold ischemia time, delayed graft function (DGF) and acute rejection were found to significantly affect outcome adversely. Transplants that did not benefit from calcineurin inhibitors had a fourfold increased risk of graft failure ($p<0.0001$). In addition, over the time of our transplant program, there was a significant lower risk for graft failure with each subsequent year ($p=0.008$). As far as HLA matching is concerned, two mismatches on HLA-A tended to be detrimental ($p=0.064$).

Kidney function (creatinine clearance) at 1 year, proteinuria (>1 g/24 h) at 1 year and the level of hemoglobin at 1 year were found to be significant predictors of graft outcome for the transplants that functioned beyond the first year. Risk of graft loss increased with the presence of proteinuria and decreased with an increase in hemoglobin level and an increase in creatinine clearance.

Variables that were not retained as predictors ($p>0.10$) of graft outcome included among others: primary kidney disease, recipient and donor gender and age, recipient and donor anthropometric parameters (weight, height, BSA, BMI), age ratio and anthropometric parameters ratio between the donor and the recipient, peak and current PRA levels, recipient and donor blood group, donor type, organ preservation solution type, CMV matching status, repeat transplant, and hypertension at transplantation and at 1 year post-transplant.

	df	HR	95% CI	p Value
Time on dialysis (years)	1	1.17	1.02-1.34	0.030
>5 Transfusions pre-Tx	1	1.82	1.12-2.97	0.016
HLA-A mismatch (2 vs. 0-1)	1	1.96	0.96-3.98	0.064
Cold ischemia time (h) (DD)				
continue variable	1	1.03	1.002-1.065	0.034
>30 h vs. ≤ 30 h	1	2.63	1.31-5.26	0.006
Warm ischemia time (min)				
as continue variable	1	1.016	0.996-1.037	0.11
>40 min vs. ≤ 40 min	1	1.66	1.02-2.71	0.042
Year of transplantation	1	0.95	0.91-0.99	0.008
Absence of calcineurin inhibitors	1	4.31	2.44-7.63	<0.0001
Dialysis in the first week post-Tx (DGF)	2			0.001
Risk graft failure within first 3 months	1	16.89	3.41-83.80	0.001
Risk graft failure after first 3 months	1	1.05	0.54-2.04	0.88
Acute rejection	1	2.61	1.55-4.40	0.0003
Proteinuria (>1 g/24 h) at 1 year	1	4.13	2.01-8.48	0.0001
Hemoglobin at 1 year (g/dl)	1	0.67	0.54-0.82	0.0002
Creatinine clearance at 1 year (ml/min/1.73 m^2)	1	0.97	0.95-0.98	<0.0001

df: degrees of freedom; HR: hazard ratio; CI: confidence interval

Table 3. Predictors of graft outcome in univariable analysis ($p<0.10$)

3.3 Multivariable analysis of factors influencing graft outcome

3.3.1 Considering all transplants - graft survival from the time of transplantation

Multivariable Cox regression analysis showed that the significant factors contributing to graft failure were: absence of calcineurin inhibitors, two mismatches on HLA-A, occurrence of acute rejection and occurrence of DGF. The need for dialysis in the first week post-transplant was linked with a very high risk for graft failure within the first three months post-transplant; beyond this period it had no significant impact on graft outcome. The hazard ratios for graft failure and their confidence intervals are given in Table 4. The other factors that were found significant in univariable analysis (multiple pre-transplant transfusions, cold and warm ischemia times, year of transplantation, duration of pre-transplant dialysis) did not significantly affect outcome when subjected to a multivariable analysis.

	df	HR	95% CI	p Value
Absence of calcineurin inhibitors	1	3.98	2.15-7.36	<0.0001
2 HLA-A mismatches	1	2.77	1.31-5.84	0.008
DGF	2			0.002
Risk graft failure within first 3 months	1	3.21	2.62-66.50	0.002
Risk graft failure after first 3 months	1	1.31	0.66- 2.61	0.44
Acute rejection	1	2.10	1.25-3.52	0.005

Likelihood ratio Chi-square 46.208, df 5, p<0.0001 (n=150)

Table 4. Multivariable Cox regression analysis of graft survival from the time of transplantation: analysis of all grafts.

3.3.2 Considering transplants with ≥ 1 year survival - graft survival after 1 year

This analysis was done on the subset of transplants that were still functioning at 1 year. Nine grafts were lost in the first year. Multivariable Cox regression analysis showed that significant risk factors contributing to graft failure after 1 year were: absence of calcineurin inhibitors, two HLA-A mismatches, kidney function (creatinine clearance) at 1 year, proteinuria at 1 year (superior to 1 g/24 h) and hemoglobin level at 1 year.
The hazard ratios for graft failure and their confidence intervals are given in Table 5.

	df	HR	95% CI	p Value
Absence of calcineurin inhibitors	1	6.73	3.19-14.21	<0.0001
2 HLA-A mismatches	1	3.25	1.45-7.27	0.004
Creatinine clearance at 1 yr (ml/min/1.73 m^2)	1	0.97	0.96-0.99	0.002
Proteinuria (>1 g/24 h) at 1 yr	1	3.13	1.44-6.81	0.004
Hemoglobin level at 1 yr (g/dl)	1	0.76	0.61-0.94	0.011

Likelihood ratio Chi-square 52.383, df 5, p<0.0001 (n=139)

Table 5. Multivariable Cox regression analysis of graft survival after 1 year post-transplantation: analysis of grafts that survived beyond the first year.

4. Discussion

This single center study investigated factors that affect renal transplant outcome in children. Numerous factors concerning recipient characteristics, donor characteristics, perioperative characteristics and post-transplant events were included in the analysis.

Univariable analysis identified a number of factors associated with outcome. Multiple blood transfusions pre-transplant, duration of dialysis pre-transplant, prolonged cold and warm ischemia times, absence of calcineurin inhibitors, occurrence of acute rejection, occurrence of delayed graft function, absence of HLA-A matching, presence of marked proteinuria at 1 year post-transplant were associated with poor outcome. Risk of graft failure decreased with higher creatinine clearance at 1 year, higher level of hemoglobin at 1 year and later year of entry in the transplant program. Certainly in term of single variable determinants, these specific factors appear familiar to professionals in renal transplantation.

The following factors remained of significance after multivariable analysis: use of calcineurin inhibitors, absence of HLA-A matching, delayed graft function defined as the need for dialysis in the first week post-transplant, occurrence of acute rejection, proteinuria superior to 1 g/24 h at 1 year, hemoglobin level at 1 year and kidney function at 1 year.

Transplants that did not benefit from **calcineurin inhibitors** had a fourfold increased risk of graft failure. Most of these transplants (14 of 16) were performed in the period 1980-1984 before CsA was introduced. As the period 1980-1984 represents also the first years of our pediatric transplant program, the lack of center experience, the so called learning curve, may be partly a confounding factor. We found CsA to impact significantly and independently both on early and long term graft survival. This is similar to the findings of two single center pediatric studies (Chavers et al., 1994; Offner et al., 1999) reporting a beneficial effect of CsA up to 5 and 8 years post-transplant. The introduction of CsA in the mid-1980s for the prevention of acute rejection has been a major breakthrough in the transplantation field. However it has been reported to impact mostly on early graft survival by lowering acute rejection rates; its effect on long term outcome being much more controversial (Chapman & Nankivell, 2006; Pascual et al., 2002; Schurman & McEnery, 1997). One of the major concerns for long term outcome is the calcineurin inhibitor-induced chronic nephrotoxicity leading to progressive nephron loss and declining renal transplant function (Chapman & Nankivell, 2006; Nankivell et al., 2004). Hence with the broadening of the immunosuppressive drugs arsenal, calcineurin inhibitor minimization, calcineurin inhibitor withdrawal or avoidance strategies have been developed. Calcineurin inhibitor withdrawal and avoidance protocols have been associated with an amelioration of the renal function, however at the cost of a higher rejection rates (Guerra et al., 2007; Höcker & Tönshoff, 2011). The long-term safety and efficacy of calcineurin inhibitor withdrawal and avoidance strategies need to be further validated in controlled clinical trials. At present the safest therapeutic strategy for pediatric renal allograft with chronic calcineurin inhibitor induced nephrotoxicity appears to be a mycophenolate based regimen with low dose calcineurin inhibitor and corticosteroids (Höcker & Tönshoff, 2011).

Two **HLA-A** mismatches was in our population a strong predictive risk factor for graft failure. Matching for HLA-DR and HLA-B has generally received priority over matching for HLA-A in children as well as in adults. Multivariable analysis of the data from the large NAPRTCS registry showed that the absence of HLA-B match and the absence of HLA-DR match were significant risk factors for graft failure (NAPRTCS, 2010). Roberts and colleagues reported that matching at the HLA-DR locus has significant effect on the survival of renal grafts from DD whereas matching at the HLA-A and B loci has only small effect (Roberts et al., 2004). However, Zantvoort and colleagues from Eurotransplant (Zantvoort et al., 1996) found an independent HLA-A matching effect on long term survival of DD kidney grafts with an increasing effect over time (up to 6 years post-transplant). This was in contrast to the strong, short-lived, effects of HLA-DR and -B matching, which could only be detected up to 6 months and 2 years after transplantation, respectively. A clear additive beneficial effect of HLA-A matching was shown in the group without B and DR mismatches. They concluded that prospective matching for the HLA-A antigens remains important for renal allograft survival and our data are in agreement with this. Data from the Collaborative Transplant Study indicated that class II HLA-DR locus has a stronger impact than the class I HLA-A and HLA-B loci during the first post-transplant year but that during subsequent years the three loci have an equivalent and additive influence on graft survival: to obtain optimal long term survival all three loci must be considered in the donor-recipient matching procedure (Opelz et al., 1999). This has been our policy through the years of our program as reflected by the very low percentage of transplants with more than 3 HLA-A,-B,-DR mismatches (14%). Obtaining the best possible HLA match for children is also an important part of the Eurotransplant allocation process. In contrast, in the United States, matching for HLA-A and -B has been abandoned and only HLA-DR is considered during the kidney allocation process. Based on an retrospective analysis of the UNOS registry data from 1585 pediatric recipients of DD kidney between 1996-2004 showing no advantage for HLA-DR matching, it has been recommended that, in the modern era of immunosuppression, the HLA match should be entirely disregarded when allocating donor kidneys to pediatric recipients (Gritsch et al., 2008). This will allow shortening the waiting time on dialysis for children. This view has been challenged in a recent report by Opelz and Döhler who examined the outcomes of 9209 pediatric recipients of DD kidneys from the CTS registry (Opelz & Döhler, 2010). Comparing two decades (1988-1997 and 1998-2007), they showed that, although overall graft survival improved over time, HLA matching remained highly significant and similarly strong despite the introduction of newer and more potent immunosuppression. A hierarchical relationship was observed for the effect of increasing number of mismatches on graft survival in both periods. Interestingly, they found a strong association between two HLA-DR mismatches and non Hodgkin lymphoma, and recommended therefore to avoid transplants with 2 HLA-DR mismatches.

In our view, a well matched first kidney is especially important in children as they have a high likelihood of needing more than one transplant during their lifetime. A poor matched kidney is more likely to result in HLA allosensitization, resulting therefore in long waiting time for a second transplant when the first graft fails and compromising the chance of a successful retransplantation (Meier-Kriesche et al., 2009).

The need for dialysis in the first week after transplantation carried in our transplant population a very high risk of graft failure within the first months post-transplant but did not impact significantly on the long term outcome. Similar findings emerged out of the analysis of the NAPRTCS registry (Tejani et al., 1999). DGF was found to be a significant independent predictor of graft failure. However, when patients whose grafts had failed during the first year were censored, no differences in graft survival were noted between patients with and without DGF for either LRD or DD recipients. Similarly DGF was not an independent predictor of long term graft survival in a large single center analysis of pediatric renal recipients (Vats et al., 2002). Good long term graft survival has also been obtained with non-heart-beating donors despite a higher incidence of DGF (Koffman & Gambaro, 2003; Sanchez-Fructuoso et al., 2004; Summers et al., 2010). Others have reported a negative influence of DGF on long term graft outcome (Gjertson, 2000; Moreira et al., 2011). It remains however difficult to determine whether this negative impact of DGF is independent of two associated known risk factors for long-term outcome: acute rejection (AR) and degree of kidney function (Geddes et al., 2002; Troppmann et al., 1996). The combination of DGF and AR seems to be the most detrimental for graft survival (Matas et al., 2000; McLaren et al., 1999).

The **occurrence of acute rejection** was an independent predictor of graft survival when all transplants were included in the analysis. When only the grafts that functioned beyond the first year were considered, acute rejection disappeared from the significant factors in the multivariable analysis. The lack of significance can be due to the reduced power as acute rejection was introduced as a time dependent covariate and most of the events (acute rejection) occurred within the first year.

Acute rejection is an important predictor of chronic rejection which is the most common cause of graft loss. Single and multicenter studies in adult and children have shown an association between acute rejection and subsequent development of chronic rejection (Dart et al., 2010; Matas, 2000; Tejani & Sullivan, 2000). It is therefore expected that a reduction in the incidence of acute rejection - in our program the incidence of acute rejection in the period 2000-2010 has dropped to 7% - should result in the reduction of chronic rejection and thus in better long term graft survival. This is supported by a NAPRTCS study (Tejani et al., 2002). Moreover some studies clearly indicate that a rejection free milieu can truly provide improved long term survival. Vats et al. in one of the largest single center study to date on long term graft outcome in pediatric renal transplant patients found freedom from acute rejection in the first year post-transplant to be the strongest independent predictor of improved graft survival (Vats et al., 2002). In an analysis of the UNOS data on 93934 adult patients, Hariharan et al. reported an increase in graft half-life from 11.9 years for patients with an episode of clinical acute rejection during the first year post-transplant to 27.1 years for those who did not have such an episode (Hariharan et al., 2000). Meier-Kriesche group, on the contrary, reported that the significant reduction in the acute rejection rates observed in the modern era has resulted in a marked improvement of the short term graft survival but in negligible progress in longer term survival as the attrition rate beyond the first year show little improvements (Lamb et al., 2011; Meier-Kriesche et al., 2004).

We found **kidney function at 1 year** to be an independent predictor of long term graft survival indicating that preservation of renal function during the first year is important and that events occurring within the first year impacting on this function are of critical importance for long term survival. Several authors have reported that renal function after transplantation has a strong impact on long term graft survival. Hariharan et al. analysing factors influencing graft survival for 105742 adult renal transplants between 1988 and 1998 reported one year creatinine and delta creatinine 6 months-1 year values to be the best predictors of long term survival and that the recent improvement in graft half-lives are related to conservation of renal function within the first year post-transplant (Hariharan et al., 2002). As it is the case in our study, when renal function within the first year and clinical acute rejection were included in their model for long term graft failure it was the creatinine at 1 year that was significant and not clinical acute rejection. Thus in the setting of acute rejection it is the preservation of renal function that is more important for graft survival. Data from a multicenter study pointed the 1 year estimated glomerular filtration rate to be the most relevant predictor of long term graft function. The impact of DGF and acute rejection on the long term graft function appeared to be fully mediated by their influence on the 1 year GFR (Salvadori et al., 2006). Similar to us, three studies found allograft function at 1 year to be a significant and independent predictor of graft outcome in children (Filler et al., 2002; Mitsnefes et al., 2003; Muscheites et al., 2009). Kidney function at one year might be thus a useful surrogate end point for renal transplant clinical trials in children.

Anemia is a significant complication of renal failure being associated with numerous adverse outcomes, including compromised renal and cardiac function, cardiovascular disease, decreased exercise tolerance, cognitive impairment, poorer quality of life, increased risk for hospitalization and mortality (Koshy & Geary, 2008; Warady & Ho, 2003). Anemia is expected to resolve after transplantation. More and more data indicate on the contrary that anemia is a common phenomenon in pediatric kidney recipients with reported prevalence rates ranging from 25% to 80% depending on the definition of anemia used and the time post-transplantation (Al-Khoury et al., 2006; Mitsnefes et al., 2005; Yorgin et al., 2002). The prevalence of anemia at 1 year (defined as hemoglobin level <11 g/dl (Al-Khoury et al., 2006; Mitsnefes et al., 2005)) was 30% among our transplanted children. The pathogenesis of post-transplant anemia is multifactorial and include iron deficiency, bone marrow suppression effects of immunosuppressive medications and other therapeutic agents, chronic inflammatory conditions caused by infections, frequent blood draws, and deteriorating renal function (Al-Uzri et al., 2003). In our multivariable analysis, hemoglobin level at 1 year post-transplant was a significant predictor of long term graft outcome, a higher level of hemoglobin being associated with a lower risk of graft failure. When hemoglobin was dichotomized at 11 g/dl, the HR for anemia in the multivariable model was 1.93 (p=0.024; 95% CI 1.09-3.42) while the HRs of the other covariates (table 5) remained in the same order of magnitude (data not shown). It was significant in the presence of "kidney function" indicating that anemia is just not merely a surrogate marker of a declining function of the allograft. Anemia is an independent risk factor for progression of renal failure in pre-dialysis adults (Kovesdy et al., 2006) and treating anemia slows down the decline of kidney function in these patients (Gouva et al., 2004). Our findings are in line with several studies in the adult population showing post-transplant anemia to be associated with increased risk for subsequent graft loss (Chhabra et al., 2008; Imoagene-Oyedeji et al., 2006; Kamar & Rostaing, 2008; Molnar et al., 2007). In these studies, anemia was also associated with impaired patient survival and with a higher proportion of cardiovascular deaths. Whether this is also the case in children remains to be determined but a cross sectional study of pediatric kidney recipients pointing anemia to be predictive of left ventricular hypertrophy - an independent predictor of cardiovascular morbidity and mortality in adults - raises concern. Post-transplant anemia has also been reported to impact on the quality of life; anemic children presenting more physical discomfort (Riano-Galan et al., 2009). For all these reasons including our findings that anemia predicts poorer graft survival, anemia deserves to be recognized early after transplantation, properly investigated and corrected.

The presence of marked **proteinuria** at 1 year was in our study population a strong and independent predictor of impaired graft outcome. This is in good agreement with several studies in adults showing increasing levels of proteinuria at 1 year post-transplant to be associated with increasing risk of graft failure (Amer et al., 2007; Fernandez-Fresnedo et al., 2004; Roodnat et al., 2001). Persistent proteinuria is also associated in these studies with increased mortality. In our population, persistent proteinuria was attributed to biopsy proven chronic allograft nephropathy, recurrence of primary kidney disease (FSGS and dense deposit disease) and de novo glomerulonephritis; this is in line with reports in adult kidney recipients (Barama, 2008). The underlying cause of proteinuria and not the proteinuria per se could thus be the factor contributing to transplant dysfunction and failure. However it is now recognized that proteinuria is not only a sensitive marker of renal disease but is directly damaging to the kidney by various mechanisms including direct mesangial toxicity, tubular overload, induction of a proinflammatory state and release of substances associated with the development of fibrogenesis and glomerulosclerosis (Baines & Brunskill, 2008). Recent reports indicate that even early (1-3 months post-transplant) very low (<0.5 g/24 h) and low grade (<1 g/24 h) proteinuria - often referred as 'subclinical' or 'negligible' - is a potent predictor of graft loss in adult kidney recipients and that short term reduction in proteinuria is associated with improved long term graft survival (Halimi et al., 2005; Sancho Calabuig et al., 2009).

While ACE inhibitors have been shown to be effective and safe in proteinuric adult kidney recipients (Barama, 2008; Hiremath et al., 2007), there is a paucity of data in the pediatric transplant population. In one retrospective study, children treated with ACEI had slightly lower proteinuria than those who did not receive such treatment (Arbeiter et al., 2004). A recent uncontrolled small prospective study showed a reduction of proteinuria in nearly all children treated with ACEI (Seeman et al., 2010).

Several factors such as donor source, donor age, recipient age and hypertension were in contrast with the literature not found significant in our study.

Large registry and single centers studies show better graft survival for recipients of LRD as compared to recipient of DD kidney (Gjertson & Cecka, 2001; Magee et al., 2008; NAPRTCS, 2010). Data from the NAPRTCS indicate that the 1 year graft survival obtained with deceased donors has reached that of the living donors. In our population, graft survival is also equivalent with both donor sources at 1 year and thereafter superior for LRD. However, this difference is not statistically significant, possibly because of the small number of LRD recipients. Another explanation is that we achieved good survival rates with the DD recipients, due to our strict policy of donor selection, good HLA matching and short ischemia times.

There are a number of reports indicating poorer results with kidney from **young donors**, essentially due to an increase incidence of vascular thrombosis, primary non function and other technical causes (Cransberg et al., 2000; Postlethwaite et al., 2002; Seikaly et al., 2001). Earlier NAPRCTS reports of poor graft survival with young donors have led to a constant decrease of the use of these donors in pediatric recipients: donor younger than 10 years represented 38% of the DD for pediatric recipients in the 1988 cohort, 13% in the 2000 cohort, 8% in the 2005 cohort and less than 5% in the 2009 cohort (NAPRTCS, 2010). We have obtained good results with young deceased donors with short and long term survival comparable to older donor (Van Damme-Lombaerts et al., 2001). Data indicate also that pediatric donor organs perform better than adult donor organs in pediatric patients (Nashan, 2004; Pape et al., 2004) and it seems thus justify that pediatric donors should preferentially be allocated to pediatric recipients. This might be stimulated by a very recent analysis of the NAPRTCS registry showing comparable 3-year graft survival and comparable kidney function in recipient of young donors (Moudgil et al., 2011).

Young recipient age (<5 yr) has been traditionally associated with poorer short term graft survival due to a high incidence of vascular thrombosis, technical complications and acute rejection (Cransberg et al., 2000; Gagnadoux et al., 1993; Kari et al., 1999; Postlethwaite et al.,

2002). However, there are a few single center reports, including ours, indicating that excellent renal transplantation results can be obtained in this high risk group of patients with careful and meticulous surgical techniques, vigilant management of fluids administration, use of low molecular weight heparin in the early postoperative period and close monitoring of immunosuppression with early diagnosis and treatment of rejection (Gagnadoux et al., 1993; Ojogho et al., 2002; Vats et al., 2002). Furthermore, past the first post-transplant year, graft survival in these youngest children has been reported to be excellent: as good or even superior to older children and adults (Gjertson & Cecka, 2001; Ojogho et al., 2002; Vats et al., 2002).

In our study **hypertension** was not a significant predictor of graft failure. This may be due to the fact that we relied on the use of antihypertensive medications and their numbers as surrogates for defining hypertension and its severity. Studies using actual blood pressure measurements found early post-transplant hypertension to be a significant and independent predictor of early allograft function and long term graft outcome in pediatric renal transplant recipients (Mitsnefes et al., 2003; Mitsnefes et al., 2001).

5. Conclusion

Despite its limitation due to the small number of patients, our study shows that several factors influence the outcome of renal allograft in our pediatric population. The introduction of CsA had a very significant impact in improving graft survival. A good HLA match remains important and matching for HLA-A locus in children should not be neglected. Early recognition, investigation and treatment of post-transplant anemia and proteinuria may play an important role in ultimately improving outcomes.

Prevention and adequate management of DGF, prevention and effective treatment of acute rejection episodes, therapeutic monitoring of calcineurin inhibitors to limit their nephrotoxicity, prevention of other injuries to the allograft by factors such as severe infection, hypertension, obstruction should contribute to the preservation of the renal function during the first year and lead to improved long term outcome.

6. Acknowledgment

We are very grateful to Dr. Steffen Fieuws from the Department of Biostatistics for his help with statistical analysis.

7. References

Al-Khoury, S., Shah, N., Afzali, B., Covic, A., Taylor, J. & Goldsmith, D. (2006). Post-transplantation anaemia in adult and paediatric renal allograft recipients-Guy's Hospital experience. *Nephrol Dial Transplant*, Vol. 21, No. 7, (July 2006), pp 1974-1980, ISSN 0931-0509

Al-Uzri, A., Yorgin, P. D. & Kling, P. J. (2003). Anemia in children after transplantation: etiology and the effect of immunosuppressive therapy on erythropoiesis. *Pediatric Transplantation*, Vol. 7, No. 4, (August 2003), pp 253-264, ISSN 1397-3142

Amer, H., Fidler, M. E., Myslak, M., Morales, P., Kremers, W. K., Larson, T. S., Stegall, M. D. & Cosio, F. G. (2007). Proteinuria After Kidney Transplantation, Relationship to

Allograft Histology and Survival. *American Journal of Transplantation*, Vol. 7, No. 12, (December 2007), pp 2748-2756, ISSN 1600-6143

Arbeiter, K., Pichler, A., Stemberger, R., Mueller, T., Ruffingshofer, D., Vargha, R., Balzar, E. & Aufricht, C. (2004). ACE inhibition in the treatment of children after renal transplantation. *Pediatric Nephrology*, Vol. 19, No. 2, (February 2004), pp 222-226, ISSN 0931-041X

Baines, R. J. & Brunskill, N. J. (2008). The molecular interactions between filtered proteins and proximal tubular cells in proteinuria. *Nephron Exp Nephrol*, Vol. 110, No. 2, (November 2008), pp e67-71, ISSN 1660-2129

Barama, A. A. (2008). Mechanisms and Management of Proteinuria in Kidney Transplant Patients. *Drugs*, Vol. 68, No. Suppl.1, pp 33-39, ISSN 0012-6667

Benfield, M. R., McDonald, R., Sullivan, E. K., Stablein, D. M.& Tejani, A. (1999). The 1997 Annual Renal Transplantation in Children Report of the North American Pediatric Renal Transplant Cooperative Study (NAPRTCS). *Pediatric Transplantation*, Vol. 3, No. 2, (May 1999), pp 152-67, ISSN 1397-3142

Chapman, J. R. & Nankivell, B. J. (2006). Nephrotoxicity of ciclosporin A: short-term gain, long-term pain? *Nephrology Dialysis Transplantation*, Vol. 21, No. 8, (August 2006), pp 2060-2063, ISSN 0931-0509

Chavers, B. M., Kim, E. M., Matas, A. J., Gillingham, K. J., Najarian, J. S. & Mauer, S. M. (1994). Causes of kidney allograft loss in a large pediatric population at a single center. *Pediatric Nephrology*, Vol. 8, No. 1, (February 1994), pp 57-61, ISSN 0931-041X

Chhabra, D., Grafals, M., Skaro, A. I., Parker, M. & Gallon, L. (2008). Impact of Anemia after Renal Transplantation on Patient and Graft Survival and on Rate of Acute Rejection. *Clinical Journal of the American Society of Nephrology*, Vol. 3, No. 4, (July 2008), pp 1168-1174, ISSN 1555-9041

Cransberg, K., van Gool, J. D., Davin, JC., De Jong, M.C.J., Darby, M., Boendermaker, M. E., De Meester, J.M.J., Stijnen, T., Wolff, E. D. & Nauta, J. (2000). Pediatric renal transplantation in the Netherlands. *Pediatric Transplantation*, Vol. 4, No. 1, (February 2000), pp 72-81, ISSN 1397-3142

Dart, A. B., Schall, A., Gibson, I. W., Blydt-Hansen, T. D. & Birk, P. E. (2010). Patterns of Chronic Injury in Pediatric Renal Allografts. *Transplantation*, Vol. 89, No. 3, (February 2010), pp 334-340, ISSN 0041-1337

Fernandez-Fresnedo, G., Plaza, J. J., Sanchez-Plumed, J., Sanz-Guajardo, A., Palomar-Fontanet, R. & Arias, M. (2004). Proteinuria: a new marker of long-term graft and patient survival in kidney transplantation. *Nephrology Dialysis Transplantation*, Vol. 19, No. suppl 3, (June 2004), pp iii47-iii51, ISSN 0931-0509

Filler, G., Trompeter, R., Webb, N. J., Watson, A. R., Milford, D. V., Tyden, G., Grenda, R., Janda, J., Hughes, D., Offner, G. et al. (2002). One-year glomerular filtration rate predicts graft survival in pediatric renal recipients: a randomized trial of tacrolimus vs cyclosporine microemulsion. *Transplantation Proceedings*, Vol. 34, No. 5, (August 2002), pp 1935-1938, ISSN 0041-1345

Gagnadoux, M. F., Charbit, M., Beurton, D., Revillon, Y., Niaudet, P. & Broyer, M. (1993). Renal transplantation in children under five years of age. Experience at the Hopital des Enfants-Malades. *Annales de Pediatrie (Paris)*, Vol. 40, No. 2, (February 1993), pp 108-111, ISSN 0066-2097

Geddes, C. C., Woo, Y. M. & Jardine, A. G. (2002). The impact of delayed graft function on the long-term outcome of renal transplantation. *Journal of Nephrology*, Vol. 15, No. 1, (January-February 2002), pp 17-21, ISSN 1121-8428

Gjertson, D. W. (2000). Impact of delayed graft function and acute rejection on kidney graft survival. *Clinical Transplantation*, pp 467-480, ISSN 0902-0063

Gjertson, D. W. & Cecka, J. M. (2001). Determinants of long-term survival of pediatric kidney grafts reported to the United Network for Organ Sharing kidney transplant registry. *Pediatric Transplantation*, Vol. 5, No. 1, (February 2001), pp 5-15, ISSN 1397-3142

Gouva, C., Nikolopoulos, P., Ioannidis, J. P. & Siamopoulos, K. C. (2004). Treating anemia early in renal failure patients slows the decline of renal function: a randomized controlled trial. *Kidney International*, Vol. 66, No. 2, (August 2004), pp 753-760, ISSN 0085-2538

Gritsch, H. A., Veale, J. L., Leichtman, A. B., Guidinger, M. K., Magee, J. C., McDonald, R. A., Harmon, W. E., Delmonico, F. L., Ettenger, R. B. & Cecka, J. M. (2008). Should Pediatric Patients Wait for HLA-DR-Matched Renal Transplants? *American Journal of Transplantation*, Vol. 8, No. 10, (October 2008), pp 2056-2061, ISSN 1600-6143,

Guerra, G., Srinivas, T. R. & Meier-Kriesche, H.-U. (2007). Calcineurin inhibitor-free immunosuppression in kidney transplantation. *Transplant International*, Vol. 20, No. 10, (October 2007), pp 813-827, ISSN 0934-0874,

Halimi, J.-M., Laouad, I., Buchler, M., Al-Najjar, A., Chatelet, V., Houssaini, T. S., Nivet, H. & Lebranchu, Y. (2005). Early Low-Grade Proteinuria: Causes, Short-Term Evolution and Long-Term Consequences in Renal Transplantation. *American Journal of Transplantation*, Vol. 5, No. 9, (September 2005), pp 2281-2288, ISSN 1600-6143

Hariharan, S., Johnson, C. P., Bresnahan, B. A., Taranto, S. E., McIntosh, M. J. & Stablein, D. (2000). Improved graft survival after renal transplantation in the United States, 1988 to 1996. *New England Journal of Medicine*, Vol. 342, No. 9, (March 2000), pp 605-612, ISSN 1533-4406

Hariharan, S., McBride, M. A., Cherikh, W. S., Tolleris, C. B., Bresnahan, B. A. & Johnson, C. P. (2002). Post-transplant renal function in the first year predicts long-term kidney transplant survival. *Kidney International*, Vol. 62, No. 1, (July 2002), pp 311-318, ISSN 0085-2538

Hiremath, S., Fergusson, D., Doucette, S., Mulay, A. V. & Knoll, G. A. (2007). Renin angiotensin system blockade in kidney transplantation: a systematic review of the evidence. *American Journal of Transplantation*, Vol. 7, No. 10, (October 2007), pp 2350-2360, ISSN 1600-6135

Höcker, B. & Tönshoff, B. (2011). Calcineurin inhibitor-free immunosuppression in pediatric renal transplantation: a viable option? *Paediatr Drugs*, Vol. 13, No. 1, (February 2011), pp 49-69, ISSN 1174-5878

Hwang, A. H., Cho, Y. W., Cicciarelli, J., Mentser, M., Iwaki, Y. & Hardy, B. E. (2005). Risk Factors for Short- and Long-term Survival of Primary Cadaveric Renal Allografts in Pediatric Recipients: A UNOS Analysis. *Transplantation*, Vol. 80, No. 4, (August 2005), pp 466-470, ISSN 0041-1337

Imoagene-Oyedeji, A. E., Rosas, S. E., Doyle, A. M., Goral, S. & Bloom, R. D. (2006). Posttransplantation Anemia at 12 Months in Kidney Recipients Treated with Mycophenolate Mofetil: Risk Factors and Implications for Mortality. *Journal of the*

American Society of Nephrology, Vol. 17, No. 11, (November 2006), pp 3240-3247, ISSN 1046-6673

Kamar, N. & Rostaing, L. (2008). Negative impact of one-year anemia on long-term patient and graft survival in kidney transplant patients receiving calcineurin inhibitors and mycophenolate mofetil. *Transplantation*, Vol. 85, No. 8, (April 2008), pp 1120-1124, ISSN 0041-1337

Kari, J. A., Romagnoli, J., Duffy, P., Fernando, O. N., Rees, L. & Trompeter, R. S. (1999). Renal transplantation in children under 5 years of age. *Pediatric Nephrology*, Vol. 13, No. 9, (November 1999), pp 730-736, ISSN 0931-041X

Koffman, G. & Gambaro, G. (2003). Renal transplantation from non-heart- beating donors: a review of the European experience. *Journal of Nephrology*, Vol. 16, No. 3, (May-June 2003), pp 334-341, ISSN 1121-8428

Koshy, S. & Geary, D. (2008). Anemia in children with chronic kidney disease. *Pediatric Nephrology*, Vol. 23, No. 2, (February 2008), pp 209-219, ISSN 0931-041X

Kovesdy, C. P., Trivedi, B. K., Kalantar-Zadeh, K. & Anderson, J. E. (2006). Association of anemia with outcomes in men with moderate and severe chronic kidney disease. *Kidney International*, Vol. 69, No. 3, (February 2006), pp 560-564, ISSN 0085-2538

Lamb, K. E., Lodhi, S. & Meier-Kriesche, H. U. (2011). Long-Term Renal Allograft Survival in the United States: A Critical Reappraisal. *American Journal of Transplantation*, Vol. 11, No. 3, (March 2011), pp 450-462, ISSN 1600-6143

Magee, J. C., Krishnan, S. M., Benfield, M. R., Hsu, D. T. & Shneider, B. L. (2008). Pediatric Transplantation in the United States, 1997–2006. *American Journal of Transplantation*, Vol. 8, No. 4p2, (August 2008), pp 935-945, ISSN 1600-6143

Matas, A. J. (2000). Impact of acute rejection on development of chronic rejection in pediatric renal transplant recipients. *Pediatric Transplantation*, Vol. 4, No. 2, (May 2000), pp 92-99, ISSN 1397-3142

Matas, A. J., Gillingham, K. J., Humar, A., Dunn, D. L., Sutherland, D. E. & Najarian, J. S. (2000). Immunologic and nonimmunologic factors: different risks for cadaver and living donor transplantation. *Transplantation*, Vol. 69, No. 1, (January 2000), pp 54-58, ISSN 0041-1337

McLaren, A. J., Jassem, W., Gray, D. W., Fuggle, S. V., Welsh, K. I. & Morris, P. J. (1999). Delayed graft function: risk factors and the relative effects of early function and acute rejection on long-term survival in cadaveric renal transplantation. *Clinical Transplantation*, Vol. 13, No. 3, (June 1999), pp 266-272, ISSN 0902-0063

Meier-Kriesche, H.-U., Scornik, J. C., Susskind, B., Rehman, S. & Schold, J. D. (2009). A Lifetime Versus a Graft Life Approach Redefines the Importance of HLA Matching in Kidney Transplant Patients. *Transplantation*, Vol. 88, No. 1, (July 2009), pp 23-29, ISSN 0041-1337

Meier-Kriesche, H. U., Schold, J. D., Srinivas, T. R. & Kaplan, B. (2004). Lack of improvement in renal allograft survival despite a marked decrease in acute rejection rates over the most recent era. *American Journal of Transplantation*, Vol. 4, No. 3, (March 2004), pp 378-383, ISSN 1600-6143

Mitsnefes, M. M., Khoury, P. R. & McEnery, P. T. (2003). Early posttransplantation hypertension and poor long-term renal allograft survival in pediatric patients. The *Journal of Pediatrics*, Vol. 143, No. 1, (July 2003), pp 98-103, ISSN 0022-3476

Mitsnefes, M. M., Omoloja, A. & McEnery, P. T. (2001). Short-term pediatric renal transplant survival: blood pressure and allograft function. *Pediatric Transplantation*, Vol. 5, No. 3, (June 2001), pp 160-165, ISSN 1397-3142

Mitsnefes, M. M., Subat-Dezulovic, M., Khoury, P. R., Goebel, J. & Strife, C. F. (2005). Increasing incidence of post-kidney transplant anemia in children. *American Journal of Transplantation*, Vol. 5, No. 7, (July 2005), pp 1713-1718, ISSN 1600-6135

Molnar, M. Z., Czira, M., Ambrus, C., Szeifert, L., Szentkiralyi, A., Beko, G., Rosivall, L., Remport, A., Novak, M. & Mucsi, I. (2007). Anemia Is Associated with Mortality in Kidney-Transplanted Patients—A Prospective Cohort Study. *American Journal of Transplantation*, Vol. 7, No. 4, (April 2007), pp 818-824, ISSN 1600-6143

Moreira, P., SÃ¡, H., Figueiredo, A. & Mota, A. (2011). Delayed Renal Graft Function: Risk Factors and Impact on the Outcome of Transplantation. *Transplantation Proceedings*, Vol. 43, No. 1, (January 2011), pp 100-105, ISSN 0041-1345

Moudgil, A., Martz, K., Stablein, D. M. & Puliyanda, D. P. (2011). Good outcome of kidney transplants in recipients of young donors: a NAPRTCS data analysis. *Pediatric Transplantation*, Vol. 15, No. 2, (March 2011), pp 167-171, ISSN1397-3142

Muscheites, J., Wigger, M., Drueckler, E., Klaassen, I., John, U., Wygoda, S., Fischer, D.-C., Kundt, G., Misselwitz, J., Müller-Wiefel, D.-E. et al. (2009). Estimated one-yr glomerular filtration rate is an excellent predictor of long-term graft survival in pediatric first kidney transplants. *Pediatric Transplantation*, Vol. 13, (May 2009), pp 365-370, ISSN 1397-3142

Nankivell, B. J., Borrows, R. J., Fung, C. L.-S., O'Connell, P. J., Chapman, J. R. & Allen, R. D. M. (2004). Calcineurin Inhibitor Nephrotoxicity: Longitudinal Assessment by Protocol Histology. *Transplantation*, Vol. 78, No. 4, (August 2004), pp 557-565, ISSN 0041-1337

NAPRTCS. (2010). NAPRTCS 2010 Annual Transplant Report ,14.04.2011, Available from https://web.emmes.com/study/ped/annlrept/2010_Report.pdf.

Nashan, B. (2004). Renal allograft allocation for children: are we penalizing children to not penalize adults? *Transplantation*, Vol. 77, No. 8, (April 2004), pp 1145-1146, ISSN 0041-1337

Offner, G., Latta, K., Hoyer, P. F., Baum, H. J., Ehrich, J. H., Pichlmayr, R. & Brodehl, J. (1999). Kidney transplanted children come of age. *Kidney International*, Vol. 55, No. 4, (April 2004), pp 1509-1517, ISSN 0085-2538

Ojogho, O., Sahney, S., Cutler, D., Abdelhalim, F., Hasan, M., Baron, P. & Concepcion, W. (2002). Superior long-term results of renal transplantation in children under 5 years of age. *Am Surg*, Vol. 68, No. 12, (December 2002), pp 1115-1119, ISSN 0002-9610

Opelz, G. & Döhler, B. (2010). Pediatric Kidney Transplantation: Analysis of Donor Age, HLA Match, and Posttransplant Non-Hodgkin Lymphoma: A Collaborative Transplant Study Report. *Transplantation*, Vol. 90, No. 3, (August 2010), pp 292-297, ISSN 0041-1337

Opelz, G., Wujciak, T., Dohler, B., Scherer, S. & Mytilineos, J. (1999). HLA compatibility and organ transplant survival. Collaborative Transplant Study. *Rev Immunogenet*, Vol. 1, No. 3, pp 334-342, ISSN 1398-1714

Pape, L., Offner, G., Ehrich, J. H., de Boer, J. & Persijn, G. G. (2004). Renal allograft function in matched pediatric and adult recipient pairs of the same donor. *Transplantation*, Vol. 77, No. 8, (April 2004), pp 1191-1194, ISSN 0041-1337

Pascual, M., Theruvath, T., Kawai, T., Tolkoff-Rubin, N. &Cosimi, A. B. (2002). Strategies to Improve Long-Term Outcomes after Renal Transplantation. *New England Journal of Medicine*, Vol. 346, No. 8, (February 2002), pp 580-590, ISSN 1533-4406

Postlethwaite, R. J., Johnson, R. J., Armstrong, S., Belger, M. A., Fuggle, S. V., Martin, S., Middleton, D., Ray, T. C., Rigden, S. P., Verrier-Jones, K. et al. (2002). The outcome of pediatric cadaveric renal transplantation in the UK and Eire. *Pediatric Transplantation*, Vol. 6, No. 5, (October 2001), pp 367-77, ISSN 1397-3142

Riano-Galan, I., Malaga, S., Rajmil, L., Ariceta, G., Navarro, M., Loris, C. & Vallo, A. (2009). Quality of life of adolescents with end-stage renal disease and kidney transplant. *Pediatric Nephrology*, Vol. 24, No. 8, (August 2009), pp 1561-1568, ISSN 0931-041X

Roberts, J. P., Wolfe, R. A., Bragg-Gresham, J. L., Rush, S. H., Wynn, J. J., Distant, D. A., Ashby, V. B., Held, P. J. & Port, F. K. (2004). Effect of changing the priority for HLA matching on the rates and outcomes of kidney transplantation in minority groups. *New England Journal of Medicine*, Vol. 350, No. 6, (February 2004), pp 545-551, ISSN 1533-4406,

Roodnat, J. I., Mulder, P. G., Rischen-Vos, J., van Riemsdijk, I. C., van Gelder, T., Zietse, R., JN, I. J. &Weimar, W. (2001). Proteinuria after renal transplantation affects not only graft survival but also patient survival. *Transplantation*, Vol. 72, No. 3, (August 2001), pp 438-444, ISSN 0041-1337

Salvadori, M., Rosati, A., Bock, A., Chapman, J., Dussol, B., Fritsche, L., Kliem, V., Lebranchu, Y., Oppenheimer, F., Pohanka, E. et al. (2006). Estimated One-Year Glomerular Filtration Rate is the Best Predictor of Long-term Graft Function Following Renal Transplant. *Transplantation*, Vol. 81, No. 2, (January 2006), pp 202-206, ISSN 0041-1337

Sanchez-Fructuoso, A., Prats Sanchez, D., Marques Vidas, M., Lopez De Novales, E. & Barrientos Guzman, A. (2004). Non-heart beating donors. *Nephrol Dial Transplant*, Vol. 19, Suppl. 3, (June 2004), pp iii26-31, ISSN 0931-0509

Sancho Calabuig, A., Pallardó Mateu, L. M., Avila Bernabeu, A. I., Gavela Martínez, E., Beltrán Catalán, S. & Crespo Albiach, J. F. (2009). Very Low-Grade Proteinuria at 3 Months Posttransplantation Is an Earlier Marker of Graft Survival. *Transplantation Proceedings*, Vol. 41, No. 6, (August 2009), pp 2122-2125, ISSN 0041-1345

Schurman, S. J. & McEnery, P. T. (1997). Factors influencing short-term and long-term pediatric renal transplant survival. *J Pediatr*, Vol. 130, No. 3, (March 1997), pp 455-462, ISSN 0022-3476

Seeman, T., Dušek, J., Vondrák, K. & Janda, J. (2010). Ramipril in the treatment of proteinuria in children after renal transplantation. *Pediatric Transplantation*, Vol. 14, No. 2, (August 2009), pp 283-287, ISSN 1397-3142

Seikaly, M., Ho, P. L., Emmett, L. & Tejani, A. (2001). The 12th Annual Report of the North American Pediatric Renal Transplant Cooperative Study: renal transplantation from 1987 through 1998. *Pediatric Transplantation*, Vol. 5, No. 3, (June 2001), pp 215-231, ISSN 1397-3142

Summers, D. M., Johnson, R. J., Allen, J., Fuggle, S. V., Collett, D., Watson, C. J. & Bradley, J. A. (2010). Analysis of factors that affect outcome after transplantation of kidneys donated after cardiac death in the UK: a cohort study. *The Lancet*, Vol. 376, No. 9749, (October 2010), pp 1303-1311, ISSN 0140-6736